Neonatal Emergencies

W0081025

Neonatal Emergencies

Meharban Singh

MD, FAMS, FIAP, FIMSA, FNNF, Hony. FAAP

Former Professor and Head
Department of Pediatrics and Neonatal Division
WHO Collaborating Center for Training and
Research in Newborn Care
All India Institute of Medical Sciences
New Delhi

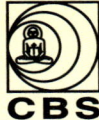

CBS

CBS Publishers & Distributors Pvt Ltd

New Delhi • Bengaluru • Chennai • Kochi • Kolkata • Mumbai
Hyderabad • Jharkhand • Nagpur • Patna • Pune • Uttarakhand

Disclaimer

Science and technology are constantly changing fields. New research and experience broaden the scope of information and knowledge. The editor has tried his best in giving information available to him while preparing the material for this book. Although all efforts have been made to ensure optimum accuracy of the material, yet it is quite possible some errors might have been left uncorrected. The publisher, the printer and the editor will not be held responsible for any inadvertent errors, omissions or inaccuracies.

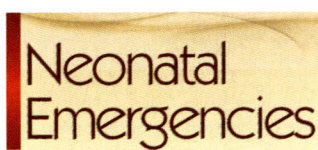

ISBN: 978-93-86478-36-8

Copyright © Meharban Singh

First Edition: 2018

All rights reserved. No part of this book may be reproduced or transmitted in any form or by any means, electronic or mechanical, including photocopying, recording, or any information storage and retrieval system without permission, in writing, from the author and the publisher.

Published by Satish Kumar Jain and produced by Varun Jain for

CBS Publishers & Distributors Pvt Ltd

4819/XI Prahlad Street, 24 Ansari Road, Daryaganj, New Delhi 110 002, India.
Ph: 23289259, 23266861, 23266867   Fax: 011-23243014   Website: www.cbspd.com
e-mail: delhi@cbspd.com; cbspubs@airtelmail.in.

Corporate Office: 204 FIE, Industrial Area, Patparganj, Delhi 110 092
Ph: 4934 4934   Fax: 4934 4935   e-mail: publishing@cbspd.com; publicity@cbspd.com

Branches

- **Bengaluru:** Seema House 2975, 17th Cross, K.R. Road, Banasankari 2nd Stage, Bengaluru 560 070, Karnataka
  Ph: +91-80-26771678/79   Fax: +91-80-26771680   e-mail: bangalore@cbspd.com
- **Chennai:** No. 7, Subbaraya Street, Shenoy Nagar, Chennai 600 030, Tamil Nadu
  Ph: +91-44-26680620, 26681266   Fax: +91-44-42032115   e-mail: chennai@cbspd.com
- **Kochi:** Ashana House, 39/1904, AM Thomas Road, Valanjambalam, Eranakulam 682 016, Kochi, Kerala
  Ph: +91-484-4059061-62-64-65   Fax: +91-484-4059065   e-mail: kochi@cbspd.com
- **Kolkata:** No. 6/B, Ground Floor, Rameswar Shaw Road, Kolkata-700014 (West Bengal)
  Ph: +91-33-2289-1126, 2289-1127, 2289-1128   e-mail: kolkata@cbspd.com
- **Mumbai:** 83-C, Dr E Moses Road, Worli, Mumbai-400018, Maharashtra
  Ph: +91-22-24902340/41   Fax: +91-22-24902342   e-mail: mumbai@cbspd.com

Representatives

• **Hyderabad**	0-9885175004	• **Jharkhand**	0-9811541605	• **Nagpur**	0-9021734563
• **Patna**	0-9334159340	• **Pune**	0-9623451994	• **Uttarakhand**	0-9716462459

Printed at: Nutech Print Services, India

to

global neonates
the foundation of human race

"*Newborn indeed is a 'seed', endowed with immense potentiality. You can't do much to alter its genome but you can provide optimal nurturing, nutrition, safe environment and tender loving care to unfold myriad of human capabilities to help him evolve as a robust citizen of the society.*"

Meharban Singh

Preface

Every neonate admitted in the neonatal intensive care unit (except those admitted for social or isolation reasons) is a medical emergency and should be handled with utmost care and high level of expertise. Just as the child is not a mini-adult, the neonate is not a mini-child. Neonates are delicate, functionally immature and vulnerable to develop a variety of life-threatening emergencies. Neonates are like flowers and they readily wither following an acute illness but bloom back rather slowly because of their physiologic immaturity and hemodynamic instability. The body homeostatic mechanisms are immature and labile, being worse in preterm compared to term babies. The knowledge and understanding of anatomical and physiological handicaps is essential for scientific, rational and evidence-based management of critical disorders in neonates.

In this comprehensive multi-author Textbook on Neonatal Emergencies, the emphasis is laid on physiologic background, etiopathogenesis, clinical spectrum, early diagnosis and management of critically sick neonates. The book has been designed to provide problem-oriented approach to medical emergencies in neonates. The organization of a NICU and stellar role of specially trained neonatal nurses for the assessment, monitoring, and humanized care of sick neonates have been discussed in detail. The common symptoms and signs encountered in critically sick neonates like hypoxia, hypothermia, cyanosis, crying, respiratory distress, fluid and electrolyte disturbances, metabolic disorders, jaundice, bleeding and shock have been covered in detail. The emergencies pertaining to dysfunction and failure of each body system and organ have been discussed. Early diagnosis and effective management of perinates with life-threatening disorders is crucial for intact survival because seeds of neuromotor disability are sown in the perinatal period. The special emphasis has been laid on the quality of care and intact survival with detailed coverage of assessment of severity of neonatal illness, follow-up of NICU graduates, ethical issues and dilemmas. Emergency procedures including transport of sick neonates, assisted ventilation and parenteral nutrition have been discussed in detail. The book is illustrated with a large of number of tables, boxes, diagrams, flowcharts and practical tips in a reader-friendly format. The distinctive feature and hallmark of the book is brevity, clarity of language and a problem-oriented approach.

I am most grateful to a large number of distinguished contributors from India and abroad, who have most willingly devoted their precious time and energy to contribute chapters pertaining to areas of their expertise. They have been kind and generous to give me the liberty to prune, revise and edit the material to produce a comprehensive textbook of a uniform format. I would like to take this opportunity to thank Mr YN Arjuna (Senior Vice-President Publishing, Editorial and Publicity), Mrs Ritu Chawla (AGM Production), Mr Kushal Pal Singh Yadav (Copyeditor), Mr Neeraj Prasad (Graphic artist), Mr Tarun Rajput and Mr Vikrant Sharma (DTP operators) for composing and inserting the manuscript in the word processor and to my friend Shri Satish Kumar Jain for his enthusiasm and commitment to publish the book.

I am confident that the book would fill a void to realise my hope and concern to provide state-of-the-art care to critically sick neonates in India and South-East Asia region.

15th August, 2017
Child Care Center
625, Sector 37, Arun Vihar, Noida
e-mail: drmbsk@gmail.com

Meharban Singh MD

Acknowledgements

I would like to express my appreciation and gratitude to a large number of distinguished contributors from India and abroad, who have most willingly devoted their precious time and energy to submit state-of-the-art chapters dealing with neonatal emergencies of their special interest and expertise. I am most appreciative of their benign gesture and concern in meeting the deadline for submission of the manuscripts despite their heavy academic commitments.

Contributors

Ramesh Agarwal MD, DM (Neonatology)
Additional Professor
Division of Neonatology
Department of Pediatrics
ICMR Center for Advanced Research in Newborn Health and WHO
Collaborating Center for Training and Research in Newborn Care
All India Institute of Medical Sciences
New Delhi-110 029
E-mail: ra.aiims@gmail.com

Emergencies at birth
Emergency procedures and life saving medications

Sriparna Basu MD, DCH, FRCPI, FRCPCH
Professor, Neonatology Unit
Department of Department, Institute of Medical Sciences
Banaras Hindu University
Varanasi-221 005
E-mail: drsriparnabasu@rediffmail.com

Neonatal meningitis
Neonatal encephalopathy

Vineet Bhandari MD, DM (Neonatology)
Professor of Pediatrics, Obstetrics and Gynecology
Drexel University College of Medicine
Chief of Neonatal–Perinatal Medicine
St. Christopher Hospital for Children/Hahnemann University
Hospital/Temple University Hospital, Philadelphia, PA, USA
E-mail: vineet.bhandari@dixelmed.edu

Assisted ventilation

B. Vishnu Bhat MD, DHA, DDE
Dean (Research)
Senior Professor and Head
Department of Pediatrics
JIPMER
Puducherry-605 006
E-mail: drvishnubhat@yahoo.com

Shock

Marsha Campbell–Yeo PhD, RN
Neonatal Nurse Practitioner
Associate Professor and Cinical Scientist
School of Nursing
Department of Pediatrics, Psychology and Neuroscience
Dalhousie University and IWK Health Center 5850/5980
University Avenue
Halifax, NS B3K 6R8
E-mail: marsha.campbellyeo@iwk.nshealth.ca

The role of nurses in the NICU

Kuntal Roy Chowdhuri MCh (Cardiothoracic and Vascular Surgery)
Associate Consultant
Department of Pediatrics and Congenital Cardiac Surgery
Fortis Escorts Heart Institute
Okhla Road, New Delhi-110 025
E-mail: kuntalroychoudhuri@gmail.com

Cardiac emergencies

Nilanjan Dutta MCh (Cardiothoracic and Vascular Surgery)
Consultant
Department of Pediatrics and Congenital Cardiac Surgery
Fortis Escorts Heart Institute
Okhla Road, New Delhi-110 025
E-mail: dr.duttanilanjan@rediffmail.com

Cardiac emergencies

Sourabh Dutta MD, PhD
Professor Neonatology
Postgraduate Institute of Medical Education and Research
Chandigarh-160 012
E-mail: sourabhdutta1@gmail.com

Fetal emergencies

Ketki Falak MSc (Nutrition)
TPN Nutritionist
KEM and Sahyadri Hospitals
Pune-411 011
E-mail: ketkifalak@gmail.com

Parenteral nutrition

Shalabh Garg MD, FRCPCH
Consultant Neonatologist
The James Cook University Hospital
Middlesbrough, Cleveland, UK
E-mail: shalabh.garg@stees.nhs.uk

Respiratory emergencies

Saurabh Kumar Gupta MD (Pediatrics), DM (Cardiology)
Associate Professor of Cardiology
Cardio-Thoracic Center
All India Institute of Medical Sciences
New Delhi-110 029
E-mail: drsaurabhmd@gmail.com

The neonate with cyanosis

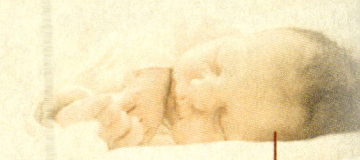

Parvathi Unninayar Iyer MD, FRCH (Melbourne)
Director
Department of Pediatrics and Congenital Cardiac Surgery
Fortis Escorts Heart Institute
Okhla Road, New Delhi-110 025
E-mail: *puiyer95@gmail.com*

Cardiac emergencies

Sandeep Kadam MD, DM (Neonatology)
Neonatologist
KEM Hospital and Ratna Memorial Hospital
Pune-411 011
E-mail: *drsandeepkadam@yahoo.com*

Fluids, electrolytes and acid-base disorders

Venkat Reddy Kallem DNB (Pediatrics), DNB (Neonatology)
Consultant
Fernandez Hospital, Hyderguda
Hyderabad-500 029
E-mail: *venkat467@gmail.com*

Severe jaundice

Geetanjli Kalyan BSN, MSN (Pediatrics)
Clinical Instructor
National Institute of Nursing Education
Postgraduate Institute of Medical Education and Research
Chandigarh-160 012
E-mail: *geetss2@gmail.com*

The role of nurses in the NICU

Japleen Kaur MD
Senior Resident
Department of Obstetrics and Gynecology
Postgraduate Institute of Medical Education and Research
Chandigarh-160 012
E-mail: *japleen18@gmail.com*

Fetal emergencies

Supreet Kaur MD
Senior Resident Neonatology
Postgraduate Institute of Medical Education and Research
Chandigarh-160 012
E-mail: *supreetkhurana85@gmail.com*

Fetal emergencies

Neelam Kler MD
Chairperson and Senior Consultant
Department of Neonatology
Institute of Child Health, Sir Ganga Ram Hospital
Rajinder Nagar
New Delhi-110 060
E-mail: *drneelamkler@gmail.com*

Transport of sick neonates

Panagiotis Kratimenos MD, PhD
Fellow in Neonatal–Perinatal Medicine
Instructor of Pediatrics
Drex University College of Medicine
St. Christopher Hospital for Children
Hahnemann University Hospital and Temple University Hospital
Philadelphia, PA, USA
E-mail: *pkratimenos@gmail.com*

Assisted ventilation

Ashok Kumar MD, FIAP, FNNF, FAMS
Professor, Neonatology Unit
Department of Pediatrics, Institute of Medical Sciences
Banaras Hindu University
Varanasi-221 005
E-mail: *ashokkumar_bhu@hotmail.com*

Neonatal meningitis
Neonatal encephalopathy

Praveen Kumar MD, DM (Neonatology)
Professor and Head
Neonatal Unit
Postgraduate Institute of Medical Education and Research
Chandigarh-160 012
E-mail: *drpkumarpgi@gmail.com*

Perinatal infections: bacterial and spirochetal

Mukta Mantan MD, DNB
Professor
Department of Pediatrics
Maulana Azad Medical College and Associated Hospitals
New Delhi-110 002
E-mail: *muktamantan@hotmail.com*

Acute kidney injury

Suja Mariam MD, DM (Neonatology)
Consultant
Division of Neonatology
Sri Ramakrishna Hospital
Coimbatore-641 044
E-mail: *sujamariam@yahoo.co.in*

Fetal emergencies
Perinatal infections: bacterial and spirochetal

NB Mathur MD
Director Professor
Department of Neonatology
Maulana Azad Medical College
New Delhi-110 002
E-mail: *drnbmathur@gmail.com*

Hypothermia and hyperthermia

SB Mathur MD
Senior Resident
Department of Pediatrics
Lady Hardinge Medical College
New Delhi-110 001
E-mail: *sbmathur05@gmail.com*

Hypothermia and hyperthermia

Neelam Mohan DNB, MNAMS, FPGN (UK), FIMSA, FACG (USA), FIAP, FRCPCH (UK)
Director
Department of Pediatric Gastroenterology, Hepatology, and Liver Transplantation
Medanta The Medicity Hospital, Sector-38
Gurugram-122 001
E-mail: *drneelam@yahoo.com*

Acute liver failure

Srinivas Murki MD, DM (Neonatology)
Chief Neonatologist
Fernandez Hospital
Hyderguda, Hyderabad-500 029
E-mail: *srinivasmurki.2001@gmail.com*

Severe jaundice

N. Karthik Nagesh MD, FRCPCH (UK), FNNF
Chairman and Head
Department of Neonatology
Manipal Hospitals Enterprises Ltd.
Chairman, Manipal Advanced Children's Centre
Manipal Hospital
Bengaluru-560 017
E-mail: *drkarthiknagesh@gmail.com*

Metabolic emergencies

Nishad Palakkal MD
Assistant Professor
Department of Neonatology
JIPMER, Puducherry-605 006
E-mail: *plakkal@gmail.com*

Shock

Ranjan K. Pejaver FRCP, FRCPCH (UK)
Professor of Neonatology
KIMS, Bangaluru
Chief Neonatologist, Meenakshi Hospital
Bangaluru-560 086
E-mail: *rpejaver@yahoo.com*

The bleeding neonate

Maneesha PH MBBS, DNB (Neonatology)
Consultant Neonatologist
Meenakshi Hospitals
Bangaluru-560 050
E-mail: *peopletreehospital@meenakshi*

The bleeding neonate

Shubha R. Phadke MD, DM (Medical Genetics)
Professor and Head
Department of Medical Genetics
Sanjay Gandhi Postgraduate Institute of Medical Sciences
Lucknow-226 014
E-mail: *shubharaophadke@gmail.com*

Neonatal emergencies due to inborn errors of metabolism

Mrinal Pillai MD, DNB (Neonatology)
Associate Consultant
SUT Hospital
Tiruvananthapuram, Pattom-695 004
E-mail: *mrinalhere@gmail.com*

Metabolic emergencies

Ratna Dua Puri MD, DM (Medical Genetics)
Professor of Genetics
GRIPMER Vice-Chairperson
Institute of Medical Genetics and Genomics
Sir Ganga Ram Hospital, Rajinder Nagar
New Delhi-110 060
E-mail: *ratnadpuri@yahoo.com*

Neonatal emergencies due to inborn errors of metabolism

Anuradha Rai MD
Fellow (NBE) Pediatrics
Gastroenterology and Hepatology
Medanta The Medicity Hospital, Sector 38
Gurugram-122 001
E-mail: *anuradharai2@gmail.com*

Acute liver failure

Swarna Rekha MD
Former Professor of Pediatrics and Neonatology
St. John's Medical College
Bengaluru-560 034
E-mail: *srekha74@rediffmail.com*

Anemia and polycythemia

Mohammed Sadique MBBS
Junior Resident
Department of Pediatrics
LLRM Medical College
Meerut (UP)-250 004

Intracranial hemorrhage

Piyush Shah MBBS, DCH, MRCPCH
Consultant Neonatologist
Cloudnine Maternity and Newborn Hospital
Siddhachal Arcade, Link Road, Malad West
Mumbai-400 064
E-mail: *doc.piyushshah@gmail.com*

Assessment of severity of neonatal sickness

Arvind Shenoi MD, DM (Neonatology)
Chief Neonatologist and Medical Director
Cloudnine Hospital, Old Airport Road, 115 Kodihalli
Bengaluru-560 017
E-mail: *arvindshenoi@gmail.com*

Neonatal infections: viral, parasitic and fungal

Meharban Singh MD, FAMS, FIAP, FIMSA, FNNF, Hony. FAAP
Former Professor and Head
Department of Pediatrics and Neonatal Division
WHO Collaborating Center for Training and Research in Newborn Care
All India Institute of Medical Sciences
New Delhi-110 029
Consultant Pediatrician
Child Care Center
625, Sector 37, Arun Vihar
Noida-201 301
E-mail: drmbsk@gmail.com

Organization of a neonatal intensive care unit
Emergencies at birth
The crying neonate
Necrotizing enterocolitis
The surgical neonate
Follow-up of NICU neonates
Ethical and legal issues in the NICU
Emergency procedures and life saving medications

Poonam Singh MD
DNB Fellow
Department of Neonatology
Institute of Child Health
Sir Ganga Ram Hospital, Rajinder Nagar
New Delhi-110 060
E-mail: drpoonamujn@gmail.com

Transport of sick neonates

Sunil Sinha MD, PhD, FRCP, FRCPCH
Professor of Pediatrics
University of Durham
Consultant Neonatologist
The James Cook University Hospital
Middlesbrough, Cleveland, UK
E-mail: sunil.sinha@stees.nhs.uk

Respiratory emergencies

Sindhu Sivanandan MD
Senior Resident
Department of Pediatrics
All India Institute of Medical Sciences
New Delhi-110 029
E-mail: drsindhusivanandan@gmail.com

Emergency procedures and life saving medications

Rhishikesh Thakre DCH, MD, DM (Neonatology), DNB, FCPS, FIAP
Director NICU, Neo Clinic and Hospital
27 Samarth Nagar
Aurangabad-431 001
E-mail: rptdoc@gmail.com

Life-threatening congenital malformations

Anup Thakur MD, DNB (Neonatology)
Associate Consultant
Department of Neonatology
Institute of Child Health, Sir Ganga Ram Hospital
Rajinder Nagar
New Delhi-110 060
E-mail: dr.thakuranup@gmail.com

Transport of sick neonates

Amit Upadhaya MD, DNB, MNAMS, DM (Neonatology)
Professor of Pediatrics
LLRM Medical College
Meerut (UP)-250 004
E-mail: au.llrm@gmail.com

Intracranial hemorrhage
Neonatal seizures

Umesh Vaidya MD, DNB
Chief Neonatologist and Incharge NICU
KEM Hospital
Pune-411 011
E-mail: kemnicu@gmail.com

Parenteral nutrition

Sanjay Wazir MD, DM (Neonatology)
Director Neonatology
Cloudnine Maternity and Newborn Hospital
Sector 47
Gurugram-122 003
E-mail: swazir21@gmail.com

Assessment of severity of neonatal sickness

Contents

Organization of a Neonatal Intensive Care Unit

Meharban Singh

Background

The organization of a neonatal intensive care unit (NICU) is essential for reducing the neonatal mortality and improving the quality of life among the survivors. During the past three decades, improvements in the diagnostic and therapeutic approaches in the care of high-risk infants have influenced their prognosis favorably. Unfortunately, many neonatal centers in the developing countries are unplanned and merely improvised. The pediatrician and nurse incharge of neonatal services should be taken into confidence during the planning stage so that the intensive care neonatal unit is based on their opinions for meeting the special needs of sick and small neonates. It is a welcome move that government of India has launched an initiative to establish special care newborn units (SCNUs) at district hospitals. The SCNU at the district hospital is envisaged to provide; (i) care at birth including resuscitation of asphyxiated newborns, (ii) management of sick newborns, (iii) referral and transport services for babies needing continuous positive airway pressure (CPAP), mechanical ventilation and major surgical intervention, (iv) postnatal care and immunization services and (v) follow-up of high-risk newborns.

Adequate space, availability of running water round-the-clock, centralized oxygen and suction facilities, maintenance of thermoneutral environment and ready availability of plenty of linen and disposables is mandatory to provide optimal level III newborn care. Facilities for prevention and management of common neonatal problems, viz. perinatal hypoxia, hypothermia, LBW babies, respiratory distress syndrome, septicemia, hyperbilirubinemia and life-threatening congenital malformations, should be established. The emphasis should be laid on developing a sound infrastructure to ensure safe delivery, promote asepsis,

provide warmth and adequate nutrition with human milk. The lop-sided enthusiasm to acquire sophisticated electronic gadgetry including ventilators, in the absence of basic infrastructural facilities, must be discouraged. At the present state of our development, level III or tertiary neonatal care should be established in a phased manner in regional centers selected on the basis of available infrastructure and professional expertise. Effective and optimal management of newborn babies at birth, prevention of hypothermia and bacterial infections and feeding of all babies with human milk should be ensured before establishing neonatal intensive care facilities. Intensive care of the newborn is highly cost-intensive and demands considerable inputs of staff, equipment and time. The philosophy of specialized conservative management of high-risk newborn babies should be fully exploited to bring down the neonatal mortality rate to less than 20 per 1000 live births before intensive care facilities are launched (Figure 1.1).

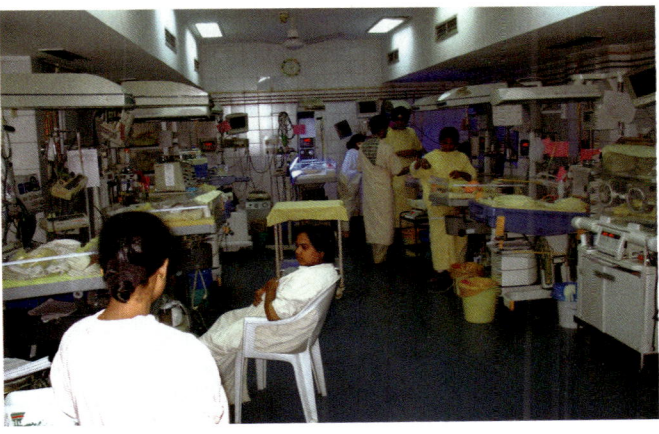

Figure 1.1 NICU of All India Institute of Medical Sciences, New Delhi.

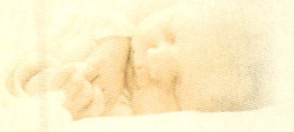

PHYSICAL FACILITIES

Space

The size of the unit is related to the expected population intended to be served. In India, about 15 to 20% of newborn babies need special care, depending upon the criteria for antenatal booking for confinement. In addition, if the center is to serve as a referral unit for the infants born outside the hospital (extramural babies), allowance should be made for additional physical facilities and space. In a maternity unit having 2,000 deliveries per year, facilities for special care of 6–8 high-risk infants should be available. Each infant should be provided with a minimum area of 100 sq. ft. or 10 M². However, additional space would be needed to provide for special facilities as outlined below in the floor plan. There should be no compromise on space because its adequacy is crucial for reduction of nosocomial infections. Space should be allocated within the nursery complex for promotion of breastfeeding, expression of breast-milk and its storage, aseptic preparation of intravenous fluids and parenteral nutrients.

Location

The neonatal unit should be located as close as possible to the labor rooms and obstetric operation theater, to facilitate prompt transfer of sick and high-risk infants. The presence of an elevator in close proximity is desirable for transport of outborn infants. In tropical countries, the nursery should not be located on the top floor of the hospital but there should be feasibility for the sunlight to peep into the nursery to enhance brightness and provide ultraviolet rays to augment asepsis.

Nursery Design

The unit design may be in a square space or a single corridor-based rectangular unit. A split unit, i.e. on either side of the hospital corridor, should be avoided for ease of mobility and for prevention of infections. A unit design occupying one side of the corridor with a nurses control room in the center, from where all the babies can be viewed, is preferred (Figure 1.2). Apart from constant surveillance of all babies, the design should ensure minimal walking distance for the staff.

Baby Care Area

The unit should be provided with areas and rooms for inborn or intramural babies, stepdown nursery, outborn or extramural babies, examination area, mother's area for breastfeeding and expression of breast-milk, preparation of intravenous fluids and parenteral nutrients, nurses station and charting area. The floor and walls should be made of washable glazed or vitrified tiles and windows should have two layers of glass panes to ensure some measure of heat and sound insulation. The obviously infected infants with open sepsis (especially those with diarrhea and abscesses) should be isolated in a septic nursery, which should be located away from the NICU and manned by different nursing and resident staff. A large number of ancillary services are needed and should be designed and earmarked during the planning stage.

Handwashing and gowning room Handwashing and gowning facility should be located at the enterance. It should be provided with abundant space with self-closing doors. A positive air pressure should be maintained in the NICU so that corridor air does not enter the NICU. Street shoes are changed with nursery slippers, followed by handwashing and gowning. The use of mask is controversial and is best avoided. Hand-free elbow or foot-operated tap fitted in a handwashing sink with liquid soap dispenser is recommended. Sink should be made of porcelain or stainless steel. Pictorial handwashing instructions should be affixed on the wall next to the sink. Hands should be dried with single use or disposable paper napkins. Air dryers are not recommended due to risk of dissemination of microbes. Walls adjacent to the sink should be made of non-porous or non-absorbent material to prevent growth of molds. Sinks should not be provided with slabs or counter-tops which are a potent source of infection. The unit should be provided with 24-hour uninterrupted water supply by having dedicated overhead tank with a capacity of 1000–2000 liters.

Examination area A small comfortable room with examination table, comfortable seating, sufficient light, and warmth is needed for assessment of baby before admission to the nursery. The baby is cleaned and provided with nursery garments in this room.

Mother area The room should be provided with comfortable seating and privacy to the mother to breastfeed and express the breast-milk with the help of a lactation nurse.

Handwashing stations Handwashing sinks should be provided within 20 feet (6 meters) of every newborn bed. The sink should be large and deep (24" wide × 16" front-back and 10" deep) and made of porcelain or stainless steel and without any counter or shelf. Single use sterile cotton napkins or disposable paper napkins should be available for drying the hands. Alternatively, antiseptic

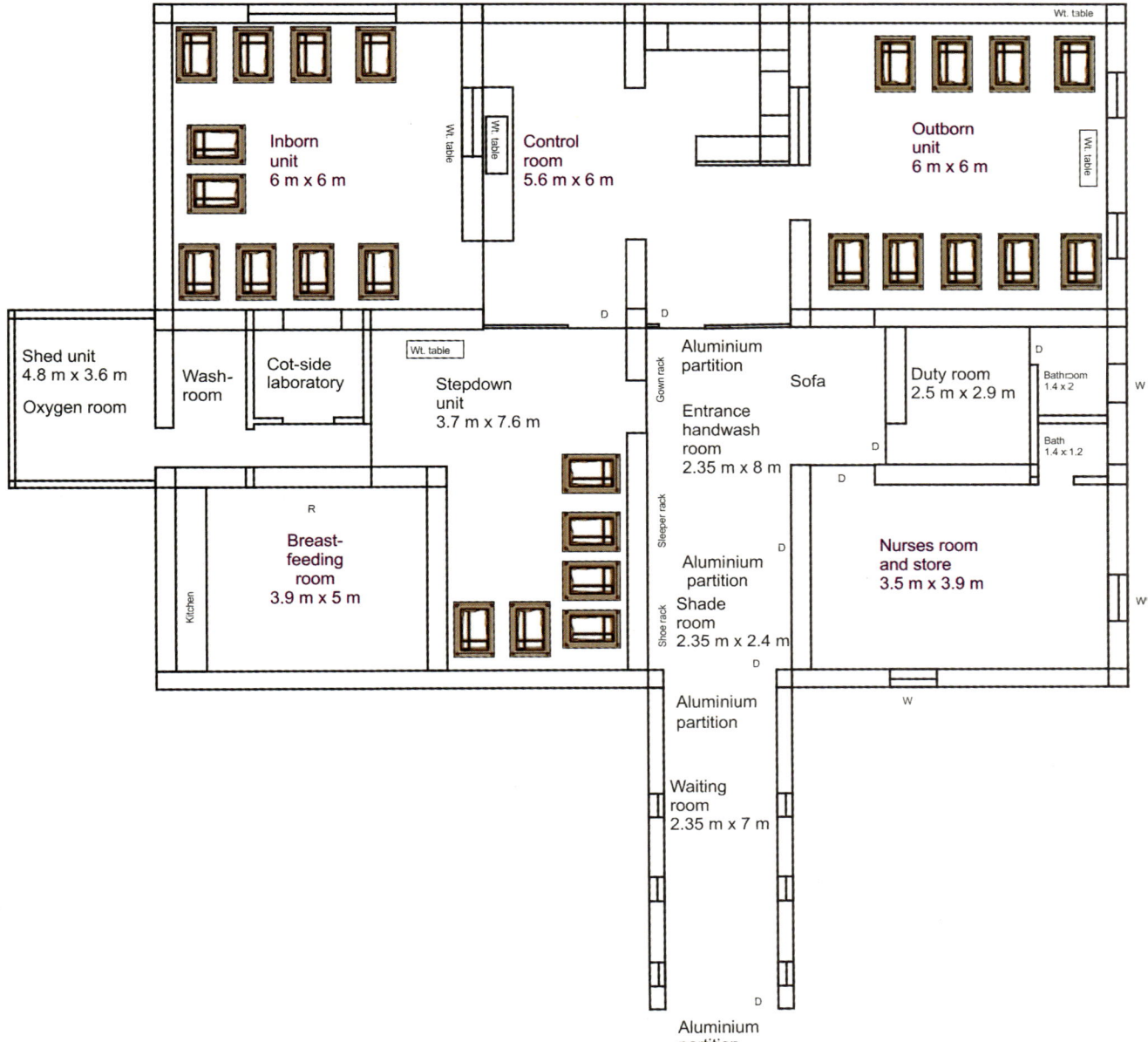

Figure 1.2 The conceptual layout for a neonatal intensive care unit for 25 babies. *Adapted from* tool kit for setting up special care neonatal unit, UNICEF.

sanitizing solution (sterillium) can be used for disinfection of hands in-between the babies.

Preparation of intravenous fluids A separate area should be earmarked and provided with a laminar flow system for preparation of intravenous fluids, parenteral nutritional formulations, enteral feeds and medications. Boiling and autoclaving facilities should be available adjacent to this area.

Nurses station Nursing station and charting area for nurses and residents should be located in a central area from where all the babies can be observed. Newborn

charts, hospital forms, computer terminals, telephone lines should be located in this area. It is preferable to use electronic medical recording of clinical notes and retrieval of laboratory reports.

Clean utility and soiled utility holding rooms There should be enough space for stocking clean utility items and sterile disposables, and for disposal of dirty linen and contaminated disposables. Built-in wall wooden cabinets with foldable covers are useful for stacking purposes. The ventilation system in the soiled utility or holding room should be engineered to have negative air pressure with all air being exhausted to the outside. The soiled utility room should be so located that it enables removal of soiled material without passing through the baby care area.

Staff rooms Space should be provided within the unit to meet the professional, personal and administrative needs of resident staff on duty. A comfortable room with intercom, telephone and computer terminal and WC facilities is mandatory. Nurse's change room is required for changing from street clothes to a smart shirt and trouser dress stipulated by the NICU.

Growing nursery A separate bay in the lying-in ward should be earmarked for transitional care of high-risk babies by their mothers before they are discharged from the hospital. The entry of visitors to this area should be restricted and it should be kept adequately warm. Facilities for monitoring asepsis and weighing the babies should be available in the transitional care room (TCR) or growing nursery (GN). The growing nursery is used with advantage for educating the mothers in child care activities and promoting the practice of exclusive breastfeeding.

Ventilation

Effective air ventilation of nursery is essential to reduce nosocomial infections. The most satisfactory ventilation is achieved with laminar airflow system which is rather expensive. When centralized air-conditioning is used, minimum of 12 changes of room air per hour are recommended. There should be no draughts of air on and near the newborn beds. The air-conditioning ducts must be provided with millipore filters (0.5 μ) to restrict the passage of microbes. A simple method to achieve satisfactory ventilation consists of provision of exhaust fan in a reverse direction near the ceiling for input of fresh uncontaminated air and fixation of another exhaust fan in the conventional manner near the floor for air exit. A constant positive air pressure should be maintained in the nursery so that contaminated air from the corridors does not gain access into the nursery. The use of chemical air disinfection and ultraviolet lamps are no more recommended.

Lighting

The nursery must be well-illuminated and painted white or slightly off-white to permit prompt and early detection of jaundice and cyanosis. It is best achieved by cool white fluorescent tubes or LED (light-emitting diodes) to provide at least 100 foot-candle, shadow-free illumination at the infant's level. The number and exact location of fixtures can be worked out taking into account size of the nursery, height of the ceiling, and availability or otherwise of sunlight. Spot illumination for various procedures can be provided by a portable angle-poise lamp having two 15 watt fluorescent bulbs which when held at a distance of about one foot from the infant, produce about 100 feet-candle intensity of light. Most open care systems are equipped with in-built source of overhead spot lights. In places where electrical failure is frequent and prolonged, the electrical system of the nursery complex must be attached to an auto-mode generator. Exposure of preterm babies to strong light has been incriminated as a risk factor for the development of retinopathy of prematurity. The nursery light should be dimmed at night to simulate day-night pattern to promote hormonal surge and growth of babies. Bedside lights with dimmer switches should be provided to create specialized micro-environment for each baby.

Environmental Temperature and Humidity

The temperature of the nursery complex must be maintained between 26–28°C (78.8–82.4°F) in order to minimize effects of thermal stress on the babies. This is best achieved by centralized air-conditioning having temperature control knobs in the nursery. The air movement should be so designed that draught is minimized. In places where air-conditioning is not feasible, room temperature can be reasonably well-maintained in winter by use of radiant heaters and hot air blowers. Portable radiant heater, infrared lamp or bakery bulb can be used to provide additional source of heat to an individual infant. The external windows of nursery should be glazed to minimize heat gain and heat loss and baby beds should be located at least 2 feet (0.6 meter) away from the wall or window. In most parts of India, relative humidity averages above 50%, which is quite satisfactory for routine needs of newborn babies. Humidity level can be raised for preterm babies nursed in an incubator. High and effective humidity level is useful to reduce insensible water loss but is associated with increased risk of nosocomial infection.

Acoustic Characteristics

The ventilation system, incubators, air compressors, suction pumps and many other devices used in the nursery produce noise. Sound intensity in the nursery should not exceed 75 dB to protect hearing of nursery personnel and infants. Excessive noise may lead to hearing loss, physiological and behavioral disturbances, such as sleep disturbances, startles and crying episodes, hypoxia, tachycardia and increased intracranial pressure. The fabrication and redesigning of nursery equipment should take into account the desirability of minimizing noise by dampening the sounds by acoustic or other means. It is desirable to have effective soundproofing of ceilings, walls, doors and floor when a NICU is designed. Telephone rings and equipment alarms should be replaced by blinking lights. Instead of air compressors, centralized sources of compressed air, oxygen and suction should be provided. Decibel meters should be installed to monitor sound levels in the nursery. The beneficial and soothing effects of meaningful sounds, such as gentle music or recordings of parent voice, should be harnessed to provide physiologic stability to the babies.

Handling and Social Contacts

Excessive and rough handling of delicate newborn babies is associated with several adverse physiological consequences, such as excessive crying, sleep disturbances, tachycardia or bradycardia, hypoxia and rise in blood pressure and intracranial pressure. Handling should be gentle and kept to the barest minimum without compromising care. Soothing words, gentle stroking and rocking should be practised after a painful procedure. Gentle caressing, cuddling and touching by the mother are desirable to provide comfort and confidence to the baby and aid the process of healing. Infants should be exposed to gentle and soothing tactile, kinesthetic, vestibular, motor, auditory and visual experiences to provide opportunities for early learning and improvement in behavior. Parents should be allowed unrestricted entry to the nursery to provide these useful sensorimotor stimuli. It enhances the process of bonding between the baby and the family.

Communication System

The nursery complex should be provided with an intercom system so that additional person can be called for help in case of emergency without leaving the sick infant. A direct line external telephone is mandatory so that parents have an easy access to inquire about welfare of their infants and in turn they can be readily contacted whenever needed. Mobile phones should not be used near the vicinity of the nursery because the electromagnetic waves are likely to interfere with the functioning of the electronic equipment. The family should be kept constantly informed about the condition of their baby including therapeutic interventions being given. They should be given emotional support and pragmatic view of the likely outcome.

Electrical Outlets

There should be adequate number (8–12 electrical points at the height of 4–5 feet) of 5 amperes and 15 amperes electrical points attached to a common ground. Each infant must be provided with at least 8 electrical outlets, 4 should be 5 amperes and another 4 of 15 amperes. The use of adapters and extension boards should be discouraged. The electrical equipment used in the nursery must be checked at least once a month for leakage of current and adequacy of grounding. If possible, special fittings with safety devices should be installed. The unit should have round-the-clock uninterrupted servo-stabilized power supply. There should be round-the-clock power back-up including provision of UPS system for the sensitive equipment.

PERSONNEL

It is important, that while allocating nursing, medical and paramedical staff to the hospital, the needs of the neonatal unit are not ignored. It is unfortunate that newborn babies are not counted as patients requiring nursing and medical care while expressing the bed strength of a hospital. The census of the hospital bed is administratively based on dieted beds. In fact, the situation is paradoxical because the neonates need rather specialized and sophisticated nursing and medical care. Therefore, the highest priority in the organization of the NICU is the availability of sufficient number of adequately trained personnel especially the nurses. The survival of newborn babies depends upon the availability of specially trained nurses. The Nursing Council of India has not outlined any special guidelines for this purpose. It has been recommended by the American Academy of Pediatrics that one nurse is needed to offer special or intermediate nursing care to 3 babies or intensive care to one infant. In countries where monitoring devices are not routinely available, relatively larger number of nurses are necessary for undertaking manual monitoring. It is generally not appreciated by the hospital administrators that a considerable time of the nurse is spent in rigorous housekeeping rituals to maintain asepsis in the nursery. The frequent toilet care, expression of breast-milk, formula preparation and feeding are time consuming and unassisted by any attendant. Whenever adequate number of nurses are not available, these rituals are compromised resulting in inadequacy of feeding and outbreak of infection in the nursery. The nursery complex must, therefore, be considered as an independent nursing unit under the charge of a fully qualified nursing sister.

The National Neonatology Forum of India has recommended that at least one trained nurse should be allocated to provide coverage to four babies in the special care neonatal unit. The allowance should be kept for additional 25% staff to provide for the exigencies of day off and leave. Therefore, for a 8-bedded SCNU or level II neonatal unit, eight nurses should be sanctioned to ensure availability of two nurses in each shift along with one additional sister incharge in the morning shift. In a NICU, the overall allocation of nurses should be one nurse for two babies, i.e. 16 nurses for 8-bedded unit. The continuity of service can be maintained, if at least 50% of the nurses are rather permanent and not transferred frequently as is the usual practice in general hospitals. There must be equal distribution of nurses in the three duty shifts during 24 hours. The nurses must be imparted continuing in-service training in the art of neonatal nursing and preventive maintenance of a variety of electronic equipment used in the NICU. They should participate in the monthly perinatal morbidity and mortality meetings. It is desirable to have services of public health nurses and social workers for follow-up and home care of low birth weight babies after their discharge from the hospital.

A pediatrician specially trained in the care of newborn babies should devote his full time to improve the existing standards of neonatal special care services in the country. The unit must also have an independent senior resident and one junior resident round-the-clock for every 4 babies requiring intensive care. The resident doctors must work in these units for at least 3 months to maintain continuity of medical care. All deliveries in the hospital should preferably be attended by a physician trained in the care of newborn. A laboratory technician should be available to operate bilirubinometer, glucometer, microcentrifuge, CRP kits and blood gas analyzer. A biomedical technician or a link person is essential to maintain a liaison with suppliers of equipment to ensure their smooth functioning, prevent breakdowns and reduce the downtime. The resident staff and nurses working in the NICU must be trained to properly handle and use the equipment. When ventilatory facilities are established, respiratory therapist is a useful member of the neonatal team to monitor ventilatory settings, provide tracheal suctioning and chest physiotherapy. A pediatric pathologist, who is specially trained for conducting and interpreting neonatal autopsies, is desirable to complement the functioning of the neonatal team.

EQUIPMENT

During the last 2–3 decades, a large number of monitoring devices for diagnostic and therapeutic use for the high-risk newborn infants have been developed. These have considerably improved the monitoring and intact survival of high-risk neonates. Several basic prerequisites must be fulfilled before any center invests in purchase of expensive equipment involving foreign exchange. The fundamental needs of the unit are availability of adequate space, round-the-clock water supply, freedom from congestion and presence of a sufficient number of adequately trained nurses. A reasonable level of asepsis must be achieved and facilities for maintaining thermoneutral environment should be established. The feeding of babies should be associated with minimal risk of aspiration.

Acquisition of new equipment does not necessarily ensure better services and outcome. *Machines cannot replace men. The best monitors with us are dedicated nurses and resident doctors involved in the care of newborn babies with their observational skills sharpened by experience.* Therefore, they need continued in-service training, teaching and encouragement for obtaining the best results. In view of the exorbitant cost of imported equipment and problems faced in their maintenance, there is a constant need to promote "make in India" concept for indigenous fabrication of equipment required for neonatal care.

The maintenance of the existing equipment in proper working condition is more important than acquiring new and sophisticated gadgets. Before placing an order, check with existent consumer/s regarding reliability of the equipment and quality of after sales service provided by the local dealer. The supplier must install the equipment and provide training to the staff for proper use and maintenance of the equipment. Date of installation and expiry of warranty period should be recorded. After expiry of mandatory warranty period, you should enter into an annual maintenance contract with the local dealer for preventive maintenance and emergency repairs in the event of breakdowns. In case of sophisticated and expensive equipment, a counter-guarantee of service should also be taken from the foreign principals. Inventory of spares should be maintained and essential spares should be purchased and kept in stock while ordering new equipment. Photocopies of working and service manuals should be available in the NICU while original documents should be kept in a safe custody. Maintain a log book containing postal and e-mail addresses, telephone and fax numbers of local dealers and suppliers of equipment. When telephonic or e-mail complaints are not heeded by the local supplier, you should send a written complaint and endorse a copy to the foreign principals.

Preventive Maintenance and Emergency Repairs

After-sales technical services including annual maintenance contract (AMC) should be a mandatory requirement at the time of purchase of the equipment. At the time of installation, the supplier should provide technical training, hands-on training for clinical use of the equipment and its proper maintenance to the nurses and resident doctors. A qualified in-house biomedical technician should be available to maintain an inventory of equipment and spares, ensure optimal preventive maintenance and take prompt action to call the service engineer to ensure maximum uptime of the life-saving medical equipment. The in-house technician should have up-to-date information regarding the proper use of the equipment, should be able to undertake first-line corrective intervention that does not require any spare parts and when required he should be able to report correctly the nature of technical malfunctioning of the equipment to the on-call service engineer of the company.

The objectives of preventive maintenance include that the equipment should be functional most of the time and should operate with accuracy, efficiency and safety. The maintenance engineer should undertake at least two technical visits per year to check the wear and tear, and performance of the device as per manufacturers technical check list. The equipment should be cleaned and defective components replaced by spare parts. He should interact with in-house technician and end-users to provide necessary guidance for correct use of the equipment to ensure effective preventive maintenance and upkeep.

Despite careful use of the equipment, the average lifetime of most electronic equipment is about 5–7 years. In the event of breakdown, when contacted the service engineer should report to the NICU without delay to ensure that the downtime of the equipment is minimum. In case the device cannot be repaired on-site and the machine is taken to the workshop, a replacement model should be provided by the company for the period of the repair.

The equipment listed and described below are by and large arranged in the order of their usefulness and priority. *The maintenance of existing equipment in proper working condition is more important than acquiring additional gadgets.*

Resuscitation Equipment

The equipments needed for resuscitation of an asphyxiated baby at birth are discussed in detail in Chapter 4. Emergency tray should be available in each infant care room of NICU containing Ambu bag and mask, infant laryngoscope, tracheal tubes of different sizes, sterile suction catheters, oral mucus suction traps, and emergency drugs.

Bag and Mask Resuscitator

Self-inflating bag of 250–750 mL capacity is ideal for resuscitation of a newborn baby. It remains inflated at all times without any compressed gas source. There are four components of self-inflating bag, i.e. air inlet, oxygen inlet, patient outlet and valve assembly (Figure 1.3). It should be provided with a pop-off valve or with a facility to attach a pressure gauge. An oxygen reservoir in the form of a corrugated tube or rubber bladder, helps to increase the oxygen concentration to 90 to 100%. When self-inflating bag is used without an oxygen reservoir, it delivers 40–60% oxygen because room air enters the bag with each inflation. A one-way valve allows delivery of oxygen at the outlet when bag is squeezed but closes as soon as the bag is released so that the exaled air cannot re-enter the bag. A peep valve can be attached to the valve assembly to deliver required PEEP. A pressure gauge can be attached to a small hole or projection located near the patient outlet. The gauge allows the person using the bag to control the pressure of air or oxygen being delivered to the baby. The self-inflating bag cannot be used for providing free-flow oxygen to the baby unless it is equipped with a closed bladder reservoir. The silicone rubber bags of Laerdal make are more sturdy and can withstand autoclaving and cleaning with antiseptic solutions. Face masks (size 0, 1 and 2) should be rigid with a cushioned rim to form a tight air-seal fit on the face enclosing the mouth and nostrils. Anatomical shaped masks are avoided due to the potential risk of causing local trauma due to pressure. Indigenously manufactured bags and masks are highly unsatisfactory due to poor quality of rubber, lack of oxygen inlet, absence of any safety features and loss of re-expansion capabilities of the bag.

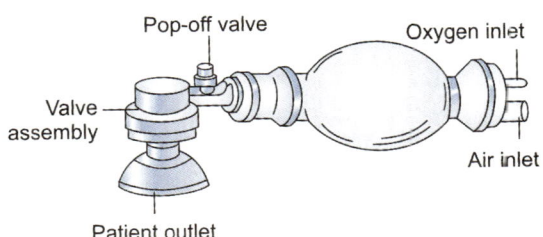

Figure 1.3 The components of self-inflating bag.

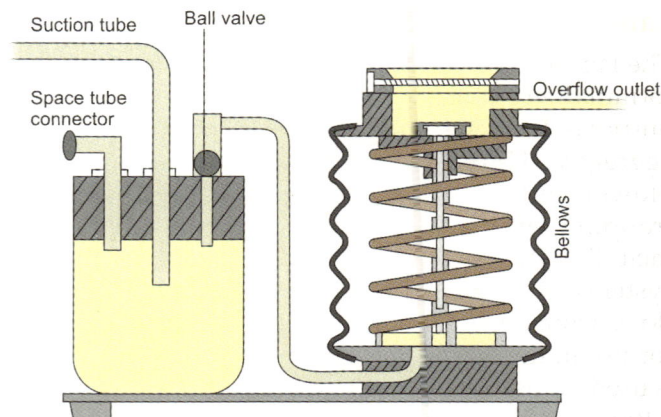

Figure 1.5 Diagrammatic sketch of a foot-operated suction machine.

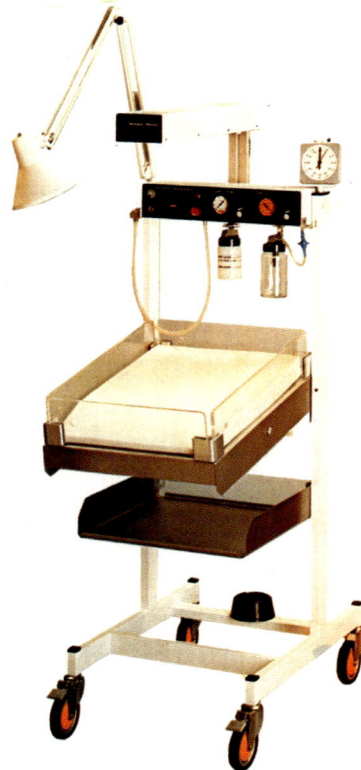

Figure 1.4 Resuscitator for receiving babies at birth. Note the stop clock which is useful to time the events during resuscitation.

A resuscitator trolley equipped with radiant warmer, timer, electrical suction, observation light and manual assisted ventilation facilities is an essential equipment for the delivery room (Figure 1.4). In-built pulse oximeter is extremely useful to monitor heart rate and oxygen saturation.

Oxygen and Suction Facilities

A centralized source of oxygen, compressed air and suction outlet consoles (50 psi) affixed on the walls is ideal. By mixing variable quantities of compressed air and oxygen, one can obtain oxygen concentrations ranging between 25% and 100%.

De Lee trap for a single use self-oral suction with 12 Fr catheter should be avoided because of potential risk of transmission of HIV infection. A soft plastic catheter or nozzle with a suction bulb is a good alternative but difficult to clean. Suction machines using recoil springs are bulky and complex to operate and difficult to clean. A foot-operated suction machine is useful in rural health care facilities because of non-availability or erratic power supply (Figure 1.5). In hospitals, centralized suction, venturi suction and electrical suction machines are used. The suction

pressure is regulated with a pressure dial. Facility should be available for intermittent suction because continuous suction may cause bradycardia and mucosal damage. The suction pressure should be limited to 60–80 cm H_2O (1.0 mm Hg = 1.3 cm H_2O). Slow suction devices are used for continuous suction of chest cavity and upper pouch of infants with esophageal atresia.

Catheters, Syringes and Needles

Nasogastric polyethylene feeding tubes (Fr 5, 6 and 8), suction catheters (Fr 10 and 12), umbilical vein catheters, small-vein infusion sets (G 23), medicaths (neoflon), and exchange transfusion sets are now freely available in India at a reasonable cost. They are prepacked sterile by a process of gamma-irradiation. These should not be reused after boiling. As relatively small volume of parenteral medications are needed for low birth weight babies, it is desirable to use tuberculin or insulin syringes for injections to ensure ease and accuracy of administration. Only single-use syringes and needles should be used. The availability of liberal supplies of disposables is crucial for reduction of nosocomial infections.

Feeding Equipment

Glass or stainless steel bowls of adequate size (120 mL capacity) should be available in the nursery for collection of expressed breast-milk, mixing and preparing the formula. A hot air autoclaving oven or a pressure sterilizer should be provided for autoclaving feeding equipment. Storage facility, like a refrigerator, should be available in the nursery. The formula room should be equipped with working shelves having laminated plastic surfaces or preferably these should be made of stainless steel so that they can be easily washed and cleaned.

Laminar Flow System

The laminar flow system is useful for safe and aseptic formulation and mixing of drugs, parenteral fluids and nutrients. It is equipped with high efficiency particulate aggregate (HEPA) filter to block entry of bacteria, a blower and plenum. HEPA filters are effective in trapping 99.97% of all the particles of >0.3 μ size including dust and bacterial pathogens. Two types of systems are available. In a vertical type system, the air flows from above downwards and it is recommended for use in the NICU. The horizontal flow type system is used for tissue culture and microbiologic techniques. Ultraviolet light source in the chamber is kept on for 30 minutes before use to make the area of operation free of bacteria. The vertical flow of bacteria-free filtered air maintains a positive pressure of 15 mm Hg to prevent entry of contaminated air into the chamber. Strict asepsis should be ensured by wearing mask, sterile gown and disposable gloves while operating the laminar flow system. The critical work area and accessible surfaces should be disinfected with bacillocid or 70% isopropyle alcohol.

Weighing Machine

Accurate weight record of babies is a sensitive index of their wellbeing and availability of a sturdy and reliable weighing machine fulfills a fundamental need. A sensitive beam-type weighing scale with a precision of ±10 g is a useful equipment in the nursery. It must be calibrated frequently against standard one kilogram weight. The chances of cross-infection should be minimized by using a sterile paper or a towel over the pan before weighing each infant. Electronic weighing machine (resolution either ±5 g or ±1 g) with a digital read-out though expensive is desirable for sake of convenience and accuracy (Figure 1.6). Availability of a reliable and sensitive electronic weighing scale is more useful and desirable than acquiring a ventilator which is kept as a show piece in the nursery.

Bassinets

A variety of bassinets are available for routine use in the nursery. It is desirable to use bassinets, which can be easily cleaned and are equipped with a locker and head tilting mechanism (Figure 1.7). The locker can be used to hold the supplies of an individual baby, such as diapers, frocks, sterile gauze, cotton, thermometer, feeding equipment, drugs, etc.

Plastic plexiglass or fiberglass bassinets with relatively low walls and placed at a convenient height are desirable for ease of observation and examination of the infant. They can be easily cleaned and disinfected by antiseptic solutions. Alcohol or organic solvents should not be used to clean the plastic or plexiglass material due to risk of opacification.

Incubators

The incubators are essential to provide an ideal micro-environment for high-risk babies. About one-third of nursery beds should comprise of incubators. The main functions of an incubator are isolation, maintenance of thermoneutral ambient temperature, desired humidity and administration of oxygen. It is desirable to nurse extremely low birth weight (<1000 g) stable babies in the incubator. The sensory stimuli, like light, sound, touch and pain, should be kept to the barest minimum without compromising the quality of care. It is essential

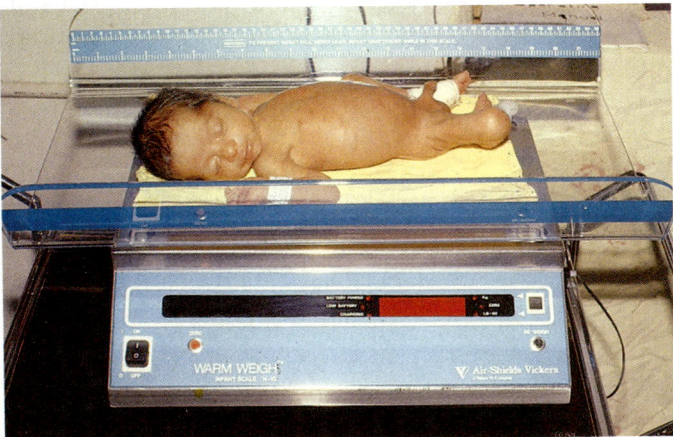

Figure 1.6 Electronic weighing scale with an accuracy of ±1.0 g.

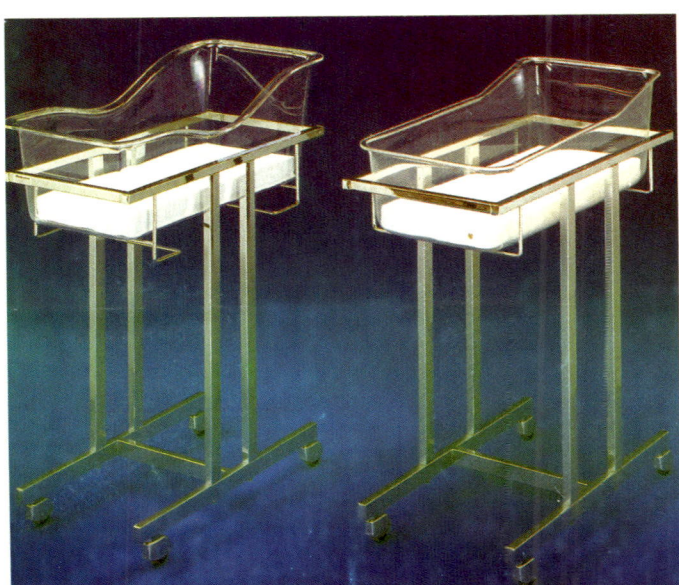

Figure 1.7 Plexiglass bassinets for keeping stable babies. They are aesthetic and easy to clean.

that an incubator should not interfere with observation of infant, should offer easy access to the baby and be readily cleanable. Even when sterile water is used in the humidity tank, incubators are a potential source of infection. The water in the humidity tank should be changed daily and 1–2 mL of glacial acetic acid or vinegar should be added to prevent bacterial colonization. Most centers are now using incubators without adding any water in the humidity chamber, while in some countries incubators are used to provide 100% humidity akin to in-utero environment.

The incubator may be of portable type for transport of sick babies or stationed in the nursery. The open box type (Armstrong) incubators are incapable of maintaining thermoneutrality due to alterations in the temperature when lid is opened. They are equipped with an inefficient thermostat and do not provide for entry of filtered air in the incubator. The intensive care or closed type (isolette) incubators are equipped with portholes for access to the infant (Figure 1.8). The front panel can also be opened and bassinet can be pulled out for unhindered access to the infant for examination and various procedures. These incubators are equipped with an air pump for circulation of filtered air for uniform distribution of heat throughout the incubator. They are also provided with partitioned circuit which allows for gradual changes in heat current as opposed to conventional on-off thermostat. A double wall incubator is preferred because radiant heat loss is reduced by 50%. A servo-control system is ideal for automatic adjustments in the ambient temperature to keep the infant homeothermic. Skin sensor or thermocouple is affixed to the abdominal skin over the liver area or right hypochondrium and incubator is set for maintenance of skin temperature at 36.5°C. The skin sensor feeds the information regarding temperature of the baby to the thermostat which automatically regulates the output of heat to maintain the desired skin temperature. Infants nursed under servo mode should be watched to ensure that skin probe is in place. If skin probe inadvertently gets dislodged, infant may get overheated because ambient temperature would approach the set temperature of 36.5°C. They should be provided with in-built audio and visual alarms for set temperature, high body temperature, air flow, probe or sensor failure, etc. When fever develops in a baby nursed on skin servo mode, there will be repeated activation of alarm unless baby is shifted to manual mode. The built-in heater output monitor provides information regarding the amount of heat generated by the incubator warmer to keep the infant homeothermic. When heater output reading is minimal or nil, it suggests that infant is capable of generating enough metabolic heat to keep himself warm and he can be taken out of the incubator and nursed in an open cot.

Radiant Warmer/Open Care System

During various procedures, the infant loses body temperature, unless he is kept warm by use of radiant heat warmer. A portable heat lamp with two 150 watt white ordinary or bakery bulbs or infrared bulb fixed on the wall about 2 to 3 feet above the level of table or trolley can serve the purpose in a rural setting. The infrared heat is preferable because it directly warms the subject without affecting the temperature of intervening environment.

Open care systems which are equipped with an overhead radiant warmer and skin thermister or thermocouple with servo-control are the most useful and popular equipment. When an overhead radiant warmer is intended to be used for a prolonged period, it should be combined with a skin sensor and a servo-control system. They are equipped with a narrow band proportional heat controllers which can rapidly cycle up and down the temperature. They are provided with audio and visual alarms for high and low temperature and heater output. Recently, talking warmers have been introduced which provide verbal warning to the nurses regarding low temperature, high temperature and out of reach temperature. The steps followed in using an open care system are summarized in Box 1.1. Unless baby is extremely small or gravely sick, open care system is preferable over an intensive care incubator because of easy access to the infant and less chances of nosocomial infection. Skin probe is applied over the liver area in the epigastrium or right hypochondrium, and shielded with a foil-covered foam adhesive pad. When a baby is nursed prone, skin probe is applied over the flank. The probe should not be allowed to come

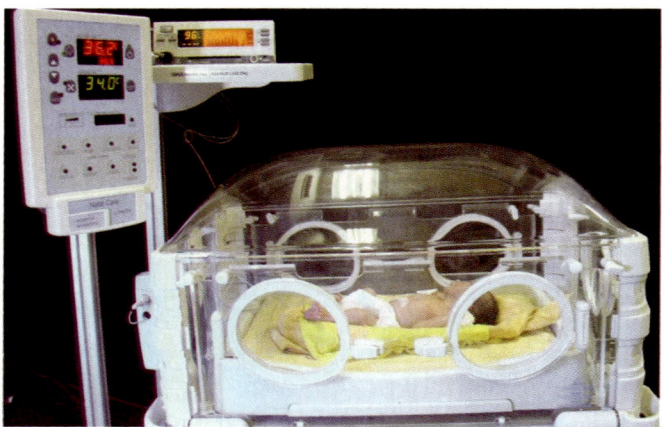

Figure 1.8 Intensive care double-walled incubator. It is provided with portholes and circulation of filtered air.

in contact with the bed. When probe is dislodged, it may lead to hyperthermia in the baby. These units also have a provision for overhead light source and phototherapy unit and are most suitable for undertaking any prolonged procedure, like assisted ventilation, exchange blood transfusion or surgery (Figures 1.9 and 1.10). Babies nursed in the open care

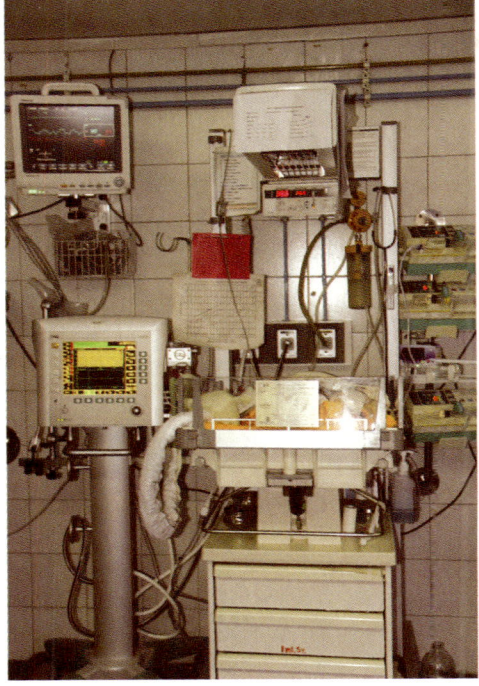

Figure 1.10 Premature infant in an open care system on ventilator and multichannel vital sign monitor.

BOX 1.1 Steps for using open care system

- Switch on the unit.
- Select manual mode with heater output of 100% for 10–15 minutes for rapid warming of the bassinet covered with linen.
- Select servo mode to maintain skin temperature of the baby at 36.5°C.
- The skin probe site (right hypochondrium in a supine baby and flank when baby is nursed prone) is prepared by using surgical spirit.
- Fix the probe with adhesive tape and cover it with a reflective pad.
- Ensure that the skin sensor is kept affixed to baby's skin at all times.
- When a hypothermic baby needs to be rapidly warmed, select the manual mode and the desired heater output.
- Record baby's axillary temperature after 30 minutes and then 2 hourly.
- Respond to alarm immediately, identify the fault and rectify it.

system have excessive evaporative fluid losses and have significantly higher metabolic rate compared to babies kept in the incubator. After stabilization of the baby kept in the open care system, it is preferable to cover the baby with clothes or thin polythene sheet to reduce evaporative fluid losses. Application of sterile liquid paraffin or non-irritating oil on the skin is associated with reduced evaporative losses from skin.

Therapeutic Cooling Devices

High technology whole baby cooling devices (Blanketrol, Tecotherm Neo, Meditherm) are equipped both for cooling and rewarming the baby by virtue of a heater, a compressor, water circulating pump and a microprocessor board. The baby is placed on a blanket which is designed to circulate cold or warm distilled water which is pumped from the unit. The equipment functions in three modes, manual mode, automatic or servo mode and monitor only mode. The water hoses of the blanket are connected to the cooling unit.

The manual control mode is used to pre-cool the blanket by circulating sterile or distilled water cooled to the set temperature of 5°C. The baby (<6 hours of age) fulfilling the inclusion criteria for whole body cooling, is placed in a supine position on the blanket to ensure that complete body including occiput is touching the blanket (Figure 1.11). The radiant warmer or any other source of exogenous heat should be put off.

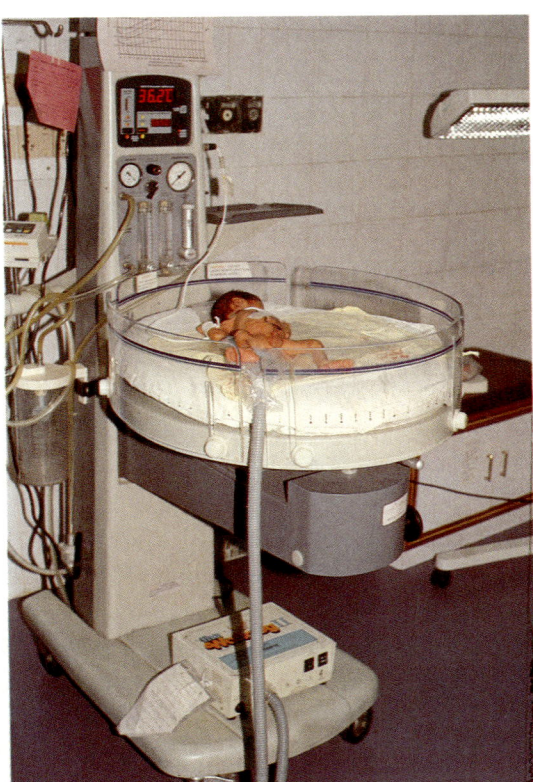

Figure 1.9 Open care system. It is equipped with overhead heat and light source along with servo-control facility.

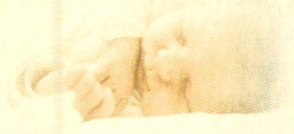

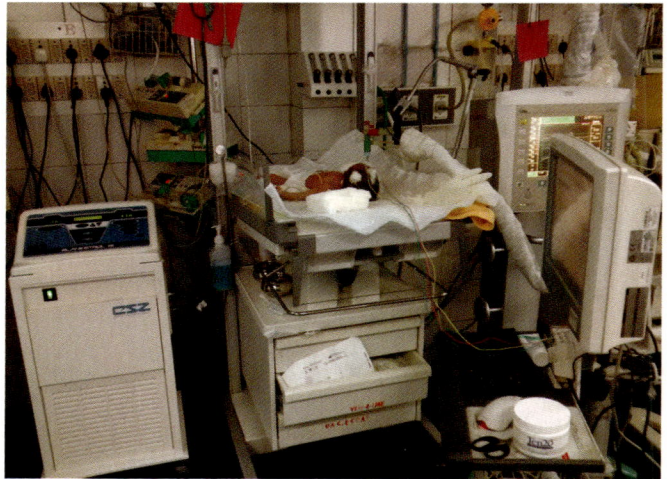

Figure 1.11 Infant with grade 3 HIE being nursed on a cooling blanket and attached with various monitoring devices.

A disposable temperature steri-probe is placed in the esophagus or rectum to automatically maintain core temperature of the baby to 33.5°C. Esophageal probe is inserted through the nose and placed in the lower third of esophagus and securely taped. During automatic or servo mode, the unit maintains the set temperature of the baby either by cooling or warming the water circulating in the blanket. After the blanket is completely filled with water, check and maintain the level of sterile water in the reservoir at the desired level. Selective head cooling devices (olympic cool cap) are available which are associated with reduced immediate adverse effects because core body temperature is maintained at a safe level by use of a radiant warmer. However, selective head cooling is less effective in improving survival and reducing the risk of neuromotor disability in neonates with severe hypoxic-ischemic encephalopathy (HIE).

The infant is provided with state-of-the-art NICU care by monitoring vital signs, biochemical parameters, maintenance of fluids and electrolytes, blood gases and acid-base parameters with the help of assisted ventilation, high-frequency oscillations (HFO) and inhaled nitric oxide (iNO). Antibiotics should be given as per the protocol of the NICU. The neurologic status is checked clinically, with the help of an aEEG and neurosonography. The infant is nursed on the cooling blanket for 72 hours and then gradually warmed by raising set temperature by 0.5°C every hour to achieve skin temperature of 36.5°C in a period of about 6 hours.

Thermometers

Low reading (30–40°C) rectal thermometer is essential to assess the severity of hypothermia. The severity of hypothermia in small babies may be overlooked, if only conventional thermometers are used. Electronic or tele thermometers with skin censors or rectal probes with an accuracy of ±0.1°C are ideal for continuous atraumatic monitoring of body temperature. These temperature monitors are also equipped with acoustic and visual alarms set at a desired low and high temperature. Simultaneous monitoring of core and toe temperature can provide useful information regarding state of peripheral perfusion. When a baby gets overheated in the incubator, both core and peripheral skin temperature rises while in an infant with circulatory failure, peripheral skin temperature may be more than 1°C lower than core temperature. This offers quantitation and objectivity to the time honored clinical observation of finding warm trunk and cold extremities in infants with septic shock. Cold extremities, in the absence of shock, suggests that the baby is under cold stress and expending extra oxygen and calories for metabolic thermogenesis and thus compromising the weight gain or growth of the baby.

Oxygen Concentrator

Portable oxygen cylinders are expensive and not readily available in a district hospital or community health center. Oxygen concentrators are being indigenously manufactured and they work both on a battery and mains. The atmospheric air is passed through a chemical zeolite (aluminium silicate) which absorbs all gases except oxygen. It can increase the concentration of oxygen in the air from 21% to about 90%. The oxygen sensor device (OSD) shows a green signal when oxygen concentration in the outlet exceed 90%. It is possible to treat simultaneously up to four infants (flow rate 0.5–1.0 liter/min) at a time by using an oxygen flow-splitting device. The equipment is provided with four filters to eliminate dust, humidity and bacteria (Figure 1.12). Depending upon the flow rate, various concentrations of oxygen can be delivered to the patient. Oxygen-air blender with an oxygen analyzer can be interposed to deliver a precise concentration of FiO_2 but it considerably enhances the price of the device. Oxygen must be warmed (36.0–36.5°C) and humidified before administration to the baby. Oxygen concentrators are cost-effective and promoted by WHO in developing countries. The unit cost is high (around INR 50,000–00) but recurrent costs are low. They are useful in domiciliary practice for administration of oxygen to preterm neonates with chronic lung disease (CLD) and children with chronic interstitial lung disease.

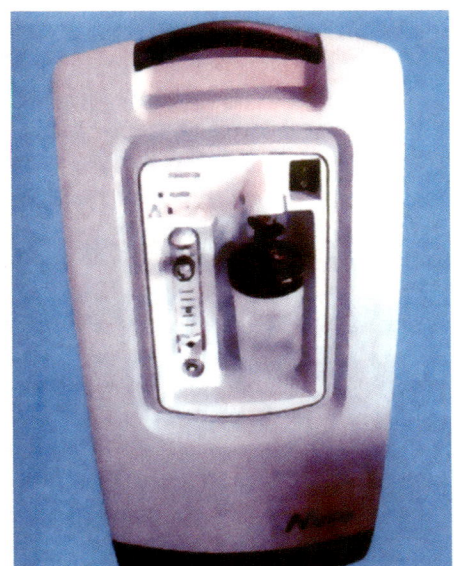

Figure 1.12 Prototype of oxygen concentrator.

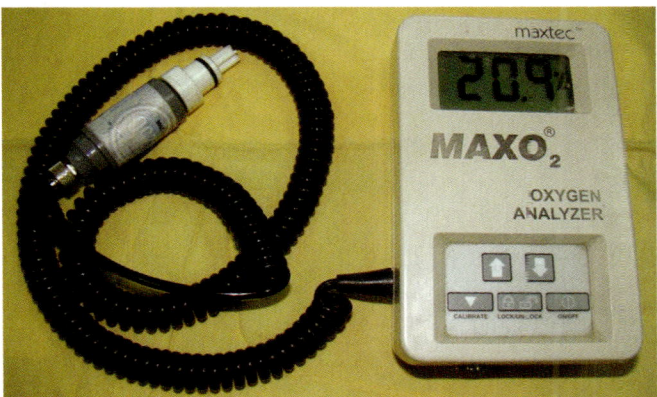

Figure 1.13 Oxygen monitor. It provides continuous digital display of ambient oxygen concentration.

Oxygen Head Box (Oxihood)

A square-shaped box made of transparent plastic or perspex which can enclose the head of the infant is useful for administration of higher concentration of oxygen. The box should be made of unbreakable material molded as a single piece without any joints. It can be used whether the baby is nursed in an open cot or incubator. It should be provided with an adjustable neck port or flexible occluding collar to create an effective seal to prevent free entry of environmental air. The oxygen concentrations which are likely to be achieved with different flow rates should be printed on the box.

Oxygen Analyzer

This is useful for monitoring ambient oxygen concentration in order to protect the infant against oxygen toxicity. It helps in regulating the flow rate of oxygen so that desired concentration of oxygen is delivered to the infant depending upon his clinical condition and oxygen requirements. The Beckman's paramagnetic oxygen analyzer of earlier days has been replaced by newer oxygen sensors which operate on galvanic cell principle. The electric current generated between two electrodes is proportional to the partial pressure of oxygen. Cathode is gold plated while anode is made of lead and filled with potassium hydroxide. The newer oxygen analyzers provide continuous digital display of oxygen concentration and trigger off audiovisual warning signal when environmental concentration of oxygen falls or rises beyond the safety levels (Figure 1.13). The instrument is calibrated by checking the oxygen concen-

tration of room air which is kept constant at 21%. The sensor life is about 9 months only and would need replacement once a year.

Perspex Heat Shield

Heat shield made of perspex or transparent plexiglass measuring 18" × 10" × 8" in a dome shape is a very simple and useful device to reduce the heat loss by radiation and evaporation. When a sick infant with respiratory distress is nursed naked in the incubator, he must be enclosed in the perspex heat shield to limit fluctuations in his body temperature. It reduces insensible water loss by about 25%. Based on this analogy, the currently available intensive care incubators are double-walled, which are credited to reduce radiant heat loss by 50%.

Transilluminator

It is a useful, cheap, non-invasive device for point-of-care use in a number of situations in NICU. Fiberoptic light source is used to provide up to 12,000 candles with a halogen quartz lamp, LED light source or xenon arc. The shorter wavelengths (up to 470 nm) of visible light which produce heat are filtered out to provide "cold light" at the tip of the cable. The efficacy of transillumination is enhanced by competence of the operator, intensity of light and by maintaining the room as dark as possible. Thermal injury to the skin can be minimized by reducing the contact of light to the skin between 15–30 seconds. The halo of light around the probe is visualized, measured and compared on two sides.

It is a useful device for point-of-care prompt diagnosis of air-leaks (pneumothorax, pneumomediastinum and pneumopericardium), hydrothorax and chylothorax. Cranial transillumination is useful for the diagnosis of subdural hematoma or effusion, hydrocephalus, hydranencephaly, cystic hygroma and craniocervical meningocele. Transillumination of abdomen and pelvis can be used for diagnosis of hypertrophic pyloric stenosis, necrotizing enterocolitis, hydronephrosis, inguinal hernia and hydrocele. It can be used for delineation of bladder for suprapubic aspiration of urine. Transillumination is a useful aid for venous and arterial cannulation in neonates.

Phototherapy Unit

Phototherapy is now generally accepted as a safe and effective method for treatment of neonatal hyperbilirubinemia. A light source designed to give an irradiance or flux of 10–30 $\mu W/cm^2/nm$ between 400–520 nm wavelength range at the mattress is ideal. Blue light is more effective than the white light but former interferes with the observation of the infant. Special blue lamps with a peak output at 425 to 475 nm are most efficient for phototherapy and these do not emit harmful ultraviolet rays. To enhance irradiance or flux, four blue compact flourescent tubes (F 20 T12/BB and Philips TL 20 W/52) and two white flourescent tubes can be used because excessive blue color makes evaluation of the baby difficult and is uncomfortable to the eyes (Figure 1.14). It is preferable to use 40 W 2 feet long tubes which are economical with reduced recurring expenses. These units provide irradiance of 20–30 $\mu W/cm^2/nm$ in the 400–520 nm range. Cooling fan is required to reduce radiant heat exposure to the baby. The nude infant may be exposed under a portable or fixed light source kept at a distance of about 18 inches (45 cm) from the skin. Double-light system, where total baby is exposed from below and above, has been used for more effective light exposure. The conventional double surface phototherapy is uncomfortable and unfriendly to the baby who is made to lie on a cold and hard perspex sheet. Instead, intensive single surface phototherapy can be given by using tubes providing greater irradiance (40 W, 2 ft, TL-52) and by reducing the distance between the tubes and the baby to 15–20 cm. The tube light should be covered with plexiglass or plastic sheet to screen out ultraviolet rays. The flux density reduces with time and average rated life of tubes vary between 1000 to 2000 hours. The tubes should be replaced when their ends become black or spectral radiant energy ('flux') at the level of skin is less than 8 $\mu W/cm^2/nm$.

Spotlight phototherapy units are available which are equipped with a 150 watt 21 volt halogen bulb with a specially coated reflector which absorbs harmful infrared waves. The latest phototherapy units are based on the principle of fiberoptics in which an illuminated blanket is wrapped around the baby. It ensures exposure of greater surface area and is ideal for providing double-surface light exposure. The baby is placed on the fiberoptic biliblanket or light-emitting diode (LED) mattress and additional phototherapy is provided with blue compact flourescent tubes from the top. The effect of phototherapy unit can be enhanced by using slings or curtains made of white cloth or aluminium to reflect light on the baby. Newer phototherapy units are equipped with dosimeter to calculate cumulative exposure to phototherapy. Recently, gallium nitride light-emitting diode units have been launched to provide intense phototherapy benefits. They produce minimal heat and provide narrow luminous spectra in the blue-green range of visible spectrum of light with massive delivery of irradiance upto 200 $\mu W/cm^2/nm$.

The efficacy of phototherapy unit is not dependent upon the intensity of light but on the irradiance or flux. Most phototherapy units in the country are suboptimal because their flux is not monitored. In a large NICU, in-house fluxmeter should be available or the supplier should be asked to periodically check the flux and replace the tubes when irradiance drops below 8 $\mu W/cm^2/nm$. The phototherapy unit is put on for at least 10 minutes. The irradiance is measured by placing the sensor probe of the fluxmeter at a distance of 50 cm. The total irradiance read-out given by the fluxmeter is averaged to $\mu W/cm^2/nm$ by dividing it by the bandwidth, i.e. for the instrument providing waveband range 425–475 nm, it is divided by 50. It is recommended to use a spectroradiometer (calibrated for 430–490 nm waveband) to measure the irradiance (Figure 1.15).

Heart Rate Monitor

Among various electronic gadgets for monitoring vital signs, cardiac monitor showing digital display of heart rate (along with audible beep) or an electrocardiographic configuration on an oscilloscope or both, is most

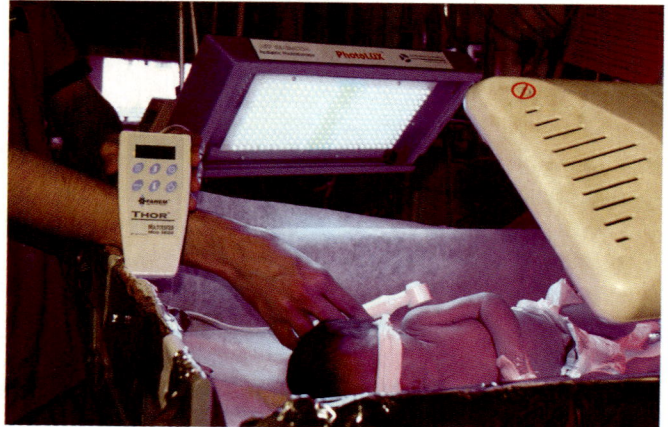

Figure 1.14 A compact fluorescent light phototherapy unit.

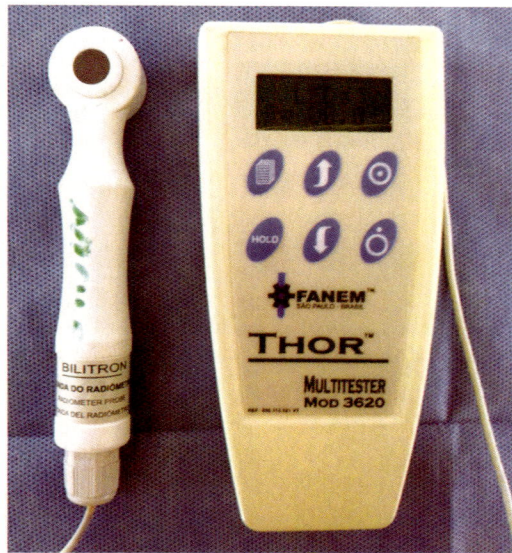

Figure 1.15 Irradiance meter.

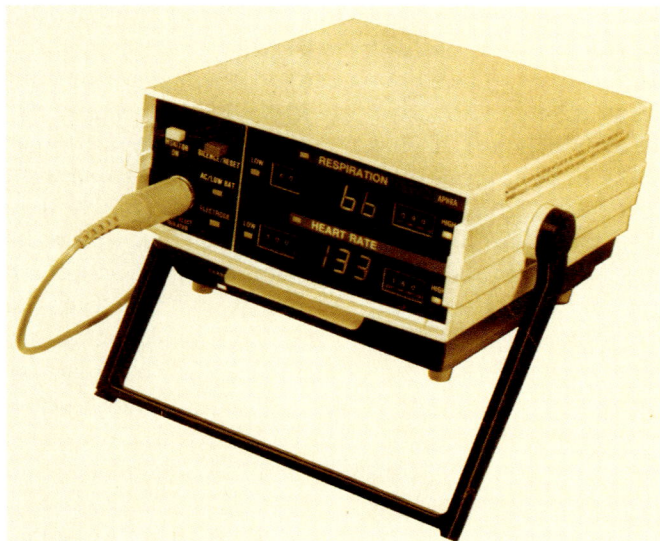

Figure 1.16 Heart rate and respiration monitor.

useful. Generally, an apneic attack is followed by bradycardia within 20 seconds so that heart rate monitor (with an alarm set at heart rate of less than 80 per minute) can be used with advantage over an apnea monitor. They are ideal to monitor high-risk infants and are especially useful during prolonged procedures, such as exchange blood transfusion and surgery (Figure 1.16).

Respiratory Rate and Apnea Monitor

The respiratory monitor based on impedance technique measures changes in the electrical resistance during breathing. The electrode is fixed on the chest wall to pick-up signals which are digitally displayed as respiratory rate. The respiratory excursions can also be displayed on the oscilloscope. The conventional apnea monitors are based on air mattress having plethysmographic sensor. The mattress is placed underneath the chest of the infant and mechanical alterations produced by the respiratory movements of the infant are recorded and displayed. When infant stops breathing, after a variable interval of 10 to 20 seconds depending upon the preset lag, the instrument emits a beep and displays red light warning signal.

A pulse oximeter in which an alarm gets activated when a baby develops bradycardia (heart rate < 100/min) or desaturation (SpO$_2$ <90%) is a useful and reliable alternative to an apnea monitor.

Blood Pressure Monitor

Recording of blood pressure by flush or conventional method is inaccurate and time consuming in newborn babies. Direct arterial pressure can be recorded by introducing a transducer into umbilical artery but this method is invasive and fraught with complications and should be reserved for critically sick VLBW babies on assisted ventilation. Doppler system based on the principle of ultrasound waves provides an accurate and non-invasive means for recording blood pressure in newborn babies. The ultrasonic waves are picked up by the transducer located in the cuff. The usual cuff size to cover two-thirds of the upper arm of a neonate varies between 2.5–4.0 cm depending upon the birth weight. The blood pressure reading may be unreliable, if baby is crying or moving. The blood pressure instruments based on oscillometric technique are more accurate and should preferably be used. They are more reliable and are not affected by the movements of the baby. The instrument provides continuous digital display of heart rate, systolic, diastolic and mean blood pressure. The mean blood pressure is based upon diastolic pressure plus one-third of the pulse pressure (systolic – diastolic pressure). Blood pressure varies depending upon the gestational age of the neonate. Means arterial blood pressure correspond to gestational age in weeks. In general, diastolic pressure lower than 25 mm Hg and mean blood pressure of less than 30 mm Hg is a cause for concern. A diastolic blood pressure of >50 mm Hg in a preterm and >60 mm Hg in a term baby is suggestive of hypertension. A pulse pressure of >20 mm Hg is suggestive of opening up of ductus arteriosus. There is a provision for alarm or warning signal when blood pressure falls or rises beyond certain preset limits (Figure 1.17). In future, finger plethysmography with the help of a small cuff and a light source may provide a constant display of mean blood pressure, heart rate and arterial oxygen saturation.

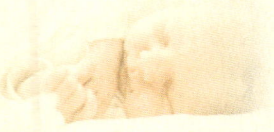

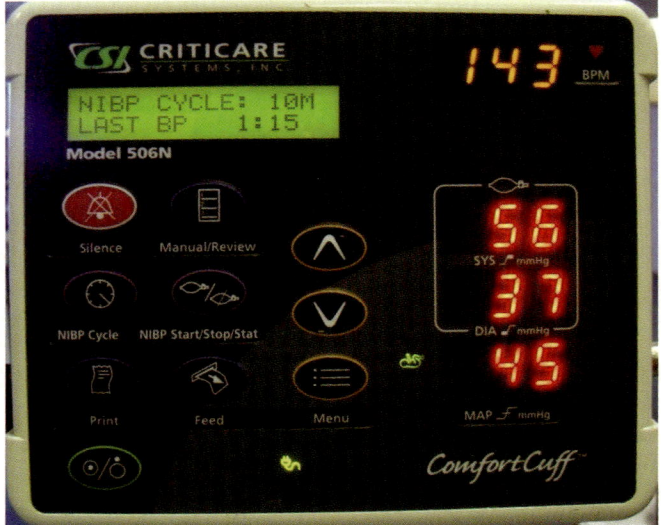

Figure 1.17 Noninvasive blood pressure monitor.

Multichannel Vital Sign Monitor

The multiple channel complex monitors are available to display and record all the vital signs on an oscilloscope. They are very useful but extremely expensive. They are equipped to record temperature at different sites, heart rate, respiratory rate with apnea alarm, invasive and noninvasive blood pressure and pulse oximetry. ECG, pulse waves and respiratogram are displayed on the oscilloscope. There is a need to have a computer based monitor to analyze all the information provided by complex vital sign monitors (Figure 1.18).

Infusion Pump

In view of the fact that relatively small quantities of fluids need to be infused and minor errors in rate of administration may prove lethal to low birth weight babies, constant infusion pumps with accurate control are essential to meet these requirements. In centers

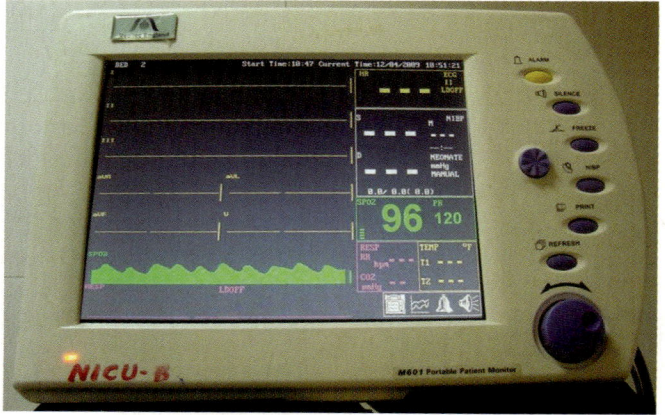

Figure 1.18 Multichannel vital sign monitor.

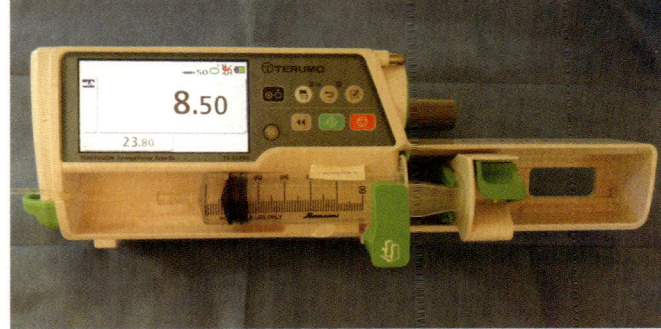

Figure 1.19 Syringe-based infusion pump. The flow rate of drip can be regulated between 1.0 and 99.9 mL/hour with this device.

where parenteral nutrition is used for the care of sick babies, the use of infusion pumps has become obligatory. The infusion pump is a sophisticated electronic micropump which displaces fluid and a microprocessor or pressure transducer controls the rate of fluid delivery. Various devices used for accurate administration of fluids in neonates include gravity-dependent drip rate regulators, volumetric infusion pump and syrings pumps accepting a wide range of syringes. The rate of infusion is either depicted as drops/minute (1–99 drops/minute) or in terms of volume (1.0–99.9 mL/hour) through a disposable cassette or plastic syringe. The syringe-based infusion pumps are ideal for administration of drugs or intralipid. It is desirable to buy an infusion pump which accepts syringes of different sizes (20, 50, 100 mL) and of all makes and should work both on mains and Ni-Cd batteries. The syringe and tubing must be changed every 24 hours to reduce the risk of nasocomial infection. The latest infusion pumps have inbuilt alarms to signal occlusion of flow, air in the system, system failure and low battery charge (Figure 1.19). The infusion site must be watched diligently for any extravasation because infusion will not stop due to the effect of pumping force. The new generation "smart" infusion pumps are available which are equipped with computerized prescriber order entry (CPOE) and automatic or programmed medication system to reduce the risk of adverse drug events.

Microcentrifuge

Centrifugation is done to separate solid particles or cells suspended in a liquid medium, like blood, urine and various body secretions, (CSF, gastric aspirate) and serosal transudates and exudates. Laboratory microcentrifuge is used for measuring hematocrit or packed cell volume (PCV) and for separation of plasma from cellular elements of blood for estimation of bilirubin in a microcapillary sample (50–70 μL). The main

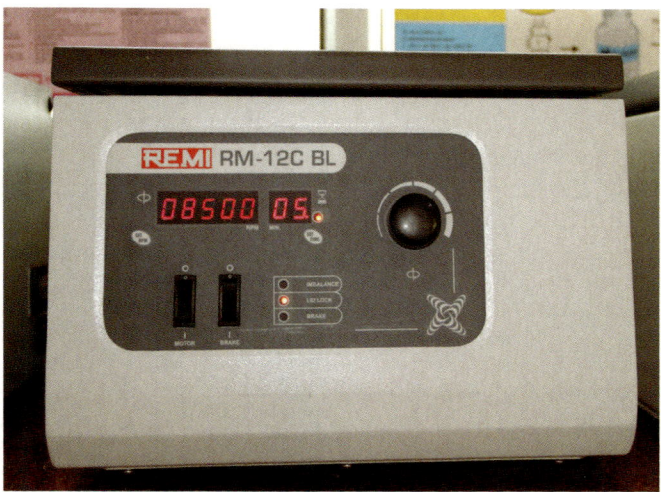

Figure 1.20 Laboratory microcentrifuge.

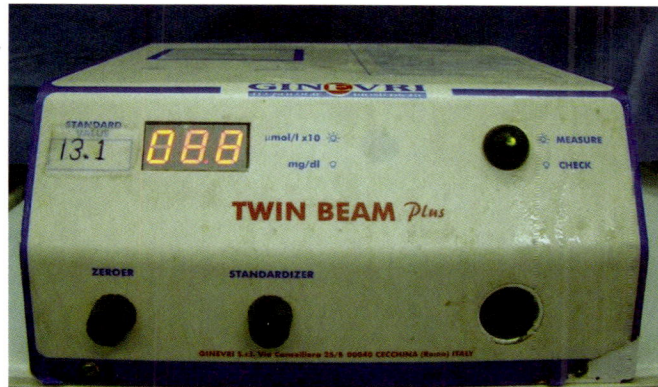

Figure 1.21 Twin beam bilirubin analyzer.

components of the centrifuge include a rotor with slots for placing capillaries, a lid with a lock, a timer and a knob for adjusting the speed. The microcapillaries made of borosilicate glass and certified for centrifugation at a high speed of 10,000–15,000 rpm are recommended for use. Heparinized microcapillaries with internal diameter of 1.0 mm and length of 7.0 cm are used. After taking the blood sample in the tube, one end is sealed with plasticine. The placement of tube/s in the slots should be balanced on two sides by placing blood or water-filled capillary tubes on the identical or corresponding slots on the opposite side of the rotor. The instrument should be kept at least 30 cm away from the wall for proper dissipation of heat. The motor is provided with a blower to ensue that the temperature of the machine is not allowed to cross 40°C. After placing the capillary tubes in slots (including balancing capillaries), the centrifuge is turned on and set to rotate at 10,000 rpm for 5 minutes (Figure 1.20). The instrument should be kept clean and any blood spills should be wiped off with a wet gauze piece or 10% bleach solution. The instrument should be kept lubricated and its motor brush should be checked every 3 months.

Bilirubin Analyzer

The spectrometric bilirubinometer works on the principle of two wavelength direct spectrometry with the help of a light source that emits a narrow beam of light at 465 nm and 540 nm. The light beam passes through a slit in the microcapillary tube holder or a couvette and the unabsorbed light is detected by a photodedector. The microcapillary tube containing 50–70 µL of baby's blood is blocked on one end with plasticene and centrifuged at 12,000 rpm for 5 minutes

to separate out the plasma or serum. The serum or plasma column should cover the entire length of the slit through which the light waves pass. The capillary slit must be kept clean of any dust or particles of plasticene to ensure accuracy of results. The instrument provides direct read-out of total serum bilirubin which is reliable for taking therapeutic decisions for the management of neonatal hyperbilirubinemia. The hematocrit can be read off from the same sample and serum can be subsequently used for determination of C-reactive protein or other biochemical tests; thus minimising the need for blood sampling (Figure 1.21).

Apart from bilirubin, there are several other components in the plasma, like oxyhemoglobin, transferrin, methemalbumin and lipids which can interfere with absorption of light. The instrument is so calibrated by using complex mathematical equations and correction factors, that the bilirubinometer gives a reliable estimate of total bilirubin. Nevertheless, beta-carotene levels of blood can interfere with test results but fortunately carotenoids are not present in the serum of newborn babies. However, after an exchange blood transfusion with adult blood, transfused carotene may provide falsely high values of bilirubin. Hemolysis does not interfere with the reliability of spectrometry method of bilirubin estimation unlike conventional Diazo method.

Transcutaneous Bilirubinometer

The yellow discoloration of skin and subcutaneous tissues can be quantitated and equated to total bilirubin value with the help of a photoprobe. The probe is pressed against, forehead or upper end of sternum. When instrument's xenon lamp flashes green, press the trigger to take the reading. Five readings should be taken and instrument displays the mean value. The light passes through inbuilt fiberoptics and reflectometer and is analyzed by computerized spectrophotometer to provide immediate digital display of total bilirubin. It is a useful bedside screening method for the young resident doctor to assess the degree of jaundice. There is a good correlation between transcutaneous and biochemically assessed bilirubin values. It gives an estimate of only total bilirubin which, however, is quite satisfactory because there is hardly any elevation of direct-reacting bilirubin during first week of life. Skin pigmentation of black babies may interfere with transcutaneous bilirubin evaluation. In such cases, photoprobe placed against a drop of blood taken on a filter paper, has given reliable estimate of serum bilirubin. The latest multi-wavelength reflectance meter (BiliChek by Norcross) or dual wavelength reflectance meter (JM-103 by Minolta/Air shields) provides reliable estimate of total serum bilirubin without any interference by skin pigmentation or gestational age of the baby. According to the guidelines of American Academy of Pediatrics, transcutaneous bilirubinometry (TcB) can be used as a surrogate of serum total bilirubin (STB) for screening of jaundice in term and near-term neonates. However, bilirubin level must be confirmed by a spectrometric bilirubin analyzer or Diazo method before starting any therapeutic intervention. During phototherapy, a small area of skin should be kept covered to serve as a reference point to reliably monitor transcutaneous bilirubin levels. Icterometer is a plastic strip depicting different shades of yellow color and can also be used to match the yellowness of the skin of the baby to roughly assess the severity of jaundice.

Transcutaneous Blood Gas Monitor

Sick preterm infants with respiratory difficulties require frequent arterial blood sampling for blood gases and acid-base analyses. Arterial electrode placed in umbilical artery has been successfully used for continuous monitoring of PaO_2 but it is complicated by inherent hazards of umbilical vessel catheterization with indwelling catheter. The availability of non-invasive transcutaneous monitor is indeed a useful technological advance in the field of bioengineering during the last decade. This has simplified constant monitoring of oxygen tension *in-vivo* with the hope that sequelae of hypoxia and hyperoxia in the newborn can be reduced. It utilizes a miniature Clarks' electrode which can be heated to 44°C. The sensor is slipped over the membrane assembly and is affixed over the chest or upper abdomen. The heated skin electrode produces local hyperthermia causing vasodilation, thus arterializing the capillary bed under the electrode. Molecular oxygen diffuses from the dilated capillaries towards the cathode (platinum) of the electrode where

it is reduced. The resultant current generated by the flow of electrode is proportional to the partial pressure of oxygen which is continuously displayed on the digital read out. The transcutaneous PO_2 values are quite reliable and comparable to simultaneous PaO_2 which should be cross-checked every 4 to 6 hours. Due to risk of skin burns, the site of sensor should be changed every 2 hourly. When the electrode becomes loose, room air may leak under the sensor to produce spuriously high $TcPO_2$ values (usually above 150 torr). Transcutaneous oxygen monitoring is essential for optimal management of infants with respiratory distress syndrome and frequent apneic attacks. It provides diagnostic information in several clinical situations. In infants with cyanotic congenital heart disease, $TcPO_2$ cannot be raised above 100 torr by administration of 100% oxygen. The right-to-left shunting at the ductal level can be suspected by using two skin sensors, one placed over the right upper chest (pre-ductal) and the other placed over left lower abdomen (post-ductal). A discrepancy of greater than 20% in $TcPO_2$ value obtained by two skin sensors is indicative of significant right-to-left shunt. Lastly, if $TcPO_2$ value is considerably lower than simultaneous PaO_2 level, it is suggestive of peripheral vasoconstriction or impending shock. Transcutaneous oxygen monitors have lost the initial enthusiasm because they are time-consuming and cumbersome to use.

Transcutaneous carbon dioxide monitors are also available though they are very expensive. The $TcPCO_2$ sensor is larger in size and work on the principle of Stowe and Severinghaus. Like the oxygen sensor, CO_2 sensor also needs to be kept heated at 44°C and its site is changed every 3 to 4 hours. Technology is also available for continuous monitoring of tissue pCO_2 with a mass spectrometer and infrared method. The continuous monitoring of tissue pH is also feasible but it is rather invasive and requires insertion of an indwelling electrode either over the surface of a muscle or in the subcutaneous tissue.

Pulse Oximeter

Pulse oximeter provides a simple, convenient and non-invasive method for continuous monitoring of hemoglobin saturated with oxygen. It has virtually replaced the transcutaneous monitors. The arterial blood oxygen saturation (SpO_2 or SaO_2) can be determined transcutaneously with an accuracy of ± 2% by measuring the absorption of two selected wavelengths of light. The light generated in the sensor (probe) passes through the blood and tissues and is converted into electronic

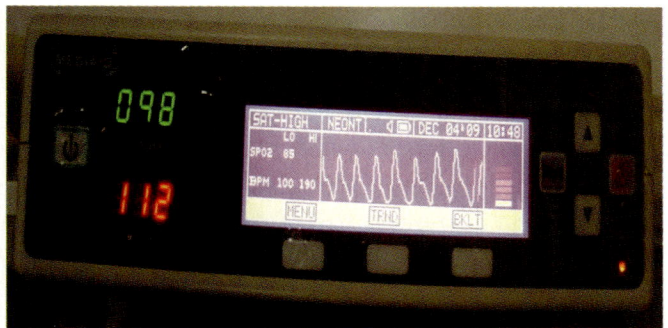

Figure 1.22 Pulse oximeter for monitoring arterial oxygen saturation and heart rate.

signals by a photodetector located in the sensor. The oxyhemoglobin and reduced hemoglobin allow different amounts of light at selected wavelengths to reach the photodetector. The monitor gives the digital display of arterial oxygen saturation, pulse rate and audible pulse tone (Figure 1.22). Most instruments have a facility to set alarm limits for SaO_2 (low and high) and for pulse rate which can provide a dual function of an apnea alarm. A hand-held pulse oximeter which runs on batteries can be used during transport of sick babies. The flex probe (sensor) can be affixed on the fingers, toes, hand and dorsum of the foot of the baby. The sensor containing the photocell is extremely sensitive to light and must be shielded from strong external light sources, like observation light and phototherapy. Do not apply cuff of blood pressure monitor on the same limb where sensor is affixed. The probe site should be periodically changed to prevent damage to skin. Pulse oximetry provides a simple, convenient and non-invasive method for continuous monitoring and display of SaO_2. It is ideal for early detection of hypoxia in critically sick newborn babies but it has its own limitations to identify hyperoxia because oxygen dissociation curve is displaced to the left in newborn babies. To safeguard against the risk of hyperoxia and retinopathy of prematurity, it is recommended that the upper limit of alarm for oxygen saturation should be set at 95%. Arterial oxygen saturation should be maintained between 90 and 95% for acute conditions and 85 and 90% for extremely preterm babies and chronic situations. Pulse oximetry is unreliable when there is poor perfusion due to shock and hypothermia, excessive movements of limb, exposure of probe to light sources, severe anemia, dyshemoglobinemias (carboxyhemoglobin and methemoglobin), and when blood pressure cuff or splint is applied proximal to the site of probe. Fetal hemoglobin and bilirubin do not affect the accuracy of pulse oximeter.

Capnography or End Tidal CO_2 (EtCO$_2$) Monitor

This is a simple, noninvasive and quick method to assess alveolar CO_2. Apart from water vapor, CO_2 is the only component of alveolar gases which absorbs infrared rays. When water vapor is eliminated, infrared analyzer provides a good measure of CO_2 concentration. Carbon dioxide, an end product of cellular metabolism, is transported from the cells via circulation, diffuses into the alveoli and exhaled through the airways. Thus $EtCO_2$ values reflect metabolism, pulmonary perfusion, alveolar diffusion and ventilatory efficacy. In normal subjects, $EtCO_2$ is an accurate approximation of "average" mixed alveolar gas composition. In spontaneously breathing infant, nasal cannula is used for air sampling while in a baby on assisted ventilation, an adaptor is placed between endotracheal tube and the ventilator circuit. It is preferable to buy the mainstream analyzer (instead of sidestream analyzer) because couvette can be mounted directly in line with the endotracheal tube without any risk of blockage.

The $EtCO_2$ range varies between 0 and 99 mmHg with an accuracy of ±2 mmHg for values between 0 and 40 mmHg and ±5 mmHg for values between 41 and 99 mmHg. It is a useful modality to assess whether endotracheal tube has gone into the esophagus or it is kinked/blocked giving $EtCO_2$ value of near zero. The gradient between arterial carbon dioxide and $EtCO_2$ ($PaCO_2 - EtCO_2$) should be calculated. In infants with normal lungs, the gradient is usually upto 5 mm Hg. In neonates with V/Q abnormalities, the gradient may be 10–20 mmHg. Even when there is a wide gradient, $EtCO_2$ is a reliable predictor of $PaCO_2$ because gradient is usually constant over a long period of time. A sudden increase in the gradient is indicative of an increase in the dead space with a decrease in pulmonary perfusion. When the gradient between $PaCO_2$ and $EtCO_2$ drops to less than 10 mmHg, it is indicative of improved lung function and feasibility of weaning. However, due to various limitations and availability of more reliable monitoring modalities, capnography is rarely used in newborn babies.

CPAP Delivery System

Continuous positive airway pressure (CPAP) is a useful and affordable technology to manage neonates with RDS and respiratory insufficiency. In contrast to assisted ventilation, it conserves surfactant, improves functional residual capacity (FRC) and reduces the risk of bronchopulmonary dysplasia. Infant on CPAP can be fed with an orogastric tube. The feeding tube is kept plugged for 20 to 30 minutes after the feed to prevent

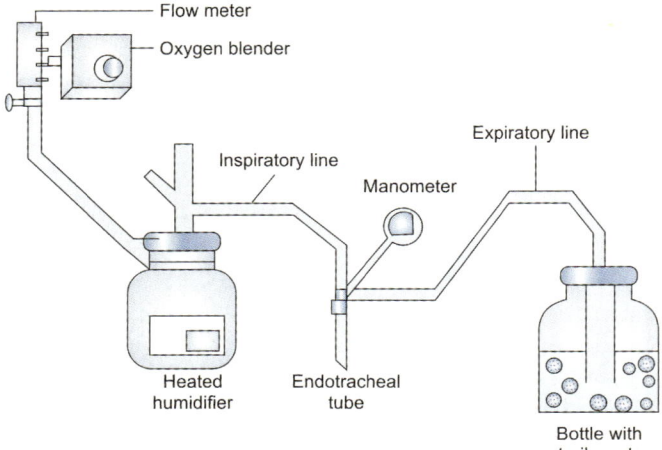

Figure 1.23 The components of bubble CPAP.

efflux of milk. However, most of the time, OG tube is kept open to prevent distension of abdomen or CPAP belly.

CPAP can be delivered through nasopharyngeal tube or face mask but is best provided through nasal prongs. The minimum requirement of CPAP include pulse oximeter (to maintain SpO_2 between 90–95%), FiO_2 monitor for mixing air and oxygen; and effective warm humidification. CPAP can be provided through a ventilator but in resource constrained situations, stand alone CPAP machine and bubble or water seal CPAP can be used. The salient components of bubble CPAP are shown in Figure 1.23. The distal end of expiratory tube is immersed in sterile water and its depth in water can be varied to provide CPAP between 5 to 10 cm of water. CPAP pressure is adjusted to control chest retractions and grunting, and maintain SpO_2 between 90 to 95%. In general CPAP pressure and FiO_2 go hand in hand, e.g. 5 cm CPAP and 50% FiO_2, 7 cm CPAP and 70% FiO_2, 10 cm CPAP and 100% FiO_2 and so on so forth. Bubble CPAP with combined effects of CPAP and pressure oscillations from the bubbles provide a lung protective, safe and effective method of providing respiratory support to spontaneously breathing sick neonates. The common complications of CPAP include abdominal distension, retention of carbon dioxide and pneumothorax.

Neonatal Ventilators

Assisted ventilation is required in several babies with respiratory failure. It is irrational to procure a ventilator unless adequate basic facilities, such as skilled nurses and residents, blood gas analyzer, monitoring devices, microchemistry and portable X-rays are available. Till such time, the financial resources may be more usefully expended in augmenting more urgent

needs of the SCNU. Centralized supply of oxygen and purified air (alternatively air compressor of 50 PSI) is mandatory for assisted ventilation. Continuous positive airway pressure (CPAP) apparatus can be readily fabricated to improve the medical care of infants with hyaline membrane disease and recurrent apneic attacks.

Ventilators are sophisticated electronic mini-air pumps. The type of ventilator being used is not as important as the level of training and experience of personnel using it. Practical experience and thorough understanding regarding the use of a particular type of ventilator is more important than having the theoretical knowledge of various ventilators. Basically there are two types of intermittent positive pressure ventilators, they are either pressure generator or flow generator modules. The pressure generator ventilators regulate the pressure gradient at the airway and flow changes are determined by the compliance and resistance of lungs. The flow generator ventilator may have a constant or variable flow rate during two phases of respiration. In flow generator ventilator, the flow of gases in the airways is predetermined while pressure changes depend upon the physical characteristics of lungs. On the basis of their in-built control principles for termination of inspiratory phase, the ventilator may be pressure-cycled, volume-cycled or time-cycled. There are mixed forms of ventilators where more than one type of cycling is utilized, viz. time-controlled, pressure-limited ventilator. All modes of ventilation should be available including intermittent positive pressure ventilation (IPPV), continuous positive airway pressure and synchronized intermittent mandatory ventilation (SIMV).

There are inherent advantages and disadvantages of various types of ventilators. A small leak in the circuit can be adequately compensated in a pressure-cycled ventilator while in a volume-cycled ventilator tidal volume can be maintained adequately even when there is severe reduction in lung compliance. A suitable infant ventilator should be able to deliver adequate gas volume and compensate for any loss of gas volume due to compression, leaks and dead space (Figures 1.24 and 1.25). It should have a sensitive patient triggering mechanism and high cycling frequency. The ventilator should be equipped to supply a wide range of air-oxygen mixtures and provided with a mechanism to vary inspiratory–expiratory ratios. The essential accessories, like humidifier, probe for recording temperature of air-oxygen mixture, air compressor, and infusion pump, must be ordered along with the ventilator. Inorder to reduce the risk of nosocomial infection, disposable patient circuits compatible with the ventilator should be used.

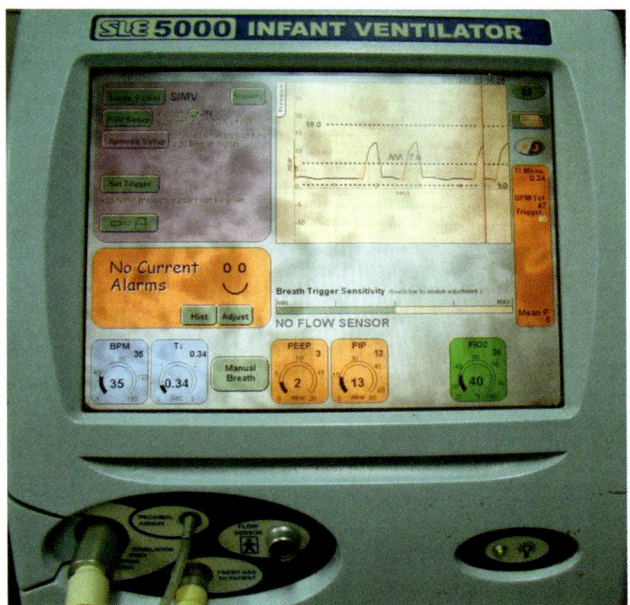

Figure 1.24 SLE 5000 infant ventilator.

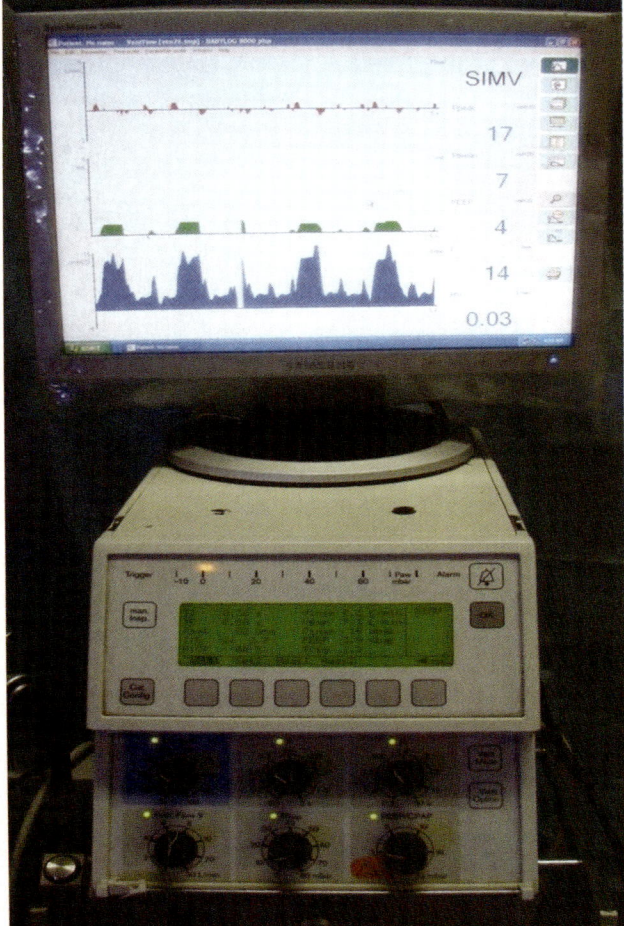

Figure 1.25 Babylog 8000 ventilator with pulmonary graphics.

When conventional ventilation fails or baby has persistent pulmonary hypertension (PPHN) and pulmonary airleaks, high frequency ventilators (HFV) are used. These ventilators use extremely low tidal volume and operate between 150 and 2,400 breaths/min. They are exorbitantly expensive and should be acquired by the state-of-the-art NICUs when their staff has achieved excellence in handling conventional ventilators.

Intermittent negative pressure ventilators are less popular due to hazards of abdominal distension. They are cumbersome and difficult to operate in very low birth weight babies and access for nursing procedures and blood sampling is difficult. The respirator is divided into two compartments to enclose the head and body with the help of sealing around neck. Intermittent negative pressure operates at chest wall resulting in the intermittent gas flow down the airway. Oxygen-air mixture is allowed to flow in the chamber enclosing the head. Endotracheal intubation may be needed in some infants.

Neonatal Pulmonary Function Tests

They are useful to assess infants with cardiopulmonary disease but are mostly used for research purposes at present. The equipment includes a pneumotach to measure airflows and volumes and an esophageal balloon catheter and transducer to measure transpulmonary pressure. These are integrated with a computer and printer. The pulmonary function profile enables the neonatologist to obtain data on tidal volume, compliance, airway resistance and work of breathing. Baseline and daily pulmonary function studies on an infant evaluates changes in lung function, adjustments in mechanical ventilation and ability to wean. It is a useful modality to monitor the therapeutic response to pharmacologic agents, such as bronchodilators, corticosteroids and diuretics in infants with bronchopulmonary dysplasia and chronic lung disease.

Cranial Ultrasonography (CUS)

Ultrasonography of brain with real-time portable ultrasound is the method of choice for evaluation of size of ventricles and possible intraventricular hemorrhage in very LBW babies. The linear-array ultrasonic scanner is used by directing ultrasound waves through anterior fontanel which serves as an acoustic window to obtain best images or echoes. A multifrequency sector probe providing 5–8 MHz resolution is ideal. It is difficult to transport high-risk LBW babies on assisted ventilation or other life supportive measures to the specialized radiodiagnosis

Routine screening cranial ultrasound (CUS) should be performed on all infants with birth weight < 1250 g or gestation of < 30 weeks at 7–14 days of age followed by a repeat ultrasound at 36–40 weeks of postmenstrual or postconceptional age. Other indications for doing CUS include (i) hypoxic–ischemic encephalopathy, (ii) neonatal seizures, (iii) suspicion of intracranial hemorrhage and (iv) enlarging head size. The neonatologist should have adequate training and skills to do cot-side cranial ultrasound evaluation. It is a useful, reliable and safe modality for diagnosis and follow-up of infants with intraventricular hemorrhage, cystic periventricular leukomalacia (PVL), ventriculomegaly and certain congenital malformations, like hydrocephalus, agenesis of corpus callosum, and AV malformation. In infants below 1000 g or < 28 weeks, cranial ultrasound may be done on day 1 to rule out severe intraventricular hemorrhage or antenatal brain injury to make a decision whether aggressive management should be given or denied.

Intracranial Pressure Monitor

Measurement of intracranial pressure in infants with birth asphyxia, intracranial hemorrhage, meningitis and hydrocephalus can provide useful information to guide therapy and predict prognosis. Several noninvasive techniques have been developed to measure intracranial pressure in the newborn. Oscillographic technique or air tonometer placed over anterior fontanel has been used with variable success. A technique based on fiberoptic system and air bellows gives reliable results with good correlation with direct intraventricular measurements. Caution is advised while placing the sensor on the anterior fontanel because excessive force can lead to spuriously high values. Most of the instruments are still experimental and are used for research purposes.

Cerebral Function Monitor

The neonatal brain or cerebral function monitor (CFM) is a point-of-care equipment for monitoring background activity of the brain by recording a single channel amplitude integrated EEG (aEEG) with the help of three electrodes, one placed over the vertex and two biparietal or bifrontal electrodes. The biparietal electrodes are commonly used because they are least affected by contraction of scalp muscles and movements of eyes. It selectively picks up < 2 and > 15 Hz frequencies of cerebral discharges by filtering out artefacts. It is preferable to use low impedance needle electrodes which are placed subdermally and secured with a tape. To ensure close contact between the

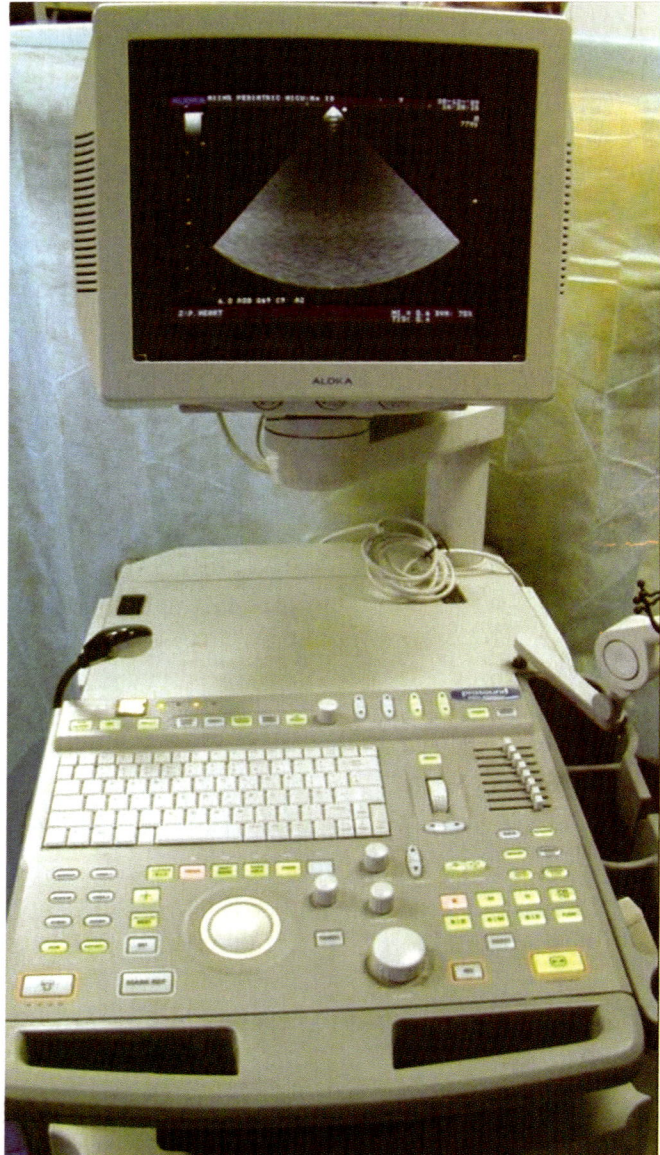

Figure 1.26 Portable ultrasound machine with color Doppler.

laboratory for CT scan or MRI studies. Instead cot-side or point-of-care testing (POCT) ultrasound in the nursery can provide equally reliable information (Figure 1.26). The second generation ultrasound machines with color Doppler facility are available which are useful to study blood flow and perfusion. It can be repeated frequently (because it is non-ionizing) as and when indicated depending upon the condition of the infant. At present, ultrasonography appears to be the safest, cheapest and most convenient technique for imaging the intracranial contents in the newborn. A single ultrasound scan performed on day 7 of life will detect almost all the infants who may have developed intraventricular hemorrhage.

electrode and brain, the impedance should be kept below 20 W. The CFM record is evaluated for amplitude, background activity, burst suppression (flat tracing between 5 and 10 µ volts) and seizure activity.

The CFM is useful to continuously monitor CNS activity in neonates with (i) perinatal asphyxia to grade the severity of HIE, assess the need for whole body cooling and therapeutic response to anticonvulsants, (ii) encephalopathy or seizures due to any cause, (iii) monitoring the effects of anticonvulsants, and (iv) assessment of prognosis. It does not replace the conventional EEG which is essential for diagnosis and management of seizures in newborns.

BERA Phone

It is a cot-side device to screen hearing of babies in the NICU by recording automated brainstem evoked response audiometry (BERA). It consists of a hand-held headphone unit having a set of three fixed touch electrodes and a preamplifier (Figure 1.27). The NICU should be noise-free and the baby should be asleep or calm and at least 34 weeks mature. The BERA phone is placed gently over one of the ear and electrodes are affixed with the help of gel. The mastoid electrode is placed below the ear lobe, the ground electrode is kept just above the ear lobe and vertex electrode is positioned higher up over the vertex. The correct position of BERA phone is checked by recording impedance which should be between 250 and 10,000 ohm for each electrode pair, i.e. mastoid-ground and vertex-ground. A USB cable connects BERA phone with a USB port of a notebook PC or desktop computer. The instrument delivers 35 dB sound stimuli or clicks to see whether wave V of automated auditory brainstem response (AABR) is present or absent. The result of screening is either PASS or REFER which is displayed on the computer. Both the ears are tested separately one after the other. When test result indicates REFER, the infant should be evaluated by an audiologist.

Extracorporeal Membrane Oxygenator (ECMO)

In seriously sick infants with persistent fetal circulation and diaphragmatic hernia, when conventional and high frequency jet ventilation have failed, ECMO has been used with variable results. The technology requires appropriate instrumentation for cardiac bypass and a membrane of an appropriate size for the infant. The blood is drawn from a catheter in the right internal jugular vein or right atrium, it is oxygenated as it crosses the membrane, and then returned to the patient via the right common carotid artery or the femoral vein. The infant is kept heparinized and ventilated at low pressures, rates and oxygen concentrations. It is highly cost-intensive modality demanding close cooperation and coordination of neonatologists with pediatric surgeons, nurses, trained technicians (perfusionists) and respiratory therapists.

Placenta Prototype

The ultimate objective of bioengineers is to fabricate a sophisticated "uteroplacental unit" so that extrauterine survival of a fetus, which is born early is assured with least hazards and greater certainty. It appears to be an extremely difficult task because placenta is not merely a membrane oxygenator and renal dialyzer but has multiple additional biological roles. Apart from passive transport of oxygen and urea, placenta actively transports a variety of substances including amino acids, calcium, glucose and maternal antibodies. The placenta also functions as an important endocrine organ, secreting hormones that effect both mother and the fetus.

COT-SIDE LABORATORY FACILITIES

Satisfactory facilities for routine radiological examination should be available in the NICU round-the-clock. A good portable 3-phase generator X-ray machine of at least 200 milliamperes with extremely short exposure time (1/120 seconds) should preferably be housed in a small room adjacent to the NICU. In-house X-ray, ultrasound, echocardiography, EKG, aEEG and BERA phone facilities should be available.

A side laboratory for routine analysis of blood, urine, amniotic fluid, gastric aspirate for shake test and cytology, Kleihauer-Betke count, glucose, bilirubin, hematocrit and blood gases and acid-base parameters should be available. Centralized facilities for micro-

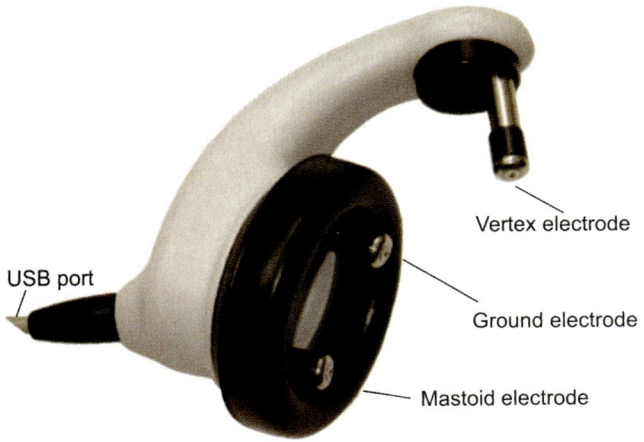

USB port

Vertex electrode

Ground electrode

Mastoid electrode

Figure 1.27 BERA phone with integrated electrodes.

biochemical techniques especially for estimation of total and direct serum bilirubin, blood glucose, arterial pO_2, pCO_2, pH and base deficit are desirable. Facilities for analysis of serum sodium, potassium, calcium and total serum proteins, and albumin should be at hand. The collection of venous blood is often difficult and hazardous in sick preterm babies. These babies often require frequent biochemical estimations. It is generally not appreciated that removal of 10 mL of blood from a 1,500 g infant amounts to about 8% of his total blood volume. This is equivalent to removal of about 400 mL of blood in an adult. Thus a micro-chemical laboratory which can carryout investigations on very small samples of blood obtained in heparinized capillary tubes or microcentrifuge tubes from heel puncture, should be considered as an essential facility for NICU.

PROCEDURE MANUAL

In view of the fact that many personnel working in the NICU are relatively floating, it is essential to have a procedure manual to establish continuity and uniformity of service. It should offer ready guidance to the new nurses and resident physicians so that the routines and policies for neonatal care are maintained at an optimal level.

The manual should outline detailed instructions regarding care of the baby in the labor room. Indications for admission to the NICU should be stated. The routines to be followed in the lying-in ward regarding bath, feeding, prophylaxis, etc. should be outlined. A detailed description of various house keeping rituals for prevention of infection in the special care nursery is most rewarding. Detailed instructions should be provided regarding temperature control of the nursery, use of open care system, incubator care, keeping babies warm, nurses observations, weight record and working knowledge of various equipments. The nurses should be conversant with various danger signs in the babies. The policy regarding mother–baby bonding, discharge, follow-up, early stimulation and what to do when a baby dies, should be clearly defined. It is essential to have various charts, such as intrauterine growth charts, postnatal growth charts, feeding routines, thermo-neutral ambient temperature ranges for low birth weight babies, drugs and dosages, etc. for ready reference. The resident doctors should be given guidelines for the management of common neonatal emergencies, such as birth asphyxia, hypothermia, respiratory distress syndrome, jaundice, metabolic disorders, sepsis and bleeding. A complete protocol and guidelines should be available for the transport team.

A computer with an internet facility should be available in the NICU. It can be used to download reports of laboratory investigations. The details of various equipment, their spares and accessories, addresses and telephone numbers of suppliers can be stored in the computer. It can be used for printing discharge summaries and analyzing the data regarding the morbidity, mortality and follow-up of NICU babies.

COOPERATION BETWEEN OBSTETRICIANS AND NEONATOLOGISTS

For effective delivery of perinatal services and to improve the management and outcome of newborn babies, the neonatologist should establish a close interaction and collaboration with a large number of specialists especially obstetrician, pediatric surgeon, pediatric cardiologist, ENT specialist, anesthetist, pediatric pathologist, pediatric radiologist, biochemist and biomedical engineer. Each one of these sub-specialists provides important and crucial links but cooperation and interaction with obstetricians is most vital to upgrade and improve the perinatal services in the teaching institutions and corporate hospitals. The neonatologists should not merely provide care to the newborn baby after their birth but must actively associate themselves with issues pertaining to fetal diagnosis, fetal therapy and over all fetal wellbeing.

The purpose of pregnancy is to produce a baby which should be healthy, good-sized, and free from any malformations. The obstetrician should ensure that this physiological function is achieved with minimal hazards to the mother. The pediatrician expends his efforts to make certain that the baby survives the hazards of delivery, cardiorespiratory adaptation, biological inadequacies and environmental insults after birth. It is often forgotten that discredit for the death of a baby or credit for his ultimate survival, usually goes to the obstetrician because mother has reposed her confidence and full faith in her obstetrician who had provided all the care to her and to her baby throughout pregnancy and during delivery. It is but natural that the obstetrician cannot suddenly sever her/his links with the baby after delivery. Indeed, the pediatricians must appreciate the magnanimity and faith that the obstetricians repose in them by handing over the baby, whom they had nurtured and tendered for nine long months. It is, therefore, desirable that pediatricians and obstetricians must join hands with each other not only to enhance neonatal survival but also to improve the quality of life among the survivors. The cooperation between obstetrician and pediatrician is particularly desired in the following areas of perinatal care.

Antenatal Care and Fetal Diagnosis

Pediatricians should be actively involved so that they can give their advice and expert guidance in the field of fetal diagnosis and fetal therapy by attending fetal medicine or high-risk mothers antenatal clinic. The responsibility for assessment of severity of rhesus isoimmunization, use of antenatal anti-D immunoglobulins, timing of delivery in various high-risk situations, assessment of the risk of continuing *in-utero* existence versus extrauterine care (on the basis of available facilities in NICU) should be jointly shared and decision taken by weighing all the pros and cons.

Perinatal Hypoxia

Adequate infrastructural facilities must be made available to the pediatrician in the delivery room and maternity OT in order to provide resuscitation facilities to all babies in each birthing room. The potentially harmful drugs, like pethidine, morphine, diazepam, etc., should be avoided during labor. The pediatricians should maintain constant liaison with expectant mothers by visiting the pre-delivery suites. Infants with fetal hypoxia must be promptly delivered and pediatrician must be informed well in time so that he/she is available at the time of delivery. The obstetricians must also be trained in the skills and art of neonatal resuscitation to handle the exigencies of unexpected or precipitate deliveries. It is important that level III perinatal facilities must evolve in paripassu with level III neonatal care services in the country by creating facilities for improved monitoring of fetus before birth and during labor. The widening gap between the quality of obstetrical and neonatal services must be narrowed. The delivery complex of the hospital should be designated as perinatal intensive care unit and administrators should be approached for adequate inputs of space, staff, and equipments.

Promotion of Feeding with Human Milk

The mother must be physically and emotionally prepared for breastfeeding during antenatal visits. The problems of retracted or cracked nipples must be managed before the baby is born. Additional room, attached to the nursery, should be available to promote the feeding of all preterm and high-risk babies with expressed breast milk (EBM). The mothers are encouraged to visit this facility round-the-clock for promotion of breastfeeding and expression of breast milk with the help and guidance of a lactation nurse. The mother should be allowed to stay in the lying-in ward as long as her baby is being managed in the NICU so that the baby is provided with all the therapeutic advantages of EBM and skin-to-skin contact. The medications which are known to produce hazards to the suckling infant should be avoided during lactation. Above all, there should be no contradiction between the advice of the obstetrician and pediatrician regarding feeding of babies to avoid any confusion in the minds of mothers. The feeding advice should be uniform and unambiguous. The policies and practices to be followed in the rooming-in ward should be finalized after mutual discussion. The policy manual should be available for the benefit of resident and nursing staff.

Supervised Care of LBW Babies

The policy of early discharge from NICU is desirable to decongest the nursery in order to reduce the risk of nosocomial infections. The extended nursery concept should be utilized by providing an area with adequate physical facilities, warmth, asepsis and weighing scale, etc. in the rooming-in ward. After initial management of life-threatening disorders, once the baby is stabilized, he/she can be managed in the "growing nursery" by the mother under the supervision and guidance of a nurse. The mother can be taught basic principles of home care of a LBW baby before she is discharged from the hospital. During follow-up, the mothers are likely to be more receptive and responsive to the pediatrician, who must share responsibility and concern to give advice and guidance to the mother regarding birth spacing and family welfare.

BIBLIOGRAPHY

Alberman E, Collingwood J, Pharoah POD, Vaizey J, Oppe TE. Arrangements for special and intensive care of the newborn. *Brit Med J* 1977, 2:1045–47.

American Academy of Pediatrics. Guidelines for Perinatal Care. 4th Ed. Illinois/Washington: *American Academy of Pediatrics and American College of Obstetricians and Gynecologists,* 2002.

American Academy of Pediatrics. Committee on Fetus and Newborn. Levels of neonatal care. *Pediatrics* 2012, 130(3):587–97.

Bergman I. Questions concerning safety and use of cranial ultrasonography in the neonate. *J Pediatr* 1983, 103:855–58.

Blix E, Kumle M, Kaergaard H, Oian P, Lindgren HE. Transfer to hospital in planned home births: a systematic review. *BMC Pregnancy and Child Birth* 2014, 14:179–90.

Deorari AK, Paul VK, Sachdeva A. Neonatal Equipment: Everything that You would Like to Know! *CBS Publishers & Distributors Pvt Ltd, New Delhi,* 5th edition, 1917.

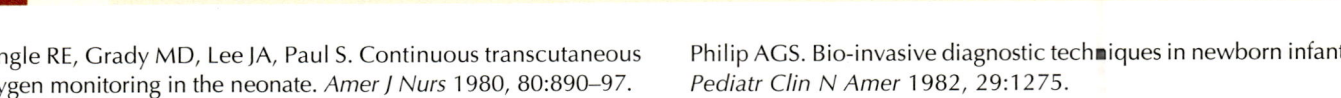

Dingle RE, Grady MD, Lee JA, Paul S. Continuous transcutaneous oxygen monitoring in the neonate. *Amer J Nurs* 1980, 80:890–97.

Easa D, Tram A, Bingham W. Non-invasive intracranial pressure measurement in the newborn. *Am J Dis Child* 1983, **137**(4): 332–35.

Gluck L (Ed.). Organization of perinatal care. *Clin Perinatol* 1976, 3:267–70.

Gluck L. Design of perinatal center. *Pediatr Clin N Amer* 1979, 17:777–91.

Hegyi T. Transcutaneous bilirubinometry: a new light on old subject. *Pediatrics* 1982, 69:124.

Lagler U, Duc G. Systolic blood pressure in normal infants during the first 6 hours of life: Transcutaneous doppler ultrasound technique. *Biol Neonate 1980,* 37:243–45.

Malhotra AK, Deorari AK, Paul VK, Bagga A, Singh M. A New transport incubator for primary care of low birth weight babies. *Indian Pediatr* 1992, 29:587–593.

Philip AGS. Bio-invasive diagnostic techniques in newborn infants. *Pediatr Clin N Amer* 1982, 29:1275.

Segal S, Pirie GE. Equipment and personnel for neonatal special care. *Pediatr Clin N Amer* 1970, 17:795–810.

Singh M, Paul VK, Deorari AK. Biomedical equipments: status and perspective. *National Neonatology Forum, New Delhi* 1990.

Singh M. Neonatal care perspectives in India (Editorial). *Indian J Pediatr* 1998, 65:243–47.

Singh M, Deorari AK. Humanized care of preterm babies. *Indian Pediatr* 2003, 40:13–20.

Steggerda S, Leijser L, Walther FJ, Van Wezel-Mei Jhu G. Neonatal cranial ultrasonography: How to optimize its performance? *Early Human Development* 2009, 85:93–99.

Vidyasagar D, Raju TNK. A simple non-invasive technique of measuring intracranial pressure in the newborn. *Pediatrics* 1977, 59 (suppl): 957.

2

The Role of Nurses in the NICU

Geetanjli Kalyan and Marsha Campbell–Yeo

Introduction

Every neonate admitted to a neonatal intensive care unit (NICU) is an emergency and needs high quality intensive care. According to American Academy of Pediatrics (AAP), the levels of neonatal care have been revised and are in accordance with levels of newborn care in India. As per the new classification, the levels are categorized as basic care (level 1), specialty care (level II), and subspecialty intensive care (level III and IV). In this chapter, we will focus primarily on the role of nurses in the subspecialty intensive care unit. The facilities are designed to provide comprehensive care to newborn infants who are considered to be extremely high-risk, critically sick and having complex medical or surgical problems. In addition to the need for medical or surgical care, all the newborns delivered at less than or equal to 32 weeks of gestation or birth weight of less than 1500 g are provided tertiary care in a level III or IV NICU. The personnel and resources are organized and effectively harnessed to provide comprehensive care and continuous life support including conventional ventilation, high-frequency ventilation, and inhaled nitric oxide. To ensure quick and safe transfer of neonates who need subspecialty care, there is a need for adequate infrastructure and availability of highly trained care providers to ensure a safe and timely transport using ground, rotor and/or fixed-wing transport services. Skilled neonatologists and neonatal nurses are the foundation of all NICUs and are of paramount importance for providing high levels of intensive care. Facilities provided at level III/IV should have round-the-clock availability of specially trained neonatologist, anesthesiologist, ophthalmologist, and surgical specialist along with access to advanced imaging (X-rays, cranial ultrasonography, computed tomography, MRI, and echocardiography) facilities on an urgent basis.

Highly skilled neonatal nurses are essential to reduce morbidity and mortality of at-risk and critically ill newborns and they constitute as critical members of the neonatal care team. As the neonate's primary care provider, neonatal nurses maintain a constant and close contact with the neonates in the NICU and play a vital role in their care, monitoring and management. Given that critically ill neonates have limited reserves, they are at high-risk of acute changes in their homeostasis and if left unattended they can succumb and collapse in a matter of minutes. The skilled neonatal nurses are trained to identify subtle changes in heath status of a neonate and stabilize him with a sense of urgency. The early identification of worsening of medical condition ensures prompt care and stabilization with improved neonatal survival. In order to ensure the provision of highly qualified nursing care to critically ill neonates, it is mandatory that neonatal nurses receive quality pre-service and in-service education, access to continuing education, and ongoing hands-on training and should have availability of resources to provide quality health care initiatives to critically sick neonates.

ROLE OF NICU NURSES

The role of neonatal nurses is complex and manifold. The components of care include ensuring the availability and maintenance of the required resources, identification of a sick neonate, receiving and stabilizing the neonate inside the facility. She should have adequate training and expertise for assessment and monitoring, thermoregulation, ensuring infection control, providing intensive care to critically ill neonates by incorporating the components of developmentally supportive care and family centered care, guiding and supervising the junior nurses and residents, dealing with loss, grief and end-of-life issues. All of these roles should be discharged while following sound ethical and legal principles.

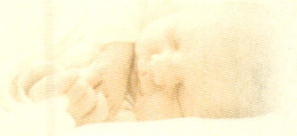

Availability of Adequate Resources

A wide range of facilities and resources are required to ensure optimal care to critically ill neonates and their families. NICU should be overseen and managed by a nurse manager/leader. Nurse managers working in collaboration with neonatologists and other members of the health care team should actively participate in team decisions related to the design and development of the unit as well as quality improvement initiatives. The leadership and decision-making initiatives should encompass the baby and family care environment including provision of appropriate temperature, humidity, sound, light, and asepsis. In addition, round-the-clock handwashing facilities must be made available to the neonatal team, subspeciality consultants, families and visitors. The design should be driven by program goals and objectives in order to deal with the medical, educational, emotional and social needs of infants, families and staff.

The unit should be located near the labor room so as to facilitate an easy access to the neonate. The ambient temperature of the delivery room should be maintained between 72°F and 78°F (24°C to 26°C) during the delivery, resuscitation and stabilization of a newborn. In addition, it should be ensured that the birthing area is isolated with the controlled access and environment. The provision of round-the-clock running water, elbow operated tap, liquid soap dispensers and handwashing sanitizer stations are a must for every NICU. It is recommended that the wash station should be located in close proximity to the patient care area to ensure direct visibility and easy access. The handwashing instructions should be displayed above the sinks. There should be a provision for availability of sterile single-use towels/paper napkins to wipe the hands. The alcohol based rubs or sanitizers are more effective than soap and water when hands are not visibly soiled.

ENSURING OPTIMAL AMBIENCE

Temperature

The NICU temperature should be maintained between 72°F to 78°F (24°C–26°C) and a relative humidity of 30 to 60%. The condensation on the walls and windows must be avoided. In one hour, minimum of six air changes should be ensured. Availability of high-efficiency particulate air (HEPA) filter in the AC ducts ensures infection control in the NICU. In addition, a regular maintenance program is necessary to maintain optimal temperature and humidity, and surveillance to ensure infection control.

Light and Sound

Maintaining desirable ambient light and sound standards help to ensure proper developmental supportive

care and comfortable environment for infants, families and health care providers. The provision of both natural and electrical light is important in a NICU. The adjustable electric light source at each bedside should be maintained between 10 to 600 lux (~1 to 60 foot candles). There should be a provision for shielding the babies from bright natural and electric light. The NICU should be designed in a way that the environmental noise is absorbed as much as possible and there should be minimum noise. The sound level should not exceed 45 to 50 dB. In addition to satisfactory ambient conditions, the nurse should ensure adequate availability of essential resources and disposables in the NICU (Table 2.1).

The last and the most important and difficult to manage resource is availability of human workforce. The nurse manager should ensure appropriate allocation of care providers. Acutely ill ventilated and

Table 2.1 Essential resources and disposables required in the NICU

1. **Oxygen and airway management**
   Suction Suction device with pressure control features, suction tubings.
   Resuscitation and ventilation Self inflating bag, masks of different sizes, laryngoscopes and blades, endotracheal and tracheostomy tubes and sets, oral and nasopharyngeal airways, stethoscope to check air entry, equipment for mechanical ventilation, portable ventilators.
   Oxygen Oxygen supply and tubings, high flow and low flow devices, humidification devices, pulse oximeter, blood gas analyzer.
   Monitoring Pulse oximeters, transcutaneous oxygen monitors.

2. **Vascular access, IV drug preparation and administration**
   Hand sanitizers, sterile/non sterile gloves, gowns, caps, masks, tape, Tegaderm, tourniquet, needles, IV catheters, three way stop cocks, central venous catheters, parenteral fluids, nutrients and drugs, cutdown sets, syringes (1 mL, 2 mL, 5 mL, 10 mL, 20 mL), umbilical catheters and tapes, betadine and alcohol, pressure lines and infusion sets, infusion pumps, laminar flow system for preparation of fluids, nutrients and drugs, sterile tray to carry the drugs to the bed side, alcohol wipes to clean the ports, etc.

3. **Diagnostic and therapeutic procedures** Arterial puncture, bronchoscopy, examination of eyes for ROP, endoscopy, heel lancing, lumbar puncture, chest physiotherapy, umbilical line insertion, dressings, adhesives, Tegaderm, nasogastric tube, bladder catheterization, suture removal, ventricular tap, drugs for pain management, phototherapy units/bili blankets, blood collection vacutainers etc.

4. **Medications** Emergency drugs, respiratory, neurologic and cardiovascular medications, antibiotics intubation medications, intravenous solutions and parenteral nutrition supplies.

5. **Additional supplies** Blood pressure cuffs, batteries and bulbs, vaseline gauze, sponges, pins, penlight, caps, socks, nappies, digital thermometers.

6. **Family support supplies** Parent sleep recliners, chairs, breastmilk expression facilities, storage containers, developmental positional aids, kangaroo care tops or wraps.

unstable infants, should be assigned 1:1 nurse-baby ratio. Infants with slightly less intensity of care could be assigned 1:2 and those close to discharge or transfer upto 1:3 nurse-baby ratio. Nurses assigned for the primary care of one or more babies should receive a verbal and/or written handover instructions prior to assuming care at the beginning of their shift. The nurse should work in partnership with the infants's primary care physician, participate in bedside rounds and maintain an open and clear communication with team members and families. The nurse should feel confident and endowed with skills and knowledge to identify a sick neonate, provide neonatal resuscitation, including ability to prepare, check and administer medications safely when needed at the time of admission and during stabilization. Maintenance of diligent charting of vitals, medical status and progress of the infant as well as ongoing verbal communication with the other members of the health care team and families and consultants is a critical role of the nurse. All members of the neonatal team should be provided ongoing continuing education related to the importance of the nursing role and need for collaborative care. The clinical parameters to identity an at-risk and sick neonate are listed in Table 2.2.

RECEIVE AND ASSESS THE NEONATE

The transfer and reception of patient indicates the handing over of the professional responsibility and accountability of all aspects of care of a patient, to the unit/organization who is at the receiving end. An inappropriate transfer and negligent reception can be life-threatening for the neonate and can lead to legal complications. The reception of the neonate in the unit should be a diligent process, where the attending nurse is required to undertake patient care responsibilities from the transferring care providers. The process of reception begins as soon the information 'Transfer the baby' is received by tertiary care NICU. Many aspects are taken into consideration while receiving a baby. An interactive inter-hospital or intra-hospital communication system is a basic requirement to transfer the neonate, as incomplete information can increase the risk of adverse outcome. Some NICU settings use locally agreed upon hand over tool known by the acronym ISBAR. It stands for Identify/introduction, Situation, Background, Assessment and Recommendation. This tool provides confidence in communication, ensures completeness of information and reduces the likelihood of missed data. This is also helpful in multidisciplinary team collaboration as it can be used between doctor-to-doctor, nurse-to-nurse, nurse- doctor, belonging to allied health system (Table 2.3). The details of transport of a sick neonate from a health care facility to a tertiary care NICU are discussed in Chapter 30.

Table 2.2 Identification of sick or at-risk neonate

1. A newborn < 32 weeks gestation, or weight <1500 g at birth, or having medical or surgical condition regardless of the gestational age.
2. A neonate who is lethargic, limp, has poor cry/inconsolable excessive crying, obtunded, poor activity and reflexes.
3. **Respiratory symptoms** Shallow breathing, apnea, bradypnea (< 20 breaths/min), tachypnea (> 60 breaths/min) gasping respiration, severe retractions of chest, nasal flaring, grunting, deep or sighing respirations, signs of impending respiratory failure.
4. **Cardiovascular symptoms** Tachycardia with weak pulses, cold extremities, capillary refill time >2 seconds, with or without pallor, pale/ashen gray color (shock/anemia), cyanosis, signs of dehydration and loss of weight. Bleeding from any site for example gastrointestinal, pulmonary, umbilical cord or IV site.
5. **Nervous system** Abnormal gaze, seizures, signs of meningeal irritation, asphyxia, encephalopathy such as opisthotonos, nuchal rigidity, photophobia, irritability, lethargy, bulging anterior fontanel, alteration in sensorium, and evidences of sepsis and meningitis.
6. **Gastrointestinal system** Abdominal distention and repeated vomitings, refusal to feed or poor sucking. Severe jaundice with staining of palms and soles and need for exchange blood transfusion.
7. **Genitourinary system** Baby who has not passed first urine for 48 hrs or the urine output is less than one mL per hour.
8. **Metabolic problems** Evidences of low blood sugar, calcium, magnesium levels, and electrolyte disturbances
9. Neonates having surgical conditions such as gastroschisis, tracheoesophageal fistula (TEF), choanal atresia, diaphragmatic hernia, neural tube defects, etc.

Note. Maintain detailed ongoing record of all the activities and observations.

Table 2.3 Steps of the ISBAR process

- **Identify/introduction** Establishing accurate identity of those who are participating in handling and ensuring that the right patient is being transferred. The health care provider who is transferring, communicates with the unit where the neonate is being referred. The one who transfers should provide the information like name, designation, ward and unit along with patients' name, age, gestational age, weight, sex, attending doctor and nurse. The one who is likely to receive the sick baby is supposed to ask who you are, your role, where you are and why are you communicating.
- **Situation** The receiver should ask for the nature of emergency, need for referral and response to various concerns.
- **Background** What are the issues that lead to this situation? Explain the reasons for hospitalization. Narrate history of present illness. State any relevant past medical, and surgical history. Ask about social background and a brief synopsis of treatment received till date.
- **Assessment** What do you think the current problem is? State the patient's current vital signs and observations on the condition of the baby. Ask the care provider who is transferring the neonate about the clinical possibilities and what has been done so far.
- **Recommendations/response** What do you recommend to correct this situation? The receiving unit can review the plan and outline revised management strategies for intact survival.

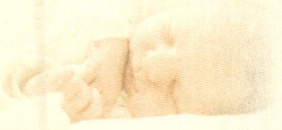

The attending nurse records complete information about the status of the neonate such as gestational age and weight, history of present illness, the current status of neonate and the interventions provided to stabilize the neonate. After confirmation about the referral, a disinfected incubator/radiant warmer (depending upon the requirement of neonate) is kept ready by using sterile linen with 100% heater output 20 min before the arrival of the neonate. All necessary equipment should be kept ready in anticipation for the admission of a sick or at-risk infant such as resuscitation kit, sterile containers with spirit and betadine swabs, separate thermometer and stethoscope. As soon as the baby is admitted, confirm the gestational age and birth weight of the neonate, check the vital signs, which include temperature, heart rate, respiratory rate, blood pressure and mean arterial pressure (Table 2.4). If the temperature of the baby is in normal range, change the

temperature control mode of the incubator/open care system from manual to servo, or else manage according to the grade of hypothermia as per WHO guidelines (Table 2.5). The blood pressure and mean arterial blood pressure guidelines for neonates are given by Dionne JM et al and Zubrow, AB et al. In general, the mean blood pressure corresponds to the gestational age of the neonate in weeks.

Table 2.4 Vital signs in neonates		
Temperature (core)	36.5–37.5°C	Normal
	36.0–36.4°C	Cold stress
	32.0–35.9°C	Moderate hypothermia
	<32.0°C	Severe hypothermia
Heart rate	120–160 beats/min	Normal
Respiratory rate	40–60 breaths/min	Normal
Mean blood pressure	Gestational age of the neonate in weeks	

Table 2.5 WHO guidelines for classification and management of hypothermia				
Category	Temperature range	Feel by touch	Clinical features	Interventions
Normal	36.5 to 37.5°C	Warm trunk and warm extremities	Normal baby	■ Cover adequately with pre-warmed linen ■ Keep the baby skin-to-skin contact with mother in upright full ventral contact ■ Encourage breastfeeding ■ Remove wet linen whenever applicable
Mild hypothermia (cold stress)	36.0 to 36.4°C	Warm trunk and cold extremities	Extremities bluish and cold. Lethargy and poor weight gain if there is chronic cold stress	■ Skin-to-skin contact (SSC) ■ Cover adequately ■ Ensure room temperature 26–28°C ■ Remove wet linen whenever applicable ■ Provide warmth* if temperature doesn't increase ■ Encourage breastfeeding
Moderate hypothermia	32.0 to 35.9°C	Cold trunk and cold extremities	Poor sucking, lethargy, weak cry and fast breathing	■ Ensure room temperature 26–28°C ■ Remove wet linen whenever applicable ■ Provide warmth* ■ Vitamin K (if not given earlier) ■ Reassess every 15 minutes ■ Administer expressed breast milk via nasogastric tube if can't breastfeed or luke warm intravenous glucose solution if neonate is having symptomatic hypoglycemia (blood glucose <40 mg/dL)
Severe hypothermia	Less than 32.0°C	Cold trunk and cold extremities	Lethargic, poor perfusion/mottling. Fast or slow breathing, slow heart rate, hardening of skin with redness and edema, bleeding, low blood sugar	■ Rapid re-warming till baby is 34°C and then slow re-warming** ■ Oxygen ■ Administer luke warm intravenous glucose solution if neonate is having symptomatic hypoglycemia ■ Inj vitamin K ■ Reassess every 15 minutes

*Keep the neonate under radiant warmer. In case radiant warmer is not available continue SSC and use extra warm clothes to cover the baby and mother to provide warmth. Avoid heat sources that can cause burn/scalds such as hot water bottles, blower, heater
**slow re-warming is done by shifting the temperature control mode from manual to servo
(Modified and adapted from Thermal protection: Newborn Nursing for Facility Based Care Level 2 Units, participatory module based learning, 3rd edition 2014, AIIMS WHO CC ENBC)

The information received, should be correlated with your observations and assessment. Document all the facts after initial stabilization of the neonate and report to the unit/facility from where the neonate is being transferred. When emergency intubation or any other life-saving measure is required, the neonatal nurse should assist the physician and document it appropriately.

STABILIZATION OF THE BABY

It is important to perform a systematic detailed assessment to evaluate and manage all possible issues requiring urgent or emergent care. Basic evaluation includes assessment of airway, breathing, circulation, temperature as well as tone and activity and blood glucose. The neonate who is lethargic, irritable, inconsolable, limp, unconscious, and unresponsive is classified as extremely sick. Potential underlying cause could include hypoxia, poor perfusion (cerebral/peripheral), sepsis, and metabolic cause such as hypoglycemia. Such neonates should be assessed and urgent attempts made to stabilize their vital parameters.

Respiratory System

Evaluate breathing and initiate immediate intermittent positive pressure ventilation if baby is not breathing (even when stimulated, i.e. apneic), has gasping respirations, or has a respiratory rate of less than 20/minute. When ventilator support is not immediately indicated, the nurse should assess the respiratory status by using the Downes–Vidyasagar score (for any gestational age group)/Silverman–Anderson score (for preterms) to evaluate risk of impending respiratory failure, and need for invasive/noninvasive ventilation (Tables 2.6 and 2.7).

Circulatory System

Palpate the pulse, if weak and fast (>160/min) and extremities are cold to touch and capillary refill time (CRT) >2 seconds with or without pallor or lethargy or unconsciousness, the neonate is likely to have shock. The etiology or cause of shock should be determined and managed appropriately. If bleeding is the likely cause, infuse 10 mL bolus physiologic saline over 10 minutes while waiting for availability of blood products. If there is a delay in obtaining blood, a second bolus of 10 mL/kg of normal saline may be considered. Administer blood (type O, Rh negative blood), stop external source of bleeding and administer vitamin K (0.5 mg if birth weight is ≤ 1000 gm; 1.0 mL if > 1000 gm). If bleeding is not the cause of shock, consider administration upto three boluses (10 mL/kg) of normal saline over one hour and try to identify the cause.

Table 2.6 Downes-Vidaysagar score for grading of respiratory distress in newborn

Sign	Score		
	0	1	2
Respiratory rate	<60	60–80	>80 or baby is having recurrent apneic attacks
Retractions	Nil	Mild	Moderate to severe
Cyanosis	Absent	Present in room air	Present in FiO$_2$ 0.4
Grunt	Absent	Audible on stethoscope	Audible without stethoscope
Auscultation	Good air entry	Breathing delayed or decreased	Breathing barely audible

Grades of severity: 1–3 mild respiratory distress, 4–6 moderate respiratory distress, >6 severe respiratory distress

Table 2.7 Silverman – Anderson score for grading of respiratory distress in preterm neonates

Sign	Score		
	0	1	2
Upper chest retractions	Synchronized	Lag on inspiration	See-saw respiration
Lower chest retractions	None	Just visible	Marked
Xiphisternum retractions	None	Just visible	Marked
Nasal flaring	Nil	Minimal	Marked
Grunt	Absent	Audible with stethoscope	Audible without stethoscope

Grades of severity: 1–3 mild respiratory distress, 4–6 moderate respiratory distress, >6 severe respiratory distress

Note: A decrease in score is not always a sign of improvement as a score may decrease if a newborn is too fatigued to retract or grunt. This causes reduction in the activity of newborn which may further indicate need for oxygen. In an extreme preterm neonate, even a score of less than 3 is an indication for respiratory support.

Nervous System

If neonate is in coma or having convulsions, assess sensorium (active, depressed, nonarousable), and perform assessment with the APU scale—**A**wake, responds to **P**ain, and **U**nresponsive. If the neonate is unresponsive and limp, treat symptoms and investigate for a cause. If the neonate is having seizures, manage the airways, check for blood glucose level, calcium level and administer anticonvulsants.

Metabolic Disorders

All critically sick neonates are at risk of a primary metabolic cause for their presenting symptoms or have an associated abnormality. Hypoglycemia is a very common and life-threatening. It is advisable to check blood glucose level of all neonates admitted to the NICU. If the blood glucose level is <45 mg/dL in plasma or less than 40 mg/dL in blood, treat for hypoglycemia. Administer 2 mL/kg of 10% dextrose IV bolus and start IV fluids. Recheck blood glucose level 15–20 minutes post bolus to ensure that glucose level is >40 mg/dL. If the glucose level remains low, give another 2 mL/kg bolus of 10% dextrose and consider an increase in the rate of administration of intravenous glucose or increase dextrose concentration to 15%.

ASSESSMENT AND MONITORING AFTER INITIAL STABILIZATION

Assessment and monitoring are the key components of nursing care provided to any patient. Neonates are at greater risk of adverse outcome as they are non-verbal (cannot convey symptoms or level of distress) and have limited capacity to handle the metabolic derangements. Hence they require more thorough assessment and monitoring as compared to children and adults. Detailed assessment and interpretation increases the possibility of early recognition of existing or potential problems and is an important component to ensure prompt treatment. Once the neonate is stabilized, perform a detailed assessment of the infant, read any accompanying information regarding neonatal or maternal history and ask the mother or father further questions if information appears to be missing or inadequate. Ensure that all information is documented clearly and updated daily on patient chart or the electronic monitoring record.

History Taking

Neonatal history includes specific questions related to the gestational age, birth weight; postnatal age, did the baby cry at birth or needed resuscitative measures to revive the baby; Apgar scores, at one and five minutes and any evidence of perinatal asphyxia which may be related to hypoxic ischemic encephalopathy; evidences of hypotonia; status of feeding; whether the baby was reported to have choking or vomiting; and whether the condition of the baby is improving or worsening.

Maternal history includes questions related to medical, past obstetrical history, social history including substance abuse, and details of pregnancy such as duration; history of fever; any medical (renal/cardiac/gestational diabetes etc.) complications during pregnancy; history of HIV; any reports of decrease in fetal movements or fetal well-being; whether the mother noted any paroxysmal rhythmic fetal movements as it has strong relationship with the seizure disorder; what medications were taken prenatally and any medications taken while breastfeeding the neonate.

Family history of cognitive impairment in other siblings, early stroke or consanguinity should be asked, as this may have implications regarding the neurologic problems due to inborn errors of metabolism.

Monitoring the Sick Neonate

The monitoring and observations of a neonate in the NICU depends upon the acuteness and severity of illness. A critically ill neonate requires detailed observations and assessment before stabilization. The integral component of nursing care is the accurate documentation of nursing observations and assessment. The sophisticated cardiopulmonary monitors have made the clinical monitoring quite easy and simple but an expert nursing observation is mandatory and cannot be replaced by machines. The skills of a trained and caring nurses are more important than the information provided by the electronic gadgets.

The standard daily monitoring sheet should include the following parameters and frequency of assessment and monitoring depends upon the severity of illness.

1. Postnatal age, length, weight (at least daily and often morning and evening for very ill infants) and weight loss/gain in past 24 hours, corrected gestational age.
2. A list of following procedures with their frequency.
   Oral suction, ET suction, position change, vital signs, glucose monitoring, abdominal girth, stomach aspirate, chest physiotherapy, urine specific gravity, and central venous pressure (CVP) monitoring.

Monitoring Parameters

The timing and frequency of assessment and monitoring in the NICU is based on the level and severity of illness of the infant. Infants who are severely compromised may require continuous observation by the care provider with ongoing monitoring and minute-to-minute documentation while less ill infants may require assessment and monitoring every 2–4 hours. In most infants requiring tertiary care in the NICU, assessment, observation and documentation is generally required at least hourly.

General Monitoring

Observe feeding behavior, color, perfusion, sensorium, sedation level and activity. Monitor vital signs such as temperature, heart rate, respiration, blood pressure and mean blood pressure because subtle changes in these parameters indicate the underlying problem. In context of temperature regulation, mention the mode selected in the radiant warmer/incubator and the temperature set for the same. It is advisable to take the skin temperature manually if there are variations in the temperature. It is important to ensure that the sensor probe is correctly affixed to the neonate's skin.

Respiratory Status

Observe movements of chest and abdomen while monitoring the respiratory rate. Always look for use of accessary, muscles of breathing, as evidenced by nasal flaring and substernal, intercostal, subclavicular retractions. Assess the severity of respiratory distress with the help of Downe's/Silverman score (Tables 2.6 and 2.7). Auscultate and describe breath sounds such as grunt, stridor, wheezing, bilateral air entry, areas of absent breath sounds and crackles. If the infant is receiving mechanical ventilator support, evaluate and record whether the baby is generating any spontaneous breaths. It is important to assess and monitor respiratory rate and spontaneous breaths over a period of full minute. The parameters which reflect adequacy of ventilation include comfortable and pink baby, adequate chest rise, synchronization, absence of retractions, CRT < 2 sec and normal blood pressure, oxygen saturation between 88–94% and normal arterial blood gases.

Assess oral and endotracheal secretions (the secretions can be documented as normal, minimal, copious, persistent, blood stained or frank blood) and determine the need for suction. Suctioning should be done only as and when necessary and will vary depending upon the need of the infant.

Record method of delivery of oxygen, note fraction of inspired oxygen (FiO$_2$), arterial oxygen saturation and the saturation alarm limits set on pulse oximeter (saturation alarm for preterm is set at 88–94%).

Remember that the reliable functioning of pulse oximeter is dependent on adequate arterial pulse. In conditions such as shock, severe edema, obstructed arterial flow (due to BP cuff), especially if pulse pressure is <10 mm Hg, pulse oximetry is not reliable. In a critically sick infant, determine partial pressure of oxygen and carbon dioxide in arterial blood by blood gas machine and transcutaneous oxygen and carbon dioxide monitors.

If the infant is receiving respiratory support, note the mode of ventilation. Monitor FiO$_2$, flow rate, peak inspiratory pressure (PIP), peak end expiratory pressure (PEEP), continuous positive airway pressure (CPAP), mean airway pressure (MAP), rate of ventilation, inspiration: expiration ratio, total volume (TV), and mean volume (MV). For infants receiving non-invasive ventilator support, it is essential that the nurse assesses the quality of the seal of the mask or whether prongs are securely fitted. Prongs or mask should be removed regularly to evaluate the skin and preventive measures should be considered such as alternative use of prongs versus mask if noninvasive support is prolonged and the use of of Tegaderm to protect pressure point areas.

Cardiovascular Status

Monitor every neonate for adequacy of cardiac output by recording heart rate, tissue perfusion, oxygenation and urine output. Tachycardia, (heart rate >180 beats per min), or bradycardia (heart rate <100 per min) are ominous. It is also important to look for cyanosis (central or peripheral), check CRT (>2 sec reflects a poor tissue perfusion), determine peripheral pulses, blood pressure, and central venous pressure. Decreased urination (because of dehydration or shock), unusual weight loss or gain, and mottled cold clammy skin are indicative of cardiovascular comprise. Look for signs of dehydration (sunken eyes, depressed anterior fontanel, loss of skin elasticity, dry tongue, and mucous membrane) and over hydration (excessive weight gain, puffy eyes, and increase in edema over the lower back). Maintain intake-output chart (type and amount of fluids administered), amount of fluids administered along with drugs, amount of oral feeds, total parenteral nutrition, volume of gastric aspirate if any, and urine output. Maintain record of serum electrolytes (sodium, potassium and calcium) and inotropes (dopamine, adrenalin, dobutamine) administered. Maintain record of blood withdrawn for various investigations especially in extremely low birth weight neonates as even a small amount of blood loss can lead to serious consequences.

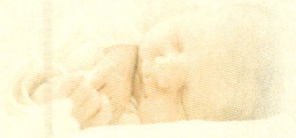

CNS Status

Assess the neonate for lethargy, weak cry, poor suck, excessive jitteriness, convulsions, and hypotonia. Assess the position of limbs (flexed or extended), and automatic reflexes (Moro, sucking, Babinski, doll's eye, tonic neck) and document the response of the neonate. Measure the occipital frontal head circumference just above the ears and eyebrows around the widest part of head. In preterm babies, the head circumference is 33 cm or less at birth and increases by 1 cm per week. Increase in head circumference >1 cm/week or >2SD and above 97th percentile should raise the suspicion of hydrocephalus/intracranial hemorrhage or a storage disorder. The head circumference below 2SD/below 3rd percentile for the gestational age and gender indicates microcephaly with increased risk of developmental delay.

Gastrointestinal System

While recording intake-output, mention the mode of feeding (nasogastric, orogastric, spoon fed, breastfed or *paladay* feed), type of milk fed (expressed breast milk, fortified breast milk, formula milk), regurgitation or vomiting, nature, color and frequency of stooling. Assessment of the abdomen includes girth, soft or firm, audible bowel sounds, and evidences of visible bowel loops. Gastric aspiration should not be performed routinely before giving the next feed. It must be done if infant displays any signs and symptoms of feed intolerance like inability to digest enteral feed leading to abdominal distension, increased gastric residuals, and/or emesis.

Genitourinary System

The urine output varies between 1–5 mL/kg/hour, the values above or below are abnormal and need reporting. Urine can be collected with a condom or test tube in a male infant and with a urine collection bag in a girl. Collect urine sample for specific gravity by aspirating with a syringe from a wet diaper as refractometer requires only one drop. Record the color, amount and pH of urine. Assess status of hydration by daily weighing on an electronic weighing scale with a resolution of ±1.0 gm.

Skin Assessment

Inspect the skin daily for discoloration, redness, primary and secondary lesions, and birth marks. Assess the areas of skin under the monitoring equipments, infusion sites and other sensors and adhesives in contact with the skin. Assess the texture (dry, flaky, smooth or shiny) and turgor of the skin. Examine the IV site at least hourly for signs of infection and infiltration (normal, red, swelling, cold or warm to touch, tender, color of hands and feet, phlebitis score). Note the location

of catheter (arterial, venous, central or umbilical), type of infusion (dextrose, saline, electrolytes, TPN solution and medications).

Thermoregulation

Preterm and low birth weight babies are at an increased risk of hypothermia due to large surface area, lack of shivering and poor quota of brown fat. During metabolic thermogenesis, oxygen and glucose are consumed. Hypothermia often leads to hypoxia, metabolic acidosis and hypoglycemia. The prevention of heat loss is essential for survival of neonates. The nurses working in the intensive care units must be competent to prevent heat loss through various avenues (Table 2.8) and must know how to maintain a thermoneutral environment

Table 2.8 Measures to prevent heat loss through all the four avenues

1. Evaporation
- High humidity reduces evaporative water loss. Incubators have a provision to circulate warm moist air that prevents evaporative and convective heat loss. The warm stagnant water increases the risk of infection because it acts as a medium for growth of bacteria. It is desirable to provide heat and humidity from external source.
- Keep infant dry and remove wet linen as early as possible.
- Don't bathe, only sponge and dry the baby as early as possible.
- Use cling wrap in incubator.

2. Conduction
- Prewarm the incubator or radiant warmer before receiving the neonate.
- Use warm items and equipment such as weighing scales, radiograph film plates, linen, intravenous fluids and blood.
- Warm your hands by rubbing before touching the baby.

3. Convection
- Use incubators with circulation of warm humidified air from outside to maintain thermoneutral temperature.
- Minimize opening the port holes and cluster the activities in order to prevent repeated opening of the incubator.
- Use cling wrap in a radiant warmer.
- When nursing in servo-controlled mode, cover head, foot and use diaper.
- Administer warm humidified oxygen
- Remove all sources of air currents.
- Maintain temperature of NICU between 24–26°C.
- Clothe the neonate appropriately when removing from the incubator.

4. Radiation
- Use double walled incubator or cover the baby with a perspex plastic shield.
- Clothe the baby appropriately if kept in a cot.
- Keep cot away from cold surfaces such as walls or iron cupboard.
- Maintain temperature of the intensive care unit between 24–26°C.

Table 2.9 Ambient temperature to be set to maintain thermo-neutral environment

Birth weight of the baby	Recommended ambient temperature for air mode at different postnatal ages			
	35°C	34°C	33°C	32°C
Less than 1500 g	1 to 10 d	11 d to 3 wk	3 wk to 5 wk	More than 5 wk
1500 to 1999 g	—	1 to 10 d	11 d to 4 wk	More than 4 wk
2000 to 2499 g	—	1 to 2 d	3 d to 3 wk old	More than 3 wk
2500 g or more	—	—	1 to 2 d	3 d old or more

(Adapted form Newborn Nursing for Facility Based Care Level 2 units, participatory module based learning, 3rd edition 2014–15, AIIMS WHO CC ENBC)

which is essential for optimal functioning of all metabolic processes. Neutral thermal environment helps to maintain a normal core body temperature with minimal oxygen and energy consumption. Optimal thermal environment helps to maintain temperature within normal range. To maintain thermoneutral temperature, it is desirable to use an incubator and set the recommended incubator temperature at air mode (Table 2.9), place the baby under radiant warmer and use cling wrap.

Rise in temperature (fever/hyperthermia) is equally detrimental to the neonatal health. The core body temperature of more than 37.5°C is referred as hyperthermia in a neonate. Fever is a normal physiologic response to infection when there is increase in the hypothalamic temperature "set point". On the other hand, in hyperthermia there is failure of normal homeostasis but hypothalamic set point is not altered. Hyperthermia occurs because of overheating and is characterised by hot flushed dry skin, dehydration, jitteriness and restlessness. To prevent hyperthermia due to overheating, ensure that the skin probe is attached securely, so that heater output occurs in response to the baby's need. In case there is a need to warm the baby with manual heater output, keep checking the temperature every 15 minutes, and once the desired temperature is attained, shift to servo mode. In case the baby has already become hyperthermic, remove the source of heat, extra clothes, consider sponging if temperature is >39°C, and recheck temperature every 15 min. Treat the underlying cause, provide adequate feeds and fluids and correct dehydration. *Antipyretics are useful to treat fever but have no role for management of hyperthermia.*

Prevention of Nosocomial Infections

The newborns are at an increased risk of acquiring infections owing to their immature immune system, and greater opportunities for exposure to infection because they are exposed to a large number of interventions and a variety of electronic gadgets. Nurses working in the NICU should be involved to take part in formulation of infection control policies including aseptic preparation of medications, parenteral nutrition solution, care of IV lines (Table 2.10), and rational use of antibiotics. Preventive strategies to reduce hospital acquired infections should be implemented by trained auxiliary staff and overseen by neonatal nurses (Table 2.11). Any person entering the NICU should remove shoes, socks, woolens, watch, bangles and rings. Strict rituals recommended before entry to the NICU should be followed. Personnel having infection should not be allowed entry to the unit and only the parents of newborns and primary care providers should be allowed entry.

Hand hygiene is the foundation of infection control in any intensive care area. A one minute handwash including arms upto the elbows before entering the neonatal unit, immediately before infant contact or if there is any visible dirt or body fluids on the hands, is recommended (Figure 2.1). Alternatively, in the absence

Table 2.10 Aseptic measures to prevent infections through intravenous cannulations

Preparation of skin before venipuncture
1. Prepare the skin to be punctured by using surgical alcohol/chlorohexidine 2% and let it dry naturally (DO NOT blow air)
2. Apply 5% betadine and let it dry (DO NOT blow air)
3. Again clean with alcohol to wipe off the betadine and let it dry (DO NOT blow air)

Infection control practices related to IV fluids and drugs
1. Keep a separate infusion bottle for each baby and label it with date and time of opening and discard it after 24 hours
2. Do not use stock IV fluids
3. Change burette sets, and IV lines every 24 hours
4. Use separate IV lines for administration of drugs
5. The expensive antibiotics can be shared among babies but an opened vial must be discarded after 24 hours
6. Do not use heparinised saline to keep the IV lines patent
7. Change the blood transfusion sets after single use

(Adapted from Newborn Nursing for Facility Based Care Level 2 Units, participatory module based learning, 3rd edition 2014–15, AIIMS WHO CC ENBC)

of visible dirt or body fluids on the hands, a NICU approved hand sanitizer can be used by effectively rubbing the solution on the hands and arms up to the elbows for 20–30 seconds before and after touching the neonate. The availability of hand sanitizers, liquid soap, running water supply, elbow operated taps, single use sterile towels or tissues to wipe hands and strict

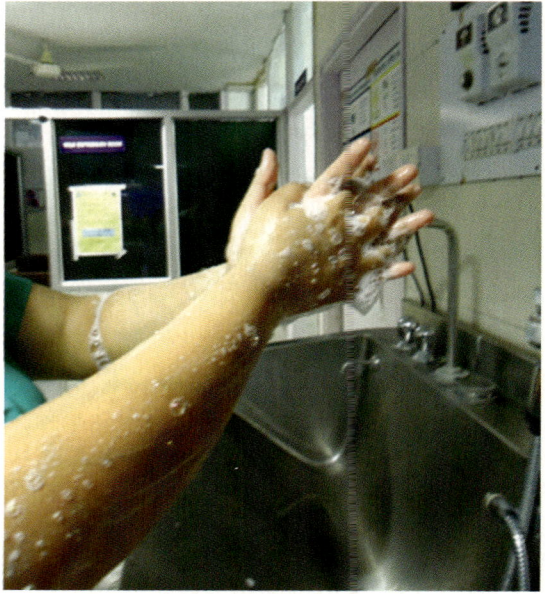

Figure 2.1 The correct technique of handwashing. Complete instructions for correct method of effective handwashing should be displayed adjacent to the wash basin.

adherence to hand hygiene norms are essential requirements for maintaining good hand hygiene. In addition, ensuring adequate nursing staff and disposables, provision of separate articles such as stethoscope, thermometer, and surgical spirit and betadine for each baby are useful to reduce the risk of hospital acquired infection (Table 2.12).

Table 2.11 House-keeping routines		
Site	*Disinfection method*	*Frequency of disinfection*
Floors	Wet mopping with phenyl	Once in each shift No dry sweeping Do not use 2% glutaraldehyde (cidex)
Walls	2% Bacillocid	Once in each shift
Fans	Wipe with clean wet cloth	Once a week
Window AC	Surface and filter to be washed with soap and water	Once a week
Refrigerator	Defrost and clean with soap and water	Once a week
Buckets	Soap and water	Daily in the morning shift
Sinks	Detergent or powdered soap	Daily in the morning shift or as required

(Adapted form Newborn Nursing for Facility Based Care Level 2 Units, participatory module based learning, 3rd edition 2014–15, AIIMS WHO CC ENBC)

Table 2.12 Asepsis routines for fomites in the NICU		
Items	*Disinfection method*	*Frequency of disinfection*
Baby linen, blanket cover	Wash and autoclave	Use autoclaved linen each time
Cotton and gauze	Autoclave	As required. Every time use autoclaved cotton and gauze
Feeding utensils (*paladay*, spoon and *katories*, etc.)	Wash with soap and water and then boil for 10 minutes	Before each use
Swab container, injection and medicine tray	Wash with soap and water / autoclave	Daily morning shift. Use separate swab container for each baby
Sets for various procedures	Autoclave	After each use; every 72 hours if not used
Cheattle forceps	Autoclave	Daily. Keep in sterile autoclaved bottle containing dry sterile cotton
Stethoscope, measuring tape, thermometer, BP cuffs, probes of radiant warmer/incubator, pulse oximeter	Clean with spirit swab	Daily and before use
Laryngoscope	Clean with spirit swabs thoroughly daily and after each use. Wrap in autoclaved cloth, put date on the cover	If used for an infected baby, wash with soap and water. Put the blade in 2% glutaraldehyde (cidex) after removing the bulb. Wash thoroughly with sterile water after removing from glutaraldehyde

(Contd...)

Table 2.12 Asepsis routines for fomites in the NICU (*Contd...*)

Items	Disinfection method	Frequency of disinfection
Syringe pumps	Clean with a wet clean cloth. If blood stained, use soap and water	Daily in the morning shift In each shift, if possible
Oxygen hood	Wash with soap and water; dry with clean linen	Daily in the morning shift
Face mask	Clean with soap and water, immerse in glutaraldehyde for 20 min, rinse in distilled running water, dry and wrap with auto-claved linen	Daily and after each use
Resuscitation bag and reservoirs, oxygen tubing, bottle and tubing of suction machine	Clean with detergent/soap and water after dismantling. Immerse in glutaraldehyde for 4–6 hours. Rinse in distilled water. Dry, wrap in autoclaved linen and put a date	Weekly for resuscitation bag and reservoir. Daily for other items
Weighing machine	Wipe with surface disinfectant	Daily in the morning shift and when required.
Radiant warmer and incubator	Clean with soap and water daily, if occupied. If not occupied, clean with 2% Bacillocid	Daily in the morning shift.

(Adapted form Newborn Nursing for Facility Based Care Level 2 Units, participatory module based learning, 3rd edition 2014–15, AIIMS WHO CC ENBC)

Promoting Adequate Nutrition and Hydration

Fluid and electrolyte imbalance can be life-threatening at any age. Neonates have higher percentage of body water as compared to adults. Moreover, their kidneys have limited capacity to excrete and conserve water and sodium, they are thus, at an increased risk of fluid and electrolyte imbalance. Total body water (TBW) includes both intracellular fluid (ICF) and extracellular fluid (ECF) compartments. Term newborns have 75% total body water (40% ECF, 35% ICF) and preterms have almost 90% water (60% ECF, 30% ICF). After birth there is efflux of fluid from ICF to ECF compartment. The neonates' kidneys gets flooded with this increase in ECF and they excrete the extra fluid in first 48–72 hours of life leading to weight loss. Term neonates lose 5–10% body weight and preterm lose 10–15% body weight as they have more ECF. If a preterm neonate fails to lose this water, he is likely to develop patent ductus arteriosus, necrotising enterocolitis, and chronic lung disease. The preterm neonates have more insensible water losses owing to thin skin, large surface area, increased respiratory rate, use of radiant warmer and phototherapy unit, increased crying and activity. All attempts should be made to prevent insensible water losses (Box 2.1).

The daily fluid requirements of preterm infants are shown in Table 2.13. The fluid of choice for initial three days is 10% dextrose. After three days, sodium (3–5 mEq/kg/day) and potassium (2 mEq/kg/d) are

BOX 2.1 Strategies to minimize insensible water loss

1. Use transparent plastic barriers (cling wrap as shown in Figure 2.2) when infant is under radiant warmer to reduce the insensible water loss by 50–70%.
2. When a baby is stable, it is preferable to nurse in an incubator to ensure better thermal control and reduced insensible water loss because of increased humidity and reduced air currents.
3. Apply liquid paraffin/coconut oil/sweet almond oil on the skin.
4. Use cap, socks and mittens.
5. Provide adequate fluids/ feeding when under radiant warmer/ phototherapy unit.
6. Administer warm humidified oxygen.
7. Prevent and manage hyperthermia.

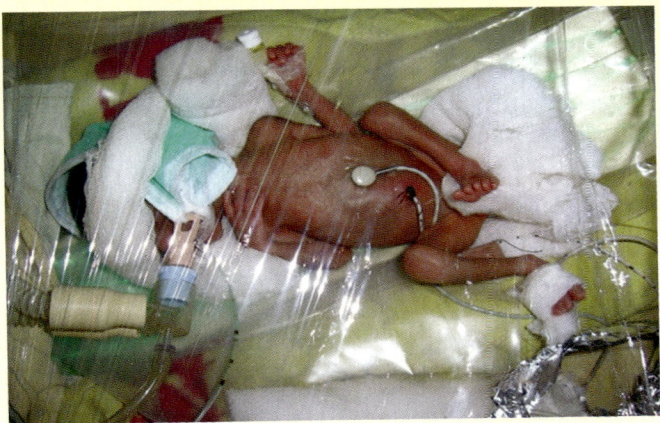

Figure 2.2 Cling wrap

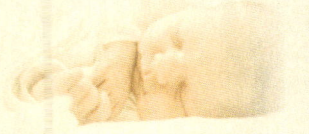

Table 2.13 Daily maintenance fluid requirements		
Day of life	Birth weight	
	≥1000 grams	<1000 grams
1	60	80
2	75	95
3	90	110
4	105	125
5	120	140
6	135	150
7	135	150

Adapted from AIIMS WHO CC STPs

added to the daily fluids because kidneys of neonates have limited capacity to reabsorb sodium and hyponatremia can lead to failure to gain weight. It is important to remember that very low birth weight (VLBW) baby needs supplementation of sodium in breast milk until 32–34 weeks of corrected age. It is important to monitor serum sodium levels and if values are deranged, sodium supplementation is modified accordingly. The baby is weaned off from IV fluids as early as possible and side by side enteral feeds are started at the rate of 10–15 mL/kg/day every 2 hourly. If there are no signs of feed intolerance (abdominal distension, increase in abdominal girth >2 cm, gastric residual volume >25% of last feed volume), the fluid intake is increased by 20–30 mL/kg/day. When volume of enteral feeds reach two-thirds of daily fluid requirements, intravenous fluids are stopped.

Monitoring of Babies Receiving Intravenous Fluids and Electrolytes

1. Assess IV insertion site at least hourly for signs of infilteration/inflammation. If present, the cannula is removed and inserted at an alternative site.

2. Check the amount of intravenous fluids and enteral feeds received and cross check with the daily requirements.

3. Monitor blood glucose in each shift, i.e. 6–8 hourly until infant's condition improves and/or value of blood glucose is stable and within normal range. If baby is born to a diabetic mother monitor blood glucose at 2, 6, 12, 24, 48, 72 hours.

4. If blood sugar is >150 mg/dL on two consecutive readings, the infant is shifted to 5% dextrose and blood glucose rechecked after 2 hours.

5. Weigh the baby daily and report any abnormalities in weight gain. If weight loss is >5% of body weight in 24 hours, the fluid intake is increased by 10 mL/kg

per day. If no weight loss occurs or there is weight gain during initial three days of life, no increment is made in the fluid intake. When daily weight gain exceeds 3 to 5% of body weight, the fluid intake is reduced by 15–20 mL/kg per day.

6. Assess for signs of over hydration or dehydration. Urine specific gravity, osmolality and sodium are checked and fluid intake is titrated accordingly.

7. Check urine output. If urine output is decreased along with excessive weight loss, fluid intake is increased. If there is increased urine output (>5 mL/kg/hr), fluid intake is reduced by 10 mL/kg per day.

CARE OF IV SITES AND LINES

In sick neonates, the parental fluids are usually administered through peripherally inserted intravenous lines (dorsal surfaces of hands and feet, antecubital, and scalp). In ELBW and sick babies, when prolonged intravenous alimentation is anticipated, central venous line through saphenous/antecubital or umbilical venous/arterial lines are established. In most NICU's in India, experienced nurses insert IV lines and maintain infusions. The lines are secured with transparent skin friendly tapes such as Tegaderm to ensure proper visualization of insertion site for signs of inflammation and infection. Proper taping of the IV site is an essential skill of a neonatal nurse to ensure visualization of the site, ensure optimal fixation with minimal risk of skin damage.

Nurses working in intensive care unit should be capable of assisting the neonatologist in initiation of noninvasive and invasive ventilation, administration of surfactant, monitoring of signs of improvement and prevention of complications. Document and monitor the nursing care provided to neonates on noninvasive ventilation (Table 2.14), note and record the signs of adequacy of CPAP therapy which include stable and comfortable neonate with minimal chest retractions, oxygen saturation between 88–94%, and blood gases within target range of PaO_2 50–60 mm Hg, $PaCO_2$ 35–45 mm Hg and pH 7.35–7.45.

When conventional ventilation is unable to stabilize the sick baby and reverse the blood gas abnormalities, infant is promoted to intensive ventilation including high frequency ventilation and inhaled nitric oxide (iNO). These infants need high level 1:1 nursing care as outline in Table 2.15.

Table 2.14 Care and monitoring of a patient on noninvasive ventilation

- **Ensure good seal** The nasal prongs need to be affixed on the nose with a good seal, mouth should be kept closed. Excessive movements interfere with a good seal, increase nasal septum irritation and it can be decreased by swaddling/nesting.
- **Close monitoring and assessment** of the effectiveness of noninvasive ventilation (NIV) is crucial to prevent, and manage complications.
- **Manage the airway** by proper positioning and suctioning. The infant should be positioned prone whenever possible, with the neck slightly extended. Alternatively, baby can be nursed supine in a sniffing position with head end slightly elevated. Airway patency should be assessed every 2–3 hours. Suction is done as and when needed.
- **Clinical and electronic monitoring** which include monitoring temperature, respiratory rate, grunt, retractions, oxygen saturation, heart rate, color, CRT, BP, activity, secretions, intake and output.
- **Ventilation report** should be prepared on hourly basis by mentioning all the parameters, e.g. PEEP/PIP, MAP, rate, FiO_2.
- **Blood gases and acid-base monitoring**.
- **Prevention of abdominal distention** Positive distending pressure (CPAP) is transmitted to the GI tract causing abdominal distension and baby may have feeding intolerance. Distinguish the benign distension from pathologic distension because of serious causes like NEC and sepsis. Nasogastric tube should be inserted and its outer end kept open to deflate the stomach.
- **Monitoring and early reporting of complications** Nasal septal irritation and necrosis, gastric distension, pneumothorax, increased intracranial pressure, difficulty in keeping the nasal prongs in place, over distension of the lungs (inadvertent PEEP), and mucous obstruction of the airway with atelectasis.

Table 2.15 Nursing responsibilities and care during invasive ventilation

1. In each shift there should be an experienced nurse on duty who is well-versed in the skills of endotracheal intubation and can assist the neonatologist to intubate the neonate and initiate invasive ventilation.
2. Keep articles ready for intubation including appropriate size straight blades (0, 1), larygocope, endotracheal tubes (<1 kg 2.5 mm, 1 kg –2 kg 3.0 mm, 2 kg –3 kg 3.5 mm, >3 kg 3.5–4 mm), suction catheters (size 2 × size of ET tube), oxygen and suction source, adhesives (Dynaplast, Tegaderm).
3. Assist in intubation and check bilateral air entry in the lungs.
4. Following intubation, obtain an X-ray chest to confirm correct tube placement (level of T 2–3).
5. Utilize various positions to optimize gas exchange
   a. Place in supine position with slight neck extension (sniffing position) to prevent blocking of airway.
   b. Prone when feasible as this improves oxygenation, helps in better tolerance of feed, and promotes better sleep rest pattern.
   c. Use semi-prone or sideling position to prevent aspiration in neonates having excessive secretions.
   d. Avoid Trendelenberg position as it can reduce lung capacity and increase ICP.

6. Observe signs of respiratory distress, and response of neonate to ventilator support.
7. Closely monitor blood gas measurements and oxygen saturation
8. Do suction as and when needed:
   a. Use proper technique to prevent infection, injury to airway, hypoxemia, bradycardia, atelectasis, mucosal trauma, infection, and pneumothorax.
   b. Length of catheter to be inserted is decided by the length of ET tube inserted + infant weight (kg) + tube left outside + length of connector (document the length of suction catheter and size to be used).
   c. Keep suction pressure <80 mmHg for preterm and 80–100 mmHg for term neonates.
   d. Some infants may require a small increase in FiO_2 prior to suctioning. This can be done by using small increments of 2–5%, instead of sudden increase upto 100% with large swings in oxygen levels with risk of development of retinopathy of prematurity.
   e. During suctioning, insert the suction catheter up to predetermined length without applying any pressure and slowly rotate the catheter while removing it when suction pressure is being applied.
   f. If secretions are thick, disconnect the ventilator, instill normal saline (don't use distilled water) to loosen the secretions and reconnect the ventilator. Allow five breaths to be delivered, then suction and reconnect within 20 seconds.
   g. Suction ET tube first followed by mouth and nose.
   h. If the baby has required an increase in inspired oxygen concentrations, wean slowly following the suction procedure. When indicated, perform chest physiotherapy (percussion, vibration, and postural drainage). Don't routinely perform chest physiotherapy if baby is <1000 g/<32 weeks in first three days, if there is air leak syndrome, persistent pulmonary hypertension (PPHN), and intraventricular hemorrhage (IVH).
9. Monitor FiO_2 to maintain target SpO_2 of 88–94%.
10. Observe carefully and act quickly if there is any sudden deterioration of the baby on ventilator. Look for ventilator malfunction, ET tube obstruction or air leaks. If there is high limits alarm, look for ventilator malfunction, ET tube kink or block. When there is low limits alarm, check for any air leak.
11. To trouble shoot sudden deterioration of the baby remember the acronym DOPE for troubleshooting.
    a. **D**isplaced tube. Absent breath sounds, no chest rise, and abdominal distension indicate tube displacement. Remove ET, provide bag and mask ventilation and re-intubate the baby.
    b. **O**bstructed airway. Decrease in oxygen saturation and increase in work of breathing indicate obstructive airway. It could be because of kink in tube, thick secretions and hyperextension /hyperflexion of neck of the baby.
    c. **P**neumothorax. It is suspected by increase in respiratory distress and shift of heart sounds to the opposite side. Inform physician and prepare for chest tube insertion to remove air from pleural space.
    d. **E**quipment failure may occur because of ventilator malfunction or disconnect. If there is no air leak, remove baby from ventilator and start bag and mask ventilation and then troubleshoot.
12. Monitor the neonate as discussed earlier.

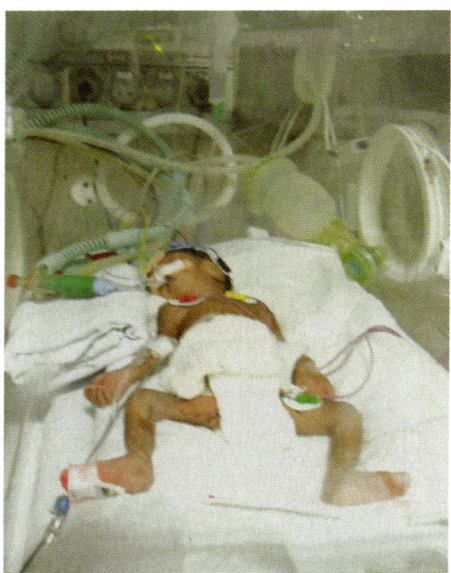

Figure 2.3 Neonate on invasive ventilation.

Developmentally Supportive Care

It has been demonstrated that all newborns, including those born preterm, respond to a variety of stimuli. The environment of intensive care unit should be stimulating and developmentally appropriate to stimulate neurodevelopment of the baby. A broad range of neuro-developmental impairments including subtle disorders of central nervous system, cognitive impairment, cerebral palsy, visual and hearing impairments, problems related to language and learning, neuromotor coordination, behavioral problems, and social-emotional difficulties have been associated with adverse NICU environment like untreated pain, improper handling and positioning, loud noise and exposure to bright light. Many neonatal care providers often overlook these concerns and consequently infants in the NICU are often subjected to inappropriate stimuli that may be harmful. Developmentally supportive care include activities that prevent the subsequent developmental and health related problems. Neurodevelopmental supportive activities are listed in Table 2.16.

Table 2.16 Neurodevelopmental supportive activities in the NICU

1. The nurses in the NICU should be allocated one or two specific babies so that they establish a bond and provide developmentally supportive care.
2. Observe the babies' behavioral patterns including sleep, reflex responses such as the startle reflex, increased movements, agitation and/or crying.
3. Look for stress signs and respond promptly
   - Fast breathing or pausing and gasping for air
   - Color turning pale, gray or blue
   - Hiccups, gagging or grunting
   - Spitting
   - Straining as if to pass stool
   - Coughing, sneezing, yawning or sighing and sticking tongue out
   - Startling, squirming, twitchings and tremors of body, limbs or face
   - Suddenly becoming limp or stiff with arching of back and neck.
4. Individualize interventions for each infant and offer them only during the period of alertness.
5. Continuously assess the infant's response by interpreting cues from the baby and provide appropriate intervention.
6. The stimulation should be stopped when infant shows signs of stress.
7. The interventions should be clustered together.
8. Assess pain using a reliable infant pain assessment tool at least once per shift and more frequently if the scores are high or if the infant is requiring some form of pain relief.
9. Minimize painful procedures and provide relief and comfort by skin-to-skin contact, swaddling, breastfeeding, pacifier or oral administration of 20% sucrose solution 2 minutes prior to the procedure (Figures 2.4 to 2.7).
10. Provide specific interventions related to five special senses
    a. Visual
    i. Ensure periods of "quiet time" in each shift and provide "day" and "night" patterns by use of dim lights at night
    ii. Cover the walls of incubator and the baby's eyes during phototherapy
    iii. Place photos of parents and differently shaped black and white objects overhead in the visual range.
    b. Auditory/vestibular
    i. Minimize noise in NICU by reducing sound level to less than 45 dB
    ii. Close portholes of incubators and drawers gently
    iii. Respond to alarm beeps promptly or use visual alarms
    iv. Encourage mother to talk to the baby
    v. Play prerecorded parent's voice (less than 45 dB at infant's ear) or soft music when baby is awake
    vi. Call infant by name at each interaction
    vii. Don'ts talk loudly during the rounds and while providing care to the babies
    viii. Don't use incubator's top as writing surfaces.
    c. Tactile
    i. Minimize handling, and promote maternal touch and skin-to-skin contact
    ii. Warm the hands before touching the baby
    iii. Provide comfort to the baby by nursing on sheep skin, and water mattress
    iv. Nesting the neonate, facilitating tucking, swaddling and ensuring midline containment
    v. Don't make sudden changes in the position of the baby.
    d. Gustatory
    i. Feeding breast milk as early as possible including small amounts of trophic feeds to provide biofactors to prevent sepsis and NEC, and promote maturity of gut
    ii. Introduce early enteral nutrition
    iii. Promote exclusive breastfeeding and use of *paladay*.
    e. Olfactory
    i. The equipment should be thoroughly washed off the disinfectant before use
    ii. Provide KMC to expose the baby to the pleasurable smell of the mother and her milk
    iii. Avoid use of strong smelling or pungent chemicals near the baby.

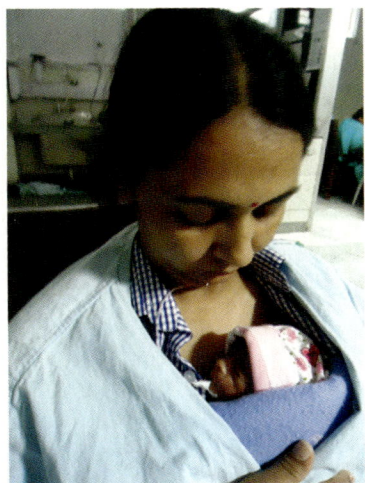

Figure 2.4 Mother providing kangaroo-mother-care.

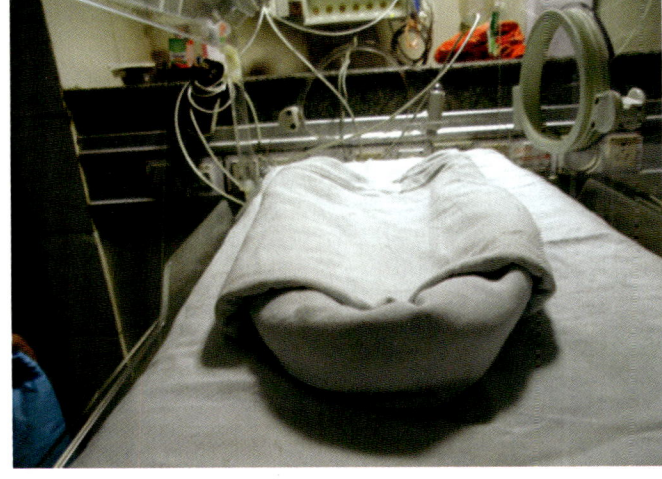

Figure 2.5 Nestled bed.

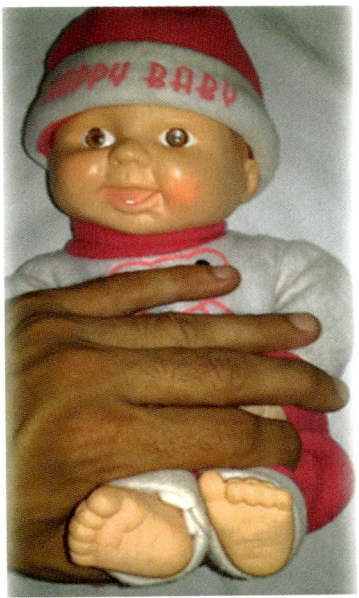

Figure 2.6 Facilitated tucking.

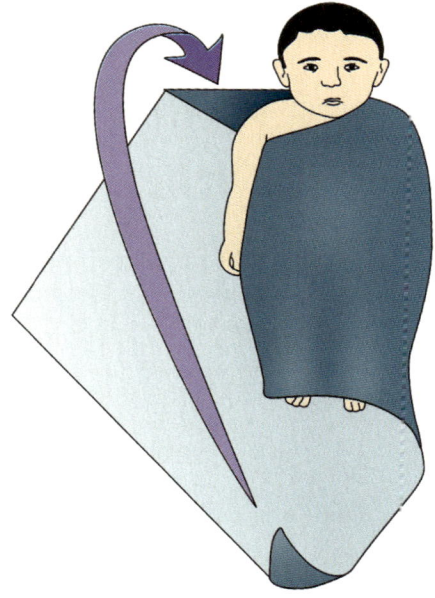

Figure 2.7 Swaddling.

Family Centered to Family Integrated Care

Birth of a preterm baby raises the concerns of viability and intact survival to the family. The family of the newborn is exposed to stress and anxiety related to inability to participate in the care of their neonate. The parents are bewildered and greatly upset to see their tiny baby attached to a variety of electronic gadgets. American Academy of Pediatrics and many other medical and nursing societies have recommended family centered and integrated care to sick neonates, receiving tertiary care. American Nurses Association and Society of Pediatric Nursing endorsed family centred care (FCC) as a useful nursing care philosophy in the NICU. As far as the child health services are concerned, family is considered as the primary source of strength and support. Further it is believed that involvement of parents in the care of their infant and in decision-making is associated with better outcomes both for the infant as well as the family. The parents should be treated as partners in the care of their infants. Information should be provided to the parents in an unbiased and honest way and it is important that the individual strengths or limitations of each family are recognized. In this system of care, most of the care is provided by the health care team, and parents play a supportive role and get used to handling the baby with due care which gives them the confidence and skills to look after the baby after discharge.

More recently, the concept of family centered care has been replaced by family integrated care. In family integrated care, parents do everything except for the most advanced medical care, parenteral medications and invasive procedures. The nurses perform the role of teachers and consultants and help parents to gain skills to handle their preterm and delicate babies with confidence. It has been clearly demonstrated that greater parent involvement is associated with a reduced length of stay of the neonate in the hospital. The principles of family integration care are given in Box 2.2.

BOX 2.2 Principles of family integrated care

- Parents should be treated with respect and dignity.
- The parents are encouraged and guided to participate in the care and stimulation of their baby (Figure 2.8).
- Families develop their strengths and capabilities by participating in experiences that enhance their confidence and independence.
- Mothers become partners and take pride in providing care to their baby.
- Parental learning is facilitated.
- Health care professionals share complete information with parents and families.
- Parents participate during the rounds and feel involved.
- Nurses are provided with tools and education to enable families to be the integral part of the team.
- Collaboration is established in policy and program development, professional education and delivery of care to neonates in the NICU.
- There is better bonding between the parents and the infant without any risk of neglect of the baby after discharge.
- The entire health care team supports the model of family integrated care.

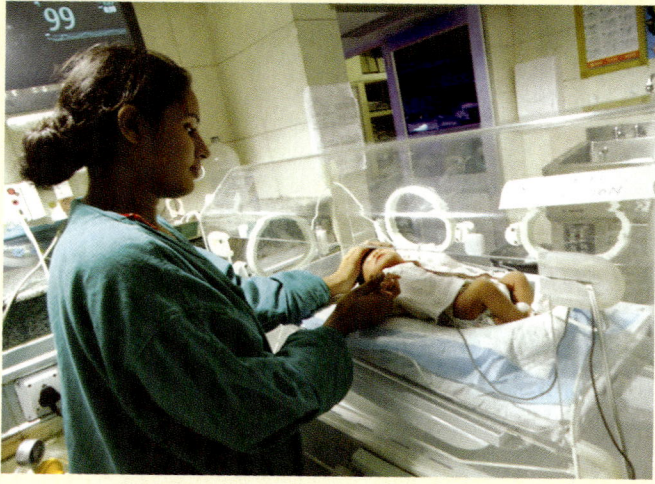

Figure 2.8 Mother caring for her preterm neonate nursed in the Isolette.

The end-of-life Issues

The parents of neonates, born extremely preterm or with a life-threatening condition that requires admission to the NICU, are exposed to physical, emotional and financial hardships and stress. When a sick neonate is destined to die despite our best intentions or survival is likely to be associated with extremely poor quality of life or vegetative state, the family should be provided with emotional support. The family should be taken into confidence and told about the likely outcome and consequences. The family should be encouraged to talk and express their concerns. The family should be made to understand that whatever was humanely possible was done for the care of their baby. When decision has been taken to withdraw life support or deny life-saving measures, they should be introduced gradually keeping in mind the acceptance level of the family and comfort of the baby. The coping of death of a neonate in the NICU is a challenging and traumatic experience both for the health care professionals and parents. The family's wishes for religious or spiritual support and request for a priest at bedside should be honored. The parents should be encouraged to hold, embrace and cuddle their baby. The family should be emotionally prepared before declaration of death. They should be allowed to name the child, take footprints and photographs for future recollection and remembrance. The family should be assisted with post death formalities with due compassion and consideration and without unnecessary delay. When autopsy has been conducted, the family must be provided with postmortem report and given guidance and counseling regarding any special care during subsequent pregnancies and newborn babies.

The Need to Build a Nursing Team

The highest priority in the organization of a tertiary care neonatal center, is the availability adequately trained personnel especially nurses. The survival of neonates in the NICU depends upon the availability of adequate number of specially trained nurses. The nursery complex must he considered as an independent nursing unit under the charge of a fully qualified and trained nurse manager or advanced nurse practitioner. The nurses posted in the NICU should not be frequently changed, they should be provided with structured orientation while joining the NICU. The neonatal nurses must be provided with continuing in-service and ongoing medical education and training in the art of neonatal nursing and preventive maintenance of a variety of electronic equipment used in the NICU. They should be integral part of neonatal health care team

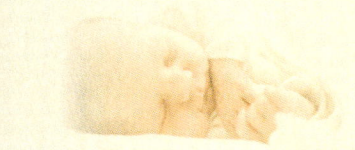

and participate in the monthly perinatal morbidity and mortality meetings. It is desirable to have services of public health nurses and medical social workers for follow-up and home care of NICU babies after their discharge from the hospital.

BIBLIOGRAPHY

Allen MC. Neurodevelopmental outcomes of preterm infants. *Curr Opin Neurol* 2008; 21(2):123–8.

Azhibekov T, Soleymani S, Lee BH, Noori S, Seri I. Hemodynamic monitoring of the critically ill neonate: An eye on the future. *Semin Fetal Neonatal Med* 2015; 20(4):246–54.

Batton B, Li L, Newman NS, Das A, Watterberg KL, Yoder BA, et al. Evolving blood pressure dynamics for extremely preterm infants. *J Perinatol* 2014; 34(4):301–5.

Belfort MB, Rifas-Shiman SL, Sullivan T, Collins CT, McPhee AJ, Ryan P, et al. Infant growth before and after term: Effects on neurodevelopment in preterm infants. *Pediatrics* 2011; 128(4): e899–906.

Chawla D, Agarwal R, Deorari AK, Paul VK. Fluid and electrolyte management in term and preterm neonates. *Indian J Pediatr* 2008; 75(3):255–59.

Cignacco E, Hamers JP, Stoffel L, et al. The efficacy of non-pharmacological interventions in the management of procedural pain in preterm and term neonates. A systematic literature review. *Eur J Pain* 2007; 11(2):139–52.

Conge–Agudelo A, Diaz-Rosello JS, Belgin JM. Kangaroo mother care to reduce morbidity and mortality in low birth weight infants. *Cochrane Database Syst Rev* 2000; (4):CD002771.

Debbie F A. Noninvasive ventilation in the neonate. *J Perinat Neonat Nurs* 2007; 21(4):349–58.

Dionne JM, Abitbol CL, Flynn JT. Hypertension in infancy: diagnosis, management and outcome. *Pediatric nephrol* 2012; 27(1):17–32.

Downes J, Vidyasagar D, Morrow G, Boggs T. Respiratory distress syndrome of newborn infants: I. New clinical scoring system (RDS score) with acid-base and blood-gas correlations. *Clinical Pediatr* 1970; 9(6):325–31.

Eden LM, Callister LC. Parent involvement in end-of-life care and decision making in the newborn intensive care unit: An integrative review. *J Perinat Educ* 2010 1; 19(1):29–39.

Fenton AC. Training of NICU nurses and paramedics in the neonatal emergency transport service (NETS). In: Neonatal Emergencies. Cambridge University Press; 2009. Available from: http://dx.doi.org/10.1017/CBO9781139010467.077

Foronda CL, Alhusen J, Budhathoki C, Lamb M, Tinsley K, MacWilliams B, et al. A mixed-methods, international, multisite study to develop and validate a measure of nurse-to-physician communication in stimulation. *Nurs Educ Perspect* 2015; 36(6):383–8.

Hladík M, Jakšová K, Sikorová L. Nurses' role in promoting relations between parents and premature newborns in accordance with the concept of family-centered care. *Cent Eur J Nurs Midwifery* 2016; 7(1):396–401.

Jesney S. A critical analysis of the role of the nurse in the implementation of skin-to-skin contact in the neonatal unit. *J Neonatal Nurs* 2016; 22(2):68–73.

Joris Lemson, Anneliese Nusmeier, and Johannes G. van der Hoeven. Advanced hemodynamic monitoring in critically ill children. *Pediatrics* 2011; 128(3):561.

Joseph RA. Neonatal care. Prolonged mechanical ventilation: challenges to nurses and outcome in extremely preterm babies. *Crit Care Nurse* 2015; 35(4):58–66.

Kalyan G, Vatsa M. Neonatal nursing: an unmet challenge in India. *Indian J Pediatr* 2014; 81(11):1205–11.

Kalyan G, Vatsa M, Paul VK, Mehta M, Srinivas M. Loss and grief response and perceived needs of parents with the experience of having their newborn at neonatal care units. *Int J Nurs Edu* 2012; 4(2):111–16.

Kenner C. The role of neonatal nurses in palliative care. *Newborn Infant Nurs Rev* 2016; 16(2):74–77.

Mari Murakami, Kyoko Yokoo, Mio Ozawa, Saori Fujimoto, Yuki Funaba, Minoru Hattori. Development of a neonatal end-of-life care education program for NICU nurses in Japan. *JOGNN J Obstet Gynecol Neonatal Nurs* 2015; 44(4):481-91.

O'Brien K, Bracht M, Robson K, Ye XY, Mirea L, Cruz M, et al. Evaluation of the family integrated care model of neonatal intensive care: a cluster randomized controlled trial in Canada and Australia. *BMC Pediatr* 2015;15:210.

Recommended standards for newborn ICU design, eighth edition — jp201310a.pdf [Internet]. [cited 2016 Jun 25]. Available from: http://www.nature.com/jp/journal/v33/n1s/pdf/jp201310a.o

Simmons D, Sherwood G. Neonatal intensive care unit and emergency department nurses' descriptions of working together: building team relationships to improve safety. *Crit Care Nurs Clin North Am* 2010; 22(2):253–60.

Spooner AJ, Aitken LM, Corley A, Fraser JF, Chaboyer W. Nursing team leader handover in the intensive care unit contains diverse and inconsistent content: An observational study. *Int J Nurs Stud* 2016; 61:165–72.

Standard Treatment Protocols for Management of Common Newborn Conditions at Small Hospitals. AIIMS WHO CC STPs. Department of Pediatrics WHO Collaborating Centre for Training And Research in Newborn Care. All India Institute of Medical Sciences, New Delhi, 3rd edition, 2014–15.

Stevens B, Yamada J, Ohlsson A, Haliburton S, Snorkey A. Sucrose for analgesia in newborn infants undergoing painful procedures. *Cochrane Database Syst Rev* 2016;7:CD001069.

Sundaram V, Chirla D, Panigrahy N, Kumar P. Current status of NICUs in India: A nationwide survey and the way forward. *Indian J Pediatr* 2014; 81(11):1198–204.

Symington J, Pinelli A. Non nutritive sucking for promotion of physiologic stability and nutrition in preterm infnts. *Cochrane Database Syst Rev* 2000; (3):CD0010.

White RD, Smith JA, Shepley MM. Recommended standards for newborn ICU design. *J Perinatol* 2013; 33(suppl 1):S2–S16.

Zubrow AB, Hulman S, Kushner H, Falkner B. Determinants of blood pressure in infants admitted to neonatal intensive care units: a prospective multicenter study. Philadelphia Neonatal Blood Pressure Study Group. *Perinatology* 1995; 15(6):470–9

3

Fetal Emergencies

Japleen Kaur, Suja Mariam, Supreet Kaur and Sourabh Dutta

Fetal emergencies include antepartum non-reassuring fetal conditions such as fetal malformations, immune hydrops, reversed end diastolic flow and abnormal non-stress test; intrapartum non-reassuring fetal status like cord prolapse; obstructed labor; uterine rupture; shoulder dystocia and entrapment of after coming head of a breech. Each of these conditions will be discussed in detail in this chapter, both regarding the obstetric and neonatal management.

ANTEPARTUM NON-REASSURING FETAL STATUS

Antepartum fetal surveillance refers to real time monitoring of fetal status to detect evidences of fetal distress. Some conditions, like fetal hydrops, abnormal non-stress test and reversed end diastolic flow in umbilical artery require immediate action.

1. Immune Fetal Hydrops

It occurs most commonly due to Rhesus or ABO iso-immunization. An Rh-negative mother with an Rh-positive fetus, is likely to form antibodies once exposed to the Rh-positive blood (e.g. through mismatched blood transfusion, sensitization in previous pregnancy, feto-maternal hemorrhage, intrauterine procedure, abruption). The Rhesus (anti-D) IgG antibodies cross transplacentally and destroy the fetal red blood cells, leading to anemia, heart failure and hydrops. Fetal anemia can be detected by rising middle cerebral artery peak systolic velocity and sonologic signs of heart failure like placentomegaly, cardiomegaly, fetal ascites and scalp edema.

Obstetric Management

a. *Fetal gestation <34 weeks.* Intrauterine transfusion is planned, with provision for immediate delivery in case of a procedure related complication.

b. *Fetal gestation 34 weeks – 37 weeks.* Intrauterine transfusion may be considered or delivery can be planned at a tertiary center, with facilities for exchange blood transfusion. Allowing enough time for adequate antenatal steroid cover is recommended, if fetal demise is not imminent as evidenced by biophysical tests.

c. *Fetal gestation >37 weeks.* Planned delivery at a tertiary center.

Neonatal Management

Resuscitation of hydropic infant requires advanced preparation and availability of skilled personnel. Resuscitation equipment should be checked well before delivery and plans for drainage of extravasated fluid must be made depending upon the location and severity of extravascular fluid collections.

Essential equipments include appropriate sized intubation tubes, laryngoscope, Ambu bag and mask, thoracocentesis/paracentesis/pericardiocentesis kits, chest tube drainage sets and umbilical catheter set. Essential drugs include availability of normal saline, adrenaline and O Rh-negative blood cross matched with mother.

Ventilatory management Intubation may be difficult due to massive edema of head and neck region. Drainage of effusion might require chest tube placement if it is not controlled by thoracocentesis. Need for surfactant administration should be considered in case of prematurity or if there is evidence of surfactant deficiency. Associated pulmonary hypoplasia, pulmonary edema, pneumothorax and barotrauma warrant judicious ventilation management.

Fluid and hemodynamic management Fluid calculation must be based on median dry weight of the baby. Intravenous fluids are started @ 40–60 mL/kg/day, until edema resolves, along with frequent monitoring of serum glucose, electrolytes, urine output, meticulous intake and output charting. Diuretics must be used with caution as these patients are hemodynamically compromised. Use of inotropes might be required in case of cardiac dysfunction.

Exchange blood transfusion Isovolumetric exchange transfusion is better tolerated in hydropic neonates. Blood used is O Rh-negative cells, suspended in AB Rh-positive plasma before delivery and crossmatched with maternal blood. After exchange transfusion, phototherapy must be continued.

2. Abnormal Non-Stress Test (NST)

Antepartum non-stress test is classified into three categories; normal, atypical and abnormal NST. Normal NST has a baseline heart rate between 110–160 bpm, with a variability of 6–25 bpm, at least 2 accelerations ≥15 bpm lasting more than 15 sec and no decelerations in a 20-minute segment (maximum 40 min). In preterm fetuses (< 32 weeks), even two accelerations of ≥10 bpm, lasting for more than 10 sec are sufficient to classify it as reassuring. Abnormal NST is of interest as it signifies fetal jeopardy, requiring urgent action. Abnormal NST is characterized by any of the following features; fetal bradycardia (<100 bpm) or fetal tachycardia (>160 bpm) for more than 30 mins, variability ≤5 bpm for 80 min, ≥25 bpm for 10 mins, sinusoidal pattern, atypical variable decelerations, late decelerations or absence of accelerations. The NST tracings require immediate assessment of maternal and fetal condition and need for emergency delivery.

Neonatal Management

Assessment of risk factors is important; category II or III fetal heart rate pattern is associated with a need for aggressive neonatal resuscitation. Appropriate preparation and availability of two qualified persons to manage the baby must be present at birth. Management at the time of birth would be identical to any newborn with birth asphyxia.

Preparation of equipment Check the availability and working status of radiant warmer, prewarmed linen; plastic wrap, exothermic mattress and woolen head cap, appropriate sized laryngoscope, resuscitation bag and mask, pulse oximeter, appropriate sized ET tubes, suction catheters and injection adrenaline.

Assessment of risk factors Pediatrician must assess gestational age, whether liquor is clear or meconium stained, multiple gestation and additional risk factors like antepartum and intrapartum fetal distress. Post birth management must follow the standard guidelines of neonatal resuscitation protocol.

3. Reversed End Diastolic Flow in Umbilical Artery (REDF)

It is a marker of uteroplacental insufficiency, when significant area of villous architecture has been involved. It is picked up in cases being monitored with umbilical artery Doppler studies.

Obstetric Management

Ensure that fetal malformations have been ruled out on ultrasound. Further management depends on period of viability, and existence of comorbid conditions of the mother.

a. *Fetal gestation <24 weeks* Termination of pregnancy by induction of labor, if indicated on the basis of maternal condition or one can wait for intrauterine fetal death after counseling the parents.

b. *Fetal gestation 24–32 weeks* Antenatal steroid cover, intensive fetal monitoring with non-stress test and biophysical profile. Termination of pregnancy (preferably via cesarean section), after steroid cover or if there is any definitive indication on the basis of biophysical tests.

c. *Fetal gestation >32 weeks* Termination of pregnancy by emergency cesarean section. Steroid cover is optional depending on local resources and unit policy.

Neonatal Management

Appropriate pre-birth preparations should be made in anticipation of perinatal asphyxia. Post birth management as per neonatal resuscitation algorithm is recommended. Neonates with reversal of end diastolic flow are at an increased risk of mortality, seizures, intraventricular hemorrhage, meconium aspiration syndrome, persistent pulmonary hypertension, hypoglycemia, necrotising enterocolitis, hematological abnormalities, retinopathy of prematurity and feed intolerance. The infant should be closely monitored for early identification and management of these conditions.

There is increased risk of necrotizing enterocolitis (NEC) in preterm infants with REDF pattern on antenatal USG Doppler studies. The enteral feeds are generally delayed in such neonates. We start feeds in REDF neonates @ 20 mL/kg per feed at 24 hours of life after examination of abdomen, auscultation of bowel sounds and enquiry about passage of stool.

INTRA-PARTUM NON-REASSURING FETAL STATUS

A variety of methods are available for intrapartum fetal surveillance, but the most commonly used is the cardiotocography (CTG). There are two guidelines for the interpretation of CTG. ACOG has adopted the three-tiered system (Category I, II, III) whereas RCOG/NICE classifies intrapartum CTG into normal, suspicious and pathological. The category III or the pathological CTG is a life-threatening fetal emergency.

Category III CTG includes any one of the following abnormalities:
1. Absence of variability with recurrent late decelerations.
2. Absence of variability with recurrent variable decelerations.
3. Absence of variability with bradycardia for at least 10 minutes.
4. Sinusoidal pattern for at least 20 minutes.

Common causes of fetal heart rate (FHR) abnormalities are listed below:
1. *Decreased variability* may occur due to fetal sleep cycle, fetal prematurity, anemia, metabolic acidemia, and medications to the mother like magnesium sulphate, codeine, benzodiazepines.
2. *Decelerations* Cord compression/occlusion, cord prolapse, uteroplacental insufficiency, head compression (early deceleration), fetal metabolic acidemia, placental abruption, and maternal shock are recognized correlates of fetal hypoxia.

Obstetric Management

When category III CTG is encountered during spontaneous labor, one must ensure that the CTG probe is properly affixed. Look for alternative causes of abnormal CTG like maternal epidural analgesia, magnesium sulphate prophylaxis, vasovagal effect due to excessive vomiting or maternal fever. Meanwhile intrauterine resuscitative measures like left lateral maternal position (to relieve aortocaval compression), oxygen by mask and intravenous hydration are instituted.

Vaginal examination is indicated at this stage. If membranes are intact, with vertex position, perform artificial rupture of the membranes. If the membranes are ruptured, rule out cord prolapse and check the color of liquor. Presence of meconium stained liquor is suggestive of fetal distress, while presence of blood stained liquor suggests placental abruption. The

urgency of delivery and the mode of delivery will depend on the exact type of CTG abnormality and other relevant maternal factors, like maternal hemodynamic stability.

It must be remembered that intrapartum CTG was introduced without any proven benefits as demonstrated by randomised controlled trials on perinatal mortality. Abnormal electronic fetal monitoring alone is not a specific indicator of neonatal acidosis because of the following reasons:
1. It has high inter and intraobserver variation.
2. It has high false positive rates. Only 50% of neonates born after an abnormal CTG have umbilical blood acidosis and only 0.5 % of them develop cerebral palsy.
3. Fetal status is dynamic and only NSTs taken within ½ to 1 hr of delivery have any correlation with fetal acidosis. However, abnormal CTG has a high sensitivity for fetal hypoxia.

Neonatal Management

Observational studies have shown that a delay of more than 20 minutes between the CTG indication of hypoxia to delivery has a higher risk of 5-minute Apgar score of <7 and increased risk of admission to NICU. Two personnels who are trained in advanced neonatal resuscitation should be present at the time of delivery. Resuscitation should be carried out as per NRP protocol. After delivery, umbilical cord arterial samples should be taken for blood gas analysis and the 1 and 5-minute Apgar scores should be recorded in the assessment sheet. If the baby requires resuscitation, the baby should receive post-resuscitation care and close observation in the NICU. If baby did not require assisted ventilation but cord blood analysis shows evidences of acidosis, the baby should be closely monitored for 6 hours for development of hypoxic-ischemic encephalopathy.

Cord Prolapse

Abnormal descent of the umbilical cord along with the fetal presenting part is defined as cord prolapse. It is classified into three varieties depending on the severity of descent.
1. *Occult cord prolapse* The cord is located by the side of the presenting part, but not felt by the examining fingers.
2. *Cord presentation* The cord pulsations are felt below the presenting part but through intact membranes.
3. *Cord prolapse* This is the most sinister variety in which membranes have ruptured and the cord is felt directly, either lying in vagina or protruding outside the vulva.

The overall incidence of cord prolapse is approximately 0.1–0.6%. There is high association of cord prolapse with non-cephalic presentations. Some other risk factors include multiparity, preterm labor, low birth weight, polyhydramnios, fetal congenital anomalies and unengaged presenting part. The importance of cord prolapse lies in the fact that it is a preventable cause of perinatal morbidity.

Diagnosis

Cord is directly felt on vaginal examination in cases of cord presentation and cord prolapse. Presence of variable decelerations on cardiotocography due to cord compression, may provide indirect evidence of occult cord prolapse.

Obstetric Management

After diagnosis, further course of action depends on whether fetus is alive, maturity of the fetus and degree of cervical dilation. If fetus is alive and cervix is fully dilated, immediate safe vaginal delivery is possible. In case of vertex presentation, delivery can be expedited with use of forceps or ventouse. In case of breech presentation, breech extraction can be attempted by an experienced obstetrician. When vaginal delivery is not imminent, the baby should be delivered by cesarean section. Certain first aid measures are adopted to alleviate pressure on the cord during transport to the operating room, but they should not cause undue delay.

a. The bladder is filled with about 500 mL normal saline and the urinary catheter is clamped, to lift the presenting part off the cord.
b. Replacement of cord in the vagina and lifting the presenting part manually by introducing two gloved fingers in the vagina until cesarean delivery.
c. Exaggerated and elevated Sims or Trendelenburg or knee chest position, but these positions may be uncomfortable for the patient. In Trendelenburg position, mother lies supine or flat on the back with feet higher than the head by 15–30 degrees.

General anesthesia is preferred due to urgency of cesarean section but regional anesthesia can be an option in expert hands. Verbal consent is adequate for undertaking an urgent cesarean section.

Neonatal Management

A neonate who is born after cord prolapse is at risk of birth asphyxia because of cord compression and vasoconstriction of umbilical vessels. The factors that increase the risk of fetal hypoxia are listed below.

- Delay between diagnosis and delivery of >30 minutes.
- Longer segment of prolapsed cord.
- Active uterine contractions.
- Cord prolapse at home or during transport.

Almost one-third of these babies require NICU admission due to prematurity, sepsis or low Apgar scores, but with modern obstetrics the incidence of neonatal encephalopathy due to cord prolapse in term otherwise uncomplicated pregnancies is less than 0.5%.

In prolonged cord prolapse secondary to premature rupture of membranes (PROM) in infants <34 weeks, intervention for delivery is not very crucial when there are no active uterine contractions compressing the cord. There is no role of prophylactic antibiotics to the neonate.

Obstructed Labor

It is diagnosed when labor is prolonged and it is not feasible to deliver the baby vaginally due to mechanical reasons.

Incidence and Risk Factors

Although the incidence of obstructed labor is decreasing in modern obstetrics, but it has been reported up to 12% in some developing countries. It is a major cause of maternal mortality and morbidity in developing countries. The common causes of obstructed labor include cephalopelvic disproportion, malposition, malpresentation, fetal congenital abnormalities like hydrocephalus, and cervical dystocia. Most women belong to low socioeconomic status and are not registered for antenatal checkups at any hospital. Perinatal mortality rates upto 66 per 1000 live births have been reported in recent studies.

Obstetric Management

The following signs indicate dystocia and should be looked for to make early decision for cesarean section.

1. Cervix is not dilating inspite of good uterine contractions.
2. There is no descent of fetal head, with increasing caput and moulding.
3. Mother appears exhausted and dehydrated.
4. Distension of lower segment and/or presence of Bandl's ring.
5. Impending uterine rupture.
6. Hematuria.

Initial management is directed towards resuscitation and wellbeing of the mother. Next step is to ensure the viability of the fetus. Abdominal and per vaginal examination are conducted to confirm the diagnosis and ascertain if at all there is any possibility of assisted vaginal delivery. The definitive management of obstructed labor, which is detected in first stage of labor, is emergency cesarean delivery. There may be a role for destructive operation in second stage of labor, if fetus is dead, maternal condition is stable and there are no signs of impending uterine rupture. Whatever the mode of delivery, antibiotic prophylaxis to the mother is mandatory.

Neonatal Management

The perinatal outcome is grave and ominous for the fetus when compared to the mother. The perinatal mortality (stillbirth and early neonatal death) varies between 25% to 92% in developing countries. More than 50% of deaths are contributed by stillbirths. Neonatal deaths occur within the first week of life secondary to birth asphyxia, septicemia and meconium aspiration syndrome.

The neonates born following obstructed labor are at risk to develop sepsis because of multiple invasive interventions, per vaginal examinations and prolonged labor. Fetal hypoxia and acidosis are common due to prolonged exposure to elevated intrauterine pressure and placental insufficiency. There is increased risk and severity of neonatal jaundice due to soft tissue bruising and hemorrhages. Facial nerve injury and limb fractures may occur. Necrosis of scalp may occur after prolonged obstructed labor due to the pressure injury by the pelvic brim.

Uterine Rupture

Disruption of all the layers of uterus including the visceral peritoneum (uterine serosa) during the course of obstructed labor is termed as uterine rupture. It can occur in a scarred (due to previous cesarean section or myomectomy) or unscarred uterus. It is a life-threatening emergency for the mother-fetus dyad. It must be differentiated from scar dehiscence, in which there is separation at the previous scar site, but serosa remains intact.

Incidence and Risk Factors

The reported incidence of uterine rupture is approximately 0.07%. The number and kind of previous cesarean deliveries, uterine anomalies, multiparity, previous myomectomy, labor induction, uterine instrumentation, obstructed labor and uterine trauma are some of the known risk factors. A single previous cesarean section increases the risk to 0.2%; whereas, in case of more than two cesarean scars, the risk approaches 2%. Grand multiparity and advanced maternal age are associated with increased risk of uterine rupture.

Clinical Importance

Uterine rupture is a catastrophic event in which both the mother and fetus are at risk. Maternal mortality goes upto 10 % in developing countries. Therefore, timely diagnosis and early delivery by cesarean section is of utmost importance. Perinatal mortality has decreased from 17% to 2% by advances in obstetrical practices.

Obstetric Management

High index of suspicion is vital, as symptoms like abdominal pain and bleeding per vaginum are nonspecific. Maternal tachycardia, hypotension, loss of uterine contractions, scar tenderness (in case of previous cesarean), recession of presenting fetal part are suggestive of impending uterine rupture. Abnormal fetal heart rate pattern like prolonged late deceleration or recurrent variable decelerations or bradycardia are recognized indicators of ruptured uterus.

Management involves resuscitation of the mother and immediate delivery of the baby by cesarean section. The maternal consequences to be kept in mind include hypovolemic shock, maternal bladder injury, need for blood transfusion and hysterectomy. Uterine repair is reserved when there is strong need for future fertility, low transverse incision rupture, good general condition of the mother and easily controllable hemorrhage. Rapid intervention may prevent neonatal death, but if cardiotocography is abnormal, there is a high likelihood of metabolic acidosis and fetal hypoxic damage.

Neonatal Management

The team must be prepared for state-of-the-art resuscitation at birth. In case the neonate is ≥ 36 weeks gestation, NICU team should be kept informed for possible requirement of NICU admission for therapeutic hypothermia. Standard guidelines of neonatal resuscitation protocol must be followed. After the baby has been resuscitated and stabilized, immediate processing of cord blood sample for acid-base studies is essential in those ≥ 36 weeks, along with weighing of the neonate and assessment of Apgar score to decide for eligibility of therapeutic hypothermia.

These neonates have an increased risk of multi-organ dysfunction; kidney being the most common organ affected (oliguria, renal failure, tubular necrosis); followed by cardiovascular dysfunction caused by myocardial ischemia mandating need for inotropes, pulmonary (pneumothorax, pulmonary hemorrhage, persistent pulmonary hypertension, asphyxial lung injury), hematological (thrombocytopenia, leucocytosis/leucopenia), hepatic (transaminitis, coagulopathy) and gastrointestinal (feed intolerance, bowel ischemia, NEC, impaired sucking and swallowing, GERD) complications. Strict monitoring of vital signs, neurological examination and maintenance of normal serum glucose, electrolytes, calcium levels, control of seizures and maintenance of intake output balance is recommended.

Long term sequelae of hypoxic-ischemic encephalopathy include cerebral palsy, hearing loss, intellectual and fine motor dysfunction, seizures, low IQ, needing multimodality approach for early diagnosis, prompt management and rehabilitation. Early magnetic resonance neuroimaging (between 7–10 days) with diffusion weighted images is desirable for prognostication.

Shoulder Dystocia

When additional obstetric maneuvers are required for delivery of shoulders, and gentle downward traction and episiotomy have failed, it is referred to as shoulder dystocia. Historically, it has also been defined as head-to-body delivery time of more than 60 sec.

Incidence and Risk Factors

The reported incidence varies from 0.6% to 1.4% worldwide. Some of the antepartum factors are macrosomia, diabetes mellitus, previous shoulder dystocia, maternal body mass index (BMI) >30 kg/m² and induction of labor. Intrapartum factors like prolonged first or second stage, secondary arrest of labor, oxytocin augmentation and assisted vaginal delivery have also been implicated.

Diagnosis

There is characteristic appearance and retraction of the head back in the perineum, while anterior shoulder lies impacted beneath the pubic symphysis (Turtle sign), akin to a turtle. Lack of restoration of the position of shoulder is also suggestive of shoulder dystocia.

Obstetric Management

Various maneuvers have been described to tackle shoulder dystocia. The 'HELPERR' mnemonic proposed by the American Life Support Organisation, is useful to remember the shoulder dystocia drill. It stands for call for **H**elp, evaluate for **E**pisiotomy, **L**egs in McRoberts maneuver, external **P**ressure-suprapubic, **E**nter; rotational maneuver, **R**emove the posterior arm, **R**oll the patient to her hands and knees. It must also be remembered to avoid fundal pressure and undue traction on fetal head.

Neonatal Management

As soon as shoulder dystocia is diagnosed, the neonatologist or a physician trained in advanced neonatal resuscitation should be intimated and should be present for resuscitation and immediate neonatal assessment. The neonatal implications of shoulder dystocia are listed below.

- Birth asphyxia.
- Brachial plexus injuries around 10–15%.
- Fractures around 5% of cases (clavicular fracture is more common than humeral fracture).
- Soft tissue injuries including contusions and lacerations.

The single most important factor which predicts the risk of these injuries is the duration of second stage of labor of more than 20 minutes and head shoulder delivery interval of more than 5 minutes. The other risk factors for injuries include birth weight >4.5 kg and maternal obesity. Direct fetal maneuvers have not been shown to increase the risk of these injuries.

Immediate Neonatal Examination

The newborn resuscitation is conducted as per standard resuscitation guidelines. After resuscitation the following observations should to be documented.

- The Apgar scores, cord blood gasometry and resuscitation details.
- The presence of soft tissue hematoma, abrasions or lacerations.
- Asymmetry of movements of upper limbs.
- Palpate both the clavicles and humerus and look for swelling, crepitus and tenderness.
- Grasp reflex in both upper limbs and symmetry of the Moro's reflex response.

Brachial Plexus Injuries

Brachial plexus injury (BPI) most commonly follows difficult labor because of shoulder dystocia. Based on the nerve root involved, brachial plexus injury can be classified as follows:

i. *Erb's palsy.* It is most common type of BPI, and has following features.
   - Roots of C5, C6 and C7 are affected.
   - Shoulder abduction, elbow flexion and supination are affected.
   - Wrist extension is limited.
   - The affected arm is kept adducted, pronated with wrist flexion giving an appearance of "waiter's tip" or "policeman bribe".
   - Grasp reflex on the affected side is present but weaker than the normal side.

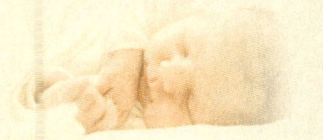

ii. *Klumpke's paralysis*
- Isolated lower root lesions are extremely rare and most often represent cases of total brachial plexus where the upper trunk nerve fibers have recovered faster.
- The lower never roots C7, C8 and T1 are affected.
- The elbow is flexed and the hand is held in a classical claw hand position.

iii. *Total paralysis of the limb* when all the roots from C5-T1 are affected. There is complete loss of movements of the involved upper limb.

iv. *Additional fndings* include involvement of
- *Sympathetic roots* of T1 leading to ipsilateral Horner's syndrome. This usually signifies trauma at the level of roots and has more grievous prognosis.
- *Diaphragmatic palsy.* The C4, C5 fibers which are involved in diaphragmatic contraction through the phrenic nerve are affected leading to ipsilateral diaphragmatic palsy. The neonate may or may not have respiratory distress. There are paradoxical chest movements on the affected side and chest X-ray shows an elevated hemidiaphragm.

Most BPIs are transient. Complete recovery is more likely to occur with Erb's palsy (90–95%) as compared to Klumpke's paralysis (60%). The recent reports suggest that 15% infants may be severely handicapped. No ancillary investigations are required to make the diagnosis. MRI scan is useful if a root avulsion is suspected.

Treatment

Strict immobilization is advised during first 15 days followed by physiotherapy to promote active and passive movements and tactile stimulation of affected limb. In infants with poor recovery, surgical repair of nerve or grafting is done after 3 months.

Fractures

i. *Clavicular fracture.* This is the second most common injury after BPI and occurs in around 9% cases of shoulder dystocia. Clavicular fractures are not associated with BPI. The movements of upper limb are reduced on the involved side with asymmetric Moro reflex. There may be crepitus, tenderness and deformity at the site of fracture. The fracture heals spontaneously with callus formation in due course of time.

ii. *Humerus fracture.* It occurs in 4–5% cases of shoulder dystocia and is usually benign. It requires immobilization alone. Malrotation is highly unlikely in the neonatal period.

Birth asphyxia

It is the most dreaded complication of shoulder dystocia. In about one-third of cases, fetal hypoxia occurs even prior to the delivery of the head. A combination of hypoxia, cerebral venous obstruction, trauma and vagal stimulation cause more damage than isolated cerebral hypoxia. It may be associated with intracranial hemorrhage, facial nerve palsy, tracheal tear and spinal cord injury due to excessive traction over the neck.

It is imperative to precisely document the following events and parameters especially for medicolegal purposes.
1. The time of delivery of the head.
2. The direction of the head after restitution.
3. Timing and sequence of the maneuvers performed.
4. The time of delivery of the baby.
5. The time of reporting by the staff for delivery and resuscitation.
6. The 1-minute and 5-minute Apgar scores of the baby, and umbilical cord blood pH.
7. Immediate neonatal examination, extent and nature of injuries.

Entrapment of Aftercoming Head during Breech Extraction

When the breech has been delivered out, whether spontaneously or with breech extraction, but the head cannot be delivered by routine measures, it is referred to as entrapment of after-coming head.

Incidence

Incidence of breech presentation varies from 25% at 28 weeks gestation to 3–4% at term. The most common complication of breech vaginal delivery is arrest of the aftercoming head (upto 8.5%), followed by cord prolapse and arrest of after-coming arms.

Risk Factors

Fetal hydrocephalus or macrocephaly, extended fetal head, occipitoposterior position of head, contracted pelvis, incomplete dilation of cervix are recognized risk factors.

Obstetric Management

Management depends on whether fetus is alive or dead, presence or absence of any gross fetal malformations. Ensure that bladder is empty and generous episiotomy is in place. Ensure adequacy of pelvis and full dilatation of cervix. Next step is to identify the cause of the delayed descent of fetal head and conservative measures should be given a fair trial.

1. *Deflexed head* Suprapubic pressure by an assistant can help to maintain flexion of the head. Delivery of the after-coming head can be facilitated by either of three methods; Mariceau-Smellie-Veit maneuver, Burns-Marshall method or the Piper's forceps. No method is proven to be better than the other. The experience and expertise of the operator are more important.

2. *Inadequately dilated cervix* This complication is mostly seen in preterm breech, where the smaller breech delivers through incompletely dilated cervix, leading to entrapment of the larger fetal head. Duhrssen's incisions have been described to facilitate delivery of head in these cases.

3. *Fetal hydrocephalus* If fetus is dead, destructive measures like craniocentesis and craniotomy are recognized options.

4. *Contracted pelvis* Emergency cesarean section should be done.

5. *Occipito-posterior presentation* The Prague maneuver is used where two fingers are placed on the fetal shoulders from behind, and the fetal body is arched over the maternal abdomen, with the occiput slipping over the perineum instead of the face.

When head entrapment occurs during cesarean section of a breech presenting baby, uterine relaxation measures like intravenous nitroglycerine (preferred mode if future fertility is required) or inverted T incision on uterus (if relaxation measures are unavailable or fail and future fertility is not desired) are recommended.

Complications

Maternal complications include increased risk of uterine rupture, increased operative interference, postpartum hemorrhage, increased cesarean delivery rate and its attendant short and long-term complications.

Neonatal Management

The neonatal morbidity and mortality varies between 4–12% in breech vaginal deliveries. The neonate is at risk of the following complications.

- *Severe birth asphyxia* Birth asphyxia is the single most important cause of perinatal mortality in these cases. Asphyxia occurs due to cord compression by the partially dilated cervix and placental separation.
- *Intracranial hemorrhage* When the aftercoming head is entrapped, there is compression of the suboccipital region of the head by the symphysis pubis. This causes rupture of the sinuses and subdural vessels causing intracranial hemorrhage. In mild cases, there is subdural hemorrhage or a combination of subdural and subarachnoid hemorrhage. In the most severe cases, there will be tears in tentorium cerebelli and massive cerebellar hemorrhage. The rapid compression and expansion of the head may cause intraventricular hemorrhage. The common symptoms include anemia, jaundice, bulging anterior fontanel, seizures and lethargy after 3–4 days of life.
- *Soft tissue and visceral trauma* There may be injury to liver, spleen and genitalia. Brachial and cervical plexus injury may occur. Fracture of bones like femur, humerus, pelvis and clavicle may occur due to various maneuvers. Spinal cord laceration and transection due to flexion and extension of the trunk is life-threatening. Gluteus maximus is the most common muscle involved in injury (67% of all cases), followed by other gluteal muscles, head and neck muscles and upper limb muscles.

Management includes immediate neonatal resuscitation by a skilled person and careful screening for injuries. Shock and low hematocrit should raise the suspicion of internal bleeding. Cranial USG should be done to exclude intracranial bleed. Complete documentation of the injuries and neurological status of the neonate should be done.

AMNIOTIC FLUID ABNORMALITIES

The amniotic fluid provides nutrients and growth factors that facilitate fetal growth. It provides mechanical cushioning and antimicrobial factors that protect the fetus. It has an important role in the development of gastrointestinal, pulmonary and musculoskeletal system and is a useful source of stem cells and diagnostic studies.

The dynamics of amniotic fluid are not well-understood. During first trimester, there is bidirectional diffusion of amniotic fluid between fetal skin and transudation of extracellular fluid from amnion, placenta and umbilical cord. After 20 weeks of gestation, when skin is keratinized, amniotic fluid is mostly contributed by fetal urine and efflux of oral, nasal and tracheal secretions. Fetus swallows liquor, absorbs and retains some and voids excess through urine. The volume of amniotic fluid is related to the gestational age and is maintained within a narrow range. Alterations in the quantity of amniotic fluid are related to certain fetal disorders which may interfere with swallowing and absorption of amniotic fluid or with production of urine, besides certain maternal conditions.

Oligohydramnios

Oligohydramnios complicates about 3–5% pregnancies. It is associated with adverse perinatal outcomes like intrauterine growth restriction, pulmonary hypoplasia, abnormal cardiotocographic patterns, meconium passage, birth asphyxia, increased risk of cesarean delivery, intrauterine or neonatal death. Therefore, amniotic fluid assessment is an essential component of antepartum fetal surveillance of high-risk pregnancies.

Diagnosis

Four quadrant amniotic fluid index (AFI) of less than 5 or mean vertical pockets of less than 2 on ultrasonography are used to define oligohydramnios. Careful assessment of fetal urinary system is recommended when pregnancy is complicated with oligohydramnios. Oligohydramnios detected in later gestation is likely to be associated with IUGR and uteroplacental insufficiency. Leakage of amniotic fluid per vaginum must be ruled out as a cause of oligohydramnios.

Obstetric Management

In oligohydramnios associated with renal anomalies or leakage per vaginum before 20 weeks of gestation, incidence of pulmonary hypoplasia is high and medical termination of pregnancy can be offered. In later gestation, close fetal surveillance is advised, with daily fetal movement count, biophysical profile and umbilical artery Doppler assessment. Antenatal steroid cover should be considered if preterm delivery is imminent. Planned delivery at term is preferable. Other indications for termination of pregnancy include poor biophysical profile, absent or reversed end diastolic flow on umbilical artery Doppler and AFI < 2 after 36 weeks of gestation. Electronic fetal monitoring during labor is recommended for prompt detection of fetal distress.

Neonatal Management

Oligohydramnios increases the risk of perinatal mortality and morbidity, particularly IUGR and its associated complications, increased risk of cord accidents, meconium staining of liquor, prematurity and perinatal asphyxia. There is greater risk of postural contractures and congenital malformations. Identification of the etiology of oligohydramnios is important for further management. PROM is one of most common causes of oligohydramnios reported across various series. In such cases, duration of rupture of membranes along with presence of risk factors for chorioamnionitis must be assessed for initiation of antibiotic therapy. Other causes that are commonly associated include urinary tract malformations in fetus such as renal agenesis, polycystic or multicystic dysplastic kidneys, posterior urethral valves. This warrants a systemic examination of the neonate for bladder and kidney palpability, evaluation of urinary stream, USG evaluation for status of kidneys and bladder, renal function parameters and metabolic acidosis. In case of renal malformations, coexistent cardiac, skeletal and central nervous system anomalies must be looked for. Maternal medication history (prostaglandin inhibitors, ACE inhibitors) and illnesses such as diabetes, and hypertension should be ruled out. Low birth weight neonates must be evaluated at birth by determining the type of IUGR (symmetric vs asymmetric) and neonate must be carefully monitored during initial days of life for occurrence of certain complications, such as hypoglycemia, hypothermia, feed intolerance, jaundice, polycythemia, hyperbilirubinemia, respiratory distress, NEC and cholestasis.

Polyhydramnios

There is excessive amount of amniotic fluid (>2 liters) and its prevalence varies between 0.2–1.6% of all pregnancies. The diagnosis is based on discrepancy between the size of fetus and the volume or size of uterus, increased amniotic fluid index (>24 cm), maximum vertical pocket of more than 8 cm, and a large gap between the fetus and the anterior and posterior uterine walls on ultrasonography. It may be associated with certain maternal disorders like pre-eclamptic toxemia, diabetes mellitus, intrauterine infections, Rhesus isoimmunization, syphilis, chronic renal or cardiac disease, and chorioangioma. Twins and hydrops fetalis are often associated with polyhydramnios. The presence of excessive amniotic fluid should alert the pediatrician for existence of a number of fetal malformations like anencephaly, high intestinal obstruction, cleft plate, omphalocele, spina bifida, gastroschisis, ectopia vesicae, diaphragmatic hernia, and Down syndrome. Around 50% cases of polyhydramnios are idiopathic.

Obstetric Management

The clinical correlates of polyhydramnios include excessive weight gain, large size of abdomen, dyspepsia, constipation, swelling of abdominal wall, vulva and legs, decreased urine output and breathing difficulty. The pregnancies complicated with polyhydramnios should be closely monitored by non-stress test, biophysical profile, fetal echocardiography and detailed ultrasonography to identify fetal malformations.

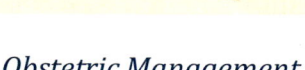

Obstetric Management

The mother is advised complete bedrest, avoidance of large or spicy meals and use of pillows and cushions to support the belly. The underlying maternal conditions should be identified and managed appropriately. The mild cases respond spontaneously on supportive management. When there is massive accumulation of amniotic fluid, amnioreduction can be done by draining excess amniotic fluid. Multiple sessions of amnioreduction may be required for keeping the amniotic fluid levels within normal range. The procedure carries risk of premature rupture of membranes, preterm labor and placental abruption. Mother can be given oral indomethacin to help reduce fetal urine production and amniotic fluid volume. Indomethacin is not recommended after 31 weeks of gestation due to increased risk of fetal heart rate abnormalities and renal dysfunction. During maternal indomethacin therapy, fetus should be closely monitored with echocardiography and Doppler ultrasound.

When there is severe polyhydramnios or excessive amniotic fluid theratens baby's wellbeing, labor may be induced around 37 weeks. The delivery should be conducted by an experienced obstetrician because of increased risk of placental abruption, cord prolapse and excessive postpartum bleeding due to decreased uterine muscle tone. The baby is delivered by an elective cesarean section if baby is lying in an atypical head down position or when there is excessive macrosomia.

Neonatal Management

The nature of fetal abnormalities should be identified by detailed ultrasonography by an experienced sonologist. In twins, twin-to-twin tranfusion is managed by endoscopic laser coagulation of placental vessels at the median gestation of 21 weeks. The delivery should be attended by a pediatrician well-trained in the art of neonatal resuscitation. Pediatric surgeon should be alerted before delivery and asked for consultation as soon as infant is shifted to NICU. Polyhydramnios resulting from severe fetal and placental malformations is likely to have poor prognosis with a case fatality rate of 60%.

FETAL ABNORMALITIES

Fetal Hemorrhage

Fetomaternal hemmorhage (FMH) is common in normal pregnancies and usually <1.0 mL fetal blood enters maternal circulation but it is enough to cause Rh-isoimmunization during the course of several pregnancies. Excessive FMH may occur following obstetrical procedures (external podalic version, chorionic villus sampling), trauma, abruption and twin-to-twin transfusion. During cesarean section, if baby is held above the level of mother without clamping the cord, significant FMH can occur leading to severe anemia. The extent of FMH can be assessed by Kleihauer-Betke test and flow cytometry on maternal blood.

Fetal hemorrhage due to vitamin-K dependent coagulation disorder may occur by maternal intake of aspirin, coumadin, anticonvulsants and antitubercular drugs during pregnancy. Maternal diseases like systemic lupus erythematosus, idiopathic thrombocytopenic purpura, pre-eclampsia, seizure disorder, excessive bruising or nose bleeds may be associated with fetal thrombocytopenia with bleeding manifestations. Fetomaternal alloimmune thrombocytopenia (FMAIT) is uncommon but a leading cause of fetal and neonatal thrombocytopenia (<1,50,000/µL). It is produced by placental transfer of maternal immunoglobulin (IgG) antibodies against fetal platelet antigens inherited from the father. Unlike erythrocyte alloimmunization (Rhesus hemolytic disease), FMAIT may appear during first pregnancy, with a high recurrence rate and with progressively more severe manifestations in subsequent pregnancies. FMAIT is the leading cause of severe thrombocytopenia in the newborns and should not be confused with autoimmune thrombocytopenia, in which both mother and fetus are affected due to maternal autoantibodies. The diagnosis of FMAIT may be suspected when neonatal thrombocytopenia is detected incidentally or when there is history of a previously affected child. The fetal manifestations usually include petechiae and superficial hemorrhages but intracranial hemorrhage may occur leading to death or long-term neuromotor disability. Intramuscular injections may be followed by hematoma or excessive bleeding may occur following circumcision.

Fetal management When mother is receiving medications which can lower vitamin K-dependent factors, she should be given 10 mg vitamin K IM before onset of labor. Fetal blood can be checked for complete blood count to diagnose anemia and thrombocytopenia. Intrauterine transfusion of RBCs is recommended to maintain fetal hemoglobin above 10 g/dL. The antenatal management of FMAIT is controversial, and therapeutic modalities include administration of intravenous immunoglobulins (IVIG) to the mother, maternal steroid administration and repeated intrauterine platelet transfusions (IUPT). Infants with fetal hemorrhage should be assessed for hemoglobin, hematocrit, platelet count, and severity of jaundice and managed accordingly.

Fetal Hydrocephalus

Background

Fetal ventriculomegaly (VM) is defined as dilatation of atrial diameter of either or both lateral ventricles (greater than 10 mm), detected on ultrasonography after 15 weeks of gestation. Reported incidence of the condition is 0.3–2%. It may be isolated anomaly or associated with other anomalies. Etiological factors include CNS malformations, CSF flow obstruction, intrauterine infections, chromosomal abnormalities, while some cases may be idiopathic.

Diagnosis

Fetal ventriculomegaly is detected on ultrasound and fetal MRI can be done for detailed evaluation. Classification as mild enlargement of ventricles (10 to 12 mm), moderate (12–15 mm) and severe (>15 mm), is of prognostic significance.

Obstetric Management

Detailed ultrasound examination to look for associated anomalies is warranted. Genetic counseling and karyotype must be offered. It is important to screen for intrauterine infections, i.e. TORCH test, especially in cases of severe ventriculomegaly, as it may be positive in up to 20% cases. Termination of pregnancy may be offered an option before 20 weeks. Fetoscopic prenatal placement of ventriculo-peritoneal shunt is an accepted treatment modality. Risk to benefit ratio of prenatal surgery must be considered prior to selection of cases. Elective cesarean delivery is indicated because of associated cephalopelvic disproportion. Alternatively, vaginal delivery can be accomplished with help of destructive procedures in case of fetal demise.

Neonatal Management

Resuscitation of the neonate must be done as per neonatal resuscitation algorithm. After stabilization, clinical examination must include assessment of head circumference, size of anterior and posterior fontanel and their fullness, and status of cranial sutures. Higher mental functions, tone abnormalities, neonatal reflexes, paralysis of cranial nerves/gaze abnormalities, signs of raised intracranial pressures must be evaluated. Careful neonatal assessment for specific etiological types include myelomeningocele associated with Arnold- Chiari type 2 malformation; thumb flexion deformity in congenital aqueductal stenosis; occipital cranial prominence in Dandy-Walker syndrome; chorioretinitis and organomegaly in intrauterine infections. USG for assessment of ventricular size and gross structure of parenchyma is helpful for assessing severity of hydrocephalus. MRI for detailed assessment of cerebral parenchyma in terms of determining size of cerebral mantle, anomalies of cerebrum (neuronal migration, cysts, calcifications) and localization of sites of CSF obstruction is imperative. Neonates with progressive increase in ventricular size or rapid head growth must undergo ventriculo-peritoneal shunt placement which remains the treatment of choice. Other surgical techniques that have been tried include endoscopic third ventriculostomy (non-communicating), cyst fenestration (arachnoid cyst) and septostomy (atresia of foramen of Monro). Short-term outcome has improved due to better neonatal care and expertise in neurosurgical techniques. Long-term prognosis of these infants depends upon disease etiology (poor if associated with holoprosencephaly, Dandy-Walker malformation with co-existent CNS anomalies, associated malformations, and surgical complications (shunt infections, shunt blockade). In a 20-year-long study Yamasaki et al reported mortality rate of 17% and among survivors, 21% had severe mental retardation while normal outcome was seen in 49% neonates diagnosed and treated for fetal hydrocephalus.

Congenital Diaphragmatic Hernia (CDH)

Background

It is characterised by a defect in the diaphragm leading to protrusion of abdominal contents into the thoracic cavity. Spectrum of defects range from posterolateral hernia (Bochdalek), anterior hernia (Morgagni and others) and rarely central defects. Although a rare condition with prevalence of less than 5 per 10,000 births, it leads to serious respiratory and cardiovascular complications in the newborn. Perinatal morbidity and mortality range from 20 to 60%.

Diagnosis

Prenatal ultrasound reveals the presence of stomach bubble, intestines or liver in the thoracic cavity, displacement of fetal heart, evidences of pulmonary hypoplasia and polyhydramnios.

Obstetric Management

Detailed ultrasound and fetal echocardiography is mandatory to look for associated anomalies. Fetal MRI can be done for further evaluation. Prognostic factors like size and location of defect, lung head ratio (for pulmonary hypoplasia), liver in the thoracic cavity and degree of pulmonary hypertension should be assessed. Genetic counseling and karyotype to rule out aneuploidies must be offered. Medical termination of pregnancy is an option before 20 weeks. Fetal endoscopic tracheal balloon placement has been tried successfully in selected cases.

Neonatal Management

After birth, the neonate must be nursed under radiant warmer and intubated. Bag and mask ventilation must be avoided as it can raise intra-abdominal pressure causing further herniation of contents. Oro-gastric tube with continuous/intermittent suction must be placed after intubation. Establish IV line after initial respiratory stabilization. X-ray chest must be obtained and the baby shifted to the NICU.

Ventilation Gentle ventilation strategy should be used, targeting pre-ductal oxygen saturation of 85–95% using peak pressures below 25 cm H_2O, PEEP of 2–5 cm H_2O; ventilator rate of 40–60/min. Arterial line placement, preferably in the right radial artery is recommended both for arterial blood gas parameters and blood pressure monitoring. SpO_2 levels as low as 70% are acceptable for first 2 hours if arterial blood pH >7.2, $PaCO_2$ <65 mmHg and gradual improvement in oxygen saturation is observed without hiking ventilation. Morphine or fentanyl infusion for maintaining adequate analgesia and sedation is desirable. High frequency ventilation is used as rescue mode for severe and refractory hypoxemia and hypercarbia on conventional mode.

Fluid and hemodynamic management Fluid and hemodynamic management must be aimed at maintaining blood pressures (≈50th centile for gestational age), predutcal SpO_2 80–95% and adequate end organ perfusion. Placement of central venous catheters in case of hypotension and evaluation of cardiac functions by echocardiography is useful in guiding management and monitoring response to therapy.

Management of pulmonary hypertension Severity of pulmonary hypertension is a major predictor of outcome of these neonates. The signs of pulmonary hypertension must be actively sought for, such as preductal to post-ductal SpO_2 difference and loud P_2. An echocardiogram must be performed within 24 hours of birth to assess the severity of pulmonary hypertension. Blood pressure must be maintained at or above 50th centile. Inhaled nitric oxide does not improve outcomes in pulmonary hypertension secondary to congenital diaphragmatic hernia. Other agents, such as sildenafil, PGE_1, endothelin antagonists and tyrosine kinase inhibitors are mostly experimental. Use of ECMO for cases with refractory hypoxemia and persistent pulmonary hypertension (PPHN) has shown reduction in short-term mortality without long-term benefits.

Surgical repair Surgical repair is recommended after hemodynamic and respiratory stabilization. Routine use of post-operative chest tube insertion is no longer recommended and can be decided on individual basis.

Feeding and nutrition Post-operative feeding should be introduced after a satisfactory abdominal examination and discussion with pediatric surgeon. Various studies have reported incidence of gastro-esophageal reflux ranging from 20–84%, which is managed with medications and at times by surgical correction.

Fetal Arrhythmias

Background

Fetal arrhythmias may be noted in up to 2% of pregnancies during routine antenatal ultrasound. Mostly transient, there can be persistent abnormalities like congenital heart block or supraventricular tachycardia. The consequences include congestive heart failure, fetal hydrops and fetal death.

Diagnosis

Spectrum of well-known fetal heart rate/rhythm abnormalities include sinus bradycardia, congenital heart block, sinus tachycardia, atrial flutter and supra-ventricular tachycardia. Four chamber view of the heart on routine ultrasound and fetal (M-mode and Doppler) echocardiography are the modalities of choice for diagnosis and characterization fetal arrhythmias. The echocardiogram also helps to identify underlying structural heart disease, associated anomalies and presence of fetal hydrops. Further evaluation is warranted in some cases like testing for maternal serum Anti Ro/La antibodies when fetus is documented to have complete congenital heart block.

Obstetric Management

Treatment modalities include close monitoring, antiarrhythmic drugs or expediting delivery. In cases of transient arrhythmias, not causing hemodynamic impairment, follow-up is a viable option. Fetal tachy-arrhythmias have been treated with maternally administered antiarrhythmic drugs like digoxin, amiodarone, sotalol and flecainide. For immune-mediated cases manifesting as congenital heart block, dexamethasone and beta adrenergic drugs (salbutamol and terbutaline) have shown promising results. Delivery by cesarean section is an option as fetal monitoring in labor is challenging in such cases.

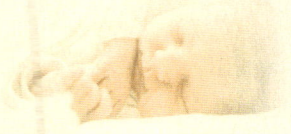

Neonatal Management

After initial stabilization at birth, the neonate with antenatal diagnosed arrhythmia must undergo a complete 12 lead ECG. Glucose and electrolyte abnormalities must be carefully looked for (Na^+, K^+, iCa^{++}, Mg^{++}), and appropriately managed.

Fetal bradycardia About 20–90% of healthy neonates experience bradycardia. Transient bradycardia resolves within 48–72 hours after birth without treatment and occurs in asscociation with stress of labor and delivery.

AV block Congenital complete AV block is commonly observed in neonates born to mothers with anti-Ro and anti- La antibodies associated with SLE/ Sjogrens syndrome and sometimes with congenital heart defects (TGA and heterotaxy syndromes). Such neonates require hemodynamic stabilization following birth and early pacemaker implantation in cases of congenital complete heart block with severe bradycardia and evidences of congestive heart failure.

Fetal tachycardias Fetal supraventricular tachycardia (SVT) caused by AV re-entry is the most common fetal tachycardia followed by fetal atrial flutter. For treatment of fetal SVT, digoxin is first line therapy, followed by sotalol, flecainide and amiodarone. SVT in neonatal period is managed by adenosine as a rapid IV bolus and vagal maneuvers (icepacks, oropharyngeal suction) if the neonate is hemodynamically stable while DC cardioversion is recommended in a neonate with hemodynamic instability (after securing airway and optimizing ventilation).

Wide QRS tachycardia This is less common in neonates. It is important to distinguish ventricular tachycardia versus SVT with wide complex as it has important prognostic implications. Response to adenosine administration might provide a useful clue to differentiate them. In case of pulseless ventricular tachycardia/ ventricular fibrillations, CPR must be initiated followed by administration of DC shock (start with 1–2 J/kg, followed by progressive increase to 4 J/kg). Adrenaline and amiodarone are considered if VT/VF persists. Treatment for pulsatile VT includes amiodarone or procainamide. In case of polymorphic pulsatile VT (Torsades de pointes) intravenous magnesium sulphate is the drug of choice.

Fetal Obstructive Uropathy

Obstruction in the lower urinary tract leading to back pressure changes in the kidneys occur due to fetal obstructive uropathy. It is usually complicated by oligohydramnios and pulmonary hypoplasia. Common causes include posterior urethral valves and urethral atresia.

Diagnosis

Ultrasonographic features include distended urinary bladder ("keyhole sign" of PUV), hydronephrosis , oligohydramnios and its sequelae.

Obstetric Management

Detailed level 2 ultrasound evaluation for associated anomalies is performed. Elective termination of pregnancy can be discussed prior to 20 weeks. For diagnosis at later gestations, if liquor is adequate, no fetal procedure may be done and baby can be reviewed after birth. If liquor is decreased, vesicocentesis is indicated to assess the degree of damage to the kidneys. Further treatment options include decompression of the obstructed system via vesicoamniotic shunting (most common), fetal cystoscopic valve ablation and vesicostomy.

Neonatal Management

Prevalence of antenatal hydronephrosis ranges from 0.6–5.4%, is bilateral in 17–54% and posterior urethral valve is etiologically recognized cause in only 1–2% cases. As per literature, 80% of fetuses diagnosed with antenatal hydronephrosis in second trimester USG, show improvement or resolution while those with moderate or severe hydronephrosis in the third trimester, are likely to require intervention after birth.

Ultrasound KUB All neonates must undergo ultrasound examination within first week, while those with severe bilateral hydronephrosis, hydronephrosis in a single kidney, suspected posterior urethral valves and oligohydroamnios on antenatal USG must get USG of KUB done after 72 hours of age. Postnatal severity of hydronephrosis is based on anteroposterior diameter of renal pelvis and classification based on the recommendations of Society for Fetal Urology. Early involvement of pediatric urologist to plan further management, prognostication and follow-up is essential.

Micturating cystourethrography (MCU) MCU must be performed as early as 24–72 hours of life in cases of suspected lower urinary tract obstruction, and at 4–6 weeks in cases of renal pelvic APD >10 mm, Society for Fetal Urology (SFU) grade 3–4 ureteric dilatation, worsening hydronephrosis, progressive parenchymal thinning and in those who develop urinary tract infection. Diuretic renography is recommended for neonates with moderate to severe unilateral/bilateral hydronephrosis or dilated ureters with no evidence of vesicoureteric reflux on MCU.

Antibiotic prophylaxis Antibiotic prophylaxis is recommended for all neonates with APD >10 mm or SFU grade 3–4 dilated ureters and those detected to have vesico-ureteric reflux (VUR). Choice of antibiotics being cephelaxin (10 mg/kg/d) for first 3 months followed by co-trimoxazole or nitrofurantoin. Urinalysis, renal functions and blood pressure monitoring is recommended for those diagnosed with hydronephrosis.

Surgical intervention Neonates with diagnosed lower urinary tract obstruction must be referred to a pediatric urologist for early surgery (cystoscopic ablation of uretheral valves) after catheterization and correction of electrolyte abnormalities. Surgical intervention is required in patients with obstructed hydronephrosis with reduced or worsening differential renal functions and those with bilateral hydronephrosis or hydronephrosis in a solitary kidney with worsening of ureteral dilatation and renal function parameters.

BIBLIOGRAPHY

Alchalabi H A, Obeidat B R, Jallad M F, et al. Induction of labor and perinatal outcome: The impact of the amniotic fluid index. *Eur J Obstet Gynecol Reprod Biol* 2006; 129:124–27.

Ayres-de-Campos D, Spong CY, Chandraharan E. FIGO consensus guidelines on intrapartum fetal monitoring: cardiotocography. *Int J Gynaecol Obstet* 2015 Oct; 131(1):13–24.

Bagolan P, Casaccia G, Crescenzi F, et al. Impact of a current treatment protocol on outcome of high-risk congenital diaphragmatic hernia. *J Pediatr Surg* 2004; 39:313.

Breeze AC, Alexander PM, Murdoch EM, Missfelder-Lobos HH, Hackett GA, Lees CC. Obstetric and neonatal outcomes in severe fetal ventriculomegaly. *Prenat Diagn* 2007; 27:124–29.

Chibber R, El-Saleh E, Al FR, Al JW, Al HJ. Uterine rupture and subsequent pregnancy outcome—how safe is it? A 25-year study. *J Matern Fetal Neonatal Med* 2010 May; 23(5):421–4.

Chiu TH, Haliza G, Lin YH, Hung TH, Hsu JJ, Hsieh TT, Lo LM. A retrospective study on the course and outcome of fetal ventriculomegaly. *Taiwan J Obstet Gynecol* 2014; 53:170–77.

Dajani NK, Magann EF. Complications of shoulder dystocia. *Semin Perinatol* 2014 Jun; 38(4):201–4.

Dilbaz B, Ozturkoglu E, Dilbaz S, Ozturk N, Sivaslioglu AA, Haberal A. Risk factors and perinatal outcomes associated with umbilical cord prolapse. *Arch Gynecol Obstet* 2006 May; 274(2):104–7.

Espinoza JP, Caradeux J, Ellanes SE. Fetal and neonatal alloimmune thrombocytopenia. *Rev Obstet Gynecol* 2013; 6(1):e15–e21.

Gherman RB. Shoulder dystocia: prevention and management. *Obstet Gynecol Clin North Am* 2005 Jun; 32(2):297–305.

Gifford DS, Morton SC, Fiske M, Kahn K. A meta-analysis of infant outcomes after breech delivery. *Obstet Gynecol* 1995 June; 85(6):1047–54.

Gupta M, Hockley C, Quigley MA, Yeh P, Impey L. Antenatal and intrapartum prediction of shoulder dystocia. *Eur J Obstet Gynecol Reprod Biol* 2010 Aug; 151(2):134–9.

Harrison MR, Mychaliska GB, Albanese CT, Jennings RW, Farrell JA, Hawgood S, Sandberg P, Levine AH, Lobo E, Filly RA. Correction of congenital diaphragmatic hernia in utero IX: fetuses with poor prognosis (liver herniation and low lung-to-head ratio) can be saved by fetoscopic temporary tracheal occlusion. *J Pediatr Surg* 1998; 33:1017–22.

Hasegawa J, Matsuoka R, Ichizuka K, et al. Intrapartum fetal heart rate pattern in oligohydramnios. *Fetal Diagn Ther* 2008; 24:267–70.

Jaeggi E., Laskin C., Hamilton R. The importance of the level of maternal anti-Ro/SSA antibodies as a prognostic marker of the development of cardiac neonatal lupus erythematosus: a prospective study of 186 antibody-exposed fetuses and infants. *J Am Coll Cardiol* 2010; 55(24):2778–84.

Ja-Y K, Han-S K, Young-H K et al. Abnormal Doppler velocimetry is related to adverse perinatal outcome for borderline amniotic fluid index during third trimester. *J Obstet Gynecol Res* 2006; 32:545–49.

Kilby MD, Morris RK. Fetal therapy for the treatment of congenital bladder neck obstruction. *Nat Rev Urol* 2014; 11:412–9.

Killen S, Fish F. Fetal and neonatal arrhytmias. *Neo Reviews* 2008; 9(6):c242–252.

Kim YA, Morkar RS. Detection of fetomaternal hemorrhage. *Am J Hematol* 2012; 87(4):417–23.

Krishna U, Bhalerao S. Placental insufficiency and fetal growth restriction. *J Obstet Gynaecol India* 2011 Oct; 61(5):505–11.

Kumar S, Regan F. Management of pregnancies with RhD alloimmunisation. *BMJ* 2005 May 28; 330(7502) 1255–8.

Lin MG. Umbilical cord prolapse. *Obstet Gynecol Surv* 2006 Apr; 61(4):269–77.

Mari G, Hanif F. Fetal Doppler: umbilical artery, middle cerebral artery, and venous system. *Semin Perinatol* 2008 Aug; 32(4):253–7.

Mari G. Middle cerebral artery peak systolic velocity: is it the standard of care for the diagnosis of fetal anemia? *J Ultrasound Med* 2005 May; 24(5):697–702.

Matsuoka S, Takeuchi K, Yamanaka Y, Kaji Y, Sugimura K, Maruo T. Comparison of magnetic resonance imaging and ultrasonography in the prenatal diagnosis of congenital thoracic abnormalities. *Fetal Diagn Ther* 2003; 18:447–53.

Mehta SH, Blackwell SC, Bujold E, Sokol RJ. What factors are associated with neonatal injury following shoulder dystocia? *J Perinatol* 2006 Feb; 26(2):85–8.

Mongiovi M, Pipitone S. Supraventricular tachycardia in fetus: how can we treat?. *Current Pharmaceutical Design* 2008 Mar 1; 14:736–42.

Murphy DJ, MacKenzie IZ. The mortality and morbidity associated with umbilical cord prolapse. *Br J Obstet Gynaecol* 1995 Oct; 102(10):826–30.

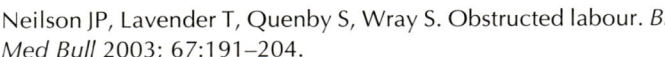

Neilson JP, Lavender T, Quenby S, Wray S. Obstructed labour. *Br Med Bull* 2003; 67:191–204.

Pedreira DA, Reece EA, Chmait RH, Kontopoulos EV, Quintero RA. Fetoscopic repair of spina bifida: safer and better? *Ultrasound Obstet Gynecol* 2016 Aug 1; 48(2):141–7.

Porcelign L, Van den Akker ES, Oepkes D. Fetal thrombocytopenia. *Semin Fetal Neonatal Med* 2008; 13:223–30.

Rahman J, Al-Sibai MH, Rahman MS. Rupture of the uterus in labor. A review of 96 cases. *Acta Obstet Gynecol Scand* 1985; 64(4):311–5.

Reiss I, Schaible T, Hout L, Capolupo I, Allegaert K, Heijst V. Standardized postnatal management of infants with congenital diaphragmatic hernia in Europe: The CDH EURO Consortium Consensus. *Neonatology* 2010; 98:354–64.

Sebring ES, Polesky HF. Fetomaternal hemorrhage; incidence, risk factors, time of occurrence, and clinical effects. *Transfusion* 1990; 30:344–57.

Sethna F, Tennant PW, Rankin J, S CR. Prevalence, natural history, and clinical outcome of mild to moderate ventriculomegaly. *Obstet Gynecol* 2011; 117:867–76.

Shenker L, Reed KL, Anderson CF et al. Significance of oligohydramnios complicating pregnancy. *Am J Obstet Gynecol* 1991; 164:1597–99.

Sinha A, Bagga A, Krishna A, Bajpai M, Srinivas M, Uppal R et al Revised guidelines on management of antenatal hydronephrosis. *Indian Pediatr* 2013; 50:215–31.

Spain JE, Frey HA, Tuuli MG, Colvin R, Macones GA, Cahill AG. Neonatal morbidity associated with shoulder dystocia maneuvers. *Am J Obstet Gynecol* 2015 Mar; 212(3):353–5.

Thomas DF. Prenatal diagnosis: what do we know of long-term outcomes? *J Pediatr Urol* 2010; 6:204–1 .

Tonni G, Vito I, Ventura A, Grisolia G, De Felice C. Fetal lower urinary tract obstruction and its management. *Arch Gynecol Obstet* 2013; 287:187–94.

van Beekhuizen HJ, Unkels R, Mmuni NS, Kaiser M. Complications of obstructed labour: pressure necrosis of neonatal scalp and vesicovaginal fistula. *Lancet* 2006 Sep 30; 368(9542):1210.

Yamasaki M , Nonaka M, Bamba Y, Teramoto C, Ban C. Diagnosis, treatment, and long-term outcomes of fetal hydrocephalus. *Semin Fetal Neonatal Med* 2012 Dec; 17(6):330–5.

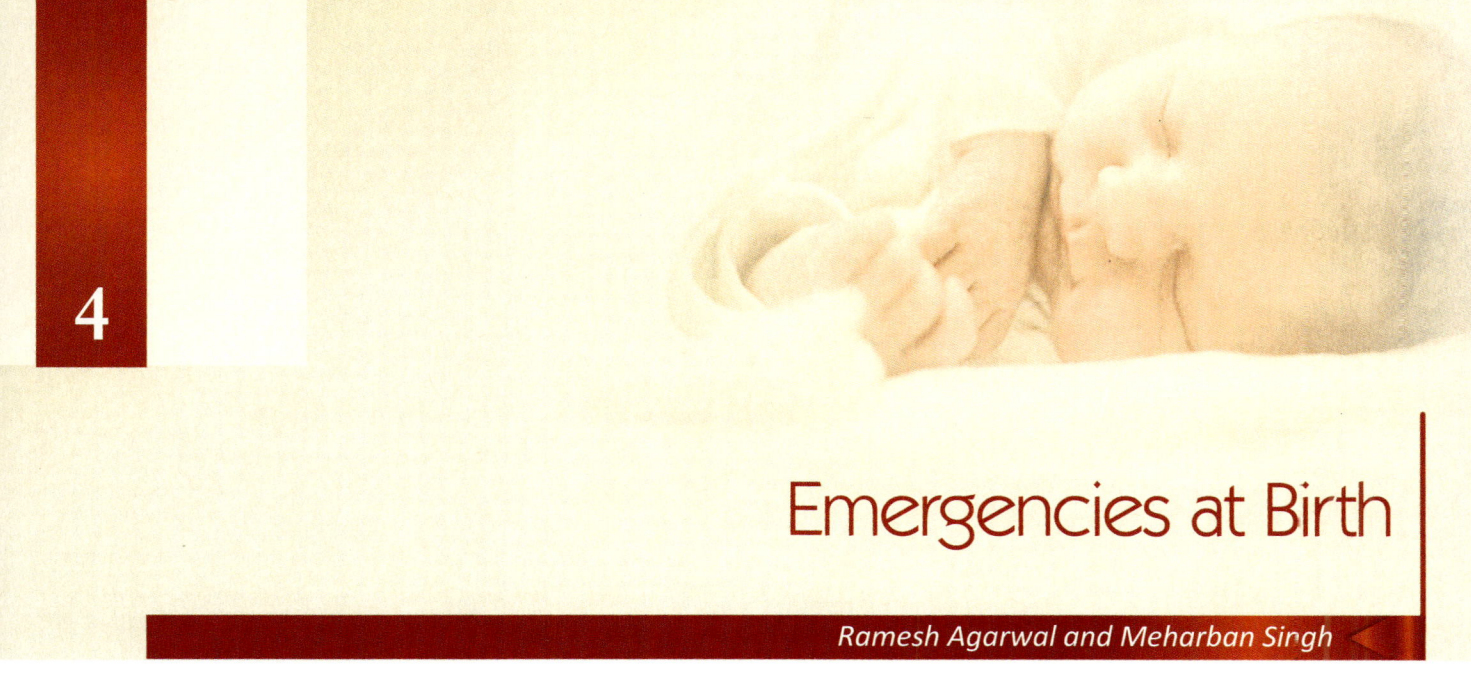

Emergencies at Birth

Ramesh Agarwal and Meharban Singh

Birthing is believed to be the most dangerous period in one's life. The process of transition from fetal to extrauterine life may be complicated by a number of life-threatening conditions, which have bearing on immediate survival as well as long-term neurological outcome. Every birth must be considered as a medical emergency and in India we should be prepared to handle 26 million emergencies every year. It is, therefore, essential for all health professionals caring for newborns to be aware of and be prepared to deal with these emergencies arising in the delivery room (DR), many of which respond favorably with appropriate timely intervention. The first step for effective management of neonatal emergencies in DR is to be adequately equipped with functional equipment, protocols, supplies and availability of skilled healthcare professionals.

The preparations to deal with emergencies in DR, should start from prenatal period itself, so that these problems can be identified in time by fetal ultrasound and other diagnostic modalities. When there is reasonable anticipation for the likely emergency to be faced at birth, adequate preparations should be made to manage it effectively at birth. Prenatal interventions exist for some disorders such as antenatal steroids for extremely preterm babies and tracheal plugging for management of diaphragmatic hernia. New NRP guidelines recommend simulation based training program for health professionals to effectively deal with DR emergencies, which significantly improves the teamwork that requires effective communication, coordination and skills. The common neonatal emergencies which may be faced in DR are listed in Table 4.1.

Table 4.1 Neonatal emergencies which can present in the labor room

- Failure to initiate or maintain effective breathing
- Multiple births and conjoined twins
- Shock and/or hypovolemia
- Severe anemia
- Pneumothorax
- Hydrops, ascites, pleural effusion or chylothorax
- Convulsions
- Birth of extremely preterm baby
- Maternal conditions/drugs affecting the fetus and neonate
- Life-threatening malformations
  a. Airways
  b. Lungs
  c. Heart
  d. Other organ systems: Neural tube defects, intestinal, and GU anomalies, and skeletal dysplasias
- Birth trauma
  a. Injuries to body organs
  b. Peripheral nerve injuries

RESUSCITATION OF AN ASPHYXIATED BABY

The most common emergency that a pediatrician confronts everyday is the infant failing to breathe and/or maintain an effective breathing at birth (perinatal asphyxia; birth asphyxia) with devastating consequences in terms of survival and subsequent neuromotor disability. According to WHO estimates, around 3% of approximately 120 million infants born every year in developing countries develop birth asphyxia requiring resuscitation. As per the latest estimates, perinatal asphyxia accounts for 9% of total under-5 mortality worldwide, being one of the three most common causes of neonatal deaths along with prematurity and bacterial infections. Apart from neonatal deaths, asphyxia is responsible for lifelong disability in a large number of children.

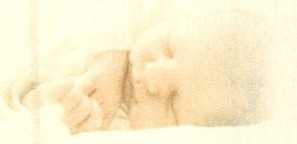

Resuscitation Alert

The existence of certain high-risk factors during pregnancy and labor serve to forewarn and alert the DR staff that they should be fully prepared to meet the challenge of an asphyxiated baby (Table 4.2). Several time honored clinical parameters of fetal distress offer useful guidelines to an experienced obstetrician.

Exaggerated Fetal Movements. The asphyxiated fetus behaves like a strangulated individual and makes desperate physical efforts followed by reduced or absent physical movements terminally.

Fetal Heart Rate. Due to release of catecholamines, initially there is tachycardia followed by bradycardia and slow-irregular heart beats. Bradycardia is a compensatory mechanism that allows longer coronary blood flow and ventricular filling because of prolonged diastole. The heart rate should be assessed during the later phase of uterine contraction.

Visceral Overactivity. The passage of meconium in a vertex presenting baby is an important and ominous sign of fetal hypoxia. It is fraught with the risk of aspiration of meconium by the gasping fetus. In preterm babies fetal diarrhea as a result of listeriosis is an uncommon cause of meconium staining of the liquor in the absence of fetal hypoxia.

Evaluation of the Infant at Birth

Despite its limitations, the Apgar scoring system is conventionally used for assessing the condition of the newborn baby at 60 seconds after birth (Table 4.3). The respiratory effort and heart beat per minute are critical components of Apgar scoring system because muscle tone, response to reflex stimulus and color are dependent upon the cardio-respiratory status of the baby.

Apgar scoring system ignores the time of cry after birth which is important to identify and differentiate between primary and terminal apnea. The peripheral cyanosis is awarded a score of one, although majority of healthy normally breathing babies are never totally pink at 1-minute. Tone and response to reflex stimulus are dependent upon gestational maturity. Moreover, centrally blue (asphyxia livida) and totally pale (asphyxia pallida) babies are given an identical score, although latter are more gravely sick due to the combined effect of cardio-respiratory failure. *Apgar scoring system is no longer used for initiating various steps of resuscitation.* However, Apgar score at 5-minutes after birth or subsequently is a useful correlate of future mental prognosis of asphyxiated babies.

Resuscitation Kit

It is a sad fact that most delivery rooms in developing countries are not adequately equipped for the resuscitation of an asphyxiated newborn baby. The procedure of carrying the newly born baby from the delivery room to another room for resuscitation is most unsatisfactory. Each delivery room must have a well-lighted and warm microenvironment to receive the newly born infant. The resuscitation kit must be

---

Table 4.2 Conditions demanding resuscitation alert

Antepartum risk factors
- Bad obstetrical history
- Young (<16 yr) or elderly (>35 yr) mother
- Maternal systemic disease or poor nutritional status
- Pregnancy-induced hypertension
- Multiple gestation
- Rhesus-isoimmunization
- Fetal malformations
- Polyhydramnios or oligohydramnios
- Fetal size to gestation discrepancy, i.e. undersized or oversized baby
- Prolonged rupture of membranes (>18 hours) and chorioamnionitis
- Drug therapy: Reserpine, lithium carbonate, magnesium sulfate, adrenergic blocking agents, maternal drug abuse, etc.

Intrapartum risk factors
- Fetal distress
- Premature or post-term gestation
- Malpresentation
- Large or macrosomic fetus
- Cord prolapse or tight nuchal cord
- APH: Placenta previa or abruptio placentae
- Prolonged labor (>24 hours) or prolonged second stage of labor (>2 hours)
- Maternal narcotics, analgesics and anesthetics
- Meconium-stained amniotic fluid
- Difficult or instrumental (forceps or vacuum-assisted) or operative (emergency cesarean section) delivery

---

Table 4.3 Apgar scoring system

Criteria	Score		
	0	1	2
1. Respiration	Nil	Slow, gasping	Crying
2. Heart rate/min	Nil	Upto 100	More than 100
3. Muscle tone	Flaccid	In-between	Flexed
4. Reflex response	Nil	Grimace	Cough, sneeze, cry
5. Color	Pale or blue	Peripheral cyanosis	Completely pink

checked by the staff nurse of every duty shift and rechecked by the physician before each delivery. The pencil-handle laryngoscope with infant (0 and 1) straight blade is preferred. Its light source and batteries should be in working condition. Gamma-irradiated disposable endotracheal tubes with internal diameters of 2.5 mm, 3.0 mm and 3.5 mm and mounted with adapters should be available. The electrical points and suction machine should be in working order. Press-type rubber bulb or oral suction mucus trap must be available to meet the exigencies of electrical failure (Figure 4.1). Oxygen cylinder should be checked for its contents. Ambu bag and mask is extremely useful and handy to resuscitate an apneic baby. The self inflatable bags are easy to use but provide only 40% to 50% oxygen. The attachment of a corrugated tube provides a reservoir for oxygen and can deliver upto 80% oxygen to the infant. The resuscitation kit should contain disposable sterile endotracheal tube and suction catheters, plastic oral airway, syringes and needles, 7.5% sodium bicarbonate, atropine, epinephrine 1:10,000, calcium gluconate 10%, neonatal nalorphine (1.0 mg/mL), naloxone hydro-chloride (0.4 mg/mL), ampoules of distilled water, physiological saline, albumin 5% solution and 5% dextrose. Sterile neonatal delivery packs containing bowl, scissors, cotton swabs and umbilical ties should be available for each delivery. The bassinet on which the baby is to be received should be kept warm and provided with an over head radiant heat source and a stopclock to accurately time the sequence of events after birth (Figure 4.2). Pulse oximetry is being increasingly used in most centers for continuous monitoring of oxygen saturation during resuscitation.

It is desirable that equipment for resuscitation should be maintained in sterile condition and baby received in sterile warm sheets with due aseptic precautions. Above all, the physician must be adept in the art of

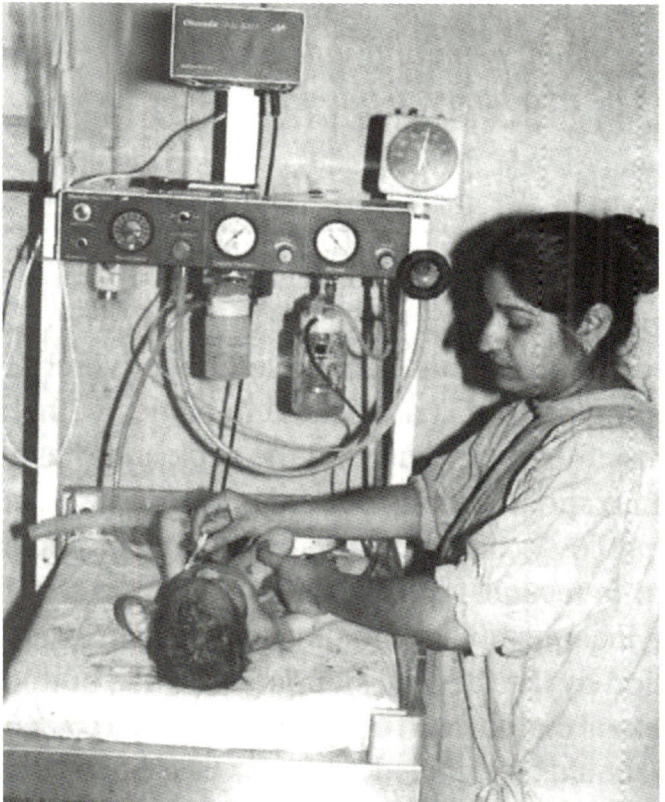

Figure 4.2 Resuscitator with overhead warmer, stopclock, and in-built facilities for suction, oxygen supply and intermittent positive pressure ventilation.

cardiopulmonary resuscitaton. The art of endotracheal intubation should be learnt and perfected by continued practice on the stillborn and dead neonates. Several life support neonatal training simulators and modules are available to learn the skills of external cardiac massage and artificial ventilation. The retention of cardio-pulmonary skills is shortlived unless they are constantly revised and practiced.

Initial Steps in Resuscitation

The resuscitation kit should be checked before the baby is born. The radiant warmer should be put on and plenty of sterile prewarmed linen should be available. Due to increasing prevalence and risk of HIV, it is desirable that the pediatrician resuscitating the baby wears the gloves. The baby should be received in a warm sheet and head kept slightly low (Figure 4.3). The conventional practice of holding the baby upside down from its feet is undesirable. The baby should be placed under the radiant warmer and both hypothermia as well as hyperthermia should be prevented. The baby should be placed supine or on its side, with the head in a neutral or slightly extended position. The infant's

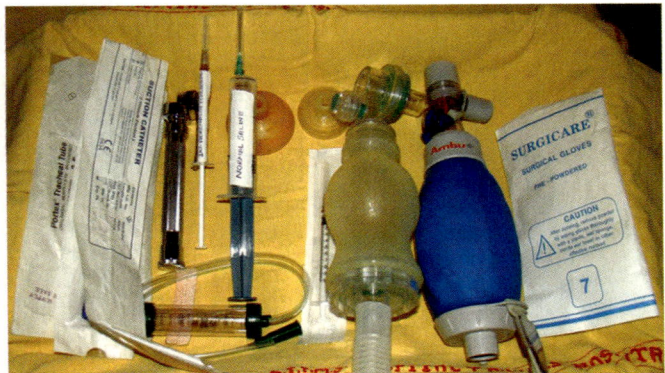

Figure 4.1 Resuscitation kit. Note corrugated tube attached at the inlet of Ambu bag to enhance concentration of oxygen delivered to the infant.

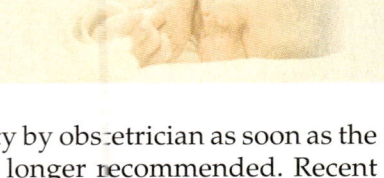

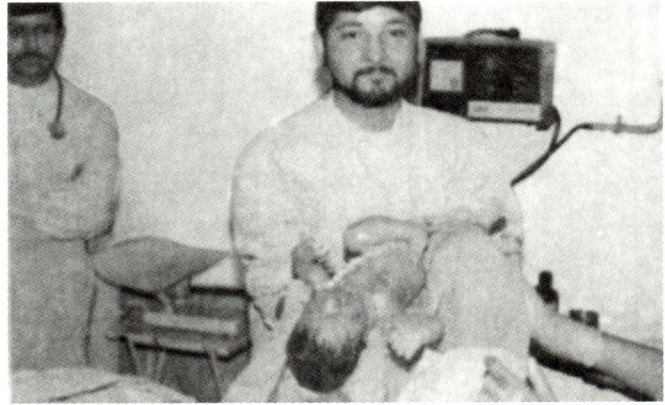

Figure 4.3 The correct method of holding the baby at birth.

mouth, oropharynx, hypopharynx and nose are sucked, in that order, using thick 10 Fr suction catheter with gentle intermittent suction. The nose should not be sucked first as it would lead to reflex breathing with the risk of aspiration of secretions contained in the oral cavity. After suction, the baby should be dried effectively and wet linen should be removed. Head constitutes a large surface area of the baby and must be effectively dried. The process of drying and suction produce enough stimulation to initiate effective breathing in most newly born babies. If an infant is not breathing or his breathing efforts are sluggish, he should be stimulated by flicking the soles or rubbing the back. The tactile stimulation should not be continued beyond 3 to 4 flicks and when it is ineffective the baby should be promptly ventilated with a bag and mask. *Evaluate the infant every 30 sec by simultaneously observing respirations, heart rate and color to decide the need for further steps in resuscitation.* Availability of a stopclock mounted on the resuscitator is essential to accurately time the sequence of events after birth.

Approach to a Meconium-stained Baby

About 10–15 percent pregnancies are complicated by passage of meconium *in utero* during labor. It is a reliable sign of fetal distress in a vertex presenting neonate with additional risk of respiratory morbidity due to meconium aspiration syndrome. The detection of *in utero* passage of meconium may be delayed if membranes are intact. Thick meconium staining of liquor (pea-soup appearance) is ominous. Yellow staining of skin, umbilical cord and nails indicate that meconium has been passed at least 4–6 hours before delivery. It is associated with increased risk of birth asphyxia and meconium aspiration syndrome. When amniotic fluid is meconium stained, the baby should be promptly delivered either by cesarean section or by forceps if cervix is adequately dilated. The practice of

suctioning the oral cavity by obstetrician as soon as the head is delivered is no longer recommended. Recent multicentric study has shown that intrapartum suctioning does not reduce the risk of meconium aspiration syndrome because babies breathe *in utero* and aspirate meconium before head is delivered.

After delivery, thorough suction of oral cavity, oropharynx and glottic area should be done under direct vision with the help of a laryngoscope. When a meconium-stained baby is depressed as evidenced by poor cry, flaccidity, or bradycardia (heart rate <100 bpm), it is recommended that endotracheal intubation should be done. The need for intubation is not based on consistency or thickness of meconium. The endotracheal tube is attached directly to a gentle intermittent suction source to suck out the meconium. The endotracheal tube is gradually withdrawn while suction is being applied. The infant may have to be intubated 2 to 3 times till all the meconium has been sucked out. At times saline lavage may be required to remove thick tenacious meconium. The meconium cannot be sucked by inserting a suction catheter through the endotracheal tube. The practice of sucking the endotracheal tube with oral negative pressure of the resuscitator, is not recommended due to the potential risk of HIV infection. The meconium stained baby should not be ventilated or bagged till air passages have been effectively cleared of all possible meconium. However, if the infant's heart rate or respiration is severely depressed, it is desirable to institute positive-pressure ventilation despite the presence of some meconium in the airway. If a meconium stained baby is vigorously crying at birth, there is no need to do endotracheal intubation. There is a potential risk of injury to the vocal cords while trying to intubate a vigorous and crying term infant. When the baby is stable, stomach wash is recommended to reduce the risk of vomiting and aspiration of meconium-stained gastric contents. Infant should be closely watched for development of respiratory distress due to meconium aspiration syndrome and onset of persistent pulmonary hypertension.

Resuscitation of an Asphyxiated Baby

American Academy of Pediatrics (AAP) and Americal Heart Association (AHS) along with several other organizations have formalized a partnership with International Liaison Committee on Resuscitation (ILCOR) to update and revise recommendations for neonatal resuscitation program (NRP). The recent Consensus On Science and Treatment Recommendations (COSTR) published in 2010 provides the latest NRP guidelines which are considered as gold standard.

Most babies have a smooth transition from fetal to neonatal life and establish spontaneous breathing at birth without any active assistance. About 5.0% to 7.5% babies in tertiary care centers are likely to have difficulty in initiating spontaneous breathing at birth and need active resuscitation. At every delivery, there should be at least one person, who is adequately trained in the art of neonatal resuscitation, to look after the needs of the newly born baby. When the delivery is high-risk, at least two trained personnel are required to perform complete resuscitation including bag and mask ventilation, endotracheal intubation, chest compressions and administration of medications. When a mother is having multiple gestations, separate teams of trained personnel and equipment should be available to handle and resuscitate each baby. The procedure of neonatal resuscitation must be carried out by skilled and experienced person with a sense of urgency but without any panic. The revised neonatal resuscitation program (NRP) guidelines of the Technical Committee of National Neonatology Forum of India recommends that the newly born baby should be assessed by asking the following question.

Is baby breathing or crying?

When answer to the above question is YES, the baby needs routine care. But when answer is NO, the baby is provided initial steps for resuscitation. During the initial steps, the baby is correctly positioned, airway is cleared and he is effectively dried and kept warm. When a baby is breathing but is cyanosed, he is administered free-flow oxygen at a rate of 5 liters/min till he becomes pink. Free-flow oxygen is administered through an oxygen mask or flow-inflating bag or a hand cupped around the oxygen tubing. If a baby is not breathing or having gasping breaths, he is provided tactile stimulation by flicking the soles or rubbing the back to promote breathing. Avoid prolonged tactile stimulation in an apneic baby, as this will waste valuable time. The baby is simultaneously assesed for respiration, heart rate and color to take further decisions for resuscitation (Figure 4.4).

Bag and Mask Ventilation

If despite stimulation, the baby is still apneic or having ineffective ventilations as evidenced by heart rate of less than 100 beats per minute, he should be given bag and mask ventilation. Position the infant supine by placing a small roll of towel under the shoulders inorder to extend the neck and open the airways (Figure 4.5). Thorough suctioning of oral cavity, hypopharynx and nose is mandatory before starting bag and mask

ventilation. The mask should tightly fit on the face enclosing nose and mouth of the baby (Figure 4.6). Supplemental oxygen (30–40%) can be given during bag and mask ventilation but there is no need to attach the oxygen reservoir to the bag to increase the concentration of oxygen. *In community setting, when oxygen is not available, infant can be successfully ventilated with room air (21% oxygen) with the help of bag and mask or tube and mask.* The infant should be ventilated at a rate of 40–60 breaths per minute. To avoid alveolar rupture and pneumothorax, the operator should train himself or herself to deliver 15–20 cm H_2O pressure with the help of a manometer. To open up the collapsed alveoli, few initial inflatory pressures of 30–40 cm H_2O pressure are recommended. There should be a noticeable rise and fall of the chest during each ventilation. Naloxone hydrochloride 0.1 mg/kg should be administered intravenously through umbilical vein if mother had received pethidine or morphine within 4 hours before delivery. If needed it can be repeated after every 2–3 minutes. During bag and mask ventilation heart rate should be closely monitored after every 30 seconds. Heart rate is assessed by auscultating the precordium or feeling pulsations at the base of the umbilical cord. To save time, heart rate is counted for 6 seconds and multiplied by 10 to get the heart rate per minute. If despite effective bag and mask ventilation, heart rate is not coming up or it further slows down and drops below 100 per minute, the infant should be intubated. *A large majority of asphyxiated babies can be effectively revived and resuscitated by using bag and mask ventilation alone and intubation is usually not required.*

In Indian setting, the use of laryngeal mask airway is currently not recommended due to the expense involved and lack of training and expertise in this procedure. In preterm neonates, a T-piece resuscitator is more useful as it can provide PEEP. There is no role of dexamethasone, atropine, calcium and respiratory stimulants like nikethamide and lobeline during resuscitation. The Apgar scoring system is not taken into consideration while taking management decisions during resuscitation of a newborn baby. The management is guided by the status of breathing, heart rate and color of the baby. Apgar score may be recorded at 1-minute, 5-minutes and subsequently (till it is more than 7) to serve as a prognostic indicator of the outcome of an asphyxiated baby.

Endotracheal Intubation

Endotracheal intubation is indicated in following situations:

- When tracheal suctioning is required in a meconium-stained depressed baby.

- If bag and mask ventilation is ineffective (heart rate remains < 100 bpm) or it is required for a prolonged period.
- When chest compressions are performed.
- Extremely preterm babies and neonates requiring administration of surfactant.
- Infants with airway anomalies, diaphragmatic hernia, and hydrops fetalis.

The art of intubation cannot be taught and must be learnt by practicing on stillborn babies, neonates dying in the nursery and baby simulators. The appropriate sized (4.0 mm in a term baby and 2.5 mm in a tiny baby) endotracheal tube should be prepared by shortening it to 13 cm and attaching a connector. Proper length of insertion of ET tube from lips can be calculated by weight of the infant in kg + 6 cm. It is easy to intubate

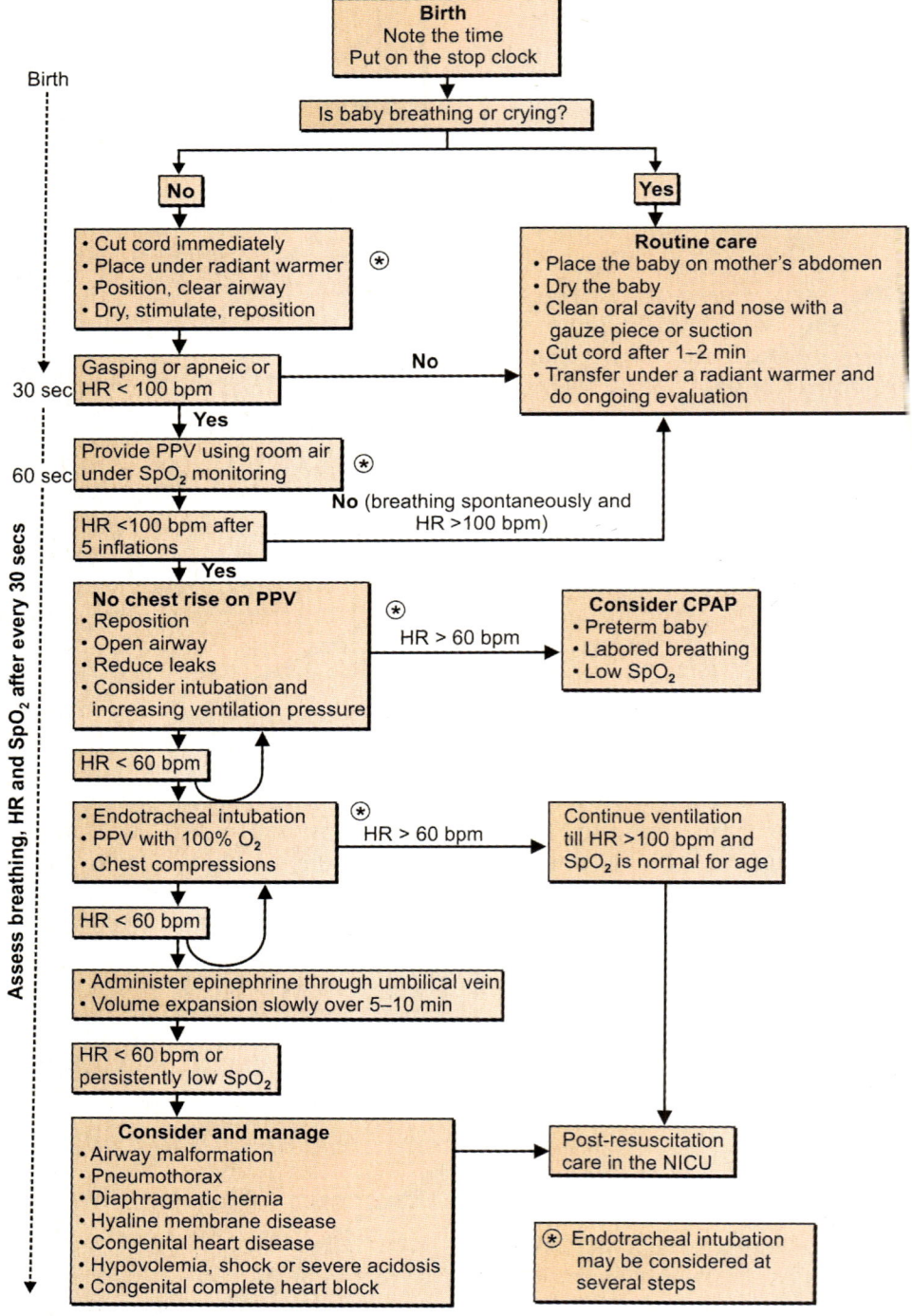

Figure 4.4 Algorithm for resuscitation of an asphyxiated baby. Adapted from NRP-India guidelines.

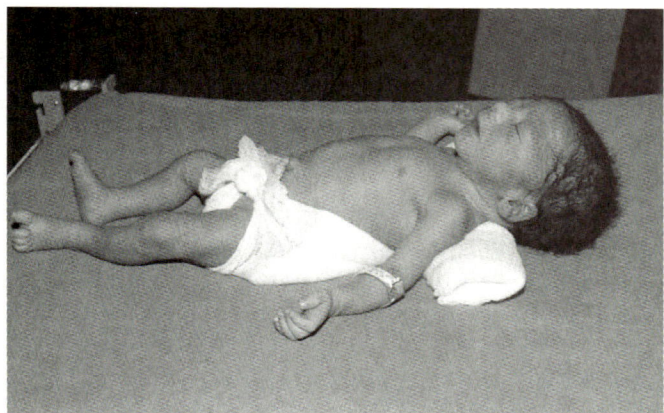

Figure 4.5 Positioning the newborn baby to maintain the patency of airways. Note the folded towel under the shoulders to extend the neck.

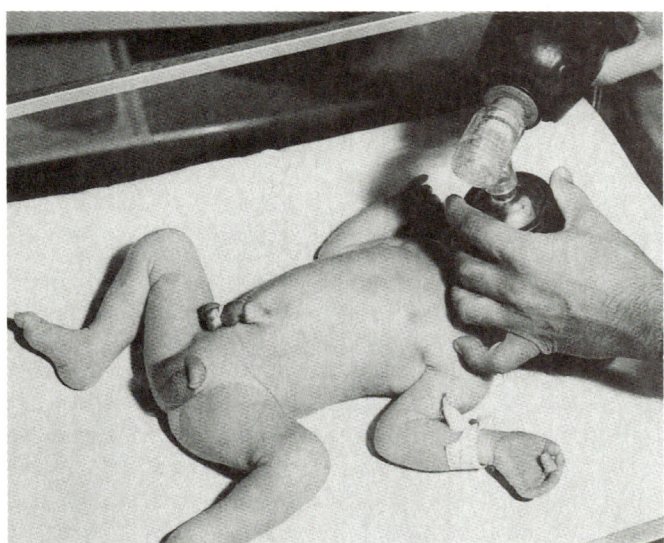

Figure 4.6 Bag and mask resuscitation. Most of the asphyxiated infants can be successfully resuscitated by this technique.

an asphyxiated baby with some practice because of lack of resistance and hypotonia. The endotracheal tube should be suctioned before starting positive pressure ventilation with a bag or machine. The laryngeal mask airway may serve as an effective alternative for establishing an airway if bag-mask ventilation is ineffective or attempts at intubation have failed. In preterm babies (< 32 weeks) T-piece resuscitator with inbuilt PEEP is useful for resuscitation. In these babies, availability of an oxygen blender and pulse oximeter is useful for resuscitation. The ventilation can be stopped as soon as the baby establishes spontaneous breathing and heart rate is maintained above 100 beats per minute.

External Cardiac Massage

External cardiac massage is indicated in babies in whom heart rate drops below 60 per minute despite effective ventilation with 100% oxygen for 30 seconds. The ventilation should be continued by an assistant and simultaneously heart should be massaged either by using two fingers of one hand or encircling the chest of the baby with both the hands and applying sternal compressions with two thumbs (Figures 4.7 and 4.8).

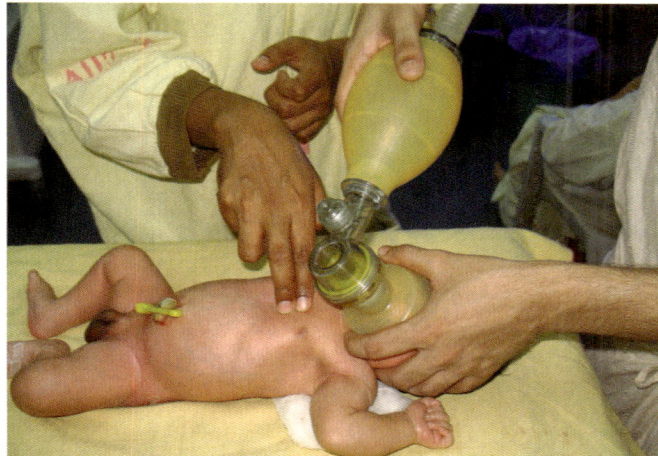

Figure 4.7 External cardiac massage with two fingers. Index and middle fingers are placed vertically over the lower third of sternum to provide cardiac compressions at a rate of 120/min. Bag and mask or bag and endotracheal tube ventilation should continue during chest compressions.

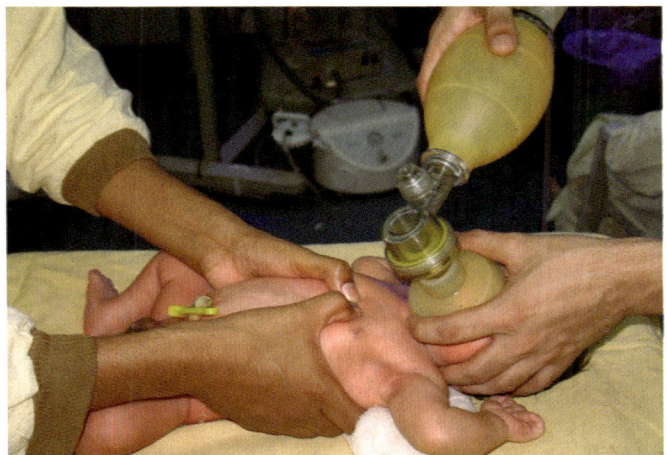

Figure 4.8 External cardiac massage with thumbs. The chest is enclosed within both hands and thumbs opposed over the lower one-third of midsternal region for providing compressions. In extremely low birth weight baby, one thumb can be placed over the other (instead of side by side) because of small size of the precordial area. Two-thumb technique is more effective in generating peak systolic and coronary perfusion pressures.

Available data suggest that the 2 thumb-encircling hand technique is more convenient and effective in generating peak systolic and coronary perfusion pressures in neonates.

Press the lower part of the sternum just above the xiphoid cartilage to a depth of one-third of the anterior-posterior diameter of the chest at a rate of 90 compressions and 30 ventilations (3:1 ratio) per minute. The thumbs and tips of fingers (depending upon the method used) should remain in contact with the sternum all the time and they should not be lifted off after each compression. Check the heart rate after every 30 seconds and chest compressions may be stopped when heart rate goes above 60 bpm.

Medications

Epinephrine is indicated when the heart rate remains below 60 bpm despite 30 seconds of assisted ventilation and another 30 seconds of coordinated chest compressions and assisted ventilation. Administer 0.1–0.3 mL/kg of 1.10,000 solution (0.01–0.03 mg/kg) of epinephrine through the umbilical vein or 0.3–1.0 mL/kg through endotracheal tube. Intracardiac route is dangerous and should be avoided due to risk of damage to the coronary vessels and development of hemopericardium. The dose of epinephrine may be repeated after every 3–5 minutes as indicated. Naloxone hydrochloride is indicated in a depressed infant whose mother received narcotics within 4 hours of delivery. Adequate ventilation must be established before administration of naloxone. The recommended dose of naloxone is 0.1 mg/kg (0.4 mg/mL solution) and can be given IV, IM or SC. If a baby is in shock, consider the use of plasma expander (ORh-negative RBCs, normal saline or Ringer's lactate) in a dose of 10 mL per kg slow intravenous push over 5 to 10 minutes. The fluids of choice for volume expansion is an isotonic crystalloid solution like physiological saline or Ringer's lactate. 5% albumin is no longer recommended for volume expansion.

Effective ventilation is followed by spontaneous correction of acidosis and alkali therapy should be guided by monitoring blood acid-base parameters. When blood gasometery facilities are not available, sodium bicarbonate 5–10 mL of 7.5% solution (adequately diluted with equal volume of distilled water or double volume of 5% dextrose) should be administered intravenously slowly at a rate of 1.0 mL/minute to infants in whom effective ventilation is not established even by 10 minutes or later (Apgar score of less than 7 at 10 minutes). Bolus administration of sodium bicarbonate should be avoided due to the risk of development of intraventricular hemorrage in preterm babies. Effective ventilation must be established before administration of sodium bicarbonate.

When to deny or stop CPR at birth?

Resuscitation at birth may be denied or abandoned when it is considered futile in terms of survival or survival is likely to be associated with gross neuromotor disability with extremely poor quality of life. It is justified and ethical to deny resuscitation to infants with gross non-correctable lethal congenital malformations and micropremies (< 750 g in developing countries). The resuscitation efforts may be abandoned in fresh still born babies (zero apgar score at one minute) if there are no signs of life at 10 minutes or if spontaneous breathing is not established by 30 minutes.

Intractable Birth Asphyxia

The conditions listed in Box 4.1 should be suspected if ventilation remains unsatisfactory even after 10 minutes of birth. Effective and thorough suctioning, endotracheal intubation and assisted ventilation are mandatory in these infants. Skiagram of chest should be taken for further management of such an infant. Blood gases, acid-base parameters, electrolytes, glucose, BUN and lactate should be monitored. Drainage of ascites and thoracocentesis would improve respiration in hydropic infants. Removal of air from pleural cavity in an infant with tension pneumothorax would be life saving. It can be promptly diagnosed in the labor room with the help of fiberoptic cold light. Oral airway facilitates breathing in infants with choanal atresia. When congenital diaphragmatic hernia is suspected, stomach should be decompressed with an orogastric

---

BOX 4.1 Causes of intractable birth asphyxia

- Meconium aspiration or tracheal plug
- Congenital malformations of airways namely choanal atresia, laryngeal web, diaphragmatic hernia, esophageal atresia with tracheoesophageal fistula, lobar emphysema or cyst, and asphyxiating thoracic dystrophy
- Pneumothorax and pneumomediastinum
- Intracranial hemorrhage
- Shock (cardiogenic or hypovolemic)
- Profound metabloic alterations
- Congenital pneumonia
- Hydrops fetalis
- Severe immaturity (<28 weeks gestation)
- Paralysis of respiratory muscles or malformation of brain
- Pulmonary hemorrhage
- Excessive maternal sedation

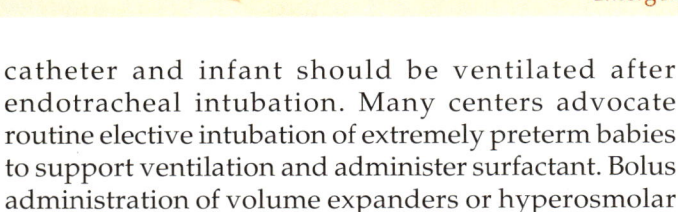

catheter and infant should be ventilated after endotracheal intubation. Many centers advocate routine elective intubation of extremely preterm babies to support ventilation and administer surfactant. Bolus administration of volume expanders or hyperosmolar solutions should be avoided due to potential risk of causing intraventricular hemorrhage.

Whole Body or Selective Brain Cooling

There is an experimental and clinical evidence to suggest that mild to moderate whole body or selective brain cooling with a cold cap is neuroprotective against the adverse effects of birth asphyxia. Cerebral hypothermia reduces ATP production and lowers metabolic rate of the brain with increase in the levels of inhibitory neuromodulators like glycine, taurine, GABA and adenosine which are neuroprotective. There is reduced alterations in ion flux and preservation of blood brain barrier. Cooling is begun within 1–6 hour after hypoxic insult by maintaining brain or core body temperature between 33–34°C for 48–72 hours.

Whole body cooling is recommended in term infants (>36 weeks and <6 hr), if three of the following five inclusion criteria are fulfilled.

   i. Apgar score ≤ 5 at 10 minutes.

   ii. pH of cord blood or infant's blood ≤ 7.0 within one hour of age.

   iii. Base deficit of cord blood or infant's blood within one hour age of ≥16 moles/L.

   iv. Need for continued assisted ventilations at birth for at least 10 minutes.

   v. History of seizures or CNS abnormalities suggestive of grade 3 or more hypoxic-ischemic encephalopathy (HIE).

These infants should be given adequate sedation and excellent supportive care. There is evidence to suggest that neuroprotective effect of moderate hypothermia can be enhanced by co-administration of topiramate. However, inadvertent excessive cooling with fall in core body temperature is associated with adverse metabolic and physiologic effects with higher risk of morbidity and mortality. It would appear that hypothermia and selective cooling of brain after perinatal asphyxia is still an experimental intervention but is being increasingly used in tertiary care centers. There is a need for more data regarding its safety and efficacy in developing countries.

Systemic Manifestations of Severe Birth Asphyxia

Seeds of neonatal morbidity and neuromotor disability are sown in the labor room. A variety of clinical problems are encountered during early neonatal period

Table 4.4 Systemic manifestations of severe birth asphyxia

Organ/system	Features
Brain	Hypoxic-ischemic encephalopathy, intra-cranial hemorrhage, apneic attacks, seizures and neuromotor disability.
Heart	Persistent fetal circulation, dys-hythmias, myocardial damage, tricuspid regurgitation, and congestive cardiac failure.
Lungs	Meconium or liquor aspiration, hyaline membrane disease, transient tachypnea, persistent pulmonary hypertension, pulmonary hemorrhage, pneumonia, pneumothorax, and shock lung.
Kidneys	Hematuria, renal failure, acute tubular necrosis, and renal vein thrombosis.
Hematologic	Coagulopathy (DIC), thrombocytopenia, hyperbilirubinemia, and sepsis.
Gastrointestinal	Necrotizing enterocolitis, GI bleeding, para-lytic ileus and and hepatic dysfunction.
Endocrinal	Syndrome of inappropriate secretion of antidiuretic hormone, adrenal hemorrhage, and transient hypoparathyroidism.
Immunologic	Septicemia
Metabolic	Acidosis, hypoglycemia, hypocalcemia, hyponatremia and hyperkalemia.

among babies who are severely asphyxiated at birth (Table 4.4). Hypoxia can cause damage to almost every tissue and organ of the baby. During hypoxia, series of protective mechanisms collectively called as 'diving sea reflex' attempt to redistribute available blood flow from lesser to more vital organs. The blood flow to brain, heart and adrenal glands of the newborn is preserved at the expense of reduction of perfusion to kidneys, lungs, gastrointestinal tract, liver, spleen and skeletal muscles.

Prognosis

Severe birth asphyxia is the most common cause of death on the first day of life. Depending upon the gestational maturity and quality of newborn care facilities, 15% to 50% of neonates exhibiting manifestations of HIE die during neonatal period. Effective management of the baby at birth with early establishment of breathing, prevention of hypothermia and hypotension are associated with improved survival and outcome. The brain of a newborn baby, especially that of a preterm, is relatively resistant to the damaging effects of hypoxia and can withstand oxygen lack upto 5 to 7 minutes without any apparent sequelae. In an individual baby it is difficult to prognosticate for future neuromotor development. It is amazing that several severely asphyxiated babies achieve fairly normal

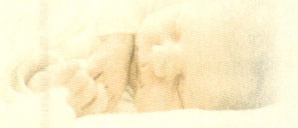

development without any neurological handicaps. Therefore, as a general policy, a guarded rather than hopeless prognosis should be communicated to the parents to cushion the anxiety and to avoid deliberate neglect of the child.

Following severe birth asphyxia, 25% infants are likely to develop evidences of HIE. Relatively adverse outcome is anticipated if the infant was in terminal apnea especially when heart beats were absent at birth or 10-minute Apgar score was less than 3. Arterial blood pH of less than 7.0, plasma lactate level of more than 60 mg/dL, hypoglycemia, occurrence of neonatal convulsions, brainstem signs (poor sucking, pooling of oral secretions, pupillary changes, etc.) or abnormal neurological behavior for more than 5 days and multiple diffuse chaotic spike pattern or isopotential amplitude integrated electroencephalogram (a-EEG) are associated with unfavorable outcome. Multiorgan failure especially development of acute renal failure is associated with poor outcome.

The American Academy of Pediatrics has proposed that the terminology of perinatal or birth asphyxia should be reserved to describe an infant who manifests all of the following features: (i) Cord umbilical artery pH < 7.0 with a base deficit of >10 mmoles/L; (ii) neonatal neurologic manifestations suggestive of hypoxic-ischemic encephalopathy (HIE); (iii) Evidences of multisystem organ dysfunction involving cardiovascular, renal, gastrointestinal, hematologic or pulmonary system.

The incidence of cerebral palsy following birth asphyxia varies between 6.5–18.5%. Infants with evidences of intraventricular or parenchymal hemorrhage and extensive areas of infarction (hypodensity) on CT scan or MRI brain during early neonatal period are often associated with neurological handicaps on follow-up. Brainstem auditory, visual and somatosensory evoked responses by and large are of limited prognostic utility. Inferior colliculi which are credited to produce wave V are specially damaged by hypoxia. In normal infants, wave V obtained during brainstem auditory evoked response is bigger in amplitude as compared to wave 1. The ratio of wave V (actually waves IV and V which are often merged) to wave 1 gets reversed when there is hypoxic damage to the inferior colliculi which is associated with increased mortality and poor late neuromotor outcome among the survivors.

SHOCK AND HYPOVOLEMIA

Shock in neonates in DR setting can occur either because of acute blood loss, myocardial dysfunction or a cardiac rhythm disorder such as complete congenital heart block (CCHB). Acute blood loss may occur because of placenta previa, vasa previa, placental abruption, tight nuchal cord (preferential occlusion of low pressure umbilical vein compared to the umbilical arteries resulting in loss of blood to placenta), or traumatic cord bleeding. Myocardial dysfunction can occur as a result of severe asphyxia, in extremely preterm babies because of inability of the left ventricular myocardium to bear the load of high resistance systemic circulation, congenital cardiac malformations and rarely in certain cardiomyopathies.

Attempts should be made to promptly search for signs of shock if an infant shows poor response to resuscitative measures. Shock manifests as tachycardia slow capillary refill (>2 sec), fast and labored breathing, low pulse volume, pale or mottled skin, cyanosis, low mean arterial pressure and metabolic acidosis.

Shock should be treated with normal saline or Ringer lactate bolus in a dose of 10 mL/kg, infused through umbilical vein over 5 to 10 minutes. The same dose can be repeated if hypovolemia is the likely cause of shock, and there has been inadequate response to the previous bolus. Randomized controlled trials in neonates have shown that isotonic crystalloid is as effective as 5% albumin for the treatment of hypovolemic shock. One may infuse ORh-negative blood (without any cross-matching) to correct for volume loss in acute hemorrhagic shock. Dopamine (5 to 20 µg per kg per min) and dobutamine (5 to 20 µg per kg per min) infusion should be considered, if the response to crystalloid bolus(es) has been suboptimal.

MULTIPLE BIRTHS

Birth of multiple babies (twins, triplets or higher order) can present as an emergency, because these babies are usually preterm, at higher risk of asphyxia, birth injury and inter-twin transfusion. The key to management is timely antenatal detection and delivery at a center equipped with independent neonatology teams with dedicated sets of equipment and supplies for each baby (Figure 4.9).

SEVERE ANEMIA

Anemia at birth constitutes an emergency requiring urgent intervention and may occur either due to acute or chronic blood loss or immune hemolysis. The common causes of acute blood loss have been mentioned *vide supra*. Chronic blood loss can occur because of twin-to-twin transfusion syndrome (TTTS), feto-maternal or feto-placental bleeding. Immune hemolysis occurs commonly as a result of Rh and ABO

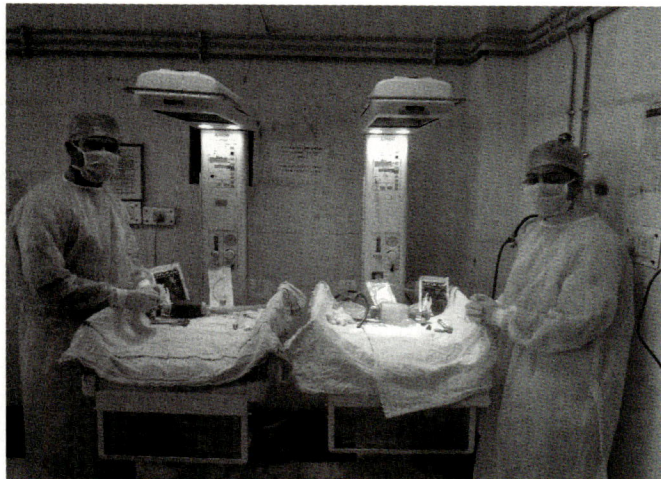

Figure 4.9 Delivery room equipped with two radiant warmers, team of health professionals, equipment and supplies to deal with a twin delivery.

blood group incompatibility, autoimmune hemolytic anemia, or rarely due to intrauterine infection with parvovirus, bone marrow hypoplasia or disorders such as hereditary spherocytosis. Long-standing severe anemia can precipitate hydrops in the baby (Figure 4.10), creating a major challenge for resuscitation. Severe anemia impairs postnatal adaptations in the infant and there may be congestive heart failure.

After establishing the airway and breathing by appropriate means, partial exchange blood transfusion using ORh-negative packed red blood cells should be undertaken to quickly improve the oxygen carrying capacity and general condition of the baby. Appropriate

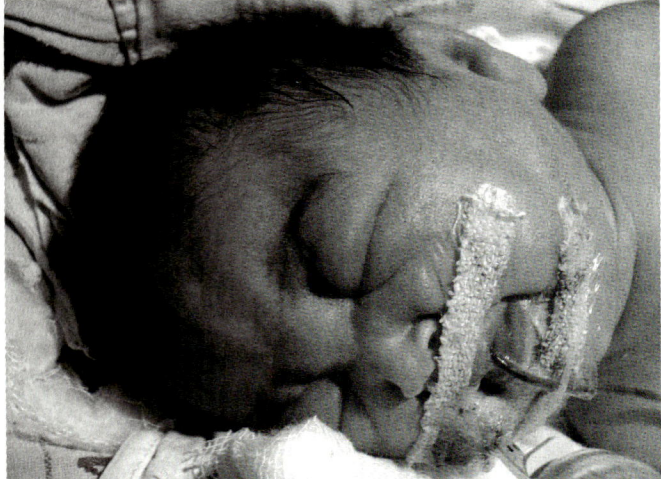

Figure 4.10 Immune hydrops fetalis secondary to severe Rh-isoimmunisation. Note marked edema of eyelids and moon facies. The baby required thoracocentesis and ascitic tap for effective ventilation and partial exchange transfusion for correction of anemia.

blood samples should be preserved before exchange transfusion to carryout investigations (Hemoglobin, reticulocyte count, DCT, peripheral smear, infection screen, etc.) to find out the cause of anemia.

PNEUMOTHORAX

Air leak into the pleural cavity (pneumothorax) can occur spontaneously in up to 3% of neonates, but often it is a complication of positive pressure ventilation (PPV). The risk is higher when the infant has been born through meconium stained amniotic fluid (MSAF) or has pulmonary hypoplasia. Small airleaks may be innocuous and can resolve on its own. However, significant amount of air can cause ventilation failure and shock because of flutter of the mediastinum and the heart, mandating immediate intervention to save life.

Pneumothorax is an important differential diagnosis in an unstable baby, particularly when there is an acute deterioration in the condition of the baby or when the baby has received positive pressure ventilation. It manifests as failure to resuscitate, desaturation, brady-cardia with or without poor perfusion. A discerning physician would be able to pick up decreased chest movements, bulging and decreased breath sounds on auscultation on the affected side.

Transillumination of the chest wall on the affected side with fiberoptic cold light is useful to make a quick diagnosis, particularly in infants with significant pneumothorax and thin chest wall. Confirmation can be done by X-ray chest, but the treatment should not be delayed. An 18–20 G angiocath should be inserted on the affected side in 4th intercostal space, above the upper margin of the lower rib, in anterior axillary line (Figure 4.11). The catheter should be attached through a three way to a 20 mL saline filled syringe. Air escaping through the saline into the syringe would confirm the

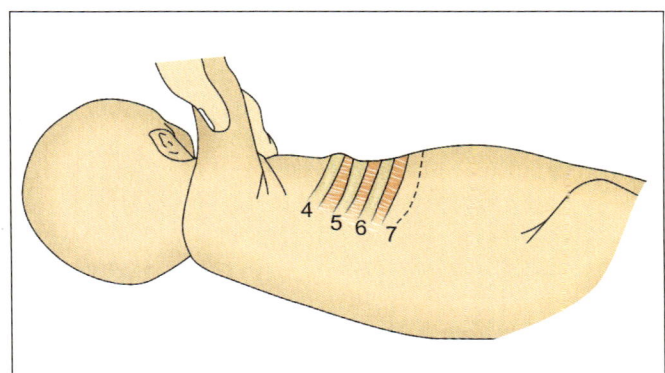

Figure 4.11 The site for needle thoracostomy or intercostal drainage (ICD) tube insertion for pneumothorax.

diagnosis of pneumothorax and would result in quick improvement of the baby. As a definitive measure, the infant requires placement of intercostal drainage (ICD) tube for continuous drainage of air until the pleural rupture gets healed.

HYDROPS, ISOLATED ASCITES OR PLEURAL EFFUSION

Birth of a hydropic infant is a life-threatening situation in the delivery room. Hydrops can result because of chronic anemia due to immune hemolysis as a result of blood group incompatibility or autoimmune hemolysis, or from a variety of other conditions such as chromosomal anomalies, congenital malformations, and developmental syndromes (non-immune hydrops). Non-immunologic hydrops fetalis may occur in association with maternal diabetes mellitus, polyhydramnios, anemia and toxemia of pregnancy. Fetal cardiac failure may occur due to congenital cardiac defects, fetal tachyarrhythmias and complete heart block. Intrauterine infections may be rarely associated with hydrops fetalis. In about one-third cases of hydrops, no cause is found.

Hydrops is characterized by widespread sub-cutaneous edema that distorts the anatomy and makes airway management including intubation rather difficult. Presence of ascites and pleural and/or pericardial effusion interferes in establishing successful ventilation and hemodynamic sufficiency. In addition, there may be severe anemia necessitating urgent transfusion of ORh-negative red blood cells for successful postnatal transition from fetal life.

Adequate preparations are needed in DR to resuscitate a hydropic baby and this includes availability of at least three health care professionals adequately trained in neonatal resuscitation, ORh-negative red blood cells and supplies for urgent thoracocentesis, pericardiocentesis and ascitic tap. These infants should be intubated in case of respiratory failure using a smaller calibre endotracheal tube rather than attempting ventilation by using a bag and mask. One should be prepared to perform urgent thoracocentesis, pericardiocentesis and/or ascitic tap, whenever indicated. No more than 20 mL/kg of fluid should be aspirated in one sitting. Partial exchange blood transfusion using ORh-negative red blood cells should be performed to correct anemia.

CONVULSIONS

The infant may rarely manifest with convulsions in DR as a result of severe hypoxic-ischemic encephalopathy (HIE), opioid withdrawal following naloxone injection, cerebral dysgenesis, inadvertent injection of local anesthetic into fetal scalp, or pyridoxine dependency. Immediate management involves securing airway and breathing by administration of glucose, calcium and anticonvulsants especially phenobarbitone. The details of management are discussed in Chapter 21.

EXTREMELY PRETERM BABY

Birth of an extremely preterm baby presents an emergency in DR and requires a coordinated teamwork for optimum outcome (Figure 4.12). Extremely low gestational age (ELGA) babies are at risk of hypothermia and respiratory failure because they have stiff and immature lungs combined with poor CNS drive for effective breathing, brain injury because of intracranial bleed and periventricular leucomalacia, hypotension and health care associated infections.

Survival of ELGA babies is inversely proportional to the gestational age of the baby, and is dependent upon the capabilities and availability of the optimal infrastructure of the neonatal unit. Apart from high death rates, these babies are at a substantial risk of development of neonatal morbidities as well as adverse neurodevelopmental outcome. Each neonatal unit should review its own survival and neuromorbidity data of ELGA babies, taking into consideration their capabilities and formulate a policy of non-initiation of resuscitation in those ELGA/ELBW babies who are unlikely to survive with the available facilities and expertise. Parental wishes must be taken into consideration in making such a decision in an

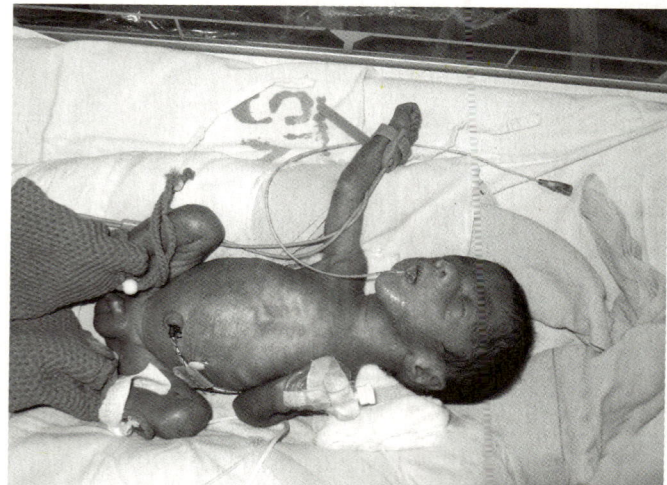

Figure 4.12 Extremely low gestational age or extremely low birth weight (ELGA/ELBW) baby on day 10 of life. The baby required early positive pressure ventilation, rescue surfactant therapy and CPAP for one week.

individual case. At AIIMS, we take a decision of non-initiation/discontinuation of resuscitation if the baby is less than 25 weeks or less than 700 gm.

The is a marked risk of hypothermia in ELGA babies owing to their large surface area to body weight ratio, low quota of brown fat, thin permeable skin and high transepidermal water loss (TEWL). Usual precautions to prevent hypothermia such as rapid drying, removing wet linen, placing baby under radiant warmer and using warm equipment and supplies are generally insufficient. There is a need for additional measures to protect the infant from hypothermia such as wrapping the baby in a plastic sheet to reduce TEWL and using warm and humidified oxygen for resuscitation.

These babies, owing to stiff and immature lungs coupled with poor respiratory drive, often require positive pressure ventilation (PPV). However, PPV can damage the immature lungs as a result of excessive tidal volumes (volutrauma), high inflating pressures (barotrauma) and high oxygen concentration (oxytrauma) culminating into acute lung injury and chronic lung disease (CLD). Therefore, extremely preterm babies should be provided with PPV using small volume breaths (low tidal volume) with positive end-expiratory pressure (PEEP). Since conventional resuscitation bag does not have the facility to provide PEEP or effectively control inflating pressures, it is preferable to use special devices (such as Neopuff, Fisher and Paykel) to deliver PPV to such babies.

It is important to avoid hyperventilation as this may produce hypocarbia with attendant risk of reducing cerebral perfusion and hyperoxia. Monitoring oxygen saturations by using pulse oximetry is recommended in ELGA babies to minimize the risk of high oxygen saturations. New resuscitation guidelines recommends use of intermediate concentration of oxygen (60%) to achieve the desired oxygen saturations.

Prophylactic surfactant replacement therapy (SRT) in such babies has been shown to improve the survival. However, recent evidence suggests that it is more beneficial to put these babies (particularly those treated with antenatal steroids) on nasal CPAP immediately after birth (delivery room CPAP) and use early rescue SRT only if the baby develops moderate to severe respiratory distress. These infants need utmost gentle handling, avoiding unnecessary fluid boluses and fiddling to prevent brain injuries like intraventricular hemorrhage (IVH) and periventricular leucomalacia (PVL).

MATERNAL CONDITIONS/DRUGS AFFECTING THE FETUS OR NEONATE

1. *Inadvertent injection of lidocaine into fetal scalp.* It can occur accidentally while injecting the drug to the mother for paracervical and pudendal block or for producing anesthesia for episiotomy. Lidocaine toxicity in the neonate would manifest as bradycardia, apnea, hypotonia and a depressed baby. The condition closely mimics hypoxic ischemic encephalopathy (HIE) because apart from the aforementioned manifestations, there may be tonic seizures that occur within minutes to hours of birth. However, it can be differentiated from HIE by presence of fixed dilated pupils and absence of doll's eye reflex, which is rarely seen in initial stages of HIE. In addition, lidocaine toxicity would improve within 24 to 48 hours of supportive care while HIE often shows clinical deterioration during the same period.

   Infants affected with lidocaine toxicity require optimum supportive care including effective ventilation. Inducing diuresis and acidification of urine promotes excretion of the drug. Exchange blood transfusion has a limited therapeutic value. The prognosis is excellent with good supportive care.

2. *Maternal myasthenia gravis* can produce a similar illness in the infant as a result of transplacentally transferred antibodies. It is a self-limiting illness, which can last for a few days to weeks, and manifests as hypotonia, areflexia, respiratory depression and bulbar involvement. The management is supportive by taking care of ventilation and ensuring optimum nutrition.

3. *Magnesium sulfate toxicity* It may occur in neonates born to mothers treated with magsulf for pre-eclampsia or arrest of preterm labor. It manifests as lethargy, apnea, respiratory depression and poor reflexes. There is no specific antidote, intravenous 10% calcium gluconate 2 mL/kg over 10 minutes may be tried. It requires supportive care including assisted ventilation at times.

4. *Opioid toxicity* can occur in infants born to mothers treated with opioids such as morphine or pethidine within 4 hours of delivery. The affected neonates show respiratory depression in the presence of normal heart rate and color. After ensuring optimum ventilation, naloxone hydrochloride 0.1 mg/kg can be administered intravenously to reverse the effect of the drug. It should be avoided in babies whose mothers have been exposed to opioids over a prolonged period of time, because of substance abuse.

LIFE-THREATENING MALFORMATIONS

Anomalies of Airways

A variety of airway anomalies, can present as an emergency in DR and include bilateral choanal atresia, pharyngeal abnormalities such as Pierre-Robin syndrome, laryngeal anomalies like bilateral vocal cord palsy, congenital laryngeal atresia, laryngo-tracheo-esophageal (LTE) cleft, and tracheal anomalies such as agenesis of trachea. These infants can be provided with temporary airway support with the help of laryngeal mask airway (LMA).

1. **Bilateral choanal atresia** Congenital choanal atresia occurs as result of abnormal persistence of bucco-nasal membrane. There is a female preponderance and nearly half of them are bilateral. It can occur as an isolated anomaly or as a part of Treacher Collins syndrome or CHARGE (colobomas of eyes, heart anomalies, atresia of choanae, retardation of physical and mental growth, genital and ear abnormalities) association.

    As the neonates are preferential nose breathers, the infant manifests with cyanosis that gets relieved on crying and reappears when baby stops crying (cyclic cyanosis). Diagnosis is suspected by inability to pass a catheter through nostrils and confirmed by CT scan. The affected neonate is treated with placement of an oral airway, as an emergency measure, and surgical reconstruction of the airways within first few days, as the definitive measure. Following surgical correction, polyvinyl tubes are sutured in the nasal passages to prevent restenosis and they can be removed after 6 weeks.

2. **Pierre Robin syndrome** The primary abnormality in Pierre Robin syndrome is mandibular hypoplasia (micrognathia) that sets in a deformation sequence resulting in posterior falling of tongue (glossoptosis), and cleft palate in 60% of cases. The narrowing of pharyngeal airway results in respiratory distress, cyanosis and apnea that gets worse in supine posture. It is managed with tracheal intubation or placement of a tracheal tube through the nose into the hypopharynx to relieve the obstruction. The infant should be kept in prone position to minimize the airway obstruction due to glossoptosis.

3. **Bilateral vocal cord palsy** A variety of central nervous system disorders such as HIE, intracranial hemorrhage, Arnold-Chiari malformation and brainstem dysgenesis may be associated with bilateral vocal cord palsy. It manifests as inspiratory stridor and breathing difficulty but cry is normal. The condition can be suspected on direct laryngo-scopy, and can be confirmed by inspecting adducted and non-mobile vocal cords on flexible bronchoscopy. It requires tracheal intubation to maintain the patency of airway, and ultimate prognosis is determined by the underlying/associated conditions.

4. **Congenital laryngeal atresia in congenital high airway obstruction syndrome (CHAOS).** The larynx is completely obstructed by a web. Typical presentation includes a resident getting frustrated by repeated failure of intubation attempts in a cyanotic baby. In most cases, a number of malformations are associated with laryngeal atresia (Figure 4.13). The condition can be suspected on antenatal ultrasound by enlarged lungs, dilated trachea and abdominal displacement of the diaphragm. There may be associated hydrops in the baby.

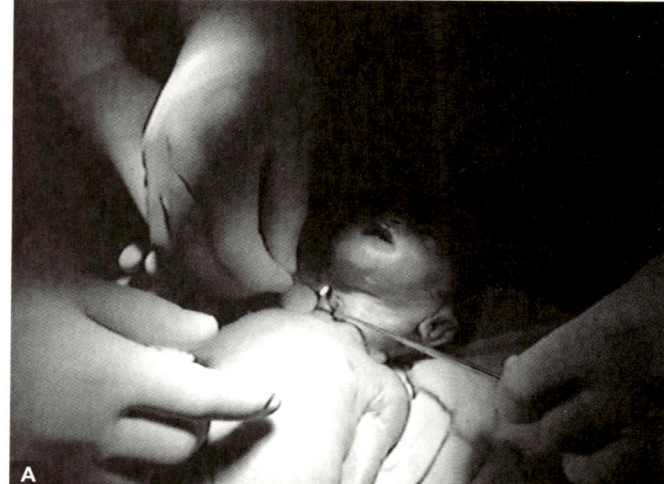

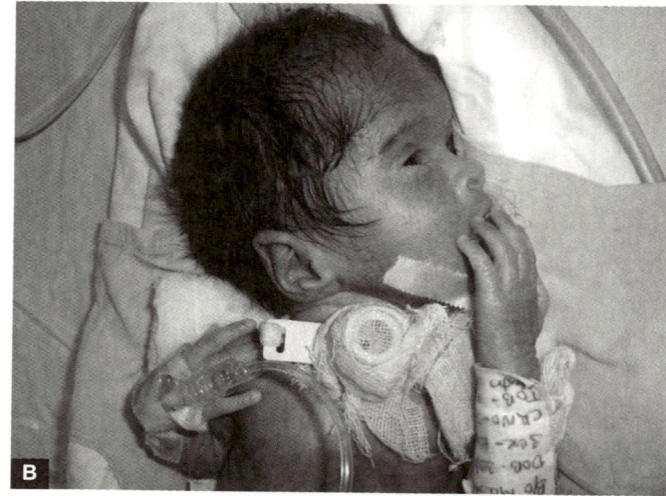

Figure 4.13 Congenital high airway obstruction syndrome (CHAOS). (A) The neonate is being tracheostomized immediately after birth, while the placental circulation is maintained by oxygenation and ventilation; (B) Baby is doing well after a couple of weeks.

At times one may be able to push the tracheal tube across the obstruction, but often it requires emergency cricothyrotomy to establish the airway. Prognosis is generally poor, because laryngeal reconstruction is extremely difficult.

5. **Laryngotracheoesophageal (LTE) cleft** The abnormality occurs as the airway and the esophagus fail to separate leaving a wide communication between two structures extending from larynx to as far down to trachea. Affected infants develop respiratory distress, stridor and cyanosis. The condition requires securing airway by tracheal intubation, as an emergency measure, followed by surgical repair. The prognosis is poor.

6. **Agenesis of trachea** In this condition, the trachea is completely atretic, resulting in severe respiratory distress and cyanosis. Associated tracheo-esophageal fistula makes it possible to achieve some ventilation through esophageal intubation. The nature of anomaly and associated malformations often lead to poor prognosis in this condition.

Anomalies of Lung Parenchyma

A variety of lung malformations can present as an emergency in DR and include congenital diaphragmatic hernia (CDH), esophageal atresia (EA) with and without tracheoesophageal fistula (TEF), bronchogenic, neuroenteric and pulmonary cysts, congenital cystic adenomatoid malformation (CCAM), bronchopulmonary agenesis, hemangiomatosis and pulmonary hypoplasia.

These conditions are rare and manifest during later part of neonatal period, infancy or even childhood but sometimes these can be severe enough to present at birth as fetal non-immune hydrops because of pressure effect on surrounding vessels.

1. **Congenital diaphragmatic hernia** Many cases of CDH may present as barrel shaped chest, scaphoid abdomen and with respiratory distress soon after birth. Most CDH are on the left side but condition may occur rarely on the right side (Figure 4.14). One may be able to auscultate bowel sounds in the chest on affected side. Nearly 40% babies have associated malformations.

If required, infants with CDH should be intubated and ventilated with endotracheal tube and bag. *Bag and mask ventilation should never be attempted because it would cause distension of gut with worsening of dyspnea.* Concomitant pulmonary hypoplasia makes lungs stiff requiring high inflating pressures for ventilation, but care should be taken to ventilate gently by limiting pressure, and using higher rates,

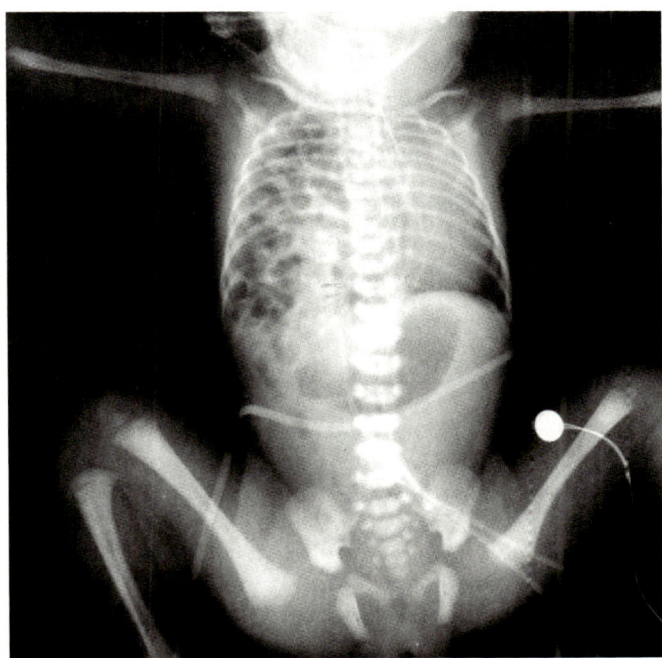

Figure 4.14 Right sided diaphragmatic hernia, detected in a baby who failed to breathe at birth and had a scaphoid abdomen.

to avoid lung injury and pneumothorax. Orogastric tube should be inserted to decompress the gut in the thoracic cavity inorder to allow the compressed lung to expand. After achieving hemodynamic stability, the defect should be corrected surgically. The condition is often complicated with PPHN and is associated with poor outcome.

2. **Esophageal atresia (EA)** Esophageal atresia can occur in isolation, but often co-exists with tracheo-esophageal fistula (TEF) in most cases. The most common variety is characterized by proximal EA and distal TEF, and babies present with respiratory distress and excessive salivation. Infants with distal EA and proximal TEF are at greatest risk of aspiration and present with severe respiratory distress due to aspiration and right upper lobe pneumonitis. Apart from initial resuscitation, these babies should be nursed in supine position with mild head elevation to prevent gastric acid aspiration into the lungs. The upper pouch of esophagus requires frequent or continuous suctioning to prevent aspiration.

3. **Cysts** Bronchogenic, neurenteric and pulmonary cysts are duplication cysts of variable sizes occurring as an aberration in fetal foregut development. They may be fluid or air filled and large enough to produce mass effect. Pulmonary cyst may be confused with tension pneumothorax, but can be differentiated by the presence of lung markings.

4. **Congenital cystic adenomatoid malformation (CCAM)** It occurs due to abnormal overgrowth of the terminal airways leading to formation of cysts of varying sizes, precluding normal alveolarization in the affected lobe, and producing mass effect. There may be associated additional malformations in about quarter of cases.

5. **Bronchopulmonary sequestration** Sequestration is characterized by abnormal lung tissue mass deriving its blood supply from systemic rather than pulmonary circulation, and does not take part in normal gas exchange process. The anomalous mass may be wrapped within the main pleural cavity (intrapulmonary) or may have its own pleural covering (extrapulmonary).

6. **Unilateral pulmonary agenesis and pulmonary hemangiomatosis** In this condition there is abnormal proliferation of vessels and it may present in DR with severe respiratory distress.

7. **Pulmonary hypoplasia** It is a relatively common condition and occurs as a deformation sequence secondary to compression of lung tissue from early fetal life by an underlying malformation such as CDH, other mass lesions described above, or by chronic leakage of amniotic fluid starting early in fetal life and continuing for a prolonged period. Renal agenesis is associated with oligohydramnios and bilateral pulmonary hypoplasia. Pulmonary hypoplasia may also occur in a variety of skeletal dysplasias such as thanatophoric dwarfism or severe myopathy, neuropathy or muscular dystrophy. The affected neonates present with respiratory distress. The hypoplastic lungs require high pressures for ventilation. The chest may be bell shaped and the babies are at risk of developing pneumothorax.

Heart Defects

Most heart defects whether cyanotic or acyanotic, do not manifest at the time of birth. However, some cardiac malformations can manifest with severe cyanosis that is unresponsive to routine resuscitative measures. A neonate should be suspected to have a cyanotic heart defect if the cyanosis does not respond to oxygen and/or ventilation. Sometimes additional clues to the diagnosis such as shock, cardiac murmur, abnormal heart sounds or associated congenital defects can be found. Some rhythm abnormalities can also present at birth namely complete congenital heart block (CCHB) as bradycardia, or supraventricular tachycardia with cardiac failure. Severely affected babies may have hydrops at birth.

The neonates with congenital heart defects may require assisted ventilation in the event of severe hypoxemia and/or respiratory distress. Prostaglandin E_1 therapy may be required to maintain the patency of duct. Bradyarrhythmias may require isoprenaline infusion to augment heart rate, while preparations are made for pacemaking. Supraventricular tachycardia may require reflex vagal maneuvers or adenosine injection to control the heart rate.

Defects of other Organ Systems

A variety of developmental defects pertaining to other organ systems may pose significant challenge in the DR. The common ones are meningomyelocele and neural tube defects (NTDs), anterior abdominal wall defects, massive tumors such as sacrococcygeal teratomas, hydronephrosis, hydrocephalus and conjoined twins.

Babies with NTDs should be provided nursing care to preserve the meningeal sac and prevent further injury and infection. The lesion should be covered with a sterile saline moist gauze. Contact with latex gloves should be avoided in case of open lesions to avoid any risk of hypersensitivity and anaphylaxis.

Anterior abdominal wall defects such as omphalocele and gastroschisis would require extreme care in resuscitation and preventing further injury to the gut. Unusual situations such as massive sacrococcygeal teratoma (Figure 4.15), conjoined twins (Figure 4.16), massive hydrocephalus, and obstructive uropathy with consequent urinary ascites are other important life-threatening conditions that require a coordinated approach by a team of trained personnel.

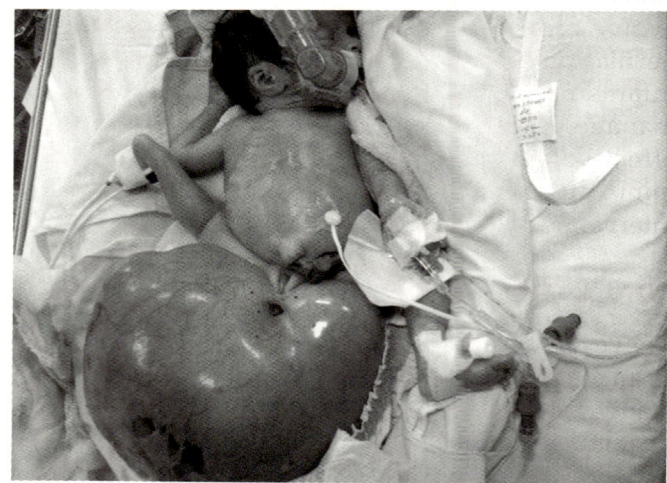

Figure 4.15 Massive sacrococcygeal teratoma leading to severe congestive heart failure in the infant.

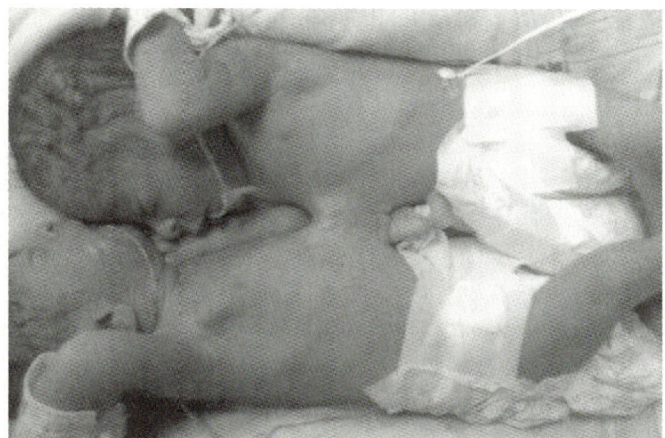

Figure 4.16 Conjoined twins can pose a major challenge to access the airway for resuscitation.

BIRTH TRAUMA

Birth trauma may at times be serious enough to present as an emergency in DR and these include spinal cord injury, subdural hemorrhage, brachial plexus injury involving C4 roots (phrenic nerve), injury to the liver or spleen, and facture of facial bones. The factors responsible for birth trauma may coexist with hypoxic-ischemic encephelopathy.

Spinal cord injury may occur following complicated breech delivery due to longitudinal, lateral or rotational traction of the neck. Often the lesion is akin to complete transection of cord and presents with marked hypotonia, weak respiratory efforts and areflexia (spinal shock), and carries a poor prognosis. Management is essentially supportive and good nursing care.

Subdural hemorrhage (SDH) results from sheer forces acting during labor and tearing apart of the dural sinuses in falx cerebri and falx cerebelli. The SDH may evolve rapidly with signs of blood loss, brainstem herniation and raised intracranial pressure. These infants are prone to develop severe jaundice. The management consists of supportive care including effective ventilation and replacing blood loss. A minority of affected infants require neurosurgical intervention.

CONCLUSIONS

Delivery room (DR) emergencies are common and can be managed effectively and carry good prognosis in many cases if managed urgently with due skills and expertise. The common DR emergencies include inability to initiate or maintain breathing, shock, anemia or multiple births. However, a variety of other developmental conditions can manifest as an emergency in DR and may require specific treatment in addition to ensuring optimum airway, oxygenation and circulation. The key to success in management of DR emergencies include adequate preparedness in terms of skilled manpower, functional equipment, supplies and ability to respond with a sense of urgency.

BIBLIOGRAPHY

Agarwal R, Deorari AK, Paul VK (Eds). AIIMS Protocols in Neonatology. 1st edition 2015, *New Delhi, CBS Publishers and Distributors Pvt. Ltd.*

American Academy of Pediatrics. American Collge of Obstetricians and Gynecologists, use and abuse of the Apgar score. *Pediatrics* 1996; 98:141–42.

Bahrami KR, MacDonal MG, Eichelberger MR. Throacostomy tubes. In: Procedures in Neonatology. MacDonald MG, Ramesethu J, 4th Ed. *Philadelphia: Lippincott Williams & Wilkins;* 2007, pp. 261–84.

Black RE, Cousens S, Johnson HL, Lawn JE, Rudan I, Bassani DG, *et al.* Child Health Epidemiology Reference Group of WHO and UNICEF. Global, regional and national causes of child mortality in 2008: a systematic analysis. *Lancet* 2010 June 5; 375 (9730): 1969–1987. Epub 2010 May 11.

Blackmon LR, Stark AR, Adamkin AR, Batton DH, Bell DG, et al. The Committee on Fetus and Newborn, American Academy of Pediatrics. Hypothermia: A neuroprotective therapy for neonatal hypoxic-ischemic encephalopathy. *Pediatrics* 2006; 117(3): 942–48.

D'souza SW, Black P, Cadman J, *et al.* Umbilical venous blood pH: a useful aid in the diagnosis of asphyxia at birth. *Arch Dis Child* 1983; 58:15.

Datta V. Therapeutic hypothermia for birth asphyxia in neonates. *Indian J Pediatr* 2017; 84(3):219–26.

Deorari AK. Newer guidelines for neonatal resuscitation: How my practice needs to change? *Indian Pediatr* 2001; 38:496–99.

Ekert P, Perlman M, Steinlin M, *et al.* Predicting the outcome of post-asphyxial hypoxic-ischemic encephalopathy within 4 hours of birth. *J Pediatr* 1997; 131:613–17.

Gluckman PD, Wyatt JS, Azzopardi D, *et al.* Selective head cooling with mild systemic hypothermia after neonatal encephalopathy: multicentre randomized trial. *Lancet* 2005; 365:663–70.

Gunn AJ, Gluckman PG, Gunn TR. Selective head cooling in newborn infants after perinatal asphyxia: a safety study. *Pediatrics* 1998, 102:885–92.

Higgins R, Raju T, Perlman J, *et al.* Hypothermia and perinatal asphyxia: executive summary of NICHD workshop. *J Pediatr* 2006; 148:170–75.

International Guidelines for Neonatal Resuscitation: An Excerpt from the Guidelines 2000 for Cardiopulmonary Resuscitation and Emergency Cardiovascular Care: International Consensus on Science. *Pediatrics* 2000; 106:1–16.

Kattwinkel J, Perlman JM, Aziz K, Colby C, Fairchild K, Gallagher J, *et al.* American Heart Association. Neonatal resuscitation 2010

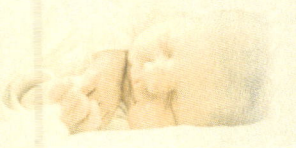

American Heart Association Guidelines for Cardiopulmonary Resuscitation and Emergency Cardiovascular Care. *Pediatrics* 2010; 126(5): e1400–13. Epub 2010, Oct 18.

Kattwinkel J. Textbook of Neonatal Resuscitation. Elk grove village, *Illinois, American Heart Association* 2000.

Levine MG, Holroyde J, Woods JR Jr, et al. Birth trauma: incidence and predisposing factors. *Obstet Gynecol* 1984, 63(6): 792–95.

Logan JW, Rice HE, Goldberg RN, Cotten CM. Congenital diaphragmatic hernia: A systematic review and summary of best-evidence practice strategies. *J Perinatol* 2007, 27:535.

Marlow N. Do we need an Apgar score? *Arch Dis Child* 1992; 67: 765–67.

Neonatal Resuscitation: India. *National Neonatology Forum of India,* second edition, 2014.

Oca MJ, Nelson M, Donn SM. Randomized trial of normal saline versus 5% albumin for the treatment of neonatal hypotension. *J Perinatol* 2003, 23:473–76.

Paneth N, Raymond IS. Cerebral palsy and mental retardation in relation to indicators of perinatal asphyxia. *Amer J Obstet Gynecol* 1983; 147:960.

Sarkar N, Agarwal R, Das AK, Deorari AK. Congenital airway abnormalities in neonates. *Indian J Pediatr* 2002, 69(11):993–95.

Thoresen M. Cooling the newborn after asphyxia: physiological and experimental background. *Semin Neonatal* 2000; 5:61–73.

Vanden Berg PP, Nelen WL, Jongsma HW, *et al*. Neonatal complications in newborn with an umbilical artery pH <7.0. *Am J Obstet Gynecol* 1996; 175:1152–57.

Volpe JJ. Neurology of the Newborn. 5th Ed. *Philadelphia: Elsevier;* 2005.

Wilkinson DJ, Casalaz D, Watkins A, Anderson CC, Duke T. Hypothermia: A neuroprotective therapy for neonatal hypoxic-ischemic encephalopathy. *Pediatrics* 2006; 119(2):422–23.

Wilkinson DJ, Singh M, Wyatt J. Ethical challenges in the use of therapeutic hypothermia in Indian neonatal units. *Indian Pediatr* 2010, 47:387–393.

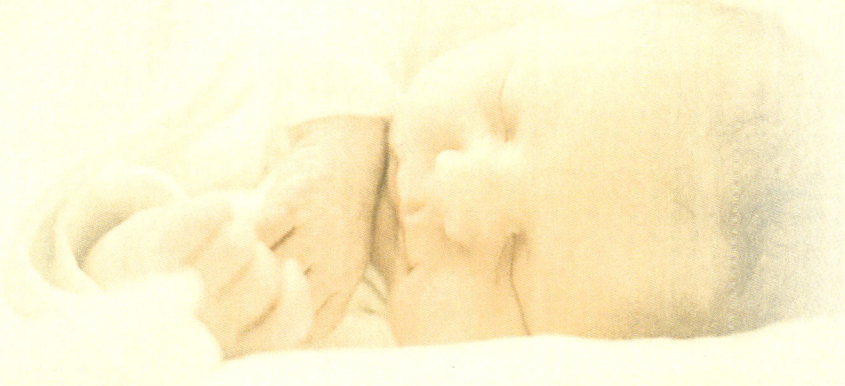

5

Life-threatening Congenital Malformations

Rhishikesh Thakre

BACKGROUND

Congenital malformation is a physical anomaly or a structural defect which is present at birth but may manifest at birth or later in life. Most of the times the anomalies are not life-threatening. Congenital malformations contribute significantly to perinatal morbidity and mortality. They can result in long-term disability, with significant impact on the affected individuals, families, healthcare system and society. The cause may be genetic, infectious, nutritional, environmental, teratogenic or multifactorial in origin. The malformation may be isolated or affect more than one system of the body. Many of these anomalies are amenable to timely surgery which can be life saving and improve long-term prognosis. This chapter identifies the common life-threatening congenital malformations and summarizes their clinical presentation, diagnosis and management. The common life-threatening malformations manifesting at birth are summarized in Table 5.1.

Table 5.1 Clinical features of common life-threatening congenital anomalies	
Malformation	*Clinical manifestations*
Choanal atresia	Respiratory distress at birth, inability to pass nasogastric tube through nose, cyanosis which is relieved on crying
Pierre Robin sequence	Micrognathia, retrognathia, cleft palate, glossoptosis and choking
Diaphragmatic hernia	Progressive respiratory distress, cyanosis, worsening on bag and mask ventilation, bowel sounds in thorax, heart sounds on right side, scaphoid abdomen, and polyhydramnios
Lung hypoplasia/Renal agenesis	Potter facies, prune-belly appearance of abdomen, unexplained pneumothorax, anuria, associated anomalies, oligohydramnios
Tracheo-esophageal fistula	Frothing at mouth, choking on feeding, inability to pass oro/nasogastric tube in stomach, single umbilical artery, and polyhydramnios
Duodenal-jeujno-ileal atresia and volvulus	Bilious vomiting, abdominal distension, constipation and dehydration
Malrotation of gut	Bilious vomiting, abdominal distension and constipation
Anorectal malformations	Non-passage of stool, absent or ectopic anal opening, passage of meconium through urethra
Gastroschisis/omphalocele	Gut herniation, intestinal obstruction, and polyhydramnios
Bladder neck obstruction	Delayed or nonpassage of urine and presence of three masses, distended urinary bladder and enlarged kidneys, oligohydramnios
Hydronephrosis	Bilateral abdominal masses in lumbar region
Meningomyelocele	Polyhydramnios, decreased fetal activity, elevated alpha-fetoprotein
Duct-dependent congenital heart disease	Cyanosis unrelieved by oxygen, cardiac murmur, and shock

AIRWAY AND RESPIRATORY ANOMALIES

Choanal Atresia

Choanal atresia is an important cause of congenital nasal airway obstruction. The usual incidence is one in 5,000–10,000 live births. There is partial or complete obliteration of posterior nares (bony, membranous or mixed) causing absent or decreased airflow from nasal cavity into the nasopharynx. It may be unilateral or bilateral, isolated or associated with other malformations and is seen more often in girls than boys. Unilateral choanal atresia occurs more frequently on the right side.

Clinical Features

Bilateral choanal atresia presents as a life-threatening emergency at birth. There is progressive cyanosis and or respiratory distress at birth, which is relieved on crying. There is inability to pass a nasal catheter (6 Fr) through the affected nare into the posterior pharynx. Feeding difficulty with choking during feeding may be seen because of inability to breathe and feed simultaneously. Absence of misting on the spatula or lack of movements on the wisp of cotton placed in front of the nares is suggestive of bilateral choanal artresia. About 50% of infants with bilateral atresia will have some the other abnormalities especially CHARGE association which is characterized by colobomas, heart defects, atresia of the choanae, growth retardation, genito-urinary abnormalities and ear deformities. Unilateral choanal atresia manifests with persistent mucoid uni-lateral nasal discharge or persistence of upper respiratory infection during first few months of life.

Investigations

CT scan of sinuses utilizing 2–5 mm cuts with prior suctioning and decongesting the nose, demonstrates narrowing of the posterior choanae to less than 34 mm.

Differential Diagnosis

Septal deviation, septal dislocation, nasal masses, and encephalocele should be excluded. Endoscopy is useful to rule out these anomalies.

Management

Bilateral choanal atresia requires immediate placement of oral airway or intubation to keep the airway patent. The newborn is nursed in a prone position. At times tracheostomy may be required. The definitive repair is done either endo-nasally or transpalatally with or without stent placement. Laser assisted surgery is increasingly used but offers no added advantage over conventional surgery. Treatment of unilateral choanal atresia is delayed beyond infancy to allow for midface growth.

Prognosis

Recurrence is seen in up to 25% of operated cases requiring repeat surgery or nasal dilatation. The prognosis is influenced by associated co-morbid conditions.

Craniofacial Syndromes

They are characterized by constellation of anomalies like enlarged tongue (e.g. Down syndrome, Beckwith-Wiedemann syndrome), small jaw (e.g. Pierre Robin sequence, Treacher Collins syndrome), or mid-face hypoplasia (e.g. Apert or Crouzon syndrome) which leads to glossoptosis manifesting with respiratory distress, cyanosis and choking on feeding. The diagnosis is generally obvious on physical examination by identification of facial dysmorphism (Figure 5.1).

Management

Nursing the baby prone, keeping the airway patent (e.g. suctioning, nasogastric tube), nasogastric feeding, respiratory support with continuous positive airway pressure (CPAP), intubation or tracheostomy are life saving options to stabilize the baby. The naso-pharyngeal tube may be left in place for weeks or even months. Most infants improve with conservative care. Additional interventions include tongue-lip adhesion surgery to hold the tongue forward and tracheostomy if a nasopharyngeal tube does not adequately relieve the obstruction.

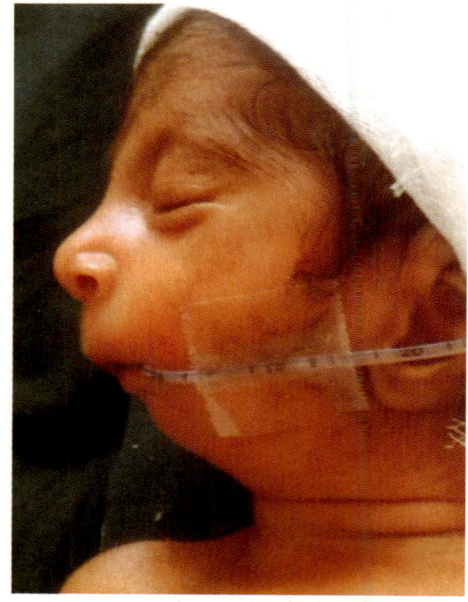

Figure 5.1 Pierre Robin syndrome showing characteristic features of micrognathia and retrognathia.

Congenital Diaphragmatic Hernia (CDH)

It is associated with a defect of the fetal diaphragm leading to herniation of abdominal contents into the thoracic cavity. It occurs due to persistence of pleuro-peritoneal canal and is seen in 1 out of every 2500–5000 live births. It is usually unilateral (98%) and mostly affects the left side of thoracic cavity (85%). It may be an isolated defect (70%) or associated with other major malformations.

The development of lung on the affected side is adversely affected with reduced number of conducting and functional airways with thickened alveolar walls, and increased interstitial tissue leading to progressive hypoplasia. There is maldevelopment of pulmonary vasculature with decreased number of vessels, adventitial thickening and medial hyperplasia. The most important factors influencing clinical presentation and outcome are primary pulmonary hypertension and pulmonary hypoplasia. Postnatally this leads to progressive hypoxia, respiratory insufficiency, pulmonary hypertension and poor pefusion of lungs. The most common form of CDH is the posterolateral Bochdalek hernia. Polyhdramnios is commonly associated.

Clinical Features

Majority of infants present at birth with progressive respiratory distress and cyanosis. During resuscitation, worsening of the condition of the baby on bag and mask ventilation should arouse the suspicion of underlying CDH. Clinical examination may reveal scaphoid abdomen, bulging hemithorax with bowel sounds on auscultation. There may be decreased air entry on the affected side and mediastinal shift to the opposite side (Figures 5.2 and 5.3). Up to 40% of affected infants have associated urinary, gastrointestinal and central nervous system anomalies. About 10% of cases have an underlying chromosomal abnormality e.g. Trisomies 13, 18 and 21. About 10% of cases may remain asymptomatic and present later in life. Bilateral diaphragmatic hernias are uncommon and are usually fatal.

Investigations

Prenatal ultrasound provides the earliest diagnosis by identification of polyhdramnios, mediastinal shift, hydrops and absence of intra-abdominal gastric air bubble. X-ry chest, posteroanterior and lateral views show bowel loops in the thorax. Abdominal and cranial sonography should be done in all cases. Echocardiography is useful to detect associated cardiac anomalies (18%).

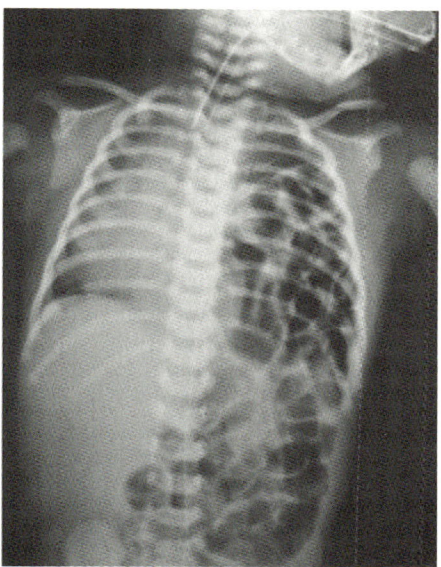

Figure 5.2 There are bowel loops in left hemithorax with shift of mediastinum to right side.

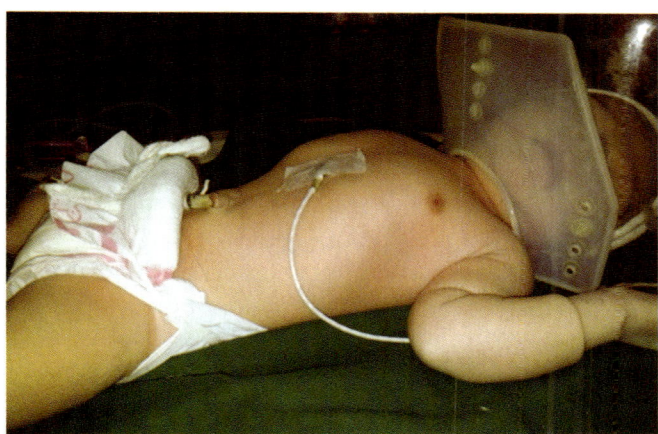

Figure 5.3 Scaphoid abdomen in an infant with congenital diaphragmatic hernia.

Differential Diagnosis

Congenital cystic adenomatoid malformation, broncho-pulmonary sequestration, and diaphragmatic eventration should be ruled out.

Management

a. **Stabilization** When diagnosis is suspected at the time of delivery, bag and mask ventilation should be avoided because it would lead to distension of herniated gut with further compromise of pulmonary functions. Elective intubation and decompression of stomach with a naso-orogastric tube is done at the earliest. Head end is raised and the infant is nursed in lateral decubitus with affected side down to reduce mediastinal displacement. During stabilization the infant is continuously monitored for thermal instability, hypoxia, hypercapnia, acidosis, perfusion and electrolyte imbalance.

Ventilation Respiratory support is provided with minimal sedation, avoidance of paralyzing agents, gentle ventilation with minimal distending pressures, allowing some degree of permissive hypercapnia and avoiding hyperventilation to minimize lung injury. High frequency ventilation is reserved for non-responsive cases. There are no data to show the superiority of high frequency ventilation over conventional ventilation. Refractory hypoxia is treated with ECMO. The administration of surfactant is controversial.

Pulmonary hypertension Pre- and postductal pulse oximetry is useful to assess the degree of PPHN because of right-to-left shunting at the level of the ductus arteriosus. Treatment options include pressor support, inhaled nitric oxide (iNO) and/or phospho-diesterase (PDE) inhibitors like sildenafil.

b. **Surgical repair** CDH is no longer considered as a dire emergency. Bowel decompression with a naso-orogastric tube and preoperative stabilization with delayed surgical repair is the current practice. The ideal time to repair congenital diaphragmatic hernia is not well-established but surgical intervention should be attempted only after stabilization of the infant. In majority of cases, primary closure of diaphragm is achieved but in others a 'patch' is used to close the defect. The most common early post-operative complications include pneumothorax or chylothorax. Thoracoscopic surgery is a useful option and is associated with reduced post-operative pain and improved cosmetic results. However, it is asso-ciated with increased risk of recurrent herniation. Attempts have been made to repair CDH *in utero* by endoscopic occlusion of fetal trachea at 26–28 weeks gestation. The trapped fetal lung secretions promotes the growth of lungs with reduced risk of pulmonary hypoplasia.

Prognosis

Surgical intervention has decreased mortality but short and long-term morbidities (e.g. chronic lung disease, recurrent respiratory infections, gastroesophageal reflux, failure to thrive, neuromotor disability, hearing and cognitive deficits) are seen in survivors. The outcome is dependent on gestational age, severity of pulmonary hypoplasia, pulmonary hypertension and associated anomalies. Prenatal scans showing liver, stomach and spleen herniation into the chest on left side, and observed to expected (O/E) lung area to head circumference ratio (LHR) of <25% are associated with poor survival. Recurrence rates are approximately 15% in the first two years of life especially in cases of large defects repaired with a patch.

Congenital Pulmonary Airway Malformation (CPAM)

Formerly called **congenital cystic adenomatoid malformation** (CCAM), the lesions are characterized by proliferation and cystic dilatation of terminal respiratory bronchioles with varying epithelial lining. They communicate with the bronchial tree and have blood supply derived from the pulmonary circulation. They account for approximately 25% of all congenital lung malformations and is seen in 1:25,000 to 1:35,000 live births. CPAMs can affect any lobe an both sides of the lungs. They commonly involve only one lobe, rarely multiple, but in 15% cases involve two or more lobes on either ipsilateral or contralateral side.

Clinical Features

Symptomatic lesions present with respiratory distress of varying severity like tachypnea, chest retractions, grunt or progressive respiratory failure in early neonatal period. The timing and severity of respiratory distress are determined by underlying pulmonary hypoplasia, mediastinal shift, air trapping, pneumothorax, and pleural effusion secondary to hydrops fetalis. In about 60% cases there are associated congenital anomalies with microcystic CPAM. Polyhydramnios may be associated in several cases. Many cases are asymptomatic and detected on routine chest radiography or are discovered because of repeated chest infections in infancy or adulthood.

Investigations

Prenatal ultrasound provides early diagnosis. The prenatally diagnosed lesions may be asymptomatic at birth (71%), and they may have normal radiographic findings (57%). Prenatal regression and complete resolution of CPAM have also been described. An air-fluid level may be seen. Symptomatic lesions require urgent chest radiography and ideally a CT scan. X-ray chest reveals a mass containing air-filled cyst but it is likely to under estimate or miss many of the lesions. There may be associated mediastinal shift, pleural and pericardial effusions, and pneumothoraces. The presence of superimposed infection may complicate the radiological appearances. CT lungs with intravenous contrast and 3D reformats showing multilocular cystic lesions with thin walls surrounded by normal lung parenchyma is diagnostic. High resolution CT is able to define lobar involvement, delineate size of cysts

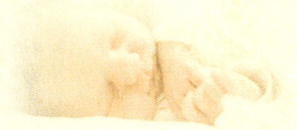

within lesions, as well as mapping of arterial and venous anatomy. Depending upon their size, the lesions are classified as macrocytic (>5 mm) and microcystic (<5 mm). Approximately 25% of lesions diagnosed as CPAM may be either pulmonary sequestration or bronchogenic cysts. The role of MRI is limited in the characterization of CPAMs, given its poor spatial resolution relative to CT. Renal and cranial ultrasound and echocardiography is done to rule out associated anomalies.

Differential Diagnosis

The conditions like congenital diaphragmatic hernia, lung sequestration, pneumothorax, pneumatocele, pleural effusion and pulmonary interstitial emphysema should be excluded.

Management

Early surgery is advocated for symptomatic babies. Surgical lobectomy is favored by many centers because of the increased risk of infection and potential for malignant transformation. Minimally invasive video-assisted thoracoscopic approach is effective in experienced hands. The conservative management is advised for lesions less than 1.0 cm in size though spontaneous resolution is rare. In stable patients, the timing of elective surgery is controversial. Fetal surgery is reserved for large lesions and hydrops.

Prognosis

Symptomatic lesions carry high morbidity. The outcome is excellent for asymptomatic cases. The recovery is complete following effective surgical excision. The outcome is poor in infants with bilateral disease, microcystic CPAMs and hydrops fetalis.

Bronchoalveolar carcinoma and rhabdomyosarcoma are potential complications seen in association with CPAM.

Bronchopulmonary Sequestrations (BPS)

These lesions are estimated to comprise up to 6% of all congenital pulmonary malformations. They are characterized by a cystic mass which may be either intralobar lung sequestration (ILS) or extralobar sequestration (ELS). ILS are contained within the lung, do not have their own pleura and drain via pulmonary veins. Extrapulmonary sequestrations are completely covered with pleura and drain via systemic veins. These areas of non-functioning lung tissue do not connect to the tracheobronchial tree. Overall, 98% of pulmonary sequestrations occur in the lower lobes. In the extrapulmonary sequestration, males are affected approximately four times more often than females.

Clinical Features

ELS are more common (75%) and have additional congenital anomalies in 65% cases. The timing of presentation depends upon associated pulmonary anomalies like congenital pulmonary adenomatoid malformation (CPAM), congenital diaphragmatic hernia, and pulmonary hypoplasia. ILS is usually isolated and presents in late childhood (Table 5.2).

Investigations

X-ray chest usually shows a radio-opaque mass. It is difficult to distinguish an intrapulmonary sequestration from extrapulmonary sequestration on plain skiagram of chest. Extralobar pulmonary sequestrations are more often solid and are associated with elevation of the ipsilateral diaphragm. Intralobar pulmonary

Table 5.2 Characteristics of two types pulmonary sequestrations		
Features	*Intralobar*	*Extralobar*
Gender	No predilection	Males are affected more often in a ratio of 4:1
Anatomy	Located within the lobe of the lung, no separate pleura	Located outside the lung lobe with a separate pleura
Bronchial communication	Present	None
Usual side	Left side in 60% cases	Left side in 90% cases
Location	Commonly located in the posterior basal segment	Usually located above the diaphragm
Age at presentation	Adolescent to young adults	Neonate in 60% cases
Symptoms	Asymptomatic or recurrent chest infections	Respiratory distress
Associated anomalies	Uncommon	Associated in more than 50% cases
Arterial supply	Single large vessel from aorta	Multiple small vessels from pulmonary circulation or aorta
Venous drainage	Inferior pulmonary vein	Azygos or hemiazygos vein; rarely portal vein

sequestration appears more cystic and may show air if a pulmonary communication exists. Ultrasonography of lung reveals solid, well-circumscribed echogenic masses. Vascular supply may be better identified with Doppler imaging. Contrast-enhanced CT remains the most widely used diagnostic modality. A hybrid lesion should be considered where features of CPAM are identified within the mass but associated with anomalous systemic arterial supply on CT. The definitive diagnosis is made by using angiography (conventional, CT angiography, or magnetic resonance angiography), which delineates the feeding vessel to the sequestrated lobe along with its venous drainage. MRI offers no advantage over CECT chest.

Differential Diagnosis

Congenital pulmonary adnomatoid malformation should be excluded because of identical clinical and imaging features.

Management

Early surgical management is advocated for symptomatic ILS lesions. Surgery involves lobectomy or non-anatomical segmentectomy. Intrapulmonary sequestrations often require lobectomy because the margins of the sequestration may not be clearly defined. Expectant management with serial imaging is offered to asymptomatic infants with ELS.

Prognosis

Prognosis depends on the degree of pulmonary hypoplasia and associated anomalies.

Congenital Lobar Overinflation (CLO)

Previously termed congenital lobar emphysema (CLE). it is characterized by hyperinflation of one or more pulmonary lobes due to partial obstruction with mucus or meconium plug. There is progressive air trapping with compression of surrounding structures. It occurs in 1 in 20,000 to 1 in 30,000 live births.

Clinical Features

The infant may be asymptomatic and the lesion may be detected incidentally on radiography. Almost 50% of cases present in neonatal period. The common features include tachypnea, respiratory distress, cyanosis, mediastinal shift or significant wheezing. At times the infant presents with sudden progressive respiratory insufficiency secondary to air leak, triggered by positive pressure ventilation. There are associated anomalies in about 40% of cases, most commonly cardiovascular anomalies like PDA and VSD.

Investigations

Fetal diagnosis can be made by prenatal ultrasonography. There is hyperlucency in the hyperinflated lobe on X-ray chest. When large, it may cause contralateral mediastinal shift and atelectasis of adjacent lobes (Figure 5.4). It occurs most commonly in the left upper lobe. Hypoplasia or agenesis of the contralateral lung may result in a marked compensatory hyperexpansion of the lung, which can closely mimic CLO. CT lungs is confirmatory while magnetic resonance imaging (MRI) is not routinely required. It can be used as an adjunct modality to evaluate the vascular supply to the affected lobe.

Treatment

Asymptomatic infants with small lesions may be observed and managed expectantly with the hope that the lesion may resolve spontaneously. Large lesions and those with sudden decompensation require thoracotomy with lobectomy to restore ventilation. The importance of careful induction of anesthesia cannot be overemphasized as these patients may not tolerate positive pressure ventilation which can lead to air trapping, air leak syndrome and rarely cardiac arrest.

Prognosis

The prognosis is favorable, but depends on the associated abnormalities.

Lung Maldevelopment

Lung maldevelopment is classified as pulmonary agenesis (total absence of the lung, bronchus, and pulmonary artery); pulmonary aplasia (total absence

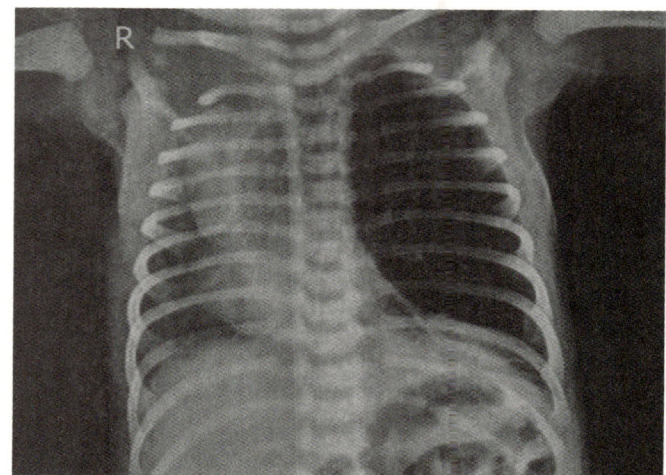

Figure 5.4 Emphysematous left upper lobe with compressed lung tissue with mediastinal displacement.

of the lung and pulmonary artery with a rudimentary blind-ending main bronchus); and pulmonary hypoplasia (hypoplastic bronchus and pulmonary artery associated with variable amounts of lung tissue). It may be unilateral or bilateral, isolated or as a consequence of other malformations. Pulmonary hypoplasia may be primary, but it is usually secondary, due to reduction in intrathoracic space, fetal breathing movements, or reduced amniotic fluid volume.

Clinical Features

The clinical profile and the time of presentation vary depending on the extent of hypoplasia and presence of associated anomalies. There may be tachypnea, respiratory distress, cyanosis or increasing need for ventilator support. The chest appears small, bell shaped, with decreased or absent air entry. There may be retractions of chest with shift of mediastinum towards the involved side. Infants with unilateral pulmonary agenesis, aplasia, and hypoplasia may be asymptomatic. There may be features to suggest the underlying cause of lung hypoplasia. Myopathic facies, with a V-shaped mouth, muscle weakness, and growth restriction suggest underlying neuromuscular disease. The Potter facies (hypertelorism, epicanthus, retrognathia, depressed nasal bridge, low set ears) suggest the possibility of lung hypoplasia secondary to renal agenesis. The condition is commonly associated with prematurity (up to 30% in <28 weeks gestation), oligohydramnios, renal dysplasia (including Potter syndrome), neuromuscular disease affecting the thoracic wall, diaphragmatic hernia, Scimitar syndrome (right-sided pulmonary hypoplasia with partial anomalous venous return) and mediastinal masses or congenital heart disease like tetralogy of Fallot. Over 50% cases are associated with VACTERL syndrome (vertebral, anorectal, cardiac, tracheoesophageal fistula, renal and limb anomalies).

Investigations

X-ray chest shows varying degree of low volume lungs. Radio-opaque lung fields are seen in neonates with lung agenesis and aplasia. There is ipsilateral elevated hemidiaphragm and mediastinal shift. There may be compensatory lung hyperinflation on the contralateral side. Ribs may be thin or slender and cave inwards. Renal profile should be checked. Doppler ultrasonography to determine pulmonary artery blood velocity waveforms, can be used to diagnose pulmonary hypoplasia in the fetus. CT is the modality of choice for differentiating pulmonary agenesis, aplasia, and hypoplasia.

Management

The treatment is directed towards the underlying cause, e.g. CDH, congenital pulmonary airway malformation (CPAM), renal impairment. Respiratory support is provided in the form of oxygen, and conventional ventilation. Refractory hypoxia may require high frequency ventilation or ECMO. Surfactant therapy has been tried with variable results. The utility of inhaled nitric oxide is marginal.

Outcome

Risk factors for a poor outcome include the presence of hydrops fetalis, pulmonary hypertension, severity of associated anomalies viz congenital diaphragmatic hernia, congenital adenomatoid malformation and renal impairment. The tetrad of pulmonary hypoplasia, positional limb deformities, Potter facies, and intrauterine growth restriction in a pregnancy complicated with oligohydramnios predicts poor outcome.

Congenital Chylothorax

Chylothorax is collection of chyle in the pleural space as a result of congenital anomaly of thoracic duct. It is the most common form of pleural effusion in neonates. It may be an isolated lesion or secondary to other anomalies.

Clinical Features

Classically there is respiratory distress at birth. The breath sounds are decreased or absent on the affected side with dullness on percussion. If severe, the fluid produces mediastinal and tracheal shift to the contralateral side. There may be associated dysmorphism, congenital anomalies or hydrops. There may be history of difficult delivery because trauma to the thoracic duct may occur because of difficult breech extraction. The common genetic conditions which may be associated with chylothorax include Down syndrome, Noonan syndrome and Turner syndrome.

Investigations

Prenatal ultrasound provides useful clues for early diagnosis. The presence of polyhydramnios, hydrops fetalis, and pleural effusion on fetal ultrasound is highly suggestive of congenital chylothorax. Postnatally, ultrasonography or skiagram of chest shows pleural effusion with or without shift of mediastinum. A diagnostic pleural tap confirms the diagnosis. Analysis reveals a milky fluid, fat content >400 mg/dL, protein >5 g/dL and plenty of lymphocytes. If the triglyceride level is above 110 mg/dL and the ratio of the pleural fluid cholesterol to serum cholesterol is <1.0, the diagnosis is confirmed. Lymphangiography and lymphoscintigraphy both require the administration of a contrast agent to study the lymphatics. CT and MRI thorax further delineate the anatomy and can identify the space occupying lesion secondary to tumors such as lymphoma, neuroblastoma and other metastatic malignancies which may cause chylothorax by obstructing the lymphatic flow in the thoracic duct.

Treatment

Most cases require respiratory support. Feeds should be restricted. A pleural drain helps to drain the effusion (Figure 5.5). Effusions may recur and take up to 6 weeks to resolve. Pleural effusion may be decreased by administration of somatostatin (continuous infusion) or octreotide (intermittent subcutaneous injection). Monitoring of serum glucose, thyroid functions, liver enzymes and indicators of cholestasis during therapy is recommended. Once the chest drainage has resolved, oral feeds are reintroduced with an MCT based formula for 3 to 6 weeks before transitioning to normal feeds. A more aggressive option is to provide complete enteric rest by using total parenteral nutrition. Whether enteral or parenteral nutrition is chosen, the calories, electrolytes, and volume must match with those lost in the chyle. If pleural drainage exceeds 10 mL/kg per day after 4 weeks of conservative management, other agents used in the treatment of chylothorax include nitric oxide and etilefrine. Surgery is rarely needed and reserved for persistent chylothorax but it is associated with variable results.

Prognosis

The complications and consequences include malnutrition, hyponatremia, fluid imbalance, increased risk of thrombosis and nosocomial infection secondary to immunodeficiency. The prognosis depends on the etiology, its response to medical/surgical therapies, and the likely complications.

Scimitar Syndrome (Hypogenetic Lung Syndrome or Pulmonary Venolobar Syndrome)

It is characterized by a hypoplastic right lung, partial anomalous venous return and unilateral pulmonary sequestration.

Clinical Features

The infant may remain asymptomatic and the condition is detected incidentally. At times these infants may develop symptoms of congestive cardiac failure. Recurrent right basal pneumonia should arouse the suspicion of this condition. The associated anomalies include cardiac (ASD, VSD, dextrocardia, patent ductus arteriosus, tetralogy of Fallot), ipsilateral diaphragmatic hernia, genitourinary tract abnormalities and vertebral anomalies (hemivertebrae).

Investigations

X-ray chest reveals low volume hyperlucent right lung (Figure 5.6). There may be ipsilateral mediastinal shift and hyperinflation of the contralateral lung. CT or MRI angiography confirms the diagnosis.

Treatment

The condition can be managed by ligation or coil embolization of systemic feeding vessel(s). When there is no satisfactory systemic feeding vessel, pneumonectomy is done if other lung is normal.

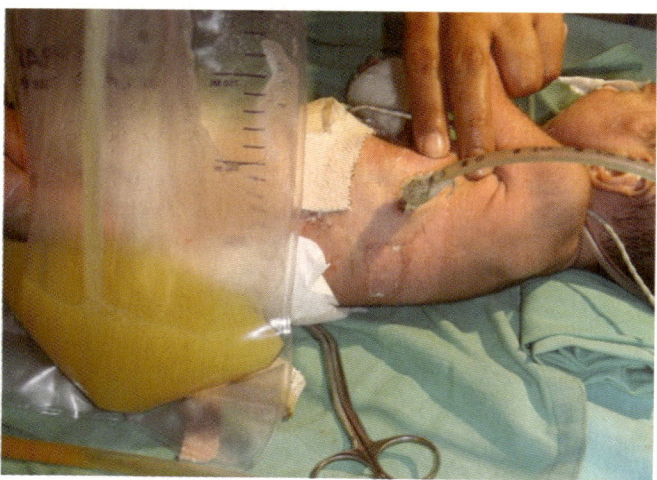

Figure 5.5 The intercostal drain in-situ for draining of chylous fluid.

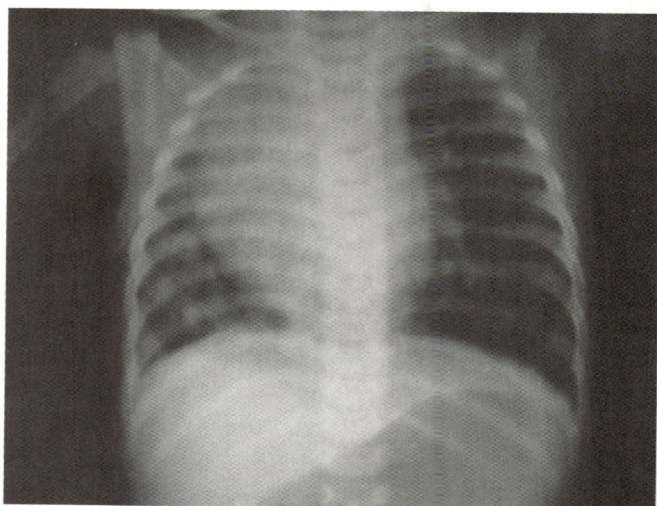

Figure 5.6 Scimitar sign. There is a small lung volume on the right side with ipsilateral mediastinal shift and anomalous draining vein seen as a tubular structure paralleling the right heart border in the shape of a Turkish sword ("scimitar").

GI MALFORMATIONS

Intestinal Obstruction

Obstruction of the gastrointestinal tract of a neonate can occur anywhere from the esophagus to the anus. The duodenum (33%) is the most frequent site of obstruction followed by ileum (25%), jejunum (15%) and colon (10%); and in the remaining 17% there are multiple sites of atresia (Figure 5.7).

Esophageal Atresia (EA)/Tracheoesophageal Fistula (TEF)

There is incomplete formation of the esophagus which ends in a blind pouch with or without a connection to trachea. Feeds and saliva may trickle into the trachea and lungs through the fistula. Five types have been described (Table 5.3). The incidence varies between 1 in 3000 to 1 in 4500 live births.

Table 5.3 Gross-Vogt classification of tracheoesophageal anomalies		
Type A	Isolated esophageal atresia	7.8%
Type B	Esophageal atresia + Proximal TEF	0.8%
Type C	Esophageal atresia + Distal TEF	85.8%
Type D	Esophageal atresia + Double TEF	1.4%
Type E	Isolated TEF (H-type fistula)	4.2%
TEF: tracheoesophageal fitula		

Clinical Features

The infant classically presents with excessive salivation and frothing during the first few hours of life with or without respiratory distress (Figure 5.8). There may be choking and cyanosis on feeding. A high index of suspicion is required because the symptoms are non-specific and vary in intensity. The abdomen appears distended if there is a fistula or scaphoid if no fistula exists. The condition is associated with other clinical defects in more than 50% of babies, notably the VACTERL sequence (vertebral, anorectal, cardiac, tracheoesophageal, renal, and limb defects) and CHARGE Association (coloboma, heart defects, atresia choanae, retarded development, genital hypoplasia, ear abnormalities) and chromosomal defects (Trisomy 18 and 21, Di George syndrome). Isolated EA without TEF is associated with a higher incidence of other malformations. Presence of unexplained chest infections, episodes of choking and cough with feeding during childhood should raise the possibility of H type fistula which is rare.

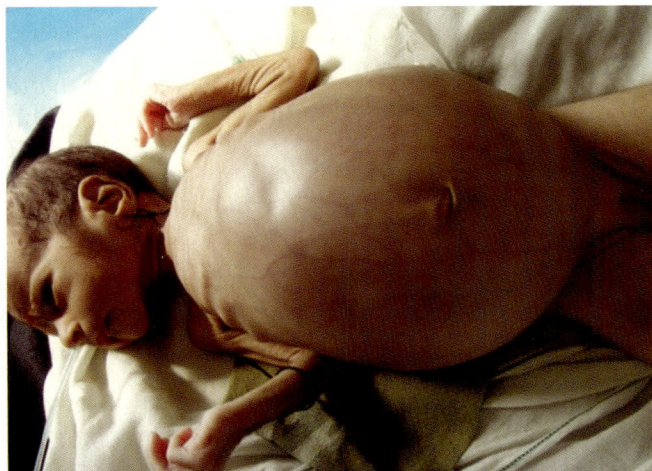

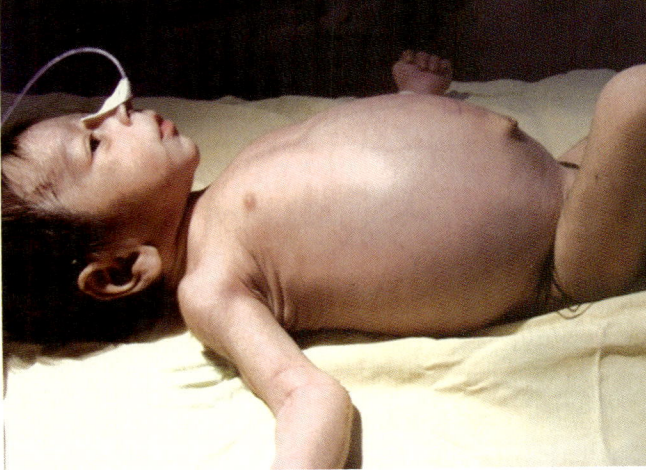

Figure 5.7 There is generalized abdominal distention with visible veins over the abdomen due to multiple atresias in ileum.

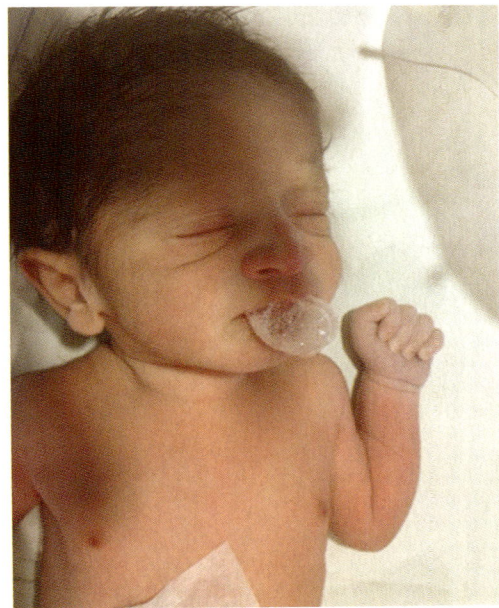

Figure 5.8 Persistent frothing and drooling in an infant with esophageal atresia and tracheoesophageal fistula.

Investigations

X-ray chest is done by including entire abdomen (postero-anterior and lateral views) after inserting a stiff red rubber catheter (8–10 Fr) through the mouth till resistance is felt in the upper esophageal pouch. In patients with esophageal atresia, the tube typically stops at 10 to 12 cm. If a soft, flexible tube is used, it may curl in the upper pouch and give a false impression that the tube has passed to the stomach (Figure 5.9). Absence of stomach shadow suggests esophageal atresia without a TEF or esophageal atresia with a proximal TEF (Figure 5.10). Chest radiographs should be evaluated carefully for skeletal abnormalities, cardio-vascular malformations, pneumonia in the right upper

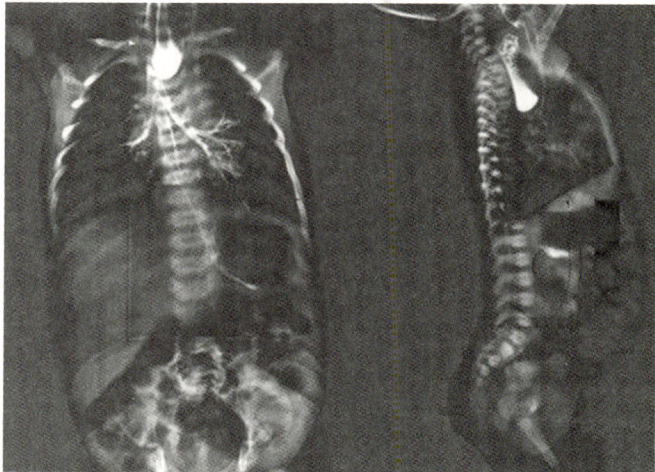

Figure 5.11 Dye study showing TEF.

lobe and a right aortic arch. The abdominal radiographic series will aid evaluation of skeletal abnormalities, intestinal obstruction and malrotation. Contrast study and fiberoptic bronchoscopy are performed if the diagnosis is in doubt (Figure 5.11). An echocardiogram and renal ultrasonogram should be obtained to rule out associated anomalies. Maternal polyhydramnios and absence of the fetal stomach bubble on prenatal ultra-sound is suggestive of TEF.

Differential Diagnosis

Laryngeal cleft, velopharyngeal incompetence, vascular ring and gastroesophageal reflux should be ruled out.

Management

Stabilization The infant is kept nil by mouth, nursed prone, with the head end raised, with frequent or continuous suctioning to maintain airway patency and reduce the risk of aspiration. Oxygen is given if there is respiratory distress. When sepsis or pulmonary infection is suspected, broad-spectrum antibiotics (ampicillin plus gentamicin) should be administered. Surgery is done at the earliest before pulmonary complications occur. Surgical repair is delayed in extre-mely preterm or LBW babies and infants with aspiration pneumonia and associated major malformations.

Surgery The standard procedure for EA-TEF is a right posterolateral (extrapleural) thoracotomy, fistula ligation, and primary esophageal anastomosis. A high leak rate, esophageal stricture, and gastroesophageal reflux are common complications seen with "long gap" repairs (more than two vertebral bodies or more than 3 cm). In isolated EA, management involves formation of a gastrostomy for feeding and suctioning of the "blind" upper pouch to keep the airway patent. Options

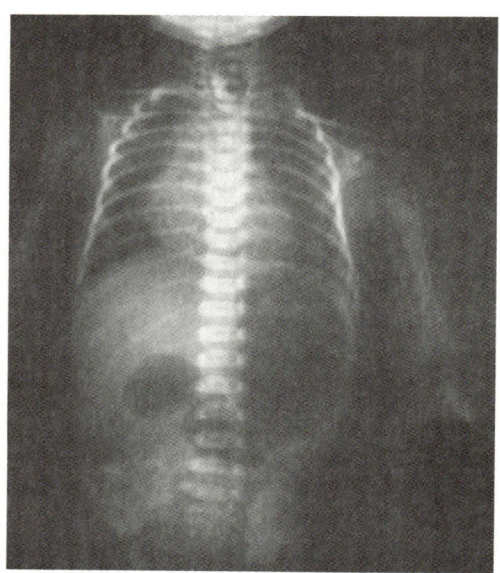

Figure 5.9 Note the coiling of tube in esophagus with double bubble shadow.

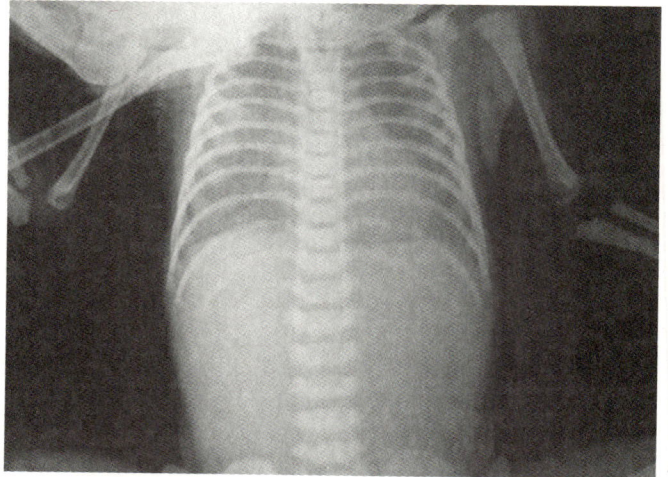

Figure 5.10 The catheter is in upper pouch with gasless abdomen in an infant with esophageal atresia without TEF.

for reconstruction include delayed primary repair using the native esophagus or replacement by using isolated colon or stomach (gastric tube or transposition). Minimally invasive thoracoscopic repair is an option in experienced hands. Antireflux medical treatments (including feed thickeners, H2 blockers, proton pump inhibitors, and prokinetic drugs) are given for 12–18 months because of high risk of gastroesophageal reflux disease (GERD).

Prognosis

The immediate survival is good if there are no co-morbid conditions (Table 5.4). Presence of gastro-esophageal reflux, anastomotic strictures, and/or esophageal dysmotility leads to feeding problems and nutritional insufficiency. Due to airway instability and tendency for alveolar collapse, these infants have repeated bouts of harsh barking "TEF cough" and recurrent chest infections in early infancy. Congenital cardiac defects and the anomalies of the VACTERL Association are major risk factors for survival (Figure 5.12). Repeated dilatations are necessary in nearly 40 % of patients who develop esophageal stricture.

Congenital Duodenal Obstruction

Duodenal obstruction may arise as a result of atresia, stenosis, web, annular pancreas or malrotation. The overall incidence is about one in 6000 births.

Clinical Features

Duodenal atresia manifests early with bile stained vomiting while stenosis may take several weeks to months to become symptomatic. There may be history of polyhydramnios in mother. These infants are usually preterm or small-for-dates. Half of the infants with duodenal atresia have associated abnormalities, such as malrotation, other bowel atresias, i.e. esophageal atresia and imperforate anus, heart defects, anomalies of the bile ducts etc. Upto 30% of cases of duodenal atresia have Down syndrome.

Investigations

Erect X-ray abdomen shows classical "double bubble" appearance (Figure 5.13). This may not be seen on a preliminary or early radiograph. Instilling 50 mL of air into the stomach through orogastric tube often provides a sufficient amount of "contrast" to establish the diagnosis in doubtful cases. Use of contrast study is rarely required. Ultrasound may show a dilated stomach and proximal duodenum as a large fluid-filled cystic mass.

Differential Diagnosis

Duodenal diverticulum, aberrant pancreas, choledochal cyst, and congenital peritoneal bands should be excluded.

Group	Criteria	Incidence (%)	Survival (%)
I	Birth weight >1500 g without major congenital cardiac defects	79	97
II	Birth weight <1500 g or >1500 g with presence of major congenital cardiac defect	19	59
III	Birth weight <1500 g and presence of major congenital cardiac defect	2	2

Table 5.4 Spitz classification for survival of TEF

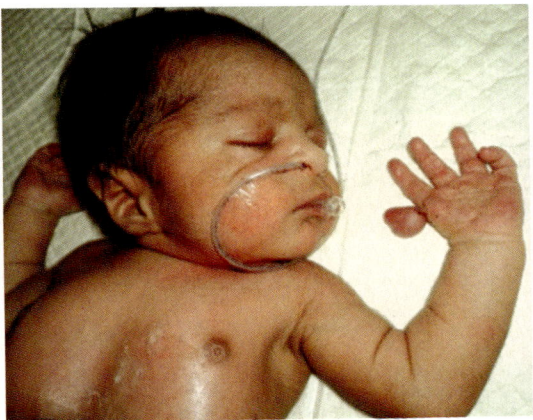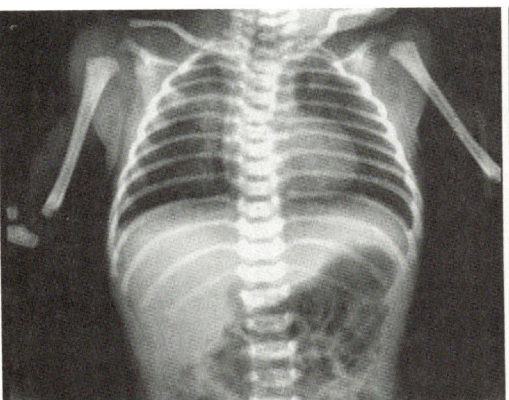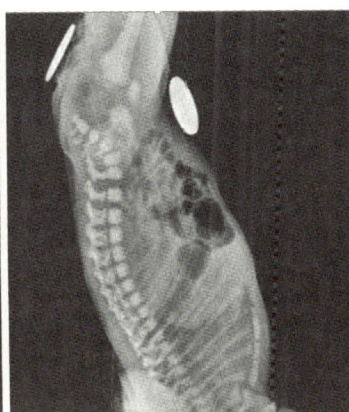

Figure 5.12 VACTERL Association. Frothing at mouth, limb anomaly, coiling of feeding tube in upper esophageal pouch, narrow based heart with egg-on-end appearance and vertebral defects.

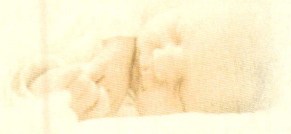

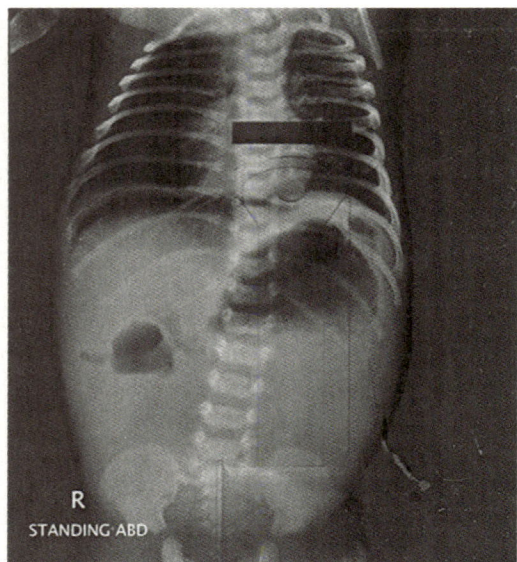

Figure 5.13 Double bubble appearance in an infant with duodenal atresia.

Management

Immediate surgical correction is carried out in infants who are stable with no associated major anomalies. Infants with obstruction due to malrotation are also operated at the earliest because of potential risk of development of volvulus. Infants with Down syndrome should also be operated. In sick patients, measures are taken to ensure, normal blood gases, euoglycemia, normotension and normothermia. The surgical procedure of choice is duodeno-duodenostomy or duodeno-jejunostomy for duodenal atresia/stenosis and annular pancreas.

Prognosis

The outcome is good in infants with isolated duodenal obstruction without any associated major malformations.

Jejunal/Ileal Obstruction

The incidence of jejunal and ileal atresia ranges from 1 in 1,500 to 12,000 live births. Atresia accounts for 95% of jejunoileal obstruction and stenosis accounts for the remaining 5% of cases. The ileum is slightly more affected than jejunum (55% vs 45%). In more than 90% of patients, there is a single site of atresia, however, multiple atresias are reported in 6–20% of cases.

Clinical Features

The hallmark of jejunal obstruction is abdominal distention. It is more marked in a case of distal atresia. The symptoms usually appear after 12–24 hours of starting enteral feeds. A normal or scaphoid abdomen in a neonate with bilious vomiting is indicative of a proximal obstruction. The vomiting is clear initially but becomes bilious by day 2–3. Jejunoileal atresia is seen in association with malrotation, meconium ileus, and gastroschisis. History of polyhydramnios during prenatal ultrasonographic evaluation is common. Most infants are likely to be preterm and low birth weight.

Investigations

Erect skiagram of abdomen shows large dilated loops of bowel with air fluid levels (Figure 5.14). The lower the atresia, greater are the number of such distended loops. In jejunal atresia, plain abdominal radiograph reveals a dilated gastric bubble and a massively dilated duodenum and proximal jejunum with a gasless abdomen distal to the level of obstruction. Barium enema helps to differentiate between small bowel and colon distention and to look for microcolon and position of cecum.

Differential Diagnosis

Malrotation with or without volvulus, meconium ileus, and Hirschsprung disease should be excluded.

Management

Laparotomy with excision and end-to-end anastomosis is performed at the earliest. A single stage repair of multiple atresias with restoration of intestinal continuity and preservation of maximal bowel length is the preferred operative procedure. Postoperative ileus and anatomic dysfunction may last up to two weeks in some cases. Special attention is given to ensure balance of fluids and electrolytes, tissue perfusion and nutrition.

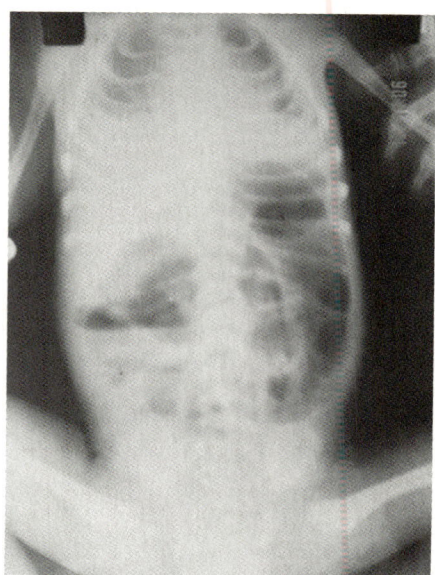

Figure 5.14 Air fluid levels with gasless distal gut in an infant with ileal atresia.

Prognosis

Early diagnosis and prompt intervention is associated with good outcome. The most common cause of death in infants with jejunoileal atresia is intercurrent infection leading to pneumonia, peritonitis, or sepsis. The common surgical complications include anastomotic leaks and functional intestinal obstruction at the level of the anastomosis in as many as 15% of patients. The overall prognosis depends upon the length of residual functional bowel. Prematurity, birth weight <2 kg, and associated anomalies are independent risk factors for prolonged hospital stay and higher case fatality rate.

Colonic Atresia

Colonic atresia is the least common type of intestinal atresias. They may occur at any site in the colon; however, atresias proximal to the splenic flexure and distal to the vascular watershed area are the most common. It is believed to be caused by an *in utero* vascular accident resulting in ischemic injury.

Clinical Features

Patients usually present with progressive abdominal distention and failure to pass meconium. The anus usually appears normal. Failure to pass any meconium suggests atresia, whereas delayed passage of meconium (>24 hours) suggests Hirschsprung's disease. At times patients with colonic atresia may pass meconium normally because the incident that caused the atresia may have occurred after the colon had become filled with meconium. Colonic atresias are frequently associated with other anomalies, including jejunoileal atresia, Hirschsprung's disease, and genitourinary malformations.

Investigations

Prenatal ultrasound provides early diagnosis. Plain abdominal radiograph reveals bowel obstruction with or without a prominent dilated loop and absence of gas in the rectum (Figure 5.15). Contrast enema is useful to rule out the presence of other atresias.

Management

Stabilization is achieved by fluid resuscitation, antibiotics and decompression of the stomach. The decision to proceed with primary resection and anastomosis or stoma diversion depends on the patient's condition. The management of colonic atresia is directed at resecting the site of obstruction and establishing intestinal continuity. This may be performed in one stage or in a phased manner depending on co-morbidities.

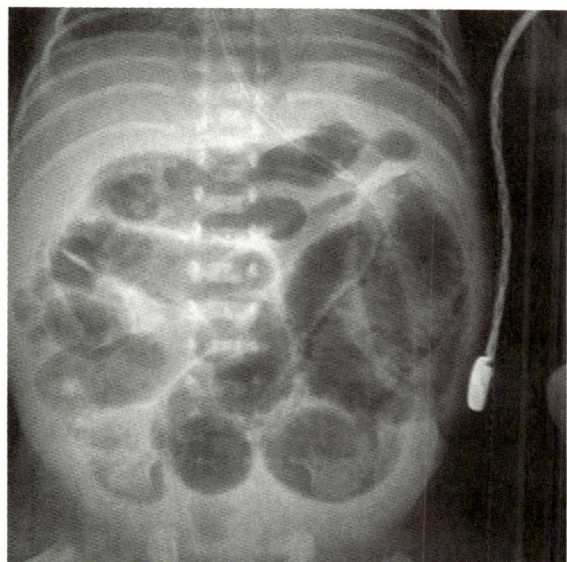

Figure 5.15 Dilated bowel loops in an infant with distal obstruction.

Malrotation

Intestinal malrotation is defined as nonrotation or incomplete rotation of the intestines around the superior mesenteric artery. It is usually associated with anomalies of intestinal fixation. Malrotation can occur at several locations and leads to either acute and subacute presentations. The incidence of intestinal malrotation is one in 500 live births. It may be an isolated problem or may be incidentally detected in association with other anomalies. The infant may have incomplete duodenal obstruction due to peritoneal (Ladd) bands compressing the duodenum. Because the mesentery is not properly fixed and attached, these infants are at risk for developing midgut volvulus.

Clinical Features

The classical presentation is bilious vomiting in a well infant which is secondary to duodenal obstruction caused by Ladd bands. A high index of suspicion is needed because some infants may have intermittent abdominal pain, vomiting, and absence of abdominal distention in the initial period. When volvulus is superimposed, the infant appears lethargic, refuses feeds and may pass altered or fresh blood per rectum. Rapid development of dehydration, hypovolemia and metabolic acidosis occurs when circulation gets compromised leading to poor perfusion. Incomplete rotation is seen in association with congenital diaphragmatic hernia as well as abdominal wall anomalies such as omphalocele and gastroschisis. Delay in diagnosis may result in extensive infarction of the bowel.

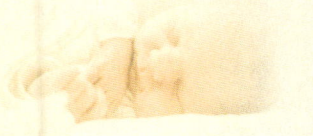

Investigations

Abdominal X-ray shows an abnormal distribution of bowel gas but appearances are variable. The classical findings are gasless abdomen with air present in the stomach and duodenum. In the stable neonate, an upper gastrointestinal contrast examination can demonstrate the duodenal rotation and determine if volvulus is present. Upper gastrointestinal contrast study remains the first line investigation for suspected malrotation (Figure 5.16). Ultrasonography has been shown to be very sensitive and presence of inversion of the superior mesenteric artery and the superior mesenteric vein is diagnostic. Use of Doppler ultrasound demonstrates the orientation of the superior mesenteric artery to the vein.

Management

In a clinically unstable neonate, investigations should not delay surgery. Surgery aims to reduce any volvulus, divide all obstructing bands of mesentery and increase the width of the base of the mesentery (Ladd's procedure) to prevent recurrence of rotation of the gut. Minimal invasive surgery is preferred as an initial approach to surgical correction of malrotation without midgut volvulus.

Prognosis

Early diagnosis and prompt intervention is associated with excellent outcome. Prognosis depends on the extent of ischemic damage due to volvulus and associated malformations.

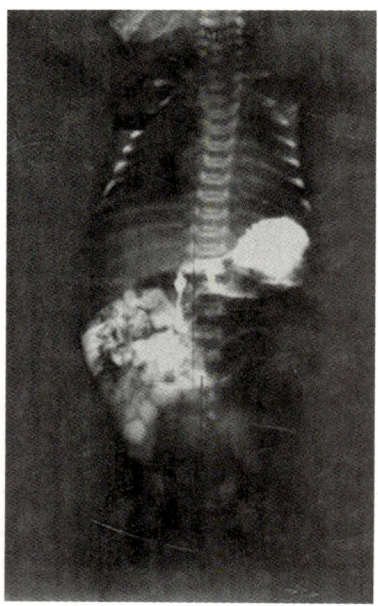

Figure 5.16 Dye study showing midgut malrotation.

Duplication of the Gut

Midgut duplications are the most common (50%) followed by foregut (38%) and hindgut (12%).

Clinical Features

The clinical presentation is variable. The newborn may have a distended abdomen and a palpable cystic mass. A small proportion of infants with duplications may present with features of subacute intestinal obstruction like vomiting, abdominal distension, colic, constipation, intestinal bleeding and peritonitis. Duplication may also act as a lead point for development of intussusception or volvulus.

Investigations

Abdominal sonography is diagnostic as it confirms the presence of cystic or tubular duplication. Plain X-rays may demonstrate obstruction and associated abnormalities of the vertebrae. Contrast studies are done to identify the level of obstruction and locate any site of compression. Isotope scans are of limited utility. At times laparotomy confirms the diagnosis.

Differential Diagnosis

Ovarian cyst, hemangioma, teratoma, lymphangioma, mesenteric cyst, meconium cyst, choledochal cyst, lower urinary tract obstruction and myelomeningocele, should be excluded.

Treatment

The treatment of duplication is surgical resection either by nucleation or excision of the affected bowel with end-to-end anastomosis.

Gastroschisis

Gastroschisis is a prenatal, paraumbilical herniation of the gut contents through a defect in the anterior abdominal wall. It is usually an isolated anomaly.

Clinical Features

Gastroschisis is usually associated with prematurity and intrauterine growth retardation. The umbilical cord is located in its normal position, and is not part of the gastroschisis defect. The herniated intestines may be shortened, dilated, matted or covered by a thickened peritoneal membrane. There may be herniation of the ovaries or testes, if the abdominal gap is large. Intestinal atresias and cryptorchidism are frequently associated. The condition is rarely associated with other congenital anomalies. These infants are prone to develop hypothermia, dehydration, sepsis and hypoglycemia.

Investigations

Prenatal ultrasound provides early diagnosis. The maternal serum alpha-fetoprotein (MSAFP) are raised and serve as a useful diagnostic marker. The diagnosis is obvious on clinical examination and investigations are needed to assess the biological and biochemical homeostasis (Figure 5.17).

Differential Diagnosis

The conditions like limb–body wall complex (LBWC), ruptured omphalocele, bladder and cloacal exstrophy, should be excluded.

Management

In utero transfer and delivery in a tertiary care center is desirable. There is no indication for elective early delivery or cesarean section. Postnatal care should be provided by a specialized neonatal surgical team.

Delivery room The bowel should be wrapped in warm moist pad and sterile plastic sheet to minimise heat loss and prevent hypothermia. Stomach should be decompressed by frequent aspirations through oro-gastric tube. Bowel should be positioned in the midline and observed continuously to ensure adequate per-fusion of the gut. Fluid resuscitation is recommended by administration of 20 mL/kg of normal saline or Ringer's lactate. The infant should be closely monitored for vital signs, difference between core and peripheral body temperature, capillary refill time, urine output and markers of sepsis. These infants should be provided maintenance fluids at twice the amount recommended for healthy infants. The steps for provision of immediate first-aid are listed in Box 5.1.

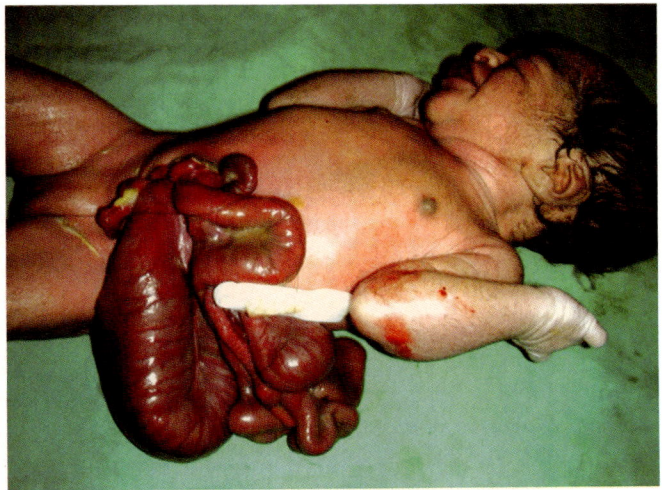

Figure 5.17 Herniation of the small and large gut through a defect in the abdominal wall below the umbilicus.

> **BOX 5.1** Immediate 'first aid' for abdominal wall defect
>
> - Cover the defect with a warm pad soaked with sterile saline.
> - Cover with a transparent plastic sheet to prevent insensible water loss.
> - Gastric decompression by oro or nasogastric tube.
> - Position and stabilize bowel in midline to avoid twisting.
> - Ensure normothermia.
> - Search for associated anomalies.
> - Nil by mouth.
> - Fluid resuscitation.
> - Surgical consultation.
> - Parental counseling.

Surgery Primary closure of skin and muscle defect is preferred. In case of larger defect, staged closure techniques may be performed. This involves enlargement of the defect and suturing a pouch (silo) to the abdominal wall around the defect to contain the herniated bowel contents. Some advocate closure by delayed primary reduction in the NICU without anesthesia. Recently, use of a preformed silo, affixed non-operatively, with gradual bowel reduction into the abdominal cavity over the next few days has been tried. Elective surgical repair may be done 4 weeks later. Special attention should be given to nutrition, tissue perfusion and pain management.

Prognosis

The hospital stay is usually prolonged for weeks or months. Outcome is excellent with timely management. Some infants may develop gastroesophageal reflux, malabsorption, poor growth, colic and constipation in infancy. Associated atresia, perforation, infarction, and short bowel syndrome lead to higher morbidity and mortality.

Omphalocele (Exomphalos)

Omphalocele is a defect in the base of the umbilical cord through which herniation of the gut and other abdominal organs occur.

Clinical Features

The defect occurs in the center of the abdominal wall. It is greater than 4 cm (defects less than 4 cm are generally called hernias of the cord) and covered by a sac that is thin and translucent with coverings of the umbilical cord (amnion, Wharton's jelly, and peritoneum). The umbilical cord inserts directly into the sac in an apical or occasionally lateral position. The salient clinical differences between gastroschisis and omphalocele are shown in Table 5.5. The sac may rupture *in utero* in 10–18% or during the process of

Features	Gastroschisis	Omphalocele
Location	Adjacent to the intact umbilicus	Through the umbilical cord
Defect	Herniation through an anatomical defect in the abdominal wall. There is no sac covering the defect	Herniation through umbilical ring, variable in size. The intestinal loops are covered with a sac
Contents	Loops of intestine and gonads but no other viscera	Loops of intestine with other abdominal organs like liver or spleen
Associated anomalies	Rare	High incidence of chromosomal, cardiac, genitourinary and/or craniofacial anomalies
Complications	Malrotation, midgut volvulus, hypoperistalsis, intestinal atresias or stenoses	Malrotation and midgut volvulus
Timing of delivery	Early if prenatal ultrasound shows evidence of bowel dilatation or bowel wall thickening	At term
Treatment	Primary repair or staged repair with silastic silo	Small: One-stage surgical repair Large: Gradual reduction with silastic silo
Outcome	Depends upon condition of the bowel and associated anomalies	Depends upon associated anomalies

Table 5.5 Salient differences between gastroschisis and omphalocele

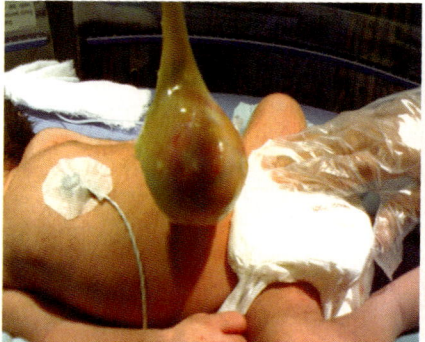
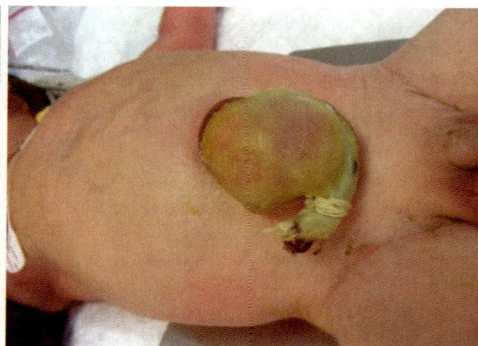
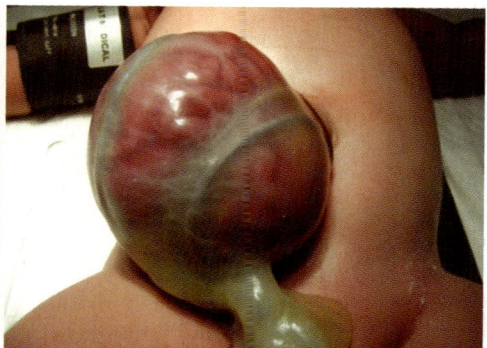

Figure 5.18 Herniation of gut through the umbilical opening. Omphalocele is covered with a sac.

delivery. Loops of intestines with or without other abdominal organs are visible in the sac (Figure 5.18). About one-half of cases have other associated cardiac and gastrointestinal tract anomalies. Common syndromes seen in association with omphalocele include Beckwith-Wiedemann syndrome, Pentalogy of Cantrell and omphalocele, exstrophy of cloaca, imperforate anus and spinal defect (OEIS) syndrome. One-third of patients have chromosomal anomalies like Trisomy 13, 18 and 21.

Investigations

Prenatal ultrasound provides early diagnosis. X-ray chest, 2D echocardiography and ultrasound abdomen are done to screen for associated anomalies. Genetic studies are done on clinical suspicion. Maternal serum alpha-fetoprotein (MSAFP) are raised and serve as a useful marker.

Management

Stabilization of the infant consists of gastric decompression by oro or nasogastric tube, covering the defect with a warm moist gauze with special attention to thermal control. These infants may require twice the amount of maintenance fluids compared to normal counterparts. They should be closely monitored for fluid and electrolyte disturbances, hypothermia, hypoglycemia and tissue perfusion.

Size of the defect, gestational age and associated anomalies determine the timing of surgery. For small defects (<5 cm) early closure is done. In a case of large defect, staged closure with or without a mesh or patch is advocated. A baby with a ruptured omphalocele is treated the same way as a baby with gastroschisis. Non-operative or escharotic therapy is used for high-risk infants with large omphaloceles and prematurity, respiratory insufficiency, congenital heart disease, or chromosomal abnormalities who cannot tolerate surgery. These are treated with topical application of Betadine® ointment or silver sulfadiazine to the intact sac. This allows secondary eschar formation and eventual epidermal ingrowth. Residual abdominal wall hernias are then repaired at one year of age.

Prognosis

Survival rates for those with isolated omphalocele are reported to vary between 75 to 95 percent. Infants with associated anomalies and giant omphaloceles have poor outcome. Potential short-term complications include necrotizing enterocolitis, prolonged ileus, and respiratory distress. Long-term complications include dependence on parenteral nutrition, gastroesophageal reflux, parenteral nutrition-related liver disease, feeding intolerance, and neurodevelopmental delay.

Imperforate Anus/Anal Atresia

Anorectal malformations (ARM) represent a wide range of complex malformations. The anomaly can be classified as high or low, depending on the level of the rectal pouch (Table 5.6). A high defect occurs when the rectum terminates above the pelvic floor musculature; lower defects occur when the incomplete descent ends below the pelvic floor musculature. About one-third of ARM are isolated and the remaining are associated with other congenital abnormalities. They occur in approximately 1 per 4000–5000 live births.

Clinical Features

ARM are often missed on initial examination and discovered after 24 hours when the newborn is observed to have distention and has not passed meconium. It is crucial to perform a good perineal examination and determine the number and location of orifices in both boys and girls. The most obvious finding is the absence of an anal opening. There may be a communication with the skin or urinary tract. "Meconuria" is indicative of a fistulous connection between the rectum and the urethral meatus (Figure 5.19). To determine the presence and location of a cutaneous fistula, one needs to observe the newborn for 24–48 hours. The presence of meconium on the perineum confirms a cutaneous fistula and a low lesion. Meconium in the urine suggests a communication between the bowel and the urinary tract (Figure 5.20).

In girls, the fistulous opening can be located either in the perineal body, as seen in an anterior anus, or more commonly in the vestibule of the vaginal vault outside the hymen (Figures 5.21 and 5.22). It is possible that it may take up to 24 hours for signs of a fistula to become evident. The presence of two orifices is indicative of a urogenital sinus. A single orifice is consistent with a cloacal anomaly which is the most complex form. A special effort should be made to look for flat bottom (higher chances of incontinence due to poor pelvic musculature), anal dimple and a presacral mass.

Table 5.6 Simplified version of International classification of anorectal anomalies		
Type of anomaly	Female	Male

High	1. Anorectal agenesis
	   a. With fistula
	     ■ Rectocloacal fistula
	     ■ Rectovaginal fistula
	   b. Without fistula
	2. Rectal atresia
		1. Anorectal agenesis
		   a. With fistula
		     ■ Rectovesical fistula
		     ■ Rectourethral fistula
		   b. Without fistula
		2. Rectal atresia

Intermediate	1. Anal agenesis without fistula or with fistula
	   a. Rectovaginal fistula
	   b. Rectovestibular fistula
	2. Anorectal stenosis
		1. Anal agenesis without fistula and with fistula
		   ■ Rectobulbar fistula
		
		2. Anorectal stenosis

Low	1. Anus at normal site
	   ■ Covered anus – complete
	   ■ Covered anal stenosis
	2. At perineal site
	   ■ Anocutaneous fistula
	   ■ Anterior perineal anus
	3. At vulvar site
	   ■ Vulvar anus
	   ■ Anovulvar fistula
	   ■ Anovestibular fistula
		1. Anus at normal site
		   ■ Covered anus – complete
		   ■ Covered anal stenosis
		2. At perineal site
		   ■ Anocutaneous fistula
		   ■ Anterior perineal anus

Miscellaneous	■ Anal membrane stenosis ■ Imperforated anal membrane ■ Perineal groove ■ Perineal canal	■ Anal membrane stenosis ■ Imperforated anal membrane ■ Perineal groove ■ Perineal canal

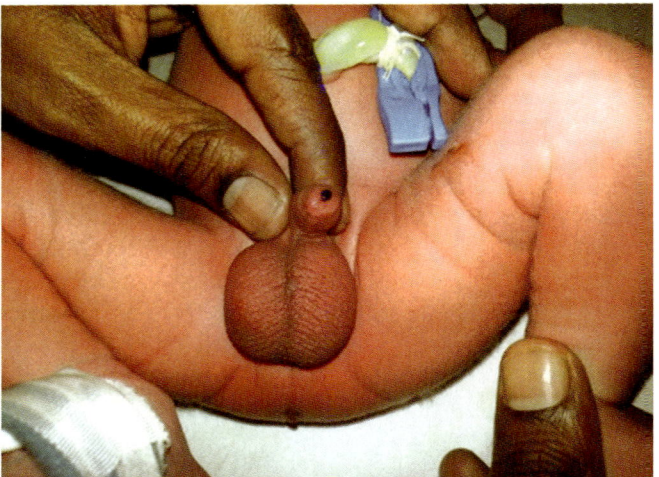

Figure 5.19 Meconuria in a male infant.

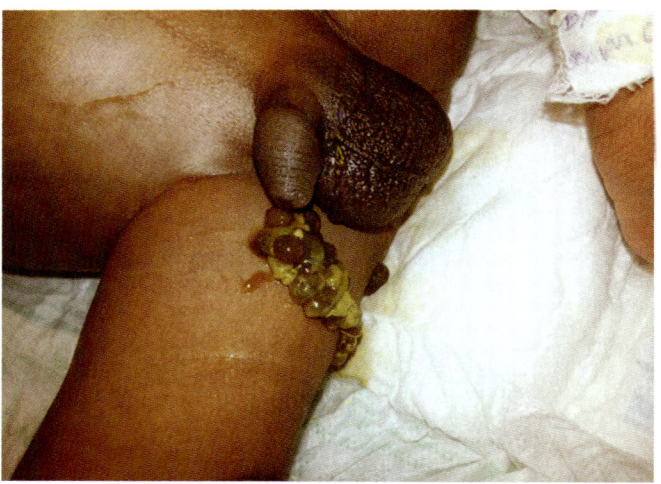

Figure 5.20 Rectourethral fistula.

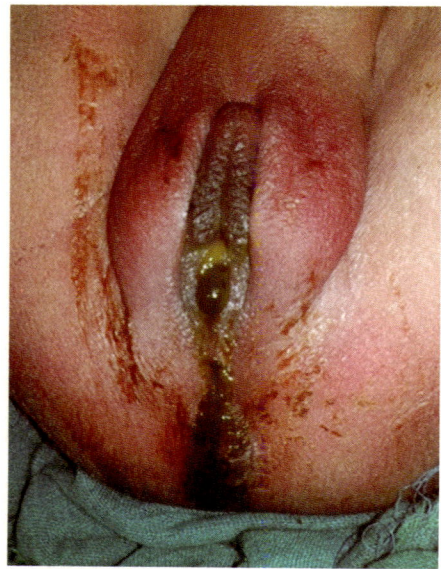

Figure 5.21 Absent anus with rectovaginal fistula.

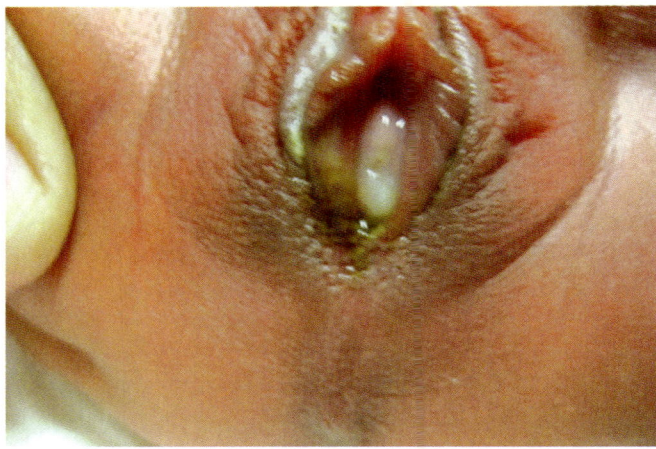

Figure 5.22 Absent anus with rectovestibular fistula.

The more severe the anorectal malformation, it is more likely to be associated with other abnormalities. The presence of an ARM should prompt an evaluation for VACTERL anomalies (vertebral anomalies, anal atresia, cardiac defects, tracheoesophageal fistula and/or esophageal atresia, renal and radial anomalies, and limb defects). The two most common cardiac anomalies associated with ARM are tetralogy of Fallot and ventricular septal defect.

Investigations

A cross-table lateral radiograph is obtained at 24 hours of birth (to allow the gas to reach the distal colon) with infant placed in a prone position, the hips and knees are flexed to the chest and a radio-opaque coin or bead is kept at anal dimple. The distance between the rectal gas and coin or bead is measured. Alternatively in a lateral radiograph, PC line (joining pubis with tip of coccyx) is a useful landmark to identify low and high ARMs. Ultrasound abdomen, X-ray chest, X-ray spine and 2D echocardiography are carried out to detect associated anomalies. Perineal ultrasound in a supine infant with a sagittal approach is used to calculate the distance between the perineum and the rectal pouch. The distance of <15 mm represent low lesions, while a distance greater than 15 mm suggests intermediate and high lesions with an accuracy of 95% and a specificity of 86% (Figure 5.23). A voiding cystourethrogram should be performed in those with upper renal tract anomalies, lumbosacral and spinal abnormalities. Postnatal MRI is most useful after surgical repair to identify the integrity of the levator sling and position of the rectal pull through. Prenatal diagnosis has both a low specificity and sensitivity.

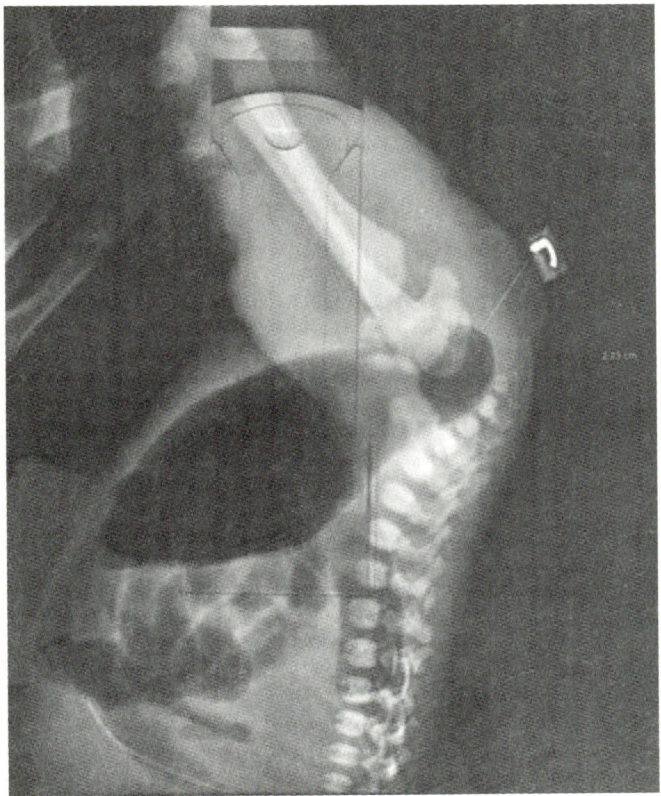

Figure 5.23 High variety of ARM.

Treatment

The timing of surgery is typically after the first 24 to 48 hours after birth. Most patients with recto-urinary fistulas undergo a diverting colostomy as the first stage operation (Figure 5.24). A high-pressure distal colostogram using water-soluble contrast is performed at 4 to 6 weeks later to determine the level of fistula with the urinary tract. Staged operations are reserved for complex, rare and life-threatening ARMs and include a colostomy for enteric diversion, definitive reconstruction, and subsequent restoration of enteric continuity by closure and reversal of colostomy.

Prognosis

Prognosis is dependent on extent and nature of malformation, associated anomalies, available expertise and infrastructure. There are concerns regarding integrity of bowel and bladder, infertility and sexual functioning on long-term follow-up. Patients with more than two missing sacral vertebrae, hemisacral defects, or tethered cord are likely to have poor bowel function scores. Certain anomalies like high cloaca (common channel >3 cm) or a recto-bladder neck fistula have a poor outcome. Patients with low defects (e.g. rectoperineal fistula, rectal atresia) and girls with rectovestibular fistulas have excellent outcomes.

CARDIAC ANOMALIES

The cardiac malformations have been discussed in detail in Chapters 8 and 24.

NEURAL ANOMALIES

Ruptured Myelomeningocele

Myelomeningocele is a localized neural tube defect with associated vertebral anomalies, malformed spinal cord, lack of skin covering, and defective functioning of nerves below the level of defect.

Clinical Features

The defect is most often seen in the lumbosacral region though it may occur at any level over the spine. Higher defects are associated with greater neural deficits. There is a gap over the spine through which the malformed spinal cord protrudes (Figure 5.25). Part of the spinal cord and nerves are present in the sac and may get damaged. CSF leaks through the protruding neural tissue predisposing to ascending intracranial infection. Associated abnormalities include hydrocephalus and Arnold Chiari II malformation, partial or complete lack of sensations, partial or complete paralysis of the legs, and feet and loss of anal reflex. Congenital dysplasia of hips and clubfeet are commonly associated.

Investigations

Prenatal ultrasound provides early diagnosis. Elevation of maternal blood or amniotic fluid alpha-fetoprotein (AFP) levels are useful screening test for neural tube defects. The cranial ultrasound is a cost-effective modality to identify the presence of associated hydrocephalus and Arnold Chiari malformation. Isolated lesions have high incidence of underlying brain

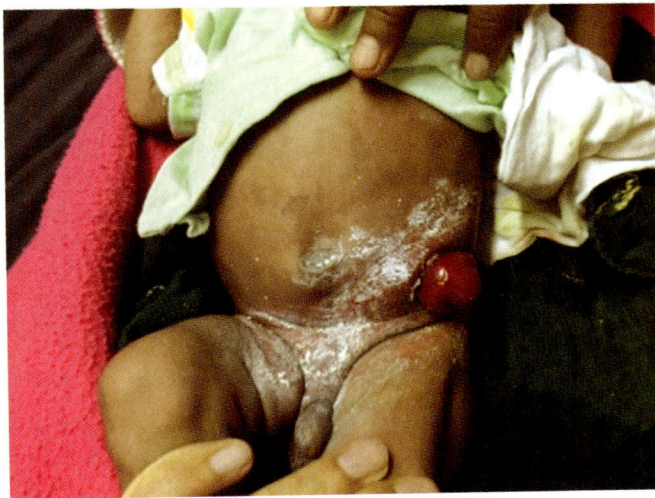

Figure 5.24 Colostomy as a stage one repair.

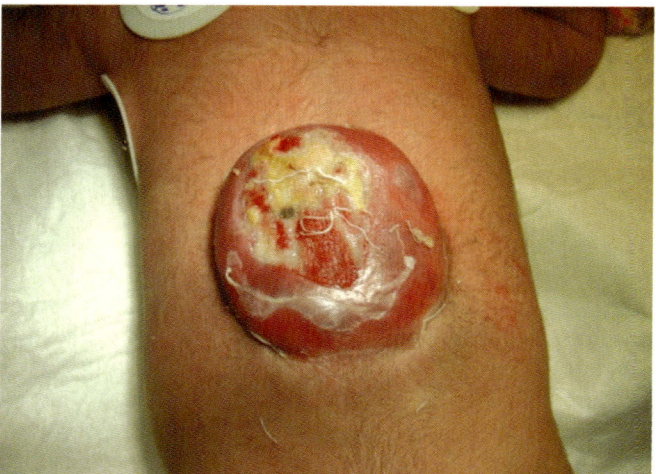

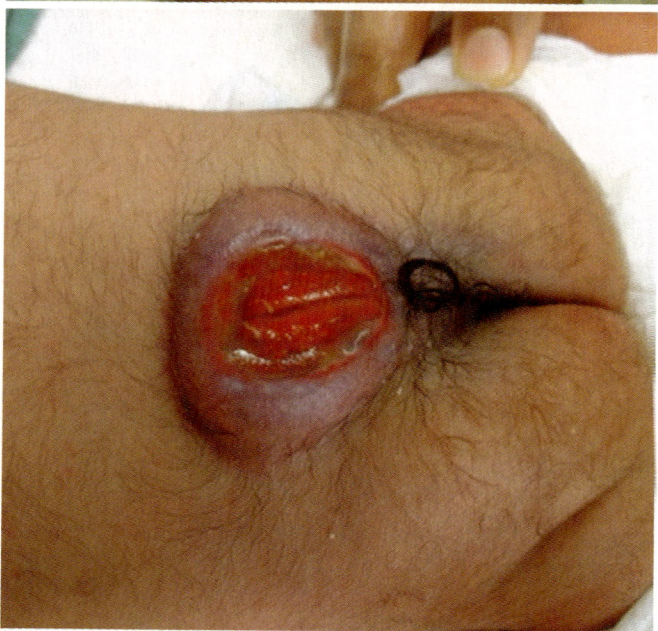

Figure 5.25 There is herniation of spinal cord, and meninges with ruptured skin covering.

malformations like cerebral heterotopias, partial agenesis of the corpus callosum, and abnormalities of the brainstem. MRI of brain should be done in all cases.

Differential Diagnosis

Meningocele and lipomyelomeningocele should be excluded.

Management

The ruptured lesion is covered with a sterile saline soaked pad, that is further covered with a non-permeable dressing. All efforts are made to prevent contamination of the lesion with urine or stool. Prophylactic antibiotics for prevention of infection are initiated prior to the surgical intervention. The surgical repair of the defect and ventriculo-peritoneal shunt for

associated hydrocephalus are done in one sitting as early as feasible. Orthopedic or physical therapy may be needed to treat musculoskeletal problems like clubfeet and dysplasia of the hips.

Prognosis

The prognosis is guarded. The outcome depends on the degree or severity of defect and associated complications like incontinence of urine and stool, hydrocephalus, hip dislocation and brain malformations. In untreated cases, the mortality may be as high as 90%. These infants need long-term follow-up and rehabilitation under the supervision of a number of specialists.

RENAL MALFORMATIONS

Bilateral Pelviureteric Junction (PUJ) Obstruction

This is the most common cause of prenatal hydronephrosis. It is defined as an obstruction at the junction of the renal pelvis and proximal ureter. The obstruction results in back pressure within the renal pelvis, which may lead to progressive hydronephrosis and renal damage. The condition is predominantly seen in boys.

Clinical Features

The clinical manifestations depend upon the severity of obstruction. Mild to moderate obstruction remains asymptomatic. Bilateral severe obstruction of pelviureteric junction is characterized by abdominal distension, palpable kidneys, tachypnea, obliguria or anuria. Ascites due to leakage of urine through ruptured pelvis, calyx or ureter is common. Obstruction of the PUJ has been associated with multicystic kidney disease as well as other anomalies including Hirschsprung's disease, cardiovascular anomalies, neural tube defects, esophageal atresia, imperforate anus, congenital dysplasia of hips, and adrenogenital syndrome.

Investigations

The vast majority of PUJ obstructions (90%) are detected on prenatal ultrasonography. Postnatally, an ultrasound of kidneys, ureters and bladder (KUB) is repeated after 72 hours of age. Isotope renography, usually a dynamic mercapto-acetyltriglycine (MAG 3) scan is useful to delineate and monitor the renal function.

Differential Diagnosis

Transient hydronephrosis, functional hydronephrosis, vesicoureteral reflux, PU valves should be excluded.

Management

Neonates with AP renal pelvic diameter of >50 mm invariably need pyeloplasty which remains the gold standard operation. Algorithm for therapeutic approach and indications for surgical intervention in

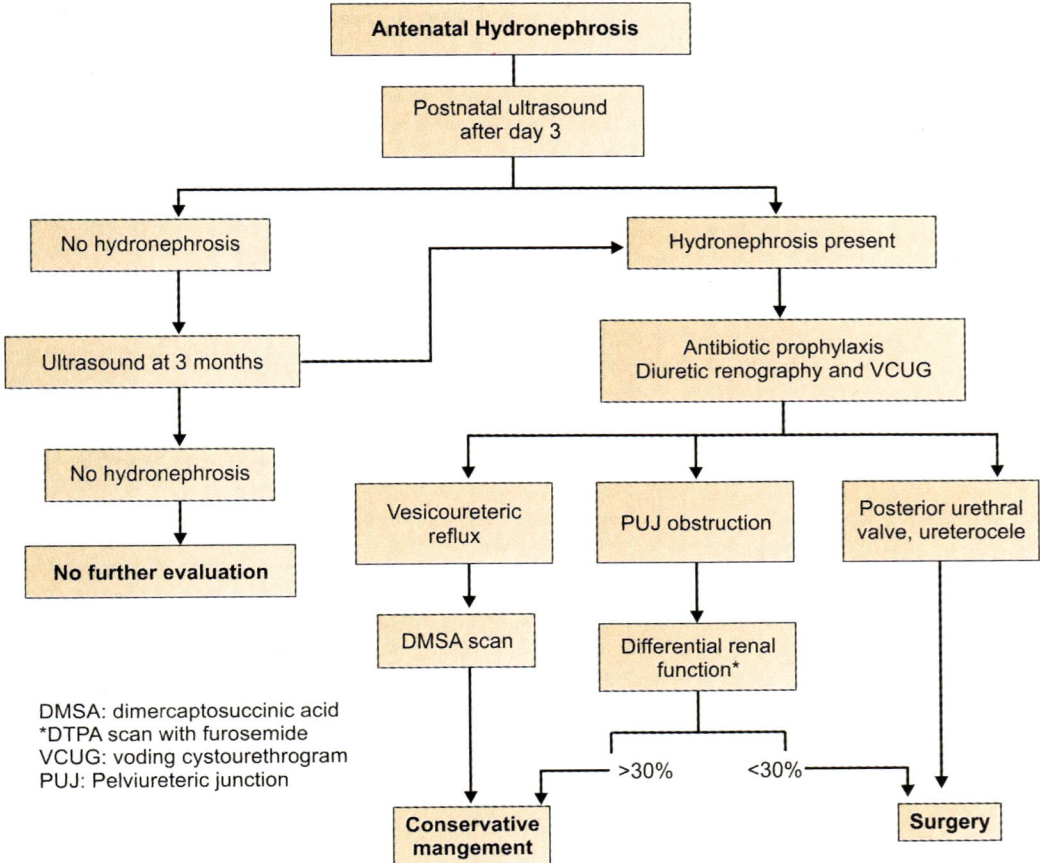

Figure 5.26 Algorithm for management of antenatally detected hydronephrosis.

infants with PUJ obstruction are shown in Figure 5.26 and Box 5.2. The alternative options include minimally invasive balloon dilatation and endopyelotomy techniques. After surgery, a repeat ultrasound on follow up shows reduced hydronephrosis and a MAG 3 renogram shows improved drainage and improvement in renal function. Complications of surgery include anastomotic leak and recurrence of obstruction. Infants with renal function of less than 10% at 4 weeks of age are candidates for nephrectomy.

BOX 5.2 Indications for surgical intervention in neonates with congenital hydronephrosis

- Bilateral hydronephrosis with AP renal pelvic diameter >30 mm
- Unilateral gross hydronephrosis, AP renal pelvic diameter of >50 mm
- Severe hydronephrosis in a solitary kidney
- Reduced differential renal function by more than 40%
- Deterioration of differential renal function greater than 10%
- Worsening renal function
- Progressive hydronephrosis

Prognosis

The prognosis for bilateral PUJ obstruction depends on the degree of obstruction. Long-term follow-up studies are needed to monitor cardiovascular and renal complications.

Multicystic Dysplastic Kidney (MCDK)

Clinical Features

The infant may present with non-specific complaints of vomiting, abdominal distention, poor feeding, respiratory difficulty with or without a palpable abdominal mass. Hypertension or malignant change is rarely seen. About 10% of patients with multicystic dysplastic kidney disease have contralateral renal agenesis or PUJ obstruction. About 10% of cases may have a family history of significant renal/urinary tract malformation.

Investigations

Prenatal ultrasound may provide clue to early diagnosis. Postnatal ultrasound shows cysts of varying sizes with no loss of normal renal architecture. The characteristic feature of MCDK is the common association with an atretic ureter. DMSA isotope scan is useful to assess renal function which is grossly affected in infants with MCDK. If the contralateral kidney is normal on ultrasound, an MCU is not required.

Differential Diagnosis

Cystic dysplastic kidney or renal dysplasia, and severe PUJ obstruction with hydronephrosis should be ruled out.

Management

Most multicystic dysplastic kidneys (MCDKs) involute over a period of time and require no intervention. Symptomatic MCDK (large mass compromising breathing or feeding) or an enlarging mass merits nephrectomy. Where expertise exists, laparoscopic nephrectomy is a suitable alternative. Elective nephrectomy of non-functioning unilateral dysplastic kidney is not warranted unless there are other complications.

Prognosis

Bilateral MCDK is incompatible with life. The larger MCDK (>6 cm) are the ones that may not involute. The prognosis depends on the integrity and functions of the contralateral kidney.

Polycystic Kidney Disease (PKD)

Autosomal recessive PKD is the the most common renal cystic disease in childhood. Autosomal dominant PKD rarely manifests in newborns.

Clinical Features

There is a wide range of clinical manifestations. The infant may be asymptomatic or have varying grades of renal dysfunction including hyponatremia and hypertension. The severely affected infants may develop "Potter" phenotype with pulmonary hypoplasia and a small chest, beaked and flattened nose, and deformities of the extremities and spine. Sepsis, and respiratory insufficiency requiring mechanical ventilation are common complications. About 15% develop periportal fibrosis and portal hypertension later in childhood.

Investigations

Parents of PKD baby should undergo ultrasonographic examination of abdomen to rule out the presence of asymptomatic PKD of autosomial dominant variant.

Management

In severely affected babies, outcome is ominous. The treatment is symptomatic by correction of electrolyte imbalance, treatment of high blood pressure, poor renal function and urinary tract infection. Dialysis and renal transplant are currently available options if renal failure sets in.

Prognosis

Respiratory failure and sepsis are leading causes of early mortality. Almost 40% progress to chronic renal insufficiency and 25% manifest with poor physical growth and need long-term follow-up with renal replacement and nutritional support.

Posterior Urethral Valves (PUV)

PU valves are a common cause of congenital bladder neck obstruction in males and is caused by a malformation of the posterior urethra. The obstruction leads to back pressure with distension of bladder, ureters, and kidneys. Wide range of anatomical abnormalities and renal dysfunction may occur.

Clinical Features

It may present as a life-threatening emergency with abdominal distension, hydrophrosis and respiratory distress due to pulmonary hypoplasia. The clinical features include three palpable masses in the abdomen (distended bladder and hydronephrotic kidneys), lethargy, poor weight gain, urosepsis, oliguria or poor urinary stream. There may be abdominal distention (ascites), Potter facies and limb deformities (skin dimpling) and indentation of the knees and elbows due to intrauterine compression because of oligohydramnios. Several affected neonates remain asymptomatic and manifest during infancy or childhood, with recurrent urinary tract infections, abnormal urinary stream, failure to thrive and progressive renal dysfunction.

Differential Diagnosis

PUJ obstruction, urethral meatal stenosis in males, neurogenic bladder, and ureterocele should be excluded.

Investigations

Prenatal ultrasound provides an early diagnosis. Renal scan may demonstrate perirenal collection of urine, echogenic kidneys, subcortical cyst, and indistinct corticomedullary junction. The diagnosis is confirmed by micturating cystourethrogram (Figure 5.27). Radionuclide studies (MAG 3) are done when either

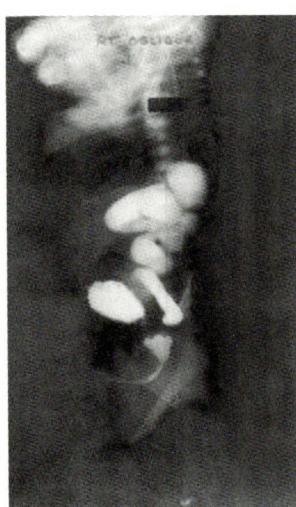

Figure 5.27 Micturating cystourethrogram showing dilated urinary system due to bladder neck obstruction.

kidney shows thin or abnormal parenchyma and in infants in whom postoperative ultrasound shows no improvement and scan is done to distinguish between persistent bladder neck obstruction and cystic dysplasia. Urodynamic evaluation provides information about storage capacity of bladder and residual urine.

Management

Management strategies include stabilization by providing adequate urinary drainage (urethral or suprapubic catheter), correction of fluids, electrolytes and acid-base imbalance and treating urinary tract infection. Cystoscopy serves both diagnostic and therapeutic functions in these infants. Valve ablation with endoscopic disruption or resection is done once infant is stabilized. At times, short-term nephrostomy drainage or surgical urinary diversion (pyelostomy, ureterostomy or cutaneous vesicostomy) is required. Bladder management after ablation of the valves is crucial to improve the outcome in patients with PUV.

Prognosis

The prognosis depends on the status of kidneys and bladder at the time of diagnosis. Predictors of a poor outcome include antenatal detection at <24 weeks gestation, marked prenatal hydroureteronephrosis, prenatal renal parenchymal damage, oligohydramnios and respiratory distress at birth. Echogenic kidney, subcortical cyst and bilateral VUR are associated with unfavorable outcome. Long-term follow-up is essential because 10–15% patients develop progressive renal failure. Approximately one-third of patients with PUV develop vesicoureteric reflux (VUR) and one-third progress to end-stage renal disease.

Renal Agenesis/Dysgenesis

Renal agenesis may affect one or both the kidneys. It can occur as an isolated anomaly or as part of a syndrome or genetic disorder.

Clinical Features

The infant is likely to be preterm or growth retarded. Oligohydramnios in the mother is invariably present. The classical presentation is of Potter syndrome with abnormal facies, beaked nose, low-set ears, receding chin and bowed legs. There is significant respiratory distress due to pulmonary hypoplasia. Pneumothorax is likely to occur following bag and mask resuscitation. Single umbilical artery on cut section of the cord should prompt screening for underlying anomalies. Musculo-skeletal anomalies (e.g. cleft palate, absent radius or fibula, congenital diaphragmatic hernia) occur in 40% of patients. About 14% of cases have coexisting cardio-vascular anomalies (tetralogy of Fallot, ventricular or atrial septal defects, hypoplastic left ventricle, coarctation of the aorta). GI anomalies occur in 19% (duodenal atresia, malrotation of the bowel, tracheo-esophageal fistula, omphalocele) of affected infants. In addition, 10% of patients with multicystic dysplastic kidney disease have contralateral renal agenesis. The absence of the kidney may be associated with absence of the ureter, but adrenal gland is usually present.

Investigations

Prenatal ultrasound provides clues for early diagnosis. Postnatal ultrasound confirms the diagnosis. The diagnosis of isolated renal agenesis is one of exclusion. Renal agenesis in a fetus should prompt a renal scan of the parents to determine the risk of recurrence.

Management

There is no definitive treatment. Renal dialysis and, later, transplantation of a kidney, are available options to prolong survival.

Prognosis

The prognosis is poor. The degree of severity of lung hypoplasia determines the outcome.

Prune Belly Syndrome

Prune-belly syndrome is a specific constellation of anomalies seen exclusively in boys.

Clinical Features

The classical feature is a large, floppy and shrivelled abdomen due to congenital deficiency of the abdominal

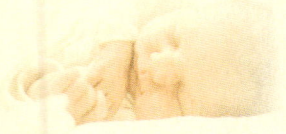

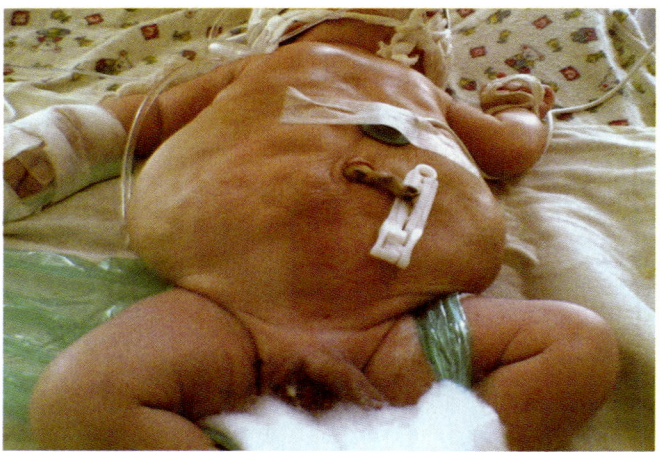

Figure 5.28 Prune belly syndrome. Note shrivelled floppy abdomen and enlarged phallus.

wall musculature. Bilateral nonpalpable undescended testes and a large phallus due to dilated urethra are usually present. A variety of skeletal, gastrointestinal, cardiac, and pulmonary anomalies are associated.

Investigations

Ultrasound abdomen reveals dilated and tortuous ureters with bilateral hydronephrosis. Kidneys show varying degrees of dysplasia and cystic changes. Micturating cystourethrography demonstrates a large, elongated bladder with an irregular contour and bilateral VUR.

Differential Diagnosis

Megacystis-microcolon-intestinal hypoperistalsis syndrome, enteric duplication cyst, urachal cyst, ureteropelvic junction obstruction, posterior urethral valve syndrome, bladder exstrophy, and ascites should be ruled out.

Management

Treatment for the syndrome depends on the severity of symptoms. Some infants may require an emergency vesicostomy to facilitate drainage of the urine. In severely affected infants extensive surgical remodeling of the abdominal wall and urinary tract and orchidopexy for undescended testes are required.

Prognosis

Infants with a functional abnormality of bladder but with no urethral obstruction survive the neonatal period but develop chronic urinary tract disease. Those with obstructive lesion of the urethra (urethral atresia or posterior urethral valve) have a high fatality rate unless early surgical intervention is done. The most common postnatal cause of death is urosepsis.

SKELETAL ANOMALIES

Osteogenesis Imperfecta (OI)

Osteogenesis imperfecta is an autosomal dominant, disorder of collagen production (mutations in the *COL1A1* and *COL1A2* genes) resulting in fragile bones that fracture easily. Fifteen types of OI have been described.

Clinical Features

The features and severity of OI vary greatly. Most infants appear short with small and short limbs and blue sclerae. Respiratory difficulty may be seen due to pulmonary hypoplasia and chest deformity. The long bones are the most common site of fractures, with bowing and angular deformities. Deformities compromise the quality of life and mobility. Type II OI is most lethal and manifests in perinatal period. Fractures occur *in utero*. Children with Type III OI bruise easily due to capillary fragility. Type I and IV present in late childhood. Family history may be present because of dominant inheritance.

Investigations

Prenatal ultrasound provides useful clues for early diagnosis. Chorionic villus sampling can be used to identify reduced or absent synthesis of collagen. Detailed studies of the skull, spine, pelvis, and long bones are recommended. Deformities range from bowing to multiple fractures of the long bones, Wormian skull bones, scoliosis and chest deformities. Infantogram is done to identify deformities, fractures and callus formation at several sites (Figure 5.29). A skin biopsy allows biochemical analysis at the molecular level.

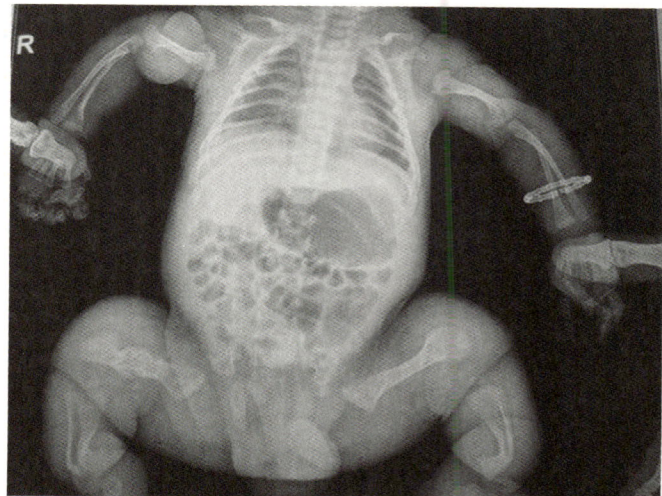

Figure 5.29 Note the short, malformed bones with callus formation due to osteogenesis imperfecta.

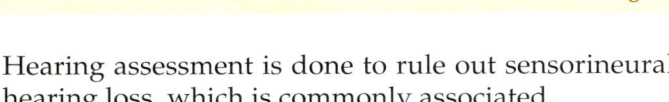
Hearing assessment is done to rule out sensorineural hearing loss, which is commonly associated.

Differential Diagnosis

Rickets, battered baby syndrome, and hypophosphatasia should be ruled out.

Management

The treatment is essentially symptomatic and supportive as there is no cure. The infant should be handled gently at birth to minimize pain and occurrence of new fractures. Lifting the infant by holding at the armpits or by the arms or legs should be strictly avoided. Foam or rubber mattress is used to minimize damage at pressure points. Care givers are taught to gently lift the infant supporting the buttocks and head with the limbs resting on forearms. Clothes should be front opening with velcro or snaps for ease of wearing and disrobing. Supervised feeding or gavage feeding may be required as these infants often have swallowing difficulty. The fractures are managed with splints rather than casts to avoid osteoporosis. Braces and splints are used to stabilize the lax joints and to prevent fractures. Hip spica may be used for fractures of femur. Pain relieving measures should be implemented round-the-clock. Paracetamol or ibuprofen are used as analgesics. Biphosphonates, calcium and phosphorus supplements help prevent fractures and bone deformities. Therapeutic efficacy of transplant of bone marrow-derived mesenchymal cells is being tried to achieve cure in osteogenesis imperfecta.

Prognosis

Type II OI has a high case fatality rate. Respiratory failure is the most frequent cause of death. Early intervention program with multidisciplinary team and long-term follow-up is mandatory. Physiotherapy, orthotic care, surgical interventions improve the overall outcome of these children.

BIBLIOGRAPHY

Andrena Kelly, Morag Liddell. The nursing care of the surgical neonate. *Semin Pediatr Surg* 2008; 17:290–96.

Bosenberg AT, Brown RA. Management of congenital diaphragmatic hernia. *Curr opin Anaesthesial* 2008; 21(3):323–31.

Dennis B Liu, William R, Armstrong I, Max Maizels. Hydronephrosis: Prenatal and postnatal evaluation and management. *Clin Perinatol* 2014; 41:661–78.

Donald J F, Richard L B. Cardiac evaluation of the newborn. *Pediatr Clin N Am* 2015; 62:471–89.

Emily F D, Aimen S. Commonly encountered surgical problems in the fetus and neonate. *Pediatr Clin N Am* 2009; 56:647–69.

Grigorios C K. Posterior urethral valves. *Essentials Pediatr Urol* 2012; 25:115–24.

Joseph VT. The management of renal conditions in the perinatal period. *Early Human Develop* 2006; 82:313–24.

Ledbetter DJ. Gastroschisis and omphalocele. *Surg Clin North Am* 2006; 86:249–60.

Lee SE, Kim HY, Jung SE, et al. Situs anomalies and gastro-intestinal abnormalities. *J Pediatr Surg* 2006; 41(7):1237–42.

Levitt MA, Pena A. Outcomes from the correction of anorectal malformations. *Curr Opin Pediatr* 2005; 17(3):394–401.

Logan JW, Rice HE, Goldberg RN and Cotton CM. Congenital diaphragmatic hernia: a systematic review and summary of best-evidence practice strategies. *J Perinatol* 2007; 27:535–49.

Samir P. Anorectal malformations. *Neo Reviews* 2016; 17;e251.

Shaw-Smith C. Oesophageal atresia, tracheo-oesophageal fistula and the VECTERL association: a review of genetics and epidemiology. *J Med Genet* 2006; 43(7):545–54.

Susan DA, Richard G, Solveig H, Amy Lee, Thomas McNalley, Niswander Lee, et al. Advances in the care of children with spina bifida. *Advances Pediatr* 2014; 61:33–74.

Whitney McBride. Congenital lesions of the lung. *Neo Reviews* 2016; 17; e263.

6

Hypothermia and Hyperthermia

NB Mathur and SB Mathur

HYPOTHERMIA

Thermal protection to the newborn is provided by the series of measures taken at birth and during early days of life to ensure that the newborn does not become either cold or overheated and maintains a normal core body temperature of 36.5–37.5°C. Hypothermia has been recognised as a significant cause of neonatal illness and death even in tropical countries. Although data are scarce, hypothermia is a common problem and it contributes to the high perinatal mortality rate seen in the developing world.

Newborns especially low birth weight babies are at increased risk of heat loss due to certain characteristics such as a large body surface area in relation to weight, large head size in proportion to the body, and scanty subcutaneous fat. When heat loss exceeds the baby's ability to produce heat, its body temperature drops below the normal range and baby becomes hypothermic. Hyperthermia mostly occurs in the neonate because of overheating during hot summer months.

Thermal Disturbances

According to WHO, the newborn with a core body temperature of 36.0–36.4°C is under cold stress (mild hypothermia) which is associated with poor weight gain including brain growth. A baby with a temperature of 32.0–35.9°C has moderate hypothermia, while a body temperature below 32°C is considered to be severe hypothermia (Figure 6.1).

Data on validation of the WHO classification on severity of hypothermia is scanty. There is evidence to suggest that in extramural sick neonates, the case fatality rate correlates with the severity of hypothermia. The presence of comorbidities, like physiological derangements and low birth weight are associated with

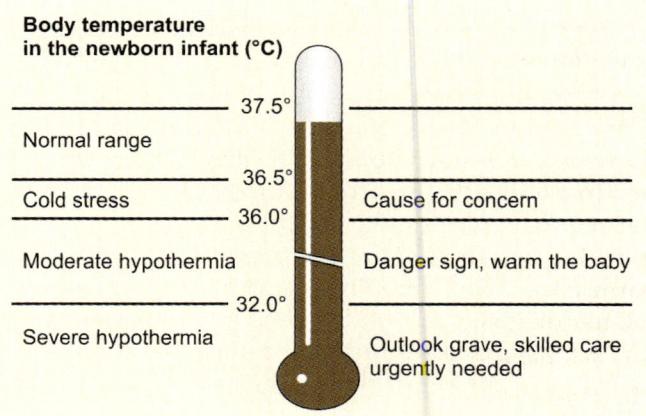

Figure 6.1 WHO classification of severity of hypothermia in the newborn.

significantly higher fatality. The WHO uses body temperature as the sole criterion for classifying severity of hypothermia. Associated illnesses (birth asphyxia, neonatal sepsis, respiratory distress), physiological derangements (hypoxia, hypoglycemia, shock) or weight less than 2000 g are recognized adverse factors and their presence should be used to classify hypothermia in the next higher category of severity. Hyperthermia is defined as a rectal temperature of greater than 37.5°C.

Physiological Response to Cold Stress

The physiologic response to cold stress is related to the oxidation of brown fat or brown adipose tissue. In full term neonates, non-shivering thermogenesis (oxidation of brown adipose tissue) is the major mechanism to increase heat production in response to cold exposure. During early stages of hypothermia increased body movements try to enhance heat production but once hypothermia is prolonged or becomes severe, the baby becomes sluggish. Brown adipose tissue can be identified around 26 weeks gestational age. It contains high concentration of stored triglycerides, a rich capillary network and is densely innervated sympathetic nerve endings on the blood vessels and on each adipocyte. Each fat cell has numerous mitochondria with respiratory chain enzymes and the uncoupling protein that is the rate limiting enzyme in the process of heat production. When fat is oxidized, heat is produced because of the oxidation of uncoupling proteins. In the presence of cold stress, noradrenaline stimulates lipolysis and metabolic activity of the uncoupling proteins thus producing heat.

The consequences of cold stress include metabolic acidosis, hypoxia and hypoglycemia. These are exaggerated in the preterm neonate compared to the full term neonate. The preterm neonate has less quota of brown fat, poor vasomotor response and less insulation to cope with a hypothermic event.

Risk Factors for Cold Stress

The newborn is most vulnerable to hypothermia during the first few hours after birth. Subsequently hypothermia may develop during bathing, on a cold night or during transportation, if measures to keep the baby warm are inadequate. The following neonates are at risk to develop cold stress.

  i. All neonates during the first 12 hours of life.
 ii. Preterm babies and neonates who are growth retarded.
iii. During transportation.
 iv. Neonates with neurologic impairment because of damage to the hypothalamus, birth asphyxia, and anesthetic medications.
  v. Neonates with hypoglycemia.
 vi. Neonates with abnormalities in their skin integrity due to neural tube defects, omphalocele, gastroschisis, and ichthyosis.
vii. Lack of awareness among care givers regarding thermal protection of the neonate.
viii. Prolonged procedure or surgery.

Assessment of Body Temperature

Skin temperature is usually measured with thermocouples or thermistor probes taped to the skin over the liver (right hypochondrium). A thermometer that reads up to a minimum of 35°C is not appropriate for routine checking of body temperature. When such a thermometer cannot record the body temperature, this is an indication of moderate to severe hypothermia. Rewarming will be better guided by knowing the exact body temperature, and this can be done by using a low reading thermometer (one that reads up to 25°C). Digital thermometers are low reading and are reliable to record the body temperature.

As a general rule, taking the axillary skin temperature is better than the rectal temperature because of safety, hygiene and relative ease. Taking the axillary temperature does not pose any risk to the neonate and if properly done it gives a good approximation of core body temperature. The clean thermometer should be placed high in the axilla, and the arm snugly held against the side of the body for at least five minutes. When hypothermia is suspected, the rectal temperature provides more accurate measure of the body temperature. For taking the rectal temperature, the thermometer should be placed in the rectum to a maximum depth of 2 cm, and kept in situ for at least three minutes. The baby should never be left alone with a thermometer in the rectum because of risk of rectal perforation.

Studies have shown that physicians and trained assistants can assess the temperature of a newborn baby by touch with reasonable accuracy. In a healthy baby, the trunk is warm to touch, and extremities are reasonably warm and pink.

Adverse Effects of Hypothermia

Prolonged hypothermia is associated with impaired growth and the newborn is more vulnerable to develop infection. Sick or low birth weight babies admitted to neonatal units with hypothermia are more likely to die than those admitted with normal body temperature.

During early stages of hypothermia, the hands and feet become cold to touch. If hypothermia is allowed to continue, the skin becomes cold and pale all over the body. After initial restlessness the baby becomes less active, suckles poorly and has a weak cry.

In severely hypothermic babies, the face and extremities may develop a bright red color. Sclerema (hardening or hidebound skin associated with reddening and edema) may occur on the trunk and extremities. The baby becomes lethargic and develops slow, shallow and irregular breathing, apnea and bradycardia. Hypoglycemia, metabolic acidosis, generalized internal bleeding (especially in the lungs) and respiratory distress may occur. Unless urgent measures are taken, these babies are likely to die.

The Warm Chain

The "warm chain" or "thermoregulation bundle" is a set of interlinked procedures which should be taken at birth and during the next few hours and days in order

> **BOX 6.1** The components of warm chain
>
> 1. Warm delivery room
> 2. Immediate drying
> 3. Warm resuscitation
> 4. Skin-to-skin contact
> 5. Breastfeeding
> 6. Bathing and weighing are postponed
> 7. Appropriate clothes/warm bedding
> 8. Mother and baby kept together
> 9. Warm transportation
> 10. Training and awareness of health care personnel

to minimize heat loss in all newborns. Failure to implement any one of these procedures will break the chain and put the newborn baby at risk of developing hypothermia. The ten steps of the "warm chain" are described in Box 6.1.

Step 1. Warm delivery room

The delivery room should be kept clean, warm (at least 26–28°C), and free from draughts from open windows and doors, or fans. If the temperature of the room is less than optimal, a heater should be available to warm the room. It is easier to warm a small area of a room rather than the whole room (warm microenvironment). In hot weather, air-conditioning or fans should be turned off or adjusted in the delivery room.

Supplies needed to keep the newborn baby warm should be prepared and kept ready before delivery. They include two absorbent towels large enough to cover a newborn baby's whole body and head, a cap, a sheet or blanket for covering mother and baby, and suitable baby clothes and bedding. In cool weather a radiant heat source should be available to prewarm the bassinet.

Step 2. Immediate drying

After birth, the baby including its head, should be immediately dried with a dry warm towel. While the newborn is being dried, the baby should be placed on a warm surface such as the mother's chest or abdomen (skin-to-skin contact), or a prewarmed sheet of the resuscitator.

The baby should then be covered with a second dry towel (discard the first towel) and head should be covered with a cap. If the room temperature is less than optimal (less than 26°C), towels and cap should be prewarmed.

Step 3. Warm resuscitation

If a newborn is not breathing after drying, resuscitation must be started immediately. It is very important that the baby is kept warm during resuscitation since newborns with asphyxia are at an increased risk of getting cold. To keep the baby warm during resuscitation, the baby should be kept under an additional source of heat such as a heating bulb or a radiant warmer. The radiant warmer should be prewarmed to 100% output by maintaining it in the manual mode for 10 minutes prior to delivery.

Step 4. Skin-to-skin contact

Skin-to-skin contact is an effective method of preventing heat loss in newborns. The mother's chest or abdomen can be used as a surface to receive the newborn as it is clean and warm, and it promotes bonding. The newborn can be dried while lying on the mother and then covered.

The baby should be uncovered as little as possible during assessment of its condition, while providing eye care, and when the cord is being tied and cut. The baby should be kept in skin-to-skin contact with the mother while she is being attended (delivery of placenta, suturing of tears), during transfer to the postnatal ward and during the first few hours after birth. Skin-to-skin contact can also be used afterwards in the NICU.

The extremely preterm (<32 weeks) babies should be protected with a cling film and covered with a warm towel immediately after birth. There is no need to dry the baby before application of cling film or plastic wrap. After resuscitation, the baby should be transferred to the NICU in a prewarmed transport incubator. A preheated radiant warmer should be available in the NICU before baby is transferred.

Step 5. Breastfeeding

Breastfeeding should begin as soon as possible after delivery, preferably within an hour. Early skin-to-skin contact with mother promotes bonding and breastfeeding. An early and adequate supply of breast milk is essential to provide the newborn with calories so that it can generate metabolic body heat. In the hours and days following birth, it is very important that the newborn be allowed to suckle at the breast "on-demand", both during day and night. This stimulates milk production and provides the baby with enough calories for heat production and for physical and mental growth.

Step 6. Bathing and weighing

Bathing the newborn soon after birth causes a drop in the baby's body temperature and is not recommended. Blood, meconium and excessive vernix can be wiped off during the process of drying at birth. The remaining vernix does not need to be removed as it is harmless, may reduce heat loss and is reabsorbed through the skin during the first few days of life. If cultural tradition demands bathing, this should be carried out after 6 hours of birth, or preferably on the second or third day of life when baby is stabilized.

Ensure that bathing is done in a warm room and by using warm water. After the bath, the baby should be immediately wrapped in a dry warm towel, dried thoroughly, dressed quickly and placed next to the mother. Baby bath during hospital stay of the baby is not mandatory and only sponging the soiled baby with a warm wet towel is the preferred option. Weighing of the baby at birth also increases the risk of heat loss and should be postponed for few hours.

Step 7. Appropriate clothing and bedding

The newborn should be protected by providing adequate clothing and bedding that are appropriate for the environmental temperature. As a general rule, newborns need one or two more layers of clothes and bedding than adults. Clothing should always include a cap, since as much as 25% of heat loss in a newborn baby may occur from an uncovered head. Mittens and socks are useful to keep the hands and feet warm.

Clothing and bedding should not be too tight as trapped air in loose garments is a very efficient insulator. Swaddling tightly reduces the efficiency of heat retention and may not allow the baby's lungs to expand fully.

Step 8. Mother and newborn are kept together

Babies born at home as well as in institutions should be roomed-in with their mothers, preferably kept on the same bed, in a warm room (at least 26°C). When mother and her baby are kept together, it is easier to keep the baby warm and promote breastfeeding on demand. Rooming-in also reduces the risk of exposure of the newborn to hospital acquired infections.

Step 9. Warm transportation

It is important to keep the baby warm during transportation. This step, if overlooked, can result in a drop of the baby's body temperature even if thermal protection measures were adequate at the time of birth.

Step 10. Training and awareness of health professionals

All health care providers involved at the time of birth and subsequent care of the newborn (physicians, midwives, maternity nurses, community health workers, traditional birth attendants) need to be adequately trained on the principles and procedures of the warm chain.

In institutions where hi-tec equipment is used (radiant heaters, incubators), there should be well-trained staff to monitor the baby's temperature and to clean and maintain the equipment. Families and communities need to be made aware of the importance of keeping newborns warm with simple common sense maneuvers as well as technology based methods.

MANAGEMENT OF HYPOTHERMIA

Rewarming

The methods used for rewarming depends on the severity of hypothermia and the availability of staff and equipment. In cases of mild hypothermia, the baby can be warmed by skin-to-skin contact, in a warm room (at least 26°C). In cases of moderate and severe hypothermia the baby may be rewarmed using the following devices.

Warm Room

Warming the room to 32–34°C is the least desirable method of rewarming as it likely to be uncomfortable for the personnel and even term neonates. The temperature of the nursery should be maintained between 26–28°C.

Radiant Warmer

It is a popular mode of warming because it provides unimpeded access to neonates requiring intensive care. However, insensible water losses are large. Covering the neonate with a plastic sheet or an acrylic shield can minimize the insensible water loss (IWL). Apneic spells do not occur during rewarming, as the air breathed is not warmed by the radiant warmer.

Incubator

In a convectively heated incubator, rewarming is done at a set air temperature of 35–36°C. The heating of incubator air can be controlled by a thermostat set to air temperature within the incubator or to the neonate's skin temperature. Little data exists in selecting the ideal skin temperature as a control point in a servo controlled system and any value between 36.5°C and 37°C is appropriate.

When a newborn is rewarmed using a non-servo warming device, the temperature should be checked frequently. Once the baby's core temperature reaches 34°C, the rewarming process in an incubator on air mode should be closely monitored to avoid overheating.

In cases of severe hypothermia, fast rewarming is preferable because slow rewarming over several days is associated with high mortality. Rapid rewarming can be achieved by using a radiant warmer with skin temperature set at 37°C (Figure 6.2) or by using an incubator on air mode with the air temperature set at

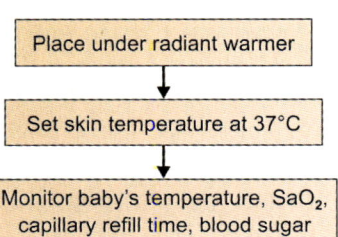

Figure 6.2 Rewarming under a radiant warmer.

35–36°C or a thermostatically controlled heated mattress set at 37–38°C.

Studies have shown that the duration of rewarming time (defined by time taken to raise the abdominal skin temperature to normal by a servo controlled radiant warmer with skin temperature set at 37°C), was 4.9 ± 0.8 min, 17.5 ± 9.5 min and 42 ± 7.9 min for mild, moderate and severe hypothermia respectively ($p = 0.021$). The duration of rewarming a baby did not differ significantly between the different weight and gestational age groups. When the rate of rewarming was expressed as rate of rise in body temperature (°C per kg body weight per hour), it was higher in smaller and more premature babies.

Supportive Management

Provide calories and fluids and prevent a drop in the blood glucose level which is a common problem in hypothermic neonates. When perfusion is poor, give an intravenous bolus of Ringer lactate or normal saline. Careful monitoring with an apnea or cardiac monitor must be done because some neonates may develop apnea during rewarming. Oxygen must be provided if the neonate is desaturating or cyanosed.

Management at Home

At home, skin-to-skin contact is the best method to rewarm a baby with mild hypothermia. The room should be warmed (at least 26°C), and the baby should be covered with a warm blanket and worn a prewarmed cap, mittens and socks. Wet clothes should be replaced by dry prewarmed clothes. There should be no draught of air. The rewarming process should be continued until the baby's temperature reaches the normal range or the baby's hands and feet are no longer cold or blue.

The cold skin of babies has poor blood circulation and is likely to burn easily by hot water bottles which should never be placed next to the baby. When used to warm a cot, hot water bottle should be removed before the baby is placed in the cot. The mother should continue breastfeeding on demand. If the baby becomes lethargic and refuses to suck, the baby should be taken to the hospital. During transport, the baby should be kept in skin-to- skin contact with the mother.

HYPERTHERMIA

Hyperthermia is defined as a rectal temperature greater than 37.5°C (99.5°F). Environmental overheating leads to peripheral vasodilatation and both trunk and peripheries become warm. During fever, peripheral vasoconstriction leads to colder extremities while the abdominal or chest temperature is raised. Thus, assessment of abdominal and peripheral temperature (by touch or thermistor probe) in a hyperthermic neonate can differentiate between hyperthermia due to raised ambient temperature and fever in a sick neonate.

Physiological Response to Hyperthermia

During a febrile state, the hypothalamic temperature set point is raised leading to hyperthermia. During fever there is peripheral vasoconstriction and extremities become cold. The neonate makes physiological and behavioral responses to reduce heat loss, and increase heat production to raise the body temperature. An overheated neonate, on the other hand, makes physiological and behavioral responses to increase heat loss. Either form of hyperthermia is associated with increased metabolic demands for the neonate. The neonate is likely to have increased oxygen requirements, apnea, dehydration, metabolic acidosis and in extreme cases, heat stroke, brain damage, shock and death.

Causes of Hyperthermia

Infection is not the only cause of a raised set point of temperature in the hypothalamic thermostat, it is also caused by a severe cerebral abnormality, either congenital (holoprosencephaly, hydranencephaly, encephalocele) or acquired (birth asphyxia). Environmental overheating is the most common cause of hyperthermia. Overheating may lead to hyperpyrexia (rectal temperature above 41°C). Mild hyperthermia occurs when an active, large neonate is overwrapped and left in a warm room, or when preterm neonates are overheated in an incubator or under a radiant warmer. Severe hyperthermia occurs when there is electrical or mechanical failure of a warming device, when an incubator is exposed to direct sunlight (creation of greenhouse effect) or thermistor probe gets dislodged when a neonate is nursed in servo-control mode. Hyperthermia may occur in infants of families with a history of malignant hyperpyrexia and anhidrotic ectodermal dysplasia.

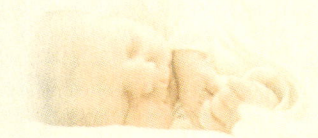

Symptoms

The signs and symptoms of hyperthermia secondary to overheating are given in Box 6.2. It is important to clinically differentiate between an overheated (hyperthermia) and a febrile neonate (Table 6.1). Mild overheating is an important predisposing factor for apnea of prematurity. Severe overheating may lead to hyperpyrexia and cause sudden death in a newborn without any prior symptoms.

Management

Overheated neonates simply need a cooler environment. The heat stressed neonate should be assisted to keep metabolic heat production to a minimum. The neonate who assumes an extended posture should be left in that position in order to promote heat loss. Shift the baby to a cooler environment and reduce the clothing if it is excessive. Skin surfaces can be left exposed to promote evaporation and heat loss. Active temperature reduction methods should be kept at a bare minimum to prevent a dramatic loss of heat, leading to cold stress and shock.

Administer intravenous fluid bolus of Ringer lactate or normal saline if shock is present. Metabolic acidosis if present should be corrected. Provide adequate fluids to maintain hydration and continue breastfeeding. Monitor baby's temperature, respiration (for apnea), capillary refill time and state of hydration. In a febrile neonate investigate for the cause of fever and treat it accordingly.

BIBLIOGRAPHY

Agarwal S, Sethi V, Srivastava K, Jha PK, Baqui AH. Human touch to detect hypothermia in neonates in Indian slum dwellings. *Indian J Pediatr* 2010; 77(7):759–62.

Castrodale V, Rinehard S. The golden hour: improving the stabilization of the very low birth weight infant. *Adv Neonatal Care* 2014; 14(1):9–14.

Cinar ND, Filiz TM. Neonatal thermoregulation. *J Neonat Nurs* 2006; 12(2):69–74.

Daga AS. Determinants of death among admissions to intensive care units for newborns. *J Trop Ped* 1991; 37:53–55.

Dagan R, Gorodischer R. Infections in hypothermic infants younger than 3 months old. *Am J Dis Child* 1984; 138:483–85.

Ellis J. Neonatal hypothermia. *J Neonat Nurs* 2005; 11(2):76–82.

Glass L, Silverman WA, Sinclair JC. Effect of the thermal environment on cold resistance and growth of small infants after the first week of life. *Pediatrics* 1968; 41:1033–46.

Godfrey K, Nativio DG, Bender CV, Schlenk EA. Occlusive bags to prevent hypothermia in premature infants: a quality improvement initiative. *Adv Neonatal Care* 2013; 13(5):311–16.

Kaplan M, Eidelman AI. Improved prognosis in severely hypothermic newborn infants treated by rapid rewarming. *J Pediatr* 1984; 105:470–74.

Kumar V, Shearer JC, Kumar A, Darmstadt GL. Neonatal hyperthermia in low resource setting: a review. *J Perinatol* 2009; 29:401–12.

Lunze K, Hamer DH. Thermal protection of the newborn in resource-limited environments. *J Perinatol* 2012; 32:317–24.

Lyon A. Temperature control in the neonate. *Paediatr Child Hlth* 2008; 18(4):155–60.

Mathur NB, Krishnamurthy S, Mishra TK. Estimation of rewarming time in transported extramural hypothermic neonates. *Indian J Pediatr* 2006; 73:395–99.

Mathur NB, Krishnamurthy S, Mishra TK. Evaluation of WHO classification of hypothermia in sick extramural neonates as a predictor of fatality. *J Trop Pediatr* 2005; 51:341–45.

Sarman I, Can G, Tunell R. Rewarming preterm babies on a heated, water filled mattress. *Arch Dis Child* 1989; 64:687–92.

Singh M, Rao G, Malhotra AK, Deorari AK. Assessment of newborn baby's temperature by human touch: A potentially useful primary care strategy. *Indian Pediatr* 1992; 29:449–52.

Tafari N, Gentz J. Aspects on rewarming newborn infants with severe accidental hypothermia. *Acta Paediatr Scand* 1974; 63: 595–600.

Thermal protection of the newborn: A practical guide. WHO/RHT/MSM/Reference No. WS 420, 1997.

BOX 6.2 Clinical features of hyperthermia

Symptoms	Signs
• Irritability or lethargy	• Flushing
• Diaphoresis	• Warm and pink extremities
• Eager to feed	• Tachycardia
• Normal, weak or rarely absent cry	• Hypotension is rare
	• Apneic attacks
	• Hypotonia with extended posture
	• No difference between skin temperature of extremities and core body temperature

Table 6.1 Differences between a healthy neonate who is overheated and a febrile sick neonate

Overheated neonate	Febrile neonate
• High rectal temperature	• High rectal temperature
• Warm and pink hands and feet	• Cold and pale hands and feet
• The difference between abdominal skin temperature and hand skin temperature is less than 2°C	• Abdominal skin temperature exceeds hand skin temperature by more than 3°C
• Tachycardia	• Tachycardia
• Irritability and restlessness	• Lethargic
• Healthy flushed appearance	• Looks unwell with circumoral cyanosis
• Keen to feed	• Refusal to feed
• No shock	• Shock may occur

7

The Crying Neonate

Meharban Singh

BACKGROUND

Crying is the most eagerly awaited signal at the time of birth of a healthy baby! When a baby fails to cry at birth, it is a cause for concern and efforts are made to resuscitate the baby and make him cry. Subsequently, crying is viewed as a nuisance and a cause for anxiety to the parents. Infants and young children who cannot speak, cry is the only signal to express their needs and draw attention to their discomfort, hunger, thirst and painful or unpleasant conditions. Certain amount of crying is physiological and desirable and is believed to be akin to "exercise period" and "letting off the steam" to give vent to their anger, frustration and to seek attention. Crying may even serve an important development purpose. Healthy infants on an average cry for 1–3 hours everyday during first 8 weeks of life. Periodic crying in infants is most commonly due to hunger, thirst, fatigue uncomfortable environment, over clothing or under clothing, wet nappies, and boredom. Most infants cry and fret while falling asleep.

An intelligent and perceptive mother can readily differentiate between the cry due to hunger and cry as a signal of discomfort. Cry of hunger is likely to be short and low-pitched while cry of pain is sudden, loud, prolonged and high-pitched. A large number of disorders during infancy can be diagnosed on the basis of nature, quality and character of crying. Most parents are quite used to episodic crying of their infants but *persistent or protracted and inconsolable crying* is frightening and presents as one of the common disorders in the emergency department. Excessive crying, especially in the absence of any predisposing conditions and localizing features, poses a great diagnostic challenge to a pediatrician. The majority of cases of infants with excessive crying are due to nonserious conditions but at times crying babies may have illnesses that may be life-threatening.

CAUSES

Excessive crying and restlessness most commonly occurs due to a painful condition originating in any of the body system (Table 7.1). Hypoxia due to cardio-respiratory disorders and shock is an important cause of restlessness and crying but the clinical picture is dominated by underlying condition and infant looks critically sick. Infant may manifest cow's milk protein allergy or allergens consumed by the mother (like cow's milk, eggs, nuts, wheat, fish) may be passed in her breast milk to cause discomfort and cramping in her suckling infant. Cow's milk allergy usually manifests with fussiness, discomfort, vomiting, wheezing, eczema, poor weight gain and blood in the stool. Visceral pain occurs due to sudden distension of viscera and stretching of their serosal coverings because internal body organs per se are not supplied by pain fibers. Excessive unexplained crying in infancy may be a marker of brain damage and development of autism and attention deficit hyperactivity disorder later in life.

Table 7.1 Causes of excessive crying in neonates

Central nervous system

Raised intracranial pressure
- Meningitis/encephalitis
- Intracranial bleeding
- Space occupying lesion
- Pseudotumor cerebri
- Brain damaged infant

Cardiovascular system
- Congestive heart failure
- Myocarditis
- Pericarditis
- Arrhythmias (paroxysmal supraventricular tachycardia)
- Vaso-occlusive disorders (sickle cell disease, vasculitis, thrombophlebitis, and acrodynia)

(Contd.)

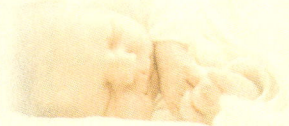

Table 7.1 Causes of excessive crying in neonates (*Contd...*)

- Abnormal origin of the left coronary artery from pulmonary artery (ALCAPA), coronary fistula and coronary stenosis

Respiratory system
- Blocked nose
- Acute suppurative otitis media
- Pneumonia
- Bronchospasm
- Foreign body in the air passages
- Pleural effusion and empyema

Gastrointestinal system
- Oral thrush
- Aphthous stomatitis
- Herpangina
- Intestinal colic (evening colic)
- Lactose intolerance
- Cow's milk allergy
- Mesenteric adenitis
- Appendicitis
- Gastroesophageal reflux disease (GERD)
- Malrotation and midgut volvulus
- Necrotizing enterocolitis
- Intussusception
- Acute intermittent porphyria
- Constipation
- Anal fissure
- Foreign body ingestion
- Pinworms

Genitourinary system
- Urinary tract infection
- Bladder neck obstruction
- Renal colic
- Torsion of testis
- Incarcerated inguinal hernia

Musculoskeletal system
- Unrecognised trauma
- Fracture
- Dislocation (elbow, shoulder)
- Osteomyelitis/arthritis
- Congenital syphilis
- Chikungunya
- Bone pains (acute leukemia)
- Scurvy
- Caffey's disease
- Battered baby syndrome

Emotional causes
- Over stimulation or neglect
- Tension in the family dynamics
- Over anxious mother or grandmother
- Postpartum depression

Miscellaneous conditions
- Temper tantrums and breath holding spells
- Over covered or exposed baby
- Foreign body in the eye or nose
- Insect bites
- Open diaper pin
- Hair tourniquet syndrome
- Scared or frightened infant
- DTwP vaccine
- Drugs

HISTORY

Detailed history should be elicited to identify preceding events and associated symptoms. Episodes of crying, fretfulness and fussiness in the evening in infants between 2–16 weeks of age with characteristic periodicity is highly suggestive of evening colic. Night crying is common during infancy (Box 7.1). It is apparent rather than real because infants are not aware of day and night, even physiological whimpering due to hunger or wet napkin appears too loud during the quietness and solitude of night. Night crying is more disturbing and troublesome to tired parents and neighbours because it interferes with their relaxation and sleep. Abnormal and excessive crying at night should alert to the possibilities of exposure to cold or hot environment, wet napkin, nappy rash, insect bites due to mosquitoes and bed bugs. In a breastfed baby, ask the mother whether her lactation is satisfactory because hunger is an important cause of crying. Episodes of crying spells with arching of back, vomiting and poor feeding due to esophagitis and heartburn are suggestive of gastroesophageal reflux disease (GERD). There may be sleeplessness, difficulty in burping, gagging, ear infection and coughing at night due to aspiration into lungs.

Some infants with perinatal distress factors, and neuromotor retardation have increased incidence of unexplained crying possibly due to cerebral irritability. Infants with acute gastroenteritis often cry due to thirst but it is commonly misinterpreted as colic. Crying or fussiness while feeding should alert to the possibility of nose block, aphthous stomatitis, thrush, and herpangina. Infants cannot vocalize to indicate the site of pain, which may be suggested by certain gestures like flexion of thighs over abdomen with passage of flatus (intestinal colic), head banging (headache), poking fingers or pulling at ears (earache), touching or rubbing genitals (UTI or balanitis), inability to move a limb (pseudoparalysis due to scurvy, osteomyelitis, congenital syphilis, fracture and dislocation, etc.), blinking, rubbing and watering of an eye due to foreign

BOX 7.1 Night crying

- Evening colic
- Nasal congestion
- Over clothing or under clothing
- Pinworms
- Diaper rash
- Insect bites (mosquitoes, bed bugs, mites)
- Excessive light or noise
- Gastroesophageal reflux disease (GERD)
- Bronchospasm

body and conjunctivitis. Excessive crying may occur in infants due to dactylitis because of congenital syphilis, sickle cell disease, chikungunya, tuberculosis and streptococcal or staphylococcal infections.

Most crying infants are quietened when picked up or gently rocked. When episodes of crying are precipitated or aggravated when the baby is picked up, it is suggestive of a painful condition in the musculo-skeletal system. Sudden pulling of an infant by forearms may lead to severe pain and inconsolable crying due to subluxation of the radial head (annular ligament displacement) which is commonly called as "nursemaid's elbow". Chronic constipation and crying while defecating are suggestive of anal fissure. *When an infant with acute gastroenteritis develops sudden constipation with passage of currant-jelly stools and episodes of inconsolable crying due to abdominal colic, it is highly suggestive of acute intussusception.* Rarely, intussusception may occur following administration of rotavirus vaccine. Unexplained episodes of severe abdominal pain and bone pains may occur due to vaso-occlusive crises of sickle cell disease and in children with acute leukemia. The conditions may at times be confused with surgical abdomen and osteomyelitis.

Presence of fever is suggestive of an infective condition and in these cases the cause of crying can be usually established. Attempt should be made to look for symptoms referable to various systems of the body; central nervous system (head banging, vomiting, photophopia, seizures), cardiorespiratory system (cough, breathing and feeding difficulty), gastro-intestinal system (vomiting, constipation, abdominal distension, diarrhea, colic) and genitourinary system (dysuria, frequency, urinary retention, abnormalities in urinary stream). Most healthy neonates may cry before passing urine due to the unpleasant sensation of a full bladder. However, they become quiet, relaxed and dazed while passing urine and start crying again after having passed urine due to wet napkins.

Specific history should be asked for inhalation or ingestion of a foreign body. Sudden episode of choking and crying in an infant who was seen to be fiddling and mouthing some objects (peanut, coin, beads, toys with loose or sharp components, etc.) is highly suggestive of inhalation or ingestion of a foreign body. Detailed enquiry should be made regarding the medications being taken. Excessive irritability and restlessness may occur due to intake of atropine derivatives, pseudoephedrine, antispasmodics and xanthine derivatives. Some infants are known to become restless following intake of sedatives, which are also known to precipitate abdominal colic in

patients with acute intermittent porphyria. Excessive crying due to pseudotumor cerebri is a recognized side effect of excessive or prolonged intake of nalidixic acid, norfloxacin, tetracyclines, corticosteroids, and vitamin A. Prolonged and excessive local application of topical anesthetic (lignocaine hydrochloride) over perianal area in an infant with anal fissure may lead to excessive irritability, restlessness and seizures. Excessive and inconsolable crying with fever and swelling at the site of injection is a recognised adverse effect due to pertussis component of DTwP vaccination. History of accidental and intentional trauma should be elicited with tact and ingenuity. Inconsolable crying of an infant is a challenge and frustrating experience for parents and may lead to infant abuse and "shaking" of a crying infant. Changes in the emotional milieu like change of environment, visit by guests, change in type and mode of feeding, tension among parents, inappropriate response on the part of mother to meet the needs of her infant are important causes of fretfulness and fussiness.

PHYSICAL EXAMINATION

A detailed physical examination of a nude baby from "top-to-toes" remains the cornerstone of evaluation of the crying infant. Crying is associated with physical and physiological responses like facial grimacing, eye-squinting and screwing, limb movements, increased heart rate, blood pressure and vagal tone. Vital signs should be recorded to exclude fever, hypothermia, shock and hypotension, tachypnea and dyspnea, tachycardia and dysrhythmia which provide useful clues to the involvement of major organ systems.

Special emphasis should be placed on general physical examination. External marks of injuries, insect bites, swellings, fracture and dislocation should be looked for. Presence of papules and wheals over the exposed parts is suggestive of mosquito or insect bites. Watch for range and strength of spontaneous movements of all the extremities. Look for swelling of hand with swelling and tenderness of carpals and metacarpals (dactylitis). Infants with "pulled elbow" (subluxation of radial head) are unable to use the arm which is kept semiflexed and supinated (nursemaid's position or Indian lady supporting her saree). Look at toes and fingers to exclude strangulation due to hair tourniquet. The diaper must be removed to exclude torsion of testis, incarcerated hernia, strangulation of penis, diaper rash and injury by diaper pin. Unilateral scrotal swelling with suffusion or blueness of overlying skin with absence of cremasteric reflex are suggestive of torsion of testis. Exclude anal fissure and look for diaper rash. Entrapment of the penis in the zipper of the trousers is easy to diagnose but at times extremely difficult to extricate.

Examine orifices, oral cavity for ulcers and thrush, ears for otitis media, anus for fissure or tear, and penis for tight phimosis or balanitis. Eyes should be examined for pupillary size and eyelids must be everted to look for any evidence of a foreign body. Oral examination should be conducted to exclude aphthous ulcers, thrush, swelling of gums due to teething, and angina of throat. Otoscopy is mandatory to visualize tympanic membrane to exclude acute otitis media. Fundus examination should be done to look for retinal hemorrhages (as an evidence of battering and vigorous shaking) and papilledema. Bulging anterior fontanel is suggestive of raised intracranial tension. Neck stiffness may be absent or insignificant in young infants with meningitis.

Systemic examination should be conducted to exclude potentially life-threatening conditions. During the bout of screaming, heart (to exclude tachyrhythmia due to PSVT) and abdomen (to look for borborygmi due to intestinal obstruction and colic) should be carefully auscultated. Evidences of congestive heart failure point to the underlying cardiac problem while tachypnea with intercostal and subcostal retractions is suggestive of pneumonia and bronchospasm. In young infants excessive and inconsolable crying may be the sole manifestation of septicemia. ALCAPA (abnormal origin of left coronary artery from pulmonary artery) is a rare cause of sudden episodes of inconsolable crying with sweating which is followed by lethargy and extreme exhaustion. The infant is likely to have evidences of cardiac failure with findings of anterolateral myocardial infarction on EKG, i.e. deep Q waves in lead 1, aVL and V1–V4. History of sudden choking, stridor and unilateral wheezing are diagnostic of a foreign body in the air passages. Look for abdominal distension and peristaltic movements to exclude intestinal obstruction. When indicated, rectal examination should be done to exclude intussusception. Urinary retention should be excluded by percussing the suprapubic area and by palpating for a distended urinary bladder. The clinical features that suggest the crying is likely to be due to a serious systemic disorder are listed in Box 7.2.

Wessel et al has proposed "the rule of three" to define infantile colic, i.e. irritability, fussing or crying lasting for more than 3 hours in a day, occuring on more than 3 days in a week and lasting for at least 3 weeks. Evening colic is the most common cause of unexplained crying in infants. It occurs in about 20 percent of "normal" infants and is characterized by paroxysmal episodes of inconsolable crying during the evening in

BOX 7.2 Ominous features in a crying neonate

- Inconsolable crying for more than 3 hours
- Infant is lethargic, cold, sick and refuses to feed
- Abnormal vital signs
- Febrile or hypothermic infant
- Vomiting, constipation or diarrhea and abdominal distension
- Difficulty in passing urine or anuria for >4 hours
- Rapid or difficult breathing with hypoxia or slow capillary refill time (>2 sec)
- Bulging anterior fontanel
- Swollen scrotum due to incarcerated inguinal hernia or torsion of testis
- Evidences of injury, swollen limb or joint with pseudoparalysis

infants between 2 to 16 weeks of age. The spell of crying occurs everyday at the same time in a clockwise regularity. The infant appears in severe discomfort, cries loudly, often flexes the legs over the abdomen, boxes the arms and may pass wind to obtain temporary relief. The condition is seen in equal frequency both in breast and bottle fed babies. The episodes of crying abort spontaneously and none of the therapeutic interventions seem to offer any definite relief. The condition disappears after the age of 12 weeks. The etiology is unknown but various postulations include intestinal colic ("blocked" wind), milk allergy, lactose intolerance, altered flora of gut, immaturity of intestinal tract or central nervous system, oversensitive wiry infant, excessive stimulation, parental anxiety, abnormal emotional tension in the family dynamics, and inappropriate response on the part of mother or grandmother to serve the needs and desires of the infant.

INVESTIGATIONS

It is difficult to assess the severity of pain in infants. Visual analog, neonatal/infant pain scale (NIPS), pain assessment in neonates (PAIN), and linear scales are used to assess the intensity of pain. The acoustic characteristics of crying can be assessed by using VOXMETRIA and GRAM softwares.

Careful history, detailed physical examination and close observation are most crucial to identify the cause of inconsolable crying in an infant. In about two-thirds of the infants, the cause of excessive crying can be identified by good history and detailed physical examinaton. No routine investigations are needed for an afebrile crying infant without any signs of illness. Investigations should be planned depending upon the clues obtained on clinical assessment. No uniform plan of investigations can be recommended for all crying infants. In the absence of any localizing symptoms and signs, physiological conditions, insect bites, abdominal colic, urinary tract infection, sepsis, episodic cardiac arrhythmia or angina equivalent and emotional causes should be seriously considered. Urine examination (routine and culture) is recommended in all infants to exclude UTI and acute intermittent porphyria. When tachypnea and dyspnea are associated, detailed cardio-respiratory work-up is indicated to diagnose underlying pulmonary and cardiac disorders. In infants with bulging anterior fontanel or retinal hemorrhages, exclude meningitis and intracranial bleeding by CSF examination and CT scan of brain. When abdominal distension is present or UTI is documented, skiagrams of abdomen should be taken and ultrasonography done. Skeletal survey is indicated to look for any clinical evidences of dactylitis, scurvy, osteomyelitis/arthritis, trauma and Caffey's disease. When corneal foreign body is suspected, flourescein staining is indicated to delineate it.

MANAGEMENT

Excessive crying in the first months of life is usually benign and self limiting. The specific management depends upon the nature of underlying disease process. Symptomatic relief should be attempted when serious life-threatening conditions have been excluded. Analgesics like paracetamol, is useful for relief of pain due to inflammatory and traumatic conditions affecting musculoskeletal system. Antispasmodics (dicyclomine hydrochloride, dill oil, fennel oil) are useful for relief of colicky visceral pain. Simethicone should be avoided in an infant receiving levothyroxine because it can adversely affect the efficacy of replacement therapy. Nothing seems to offer consistent benefit to infants with evening colic. Temporary relief is obtained by rhythmic rocking, crib vibrator, playing some soft music, positioning the baby prone and patting on the back, abdominal massage, warm water bath, giving lift in a car or stroller. Swaddling or carrying the baby by using a sling or front carrier may provide respite to some babies. At times white noise (monotonous sound produced by amalgamation of different frequencies) produced by off-tuned radio, off-channel TV sound, shaver, hair dryer, vacuum cleaner, washing machine, etc. may provide relief by distraction and its sedative or sporofic effect.

Mother should not follow the policy of 'cry it out' (CIO) to manage a cranky neonate because it does not work and may lead to insecurity, behavior disorder and disturbed parent-child relationship. She must respond promptly to her child in discomfort by picking and cuddling him without any fear of spoiling the child.

Diaper should be checked for soiling and feed given if child is hungry. Application of *hing* (asfoetida) dissolved in warm water over the periumbilical area and giving decoction of *ajwain* (carom seeds) and *sonf* (anethi seeds) provides prompt relief against intestinal colic. Gripe water formulated without alcohol may be given. Dicyclomine hydrochloride (2–3 mg/dose) 30 minutes before the anticipated time of evening colic may offer relief to some infants but it is not without side effects. In a randomized placebo-controlled, double-blind study, administration of probiotics (*Lactobocillus reuteri*) for 21 days was associated with reduction in the severity and duration of colic. There is no need to change the type and mode of feeding and attempts should be made to reduce environmental tension and decrease stimulation to the child. When milk allergy is strongly suspected, the formula may be replaced with whey hydrolysate milk, soya-based milk or hypoallergenic formula. Excessive crying and sleep disturbances have been treated by chiropractic practices like gentle touch, pressure and spinal manipulations. The evening colic gradually resolves and spontaneously disappears by the age of 3 months.

Use of mosquito net and mebendazole for pinworms may relieve spells of night crying. Night crying due to GERD can be managed by positioning the infant with head raised, administration of proton pump inhibitor (ranitidine, lansoprazole) and prokinetics (domperidone, metoclopramide) before feeds. Lansoprazole is given in a dose of 1.0 mg/kg q 12 hr for 8–12 weeks. Excessive crying during acute gastroenteritis is often due to thirst and promptly responds to administration of ORS. Infants who continue to cry excessively during the prolonged period of observation are likely to have a serious cause for crying. Some of the conditions listed in Table 7.1 would need urgent surgical intervention.

Anal fissure is managed by local application of anesthetic cream and relief of constipation by use of fruit juice, honey and extra sugar in formula feed. Subluxation of radial head can be readily corrected in the emergency department by "hand shake" or "supination-flexion" maneuver. In the former procedure, child's hand is held as if to shake it and the affected elbow is enclosed by the physician in the other hand. Abruptly the forearm is pronated while increasing flexion at the elbow. Alternatively, hold the affected elbow of the child in your left hand by placing thumb over the radial head. With your right hand, quickly supinate the forearm while slightly flexing the elbow. The subluxation is promptly corrected and a palpable click may be felt by your thumb. There is no need to take any skiagrams before and after the procedure. Recurrence of nursemaid's elbow may occur in 5%–39% cases and has been successfully treated by giving instructions on telephone.

Crying due to raised intracranial tension caused by medications responds promptly on discontinuation of the offending drug. Restlessness and crying due to cerebral irritability in brain damaged children may be treated by administration of diphenhydramine hydrochloride (5 mg/kg/day q 8 hr). For management of life-threatening disorders associated with excessive inconsolable crying, refer to the appropriate sections of the book.

BIBLIOGRAPHY

Balapatabendi M, Harris D, Shenoy SD. Drug interaction of levo-thyroxine with infant colic drops. *Arch Dis Child* 2011, 96:888.

Bhatia J, Parish A. GERD or not GERD: The fussy infant. *J Perinatol* 2009, 29 (Suppl 2): S7–S11.

Branco A, Feketes, Rugolo L, Rehder MI. The newborn pain cry: Descriptive acoustic spectrographic analysis. *Int J Pediatr Otorhinolaryngol* 2007; 71(4):539–46.

Brazelton TBA. Crying in infancy. *Pediatrics* 1962; 29:579–88.

Bruce JW. Infantile colic. *Pediatr Clin North Amer* 1961; 8:143–45.

Corwin MJ, Lester BM, Golub HL. The infant cry: What can it tell us? *Curr Prob Pediatr* 1996; 26:325–34.

Ferber R. Sleeplessness, night awakening and night crying in the infant to toddler. *Pediatr Rev* 1987; 9:69–82.

Freedman SB, Al-Harthy N, Thull-Freedman J. The crying infant: Diagnostic testing and frequency of serious underlying disease. *Pediatrics* 2009, 123: 841–48.

Hall B, Chesters J, Robinson A. Infantile colic: a systematic review of medical and conventional therapies. *J Paediatr Child Health* 2012, 48:128.

Huhtala V, Lehtonen L, Heinonen R, Korvenrant H. Infant massage compared with crib vibrator in the treatment of colicky infants. *Pediatrics* 2000, 105 (6): E84.

Illingworth RS. Crying in infants and children. *Brit Med J* 1955; 1:75.

Illingworth RS. Infantile colic revisited. *Arch Dis Child* 1985; 60: 981–85.

Illingworth RS. Three months colic. *Arch Dis Child* 1954; 29:165–74.

Lee JH, Kim MJ, Lee JS, Chol YH. The effects of three alternative treatment strategies after 8 weeks of proton pump inhibitor therapy for GERD children. *Arch Dis Child* 2011, 96: 9–13

McKenzile S. Troublesome crying in infants: effect of advice to reduce stimulation. *Arch Dis Child* 1991; 66:1416–20.

Poole SR. The infant with acute unexplained excessive crying. *Pediatrics* 1991; 88:450–55.

Ruis-Conteraras J, Urquio L, Bastero R. Persistent crying as predominant manifestation of sepsis in infants and newborns. *Pediatr Emerg Care* 1999; 15:113–15.

Samira Akhnikh, Engelberts AC, Van Sleuwen BE, et al. The excessively crying infant: etiology and treatment. *Pediatr Annals* 2014, 43(4): e69–75.

Schunk JE. Radial head subluxation: epidemiology and treatment of 87 episodes. *Ann Emerg Med* 1990; 19:1019–23.

Singh M. The 'windy' baby. In: The Art and Science of Baby and Child Care. *CBS Publishers & Distributors Pvt Ltd, New Delhi*, 4th edition 2015; p 65.

St. James-Roberts I. Persistent crying in infancy. *J Child Psychol Psychiatry* 1989; 3:189–95.

St. James-Roberts I, Halil T. Infant crying patterns in the first year: Normative and clinical findings. *J Child Psychol Psychiatry* 1991; 32: 951–68.

St. James-Roberts I. Persistent infant crying. *Arch Dis Child* 1991; 66:653–55.

Valman HB. The first year of life: crying babies. *Brit Med J* 1980; 280:1522–55.

Wessel MA, Cobb JC, Jackson EB, et al. Paroxysmal fussing in infancy, sometimes called "colic". *Pediatrics* 1954; 14:421–34.

8

The Neonate with Cyanosis

Saurabh Kumar Gupta

Cyanosis is a clinical correlate of hypoxemia and result from a variety of physiological alterations, most common being cardiac and respiratory. Neonatal cyanosis, especially after initial 10–15 minutes of birth, is almost always pathological and necessitates detailed evaluation. Understanding the physiologic basis is essential for early stabilization and definitive management of a cyanotic neonate. The distinction of cardiac from the respiratory causes of cyanosis is extremely important. A systematic approach of clinical examination, electrocardiography and chest X-ray (CXR) allows this distinction and permits classification of underlying congenital heart disease (CHD). This chapter presents a clinical approach to a cyanotic neonate with emphasis on the identification and management of cyanotic CHD.

Cyanosis, derived from the Greek word *kuaneos* meaning 'dark blue', refers to the bluish discoloration of the skin, nail beds or mucous membranes. While oxyhemoglobin (OxyHb) is bright red, deoxyhemoglobin (DeoxyHb) imparts dark blue or purple color to blood producing cyanosis. Cyanosis, however, is discernible to human eyes only when DeoxyHb exceeds 3 g/dL in arterial blood.

HYPOXEMIA, HYPOXIA AND CYANOSIS

Although used interchangeably, it is important to distinguish the terms "hypoxemia", "hypoxia", and "cyanosis". Hypoxemia exists when arterial oxygen content is low. It is usually defined as reduced partial pressure of oxygen in systemic artery (PaO_2) to less than 80–100 mmHg. Hypoxemia usually, but not always, manifests as systemic arterial desaturation. Owing to the sigmoid shape of the oxygen dissociation curve (ODC), hemoglobin (Hb) is nearly fully saturated at low levels of hypoxemia. Hypoxia is failure of the oxygenation of tissues and usually manifests as

metabolic acidosis due to anerobic metabolism. Cyanosis, on the other hand, is bluish discoloration of skin and mucous membranes, mostly but not always, due to hypoxemia.

Although interrelated, all these conditions can exist independent of each other. For example, an infant or a child with cyanotic CHD could have hypoxemia and cyanosis but no hypoxia as long as the cardiac output or Hb level is maintained. On the other hand, an infant or a child with severe anemia or reduced cardiac contractility may have normal saturation and no hypoxemia or cyanosis but shows evidences of tissue hypoxia due to reduced tissue oxygen delivery. Children with defective Hb or methemoglobinemia can have cyanosis and hypoxia but no hypoxemia or arterial desaturation on blood gas analysis.

Cyanosis, like other clinical signs, relies on many variables and therefore is an imperfect surrogate of hypoxemia. Cyanosis has high specificity and positive predictive value but poor sensitivity and negative predictive value especially at low levels of hypoxemia. The determination of PaO_2 in arterial blood gas (ABG) remains the gold standard for the diagnosis of hypoxemia. ABG, however, is not performed routinely as it is invasive and is not widely available. Also since majority of the oxygen is carried in the blood bound to Hb, oxygen saturation is used as a common correlate of cyanosis. ABG derived oxygen saturation (SaO_2) is not directly measured but is calculated from PaO_2 and pH. Blood gas analyzers assumes the ODC to be normal and therefore may not reflect true oxygen saturation especially in hospitalized infants with altered physiology. On the other hand, direct measurement of oxygen saturation by pulse oximetry (SpO_2) provides much easier, non-invasive and reliable estimate of hypoxemia. Routine pulse oximetry has been shown to improve sensitivity in detecting cyanotic CHD in neonates and infants especially if the cyanosis is mild. Broadly, SpO$_2$ of less than 95% is considered to represent hypoxemia and at this cut-off value, pulse oximetry reaches high specificity of more than 99% and a sensitivity of 75%. All children with suspicion of hypoxemia should undergo pulse oximetry before they are declared free of hypoxemia.

Factors Determining Clinical Detection of Cyanosis

Hemoglobin Concentration

The appearance of cyanosis is related to the absolute concentration of DeoxyHb which in turn is dependent on total Hb. For a given degree of arterial desaturation, higher is the amount of total Hb, there is likely to be more DeoxyHb and easier to detect cyanosis. For example, an infant or a child with Hb 20 g/dL will exhibit cyanosis at a saturation of 85%, whereas an infant or a child with Hb 10 g/dL will not exhibit clinical cyanosis until saturation drops to as low as 70%. Consequently, even clinically relevant hypoxemia may remain masked in an anemic child while it may be easily apparent in the presence of polycythemia (Figure 8.1).

Type of Hemoglobin

Fetal hemoglobin Fetal hemoglobin (HbF), the predominant form of Hb in neonates, binds to oxygen more avidly than adult hemoglobin (HbA) for easy uptake of oxygen from the placenta. Owing to reduced affinity of 2, 3 Diphosphoglycerate (2,3 DPG), the ODC of HbF is shifted to the left (Figure 8.2) and as a result, for a given level of PaO$_2$, the arterial SaO$_2$ is higher in newborns than older infants or adults. Milder forms of hypoxemia may therefore be missed in neonates if cyanosis alone is used for oxygen desaturation. In other words, neonates and young infants with a high proportion of Hb may have a serious reduction in oxygenation before cyanosis is apparent.

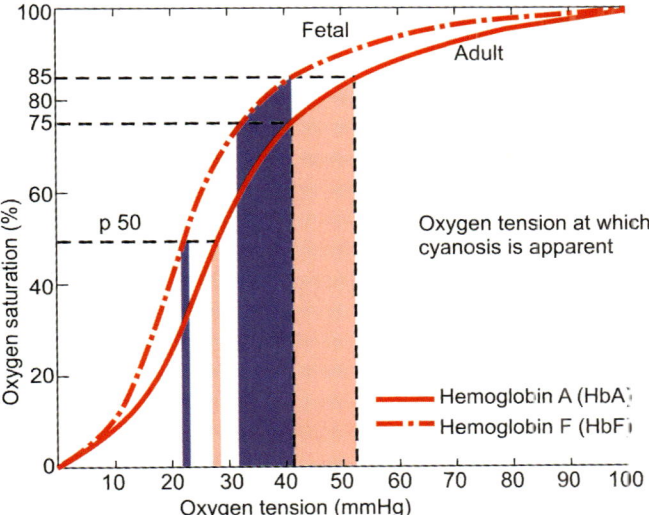

Figure 8.2 Oxygen dissociation curve of HbF and HbA. Note that the p50 of HbF is lower than the p50 of HbA. At a given level of PaO$_2$, this results in higher oxygen saturation in neonates than children and adults.

Abnormal hemoglobin Some neonates have high concentration of oxidized form of Hb, wherein iron is present in its ferric form instead of normal ferrous form, commonly known as methemoglobin (MetHb). This abnormality can be congenital due to deficiency of NADH-cytochrome reductase or acquired in various conditions producing oxidative stress. HbF is more susceptible to this oxidative transformation, thus neonates are at a greater risk to develop methemoglobinemia. In these infants, PaO$_2$ is normal because of normal oxygenation in the lungs. SaO$_2$ as assessed by ABG also turns out to be normal as this is calculated from PaO$_2$ assuming normal ODC. Interestingly, SpO$_2$ is typically fixed at about 85%. This is the result of optical interference of light by MetHb at both the wave lengths, i.e. 660 nm and 940 nm, which is used to differentiate OxyHb and DeoxyHb during pulse oximetry. *This 'saturation gap', defined as normal PaO$_2$ but reduced SpO$_2$, is diagnostic of methemoglobinemia.*

Other Physiologic Factors

Several factors, many of which are common in sick neonates, lead to shift of ODC by causing alteration in the oxygen affinity of Hb. The presence of alkalosis, low PaCO$_2$ due to hyperventilation, hypothermia and low level of 2, 3 Diphosphoglycerate (2, 3 DPG) leads to shift of ODC to the left. This decreases the amount of DeoxyHb at a given PaO$_2$ and lowers the PaO$_2$ at which cyanosis first appears. In contrast, acidosis and fever shift the ODC to the right. As a result, at a given PaO$_2$, there is increase in oxygen delivery to the tissues in these conditions, resulting in greater concentration of DeoxyHb allowing cyanosis to occur at a higher PaO$_2$.

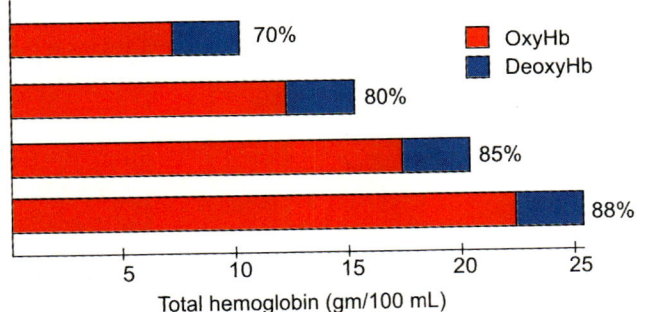

Figure 8.1 Impact of hemoglobin level on the detection of cyanosis. Higher is the hemoglobin concentration easier it is to detect cyanosis at lower levels of desaturation.

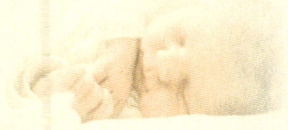

Skin Color and Experience of the Clinician

Cyanosis is usually less apparent in infants with darker skin pigmentation. Clinical examination should include evaluation of nail beds, tongue and mucous membranes. In addition, the importance of appropriate lighting and the experience of the clinician cannot be over emphasized.

Classification of Cyanosis

Based on the extent of involvement, cyanosis is classified as acrocyanosis, central cyanosis and differential cyanosis.

Acrocyanosis

Bluish discoloration in acrocyanosis or peripheral cyanosis is limited to the extremities and lips. The oxygen saturation as well as arterial PaO_2 are normal. It is commonly seen in conditions with hypothermia, local vasoconstriction and sluggish circulation and occurs as a consequence of exaggerated oxygen extraction. This results in an increased concentration of DeoxyHb on the venous side of the capillaries imparting bluish color to skin in the peripheries. Although a benign condition, especially in neonates in their first 24 to 48 hours, it may indicate the presence of serious pathologic conditions such as polycythemia, hypothermia, venous thrombosis, sepsis and shock.

Central Cyanosis

Central cyanosis is present on the cutaneous and mucosal surfaces throughout the body. Normal neonates may have central cyanosis for initial 5 to 10 minutes after birth coinciding with the adaptive changes in respiration and circulation. Oliver and colleagues by performing serial blood gases found that calculated mean percentages of oxygen saturation were 27%, 90%, 92% and 95% at 2 to 5 minutes, 6 to 10 minutes, 11 to 20 minutes and 40 to 60 minutes of age respectively. Persistent central cyanosis anytime thereafter is always pathological and should be evaluated promptly.

Differential Cyanosis

Sometimes, cyanosis is not uniform with dissimilar oxygen saturation in upper and lower half of the body. When cyanosis is more pronounced in lower limbs, it is labelled as 'differential cyanosis'. This results from different bloodstreams supplying upper and lower part of the body as a result of reversal of flow across patent ductus arteriosus (PDA) either in the setting of persistent pulmonary hypertension of newborn (PPHN) or obstruction to the aortic flow, as in cases with coarctation of aorta (CoA) or interrupted aortic arch (IAA). In the absence of PPHN, differential cyanosis is virtually diagnostic of CHD with PDA as part of the hemodynamic circuit.

In infants with PPHN or CoA and PDA, but with transposition of great arteries (TGA), lower limbs are less cyanosed than the upper limbs. This pattern is due to more oxygenated blood from the left ventricle (LV) reaching lower limbs and is known as 'reverse differential cyanosis'.

Causes of Central Cyanosis

Neonates with cyanosis are encountered in emergency department, neonatal intensive care unit and outpatient department of pediatrics and cardiology. An acronym ABCD (Airway, Breathing, Circulation and Defective Hb) allows quick evaluation of common etiologies of cyanosis (Table 8.1). Respiratory and cardiac pathologies are the most common cause of persistent cyanosis. While pulmonary venous desaturation is the underlying mechanism of cyanosis in respiratory diseases and neurological disorders causing respiratory depression, it is the right-to-left shunt, diverting blood away from lungs, that is responsible for cyanosis in CHDs. Defective Hb interferes with oxygen transport, resulting in tissue hypoxia and cyanosis but without any hypoxemia.

Table 8.1 Causes of cyanosis in neonates	
Airway	Choanal atresia
	Micrognathia, Pierre Robin sequence
	Laryngomalacia, vocal cord palsy, tracheal stenosis, vascular ring or sling
	Cystic hygroma or other neck masses
	Absent pulmonary valve syndrome with a large PA compressing the airway
Breathing	*Parenchymal*
	Hyaline membrane disease (HMD)
	Aspiration (meconium amniotic fluid, blood or milk), pneumonia (congenital or acquired)
	Pulmonary hemorrhage, lymphangiectasia
	Pulmonary edema
	Non-parenchymal
	Pneumothorax
	Congenital diaphragmatic hernia
	Congenital cystic adenomatoid malformation, pulmonary sequestration
	Pleural effusion, chylothorax, congenital lobar emphysema
	Diaphragmatic palsy

(Contd...)

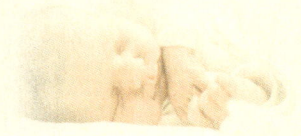

Table 8.1 Causes of cyanosis in neonates (*Contd...*)	
Circulation	Persistent pulmonary hypertension of newborn (PPHN)
	Pulmonary arteriovenous fistula
	Cyanotic congenital heart diseases
	Reduced PBF
	Increased PBF
	Transposition physiology
	Admixture physiology
	Absence of pulmonary stenosis with normal pulmonary blood flow
	Normal PBF with normal PA pressure
	Pulmonary venous hypertension
	Low cardiac output state
Defective Hb	Methemoglobinemia, sulfhemoglobinemia, hemoglobin M
Miscellaneous conditions	Sepsis, hypoglycemia, polycythemia
	CNS depression—asphyxia/ maternal sedation, apnea of prematurity

CNS: central nervous system; Hb: Hemoglobin; PA: pulmonary artery; PBF: pulmonary blood flow

Source: Gupta SK. *Indian J Pediatr* 2015; 82:1050–60.

Clinical Approach to Cyanosis in a Neonate

Clinical evaluation is aimed at identifying neonates with hypoxemia with or without cyanosis. Once the presence of hypoxemia is ascertained, it is important to arrive at the most likely cause of cyanosis. The distinction between respiratory and cardiac pathologies is an important initial step. In addition, detailed assessment is often helpful in classifying the CHD on the basis of cyanosis.

Clinical History

The evaluation begins with detailed clinical history. The importance of antenatal exposure to teratogens, viral exanthems, radiation or occurrence of gestational hypertension, intrauterine growth retardation, and suspected CHD on fetal echocardiogram cannot be overstated. There is higher incidence of transient tachypnea of newborn (TTN), hyaline membrane disease (HMD), and hypoglycemia in infants born to mothers with diabetes mellitus. History of oligohydramnios in the mother is associated with fetal renal and airway abnormalities. Prolonged rupture of membranes and maternal fever are associated with early-onset sepsis and penumonia. Maternal administration of narcotic analgesis may cause respiratory depression of the fetus and neonate at birth.

The time of onset of respiratory distress and cyanosis provide useful clues to the diagnosis. Neonates who become symptomatic at birth are more likely to have respiratory problems such as TTN, HMD, pneumothorax, meconium aspiration syndrome and congenital diaphragmatic hernia (CDH). Cyanosis while feeding can occur due to uncoordinated sucking and swallowing, vocal cord palsy or laryngeal cleft, esophageal atresia with tracheoesophageal fistula.

If the newborn develops respiratory distress and cyanosis several hours after birth, it is most likely to be due to cyanotic CHD, postnatal aspiration syndrome, or tracheoesophageal fistula. However, some cases of CHD and congenital lobar emphysema may not be symptomatic for several hours to days after birth and some cyanotic CHDs may have clinically apparent cyanosis immediately after birth. Late onset cyanosis is typically seen in patients with tetralogy of Fallot (TOF). The timing of onset of cyanosis, therefore, must be interpreted with caution while considering other related factors.

Physical Examination

The physical examination should be performed when the infant is appropriately warm and quiet. The primary focus should be on the assessment of respiratory distress, as its absence generally indicates CHD as the underlying cause. Respiratory distress, due to pulmonary conditions, on the other hand, is characterized by rapid breathing, retractions, use of accessory muscles and crackles. A child with cyanotic CHD and increased pulmonary blood flow (PBF) may also have tachypnea but with fewer retractions and generally no adventitious sounds. Neurological pathologies must be suspected if cyanosis is accompanied by slow and shallow breathing with apneic attacks. It is also important to evaluate the child's tone and activity, and to look for periodic breathing and apneic spells (Box 8.1).

BOX 8.1 Physical examination in neonates with suspected cyanotic CHD

1. Lethargy, hypotonia and poor feeding
2. Evaluate airway, breathing and circulation and defective hemoglobin
3. Presence and pattern of respiratory distress and apneic attacks
4. Heart rate and rhythm, and peripheral pulses
5. Dysmorphism or any other associated anomalies
6. Evidences of heart failure, excessive or poor weight gain, puffiness or sacral edema, tachycardia, and tachypnea
7. Location of liver (to assess situs) and hepatomegaly
8. Examine pulse, capillary refill, SpO$_2$ and blood pressure in both pre and postductal locations
9. Precordial impulse to assess location of the heart, heart sounds, mainly S$_2$
10. Murmur and thrill: timing, site, intensity and radiation

The cardiac examination includes assessment of the heart rate, peripheral pulses, tissue perfusion and evidences of heart failure. Both brachial and femoral pulses should be palpated for their character, timing and volume. The blood pressure must be recorded in all four limbs. The siddeness of liver and spleen, and location of the cardiac impulse help in deciding situs. Palpation and percussion of cardiac silhouette has a limited role in cardiac examination in a neonate. During auscultation, the focus should be on the second heart sound (S_2) which is loud and single in patients with pulmonary arterial hypertension (PAH). In contrast, S_2 is single with inaudible pulmonic component (P_2) in cardiac lesions with reduced PBF. Contrary to common belief, auscultation of cardiac murmurs is not often useful in neonates. Serious lesions such as TGA and total anomalous pulmonary venous connection (TAPVC) are not associated with murmurs while loud murmurs are frequently heard in otherwise benign lesions such as small ventricular septal defect (VSD) and mild pulmonary stenosis (PS). An occasional neonate may present with murmur of functional peripheral PS. Nevertheless, due to high likelihood of CHD, detailed cardiac evaluation by a trained pediatric cardiologist is recommended in all newborns with cardiac murmur. Approximately 1% of newborns have a heart murmur, and of these 31–86% have structural heart disease. Although a carefully conducted clinical examination by a trained pediatric cardiologist is sufficient to distinguish pathological and innocent murmur, the inter and intraobserver variability, especially among neonatologists and pediatricians is high. As a guide, the presence of one major or two minor Nada's criteria (Table 8.2), is highly suggestive of an underlying CHD. Similarly, the presence of any of the red flag signs mandates referral to a pediatric cardiologist (Box 8.2). Moreover, some of the physical signs, if present, indicate the presence of specific cardiac lesions and may allow early diagnosis and timely management (Table 8.3).

Pulse Oximetry

Pulse oximeter is an excellent noninvasive tool for monitoring oxygen saturation and has become standard of care. Unlike cyanosis, pulse oximetry is highly sensitive for the detection of hypoxemia. Moreover, pulse oximetry measurements rely on the relative and not the absolute concentration of DeoxyHb, it is not dependent on total Hb concentration as is the case with cyanosis. It is inexpensive, noninvasive and increasingly being used as point-of-care screening test. Current generation pulse oximeters work well even in

Table 8.2 Nada's criteria for the diagnosis of congenital heart disease

Major criteria
1. Systolic murmur grade 3 or more
2. Diastolic murmur
3. Cyanosis
4. Congestive heart failure

Minor criteria
1. Systolic murmur < grade 3
2. Abnormal S_2
3. Abnormal ECG
4. Abnormal X-ray chest
5. Abnormal blood pressure

1 major or 2 minor criteria suggest high likelihood of structural heart disease

BOX 8.2 Red flag signs for early referral to a pediatric cardiologist
1. Diastolic murmur
2. Pansystolic murmur (OR 5.4)
3. Any systolic murmur > grade 3 (OR 4.8)
4. Harsh murmur (OR 2.4)
5. Abnormal S_2 (OR 4.1)
6. Maximum intensity of murmur at the left upper sternal border (OR 4.2)
7. Systolic click (OR 8.3)
   OR: odds ratio

Table 8.3 Physical findings indicative of specific cardiac malformation

Clinical features	Likely diagnosis
Left ventricle (LV) type of apex beat	Tricuspid atresia Single ventricle of LV morphology DORV with restrictive VSD
Pulsations in 2nd left intercostal space due to left and anterior position of aorta	ccTGA
Pansystolic murmur of AV valve regurgitation	AV septal defect ccTGA
Early diastolic murmur at LUSB	Truncus arteriosus with regurgitation
Sea saw (systolo-diastolic) murmur at LUSB	TOF with absent pulmonary valve
Complete heart block	ccTGA Heterotaxy syndrome

AV: atrioventricular; ccTGA: congenitally corrected transposition of great arteries; DORV: double outlet right ventricle; LUSB: left upper sternal border; LV: left ventricle; PS: pulmonary stenosis; TOF: tetralogy of Fallot; VSD: ventricular septal defect the setting of poor peripheral perfusion and at low saturation level. The availability of pocket pulse oximeters has revolutionized the clinical detection of mild hypoxemia. Measurement of saturation in right hand (preductal) and either foot (postductal) is helpful in identifying differential cyanosis. The left subclavian artery may arise before or after the PDA and therefore left hand is best avoided while assessing upper body saturation. Similarly, postductal origin of umbilical artery must be kept in mind. Pulse oximetry has established itself as the screening tool for CHDs, in particular for critical cyanotic CHDs such as hypoplastic left heart syndrome, pulmonary atresia (with intact ventricular septum), tetralogy of Fallot, total anomalous pulmonary venous return, transposition of great arteries, tricuspid atresia and truncus arteriosus. As per the recent recommendations of American Academy of Pediatrics (AAP), all newborns should undergo pulse oximetry screening. The screening should begin after 24 hours of age or shortly before discharge if the baby is less than 24 hours of age. Waiting until 24 hours of life decreases the risk of false-positive results. This screening should include measurement of saturation in both the right hand and either of the foot. The screening is considered 'negative' and the baby is declared 'passed', if the oxygen saturation is 95% or greater in both right hand and foot and the difference is ≤3% between the right hand and foot. The screening is 'positive' and the baby declared 'failed', if the saturation is less than 90% in any one extremity, or is less than 95% in both extremities, or an absolute saturation difference of >3% between the right hand and either foot on three consecutive measurements taken one hour apart.

Though pulse oximetry has largely replaced ABG analysis for evaluation of hypoxia, the latter remains useful for assessment of adverse effects of hypoxia by measuring blood pH and lactate levels. Analysis of venous blood sample is equally effective in this regard albeit with limited utility in interpreting partial pressure of carbon dioxide ($PaCO_2$) levels.

Hyperoxia Test

Usually it is not difficult to differentiate between cardiac and respiratory cause of cyanosis especially when clinical data is combined with electrocardiogram (ECG) and X-ray chest. Some cases, nonetheless, remain challenging and in them hyperoxia test may be useful.

ABG or transcutaneous oxygen tension monitor should be used for hyperoxia test. ABG is performed preferably from the right radial artery while infant is receiving room air. The ABG is repeated after administration of 100% oxygen for 10 minutes. It is expected that PaO_2 rises substantially if there is no right-to-left shunt. A PaO_2 of more than 160 mmHg after 100% oxygen administration suggests that the cardiac cause of cyanosis is unlikely while a value of >250 mmHg (passed hyperoxia test) excludes it. An arterial PaO_2 of < 100 mmHg (failed hyperoxia test), and/ or rise in PaO_2 of less than 30 mmHg, in the absence of lung pathology is virtually diagnostic of cyanotic CHD. In neonates with PPHN, a similar response is observed despite absence of cyanotic CHD. Differential cyanosis, and a favorable response to various therapeutic strategies to reduce PAH favors the diagnosis of PPHN. In some cases of cyanotic CHD with increased pulmonary blood flow (PBF) such as TAPVC and truncus arteriosus, arterial PaO_2 may increase beyond 100 mmHg due to pulmonary vasodilation. Conversely, infants with a massive intrapulmonary right-to-left shunt as is seen in severe pneumonia or pulmonary arterio-venous fistula may not show significant rise in PaO_2 despite structurally normal heart. The hyperoxia test, therefore, must be interpreted with caution (Table 8.4). In the era of easy availability of echocardiography; the hyperoxia test has lost its relevance.

X-ray Chest

Chest X-ray (CXR) is useful while evaluating newborns with cyanosis and respiratory distress: Special attention should be paid to cardiomegaly and pulmonary blood flow (Figure 8.3). The role of CXR in excluding lung parenchymal pathology is well-established. The expansion of lungs on both sides should be checked. Normal inspiratory films should have eight intercostal spaces of lung fields on both sides. Diaphragmatic paralysis manifests as elevation of hemidiaphragm by more than two intercostal spaces. Hyperinflated lung fields are seen occasionally in lobar emphysema or cystic lesions of lungs. Spontaneous air leak causing pneumothorax and pneumomediastinum in a newborn are rare. HMD after progression shows the characteristic reticular granular pattern and air bronchogram. The ground glass appearance of HMD mimics severe pulmonary venous hypertension (PVH) and is seen in children with obstructed TAPVC. In meconium aspiration syndrome, fluffy infiltrates may be visible; it may also manifest as patchy areas of atelectasis and areas of hyperinflation caused by air trapping. Pulmonary interstitial emphysema may appear as honeycomb appearance of the lung fields. Pleural effusion is visible on the lateral aspect of the lung fields as linear opacity, while large effusions may cause mediastinal shift to the other side. In lobar atelectasis, there is mediastinal shift toward the ipsilateral side. In

Table 8.4 Interpretation of hyperoxia test in different clinical scenarios

	$PaO_2(SpO_2)$ @ FIO_2 0.21	$PaO_2(SpO_2)$ @ FIO_2 1.0	$PaCO_2$
Normal	70 (95%)	>200 (100%)	35–45
Pulmonary/neurologic disease	50 (85%)	>150 (100%)	50
Methemoglobinemia	70 (95%)	>200 (100%)	35
Cardiac disease			
Transposition physiology	<40 (<75%)	<50 (<85%)	35
Reduced PBF	<40 (<75%)	<50 (<85%)	35
Admixture with no PS	50–55 (85–95%)	<150 (<100%)	35
PPHN			
PFO	Pre PDA: <40 (<75%) Post PDA: <40 (<75%)	variable	35–50
PDA	Pre PDA: 70 (95%) Post PDA: <40 (<75%)	variable	35–50

PFO: patent foramen ovale; PDA: patent ductus arteriosus; PS: pulmonary stenosis; PPHN: Persistent pulmonary hypertension of newborn

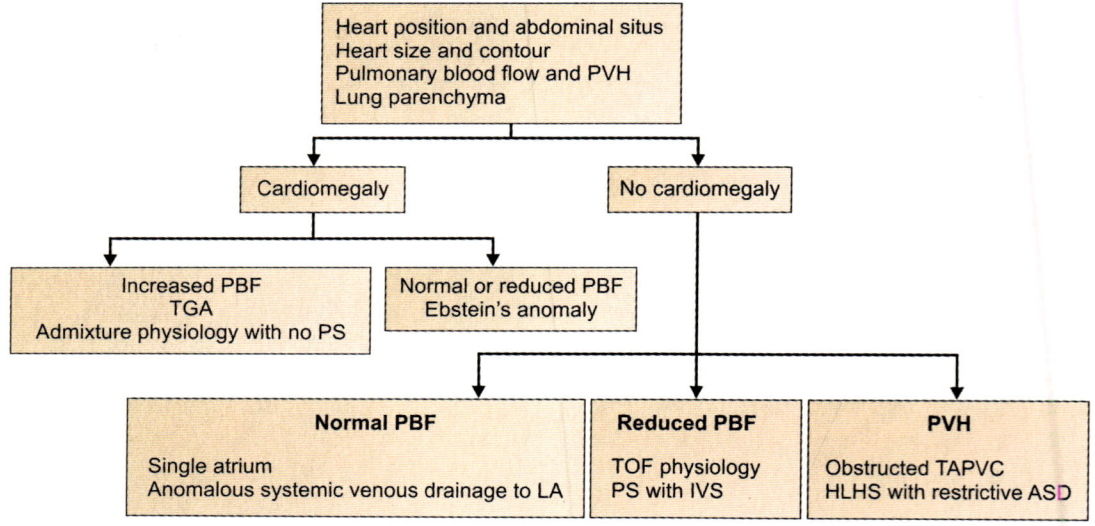

ASD: atrial septal defect; HLHS: hypoplastic left heart syndrome; IVS: intact ventricular septum; LA: left atrium; PBF: pulmonary blood flow; PS: pulmonary stenosis; PVH: pulmonary venous hypertension; TAPVC: total anomalous pulmonary venous connection; TGA: transposition of great arteries; TOF: tetralogy of Fallot

Figure 8.3 Algorithm for evaluation of X-ray chest in a neonate with cyanosis.

pneumonic consolidation, which may simulate atelectasis, there is no mediastinal shift. Soon after birth, a large area of opacity may at times be the only finding in diaphragmatic hernia instead of classical finding of bowel gas in the thorax. CXR in neonates with secondary PPHN may show a variety of parenchymal pathologies with normal cardiac silhouette.

CXR is useful for diagnosis of cyanotic CHD (Figure 8.4). The location of stomach, liver, and heart should be determined to rule out dextrocardia and situs inversus. A small heart and pulmonary oligemia suggest a malformation with reduced PBF while an enlarged heart and increased pulmonary vascular markings is suggestive of increased PBF. Cardiomegaly in patients with critical PS and Ebstein's anomaly of tricuspid valve is an exception to this rule. Some typical appearances are specific for various cardiac lesions as exemplified by ground glass appearance of obstructed TAPVC; 'egg-on-side' appearance in which cardiomegaly exists with narrow pedicle is seen in TGA; 'snowman' or 'figure of 8' appearance in cases with TAPVC and 'boot-shaped heart' of TOF. However, these typical radiological appearances may appear late and may not be apparent in the neonatal period.

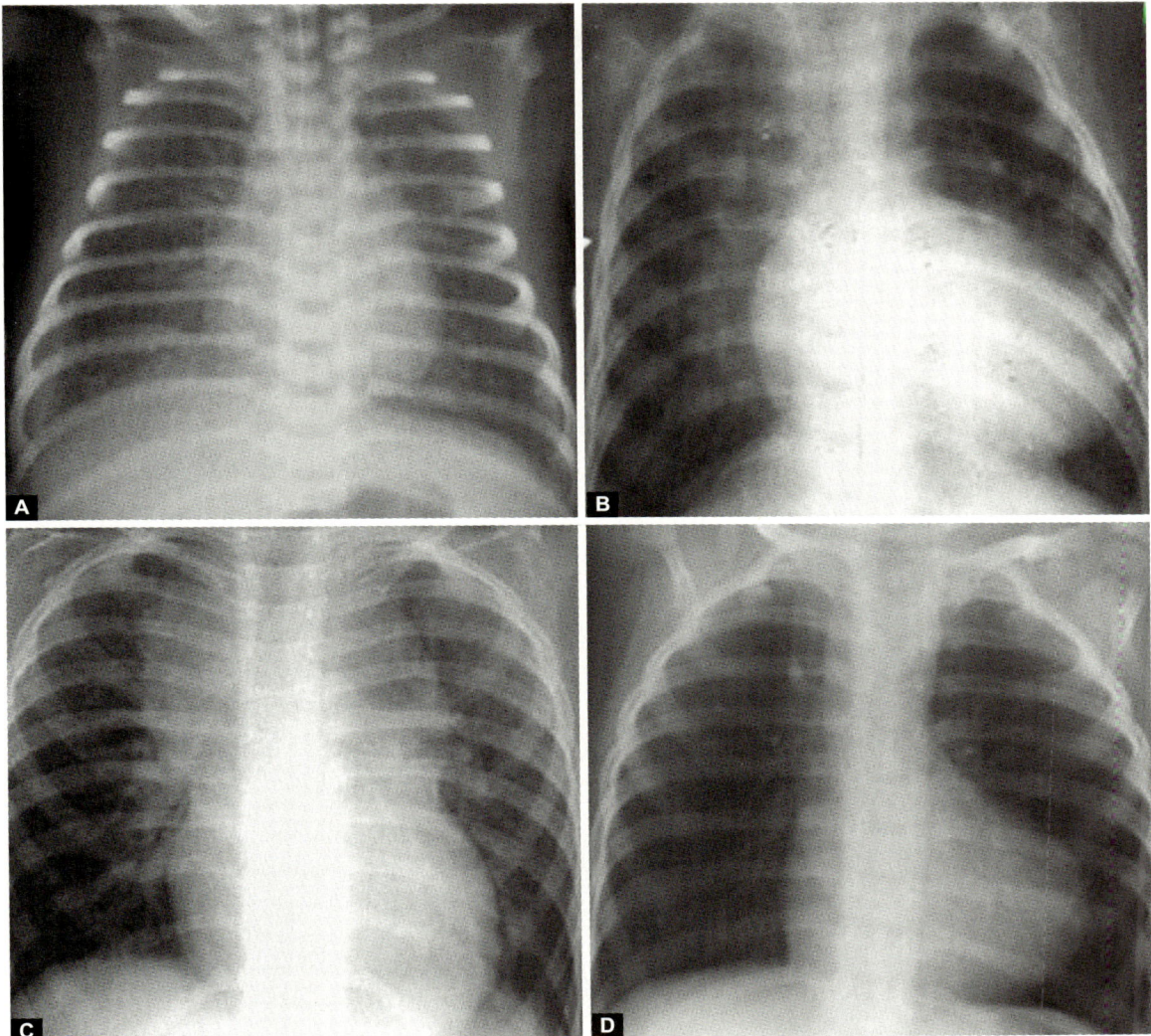

Figure 8.4 Classical appearance of several cyanotic CHDs on skiagram of chest.

(A) Obstructed TAPVC showing no cardiomegaly and severe pulmonary venous hypertension; (B) Transposition of great arteries showing cardiomegaly, narrow pedicle with pulmonary plethora, i.e. egg-on-side appearance; (C) Supracardiac TAPVC showing typical 'snowman' or 'figure of 8' appearance and (D) Tetralogy of Fallot is characterized by absence of cardiomegaly, oligemic lung fields and boot shaped heart.

Electrocardiography

Normal neonatal dominance of RV presents as right axis deviation (RAD) and right ventricular hypertrophy (RVH) on ECG. Many cyanotic CHDs, including serious malformations like TGA have similar ECG appearances and, therefore, even serious CHDs may be missed if ECG alone is relied for the diagnosis. Serial ECGs to evaluate changes in the QRS axis and chamber enlargement improve the diagnostic yield.

Despite limited sensitivity, certain ECG patterns have high specificity for precise anatomic diagnosis and, therefore, ECG must be performed in all children with suspected CHD (Table 8.5). The presence of early and sudden precordial transition is highly suggestive of typical TOF and can differentiate it from other pathologies grouped as TOF physiology (Figure 8.5). Complete heart block (CHB) in a patient with cyanotic CHD strongly point towards congenitally corrected transposition of great arteries (ccTGA) or atrioventricular septal defect (AVSD). Inverted ventricular chambers in ccTGA also produce an interesting pattern of absent septal q wave in leads V5-6. Similarly, presence of left axis deviation in neonates has high specificity for the diagnosis of tricuspid atresia, if the ECG shows LV hypertrophy (Figure 8.6) or AVSD if it shows RV hypertrophy. ECG with polyphasic QRS complexes with tall 'Himalayan' P waves is highly suggestive of Ebstein's anomaly.

Table 8.5 Typical ECG findings in various cyanotic congenital heart diseases

ECG finding	Likely CCHD	Remarks
RAD with RVH	TOF	Early and sudden R to S transition from V1 to V2
	ccTGA with VSD and PS	CHB, absent septal q wave in V5-6
	Critical PS with IVS	RV strain (ST- T changes in V1-3, II, III, aVF)
	TGA with IVS	
LAD	AVSD with PS	RVH
	Tricuspid atresia	LVH
Monomorphic QRS in V1-6	Single ventricle with PS	Tall p waves, prominent q waves and RVH
IRBBB	Ebstein's anomaly	Polyphasic QRS complexes

AVSD: atrioventricular septal defect; ccTGA: congenitally corrected transposition of great arteries; CHB: complete heart block; IRBBB: incomplete right bundle branch block; IVS: intact ventricular septum; LAD: left axis deviation; LVH: left ventricular hypertrophy; PDA: patent ductus arteriosus; PS: pulmonary stenosis; RAD: right axis deviation; RVH: right ventricular hypertrophy; TAPVC: total anomalous pulmonary venous connection; TGA: transposition of great arteries; TOF: tetralogy of Fallot; VSD: ventricular septal defect

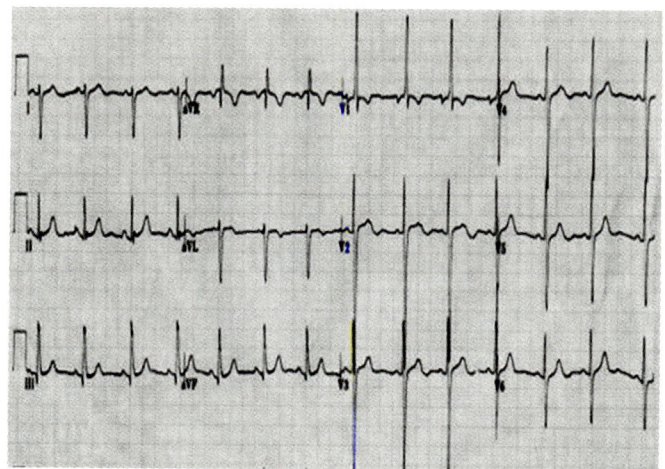

Figure 8.5 12-lead ECG in a neonate with tetralogy of Fallot (TOF) showing right ventricular hypertrophy, right axis deviation and early precordial transition. Note sudden change in QRS morphology with prominent R wave in lead V1 to prominent S wave in lead V2. Normally, this transition occurs in lead V3-4.

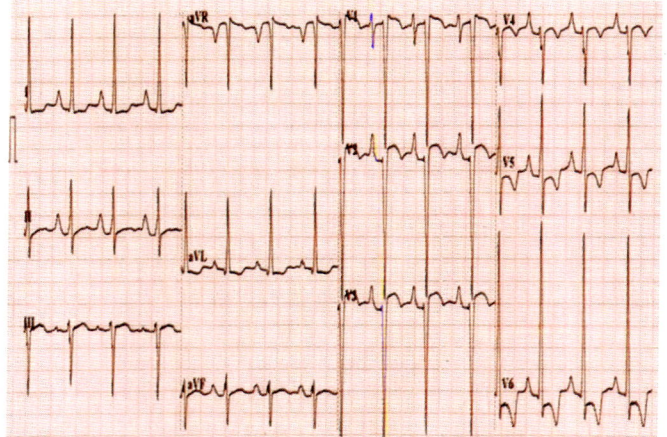

Figure 8.6 12-lead ECG from a child with tricuspid atresia, VSD with PS is characterized by left axis deviation, left ventricular hypertrophy and tall P waves.

Echocardiography

Echocardiography is the gold standard for the diagnosis of CHD. In addition to providing anatomic information, echocardiography allows detection of various physiological alterations. Combined assessment of anatomic and physiologic aberrations is the basis for rational and definitive management of CHDs. With easier availability of point-of-care echocardiography, it has become a common practice to obtain echocardiographic confirmation of CHD. Nevertheless, accurate diagnosis is seldom necessary for immediate stabilization and, therefore, focus should be on determining the hemodynamics of underlying CHD.

A stepwise approach allows easy determination of the cause of cyanosis and also helps in detecting potentially serious cardiac malformations. Figure 8.7 depicts an algorithmic clinical approach to a neonate with cyanosis.

Classification of Cyanotic CHD

Cyanotic CHDs presenting in newborn period are generally more severe and require early stabilization. The incidence of various cardiac lesions is different in neonates from adolescents and adults with TGA being the most common cyanotic CHD in neonatal period. The management is largely based on the hemodynamic subtype of the underlying cardiac lesion and this determination is the key management strategy. Based on the pulmonary blood flow (PBF) and pulmonary artery pressure, cyanotic CHDs are classified as follows.

1. Reduced Pulmonary Blood Flow with Low Pulmonary Artery Pressure

Cardiac malformations in this group are characterized by reduced PBF due to PS. Cyanosis results from right-to-left shunt across atrial or ventricular septal defect. Based on the site of of communication, this group can be broadly divided into two subgroups.

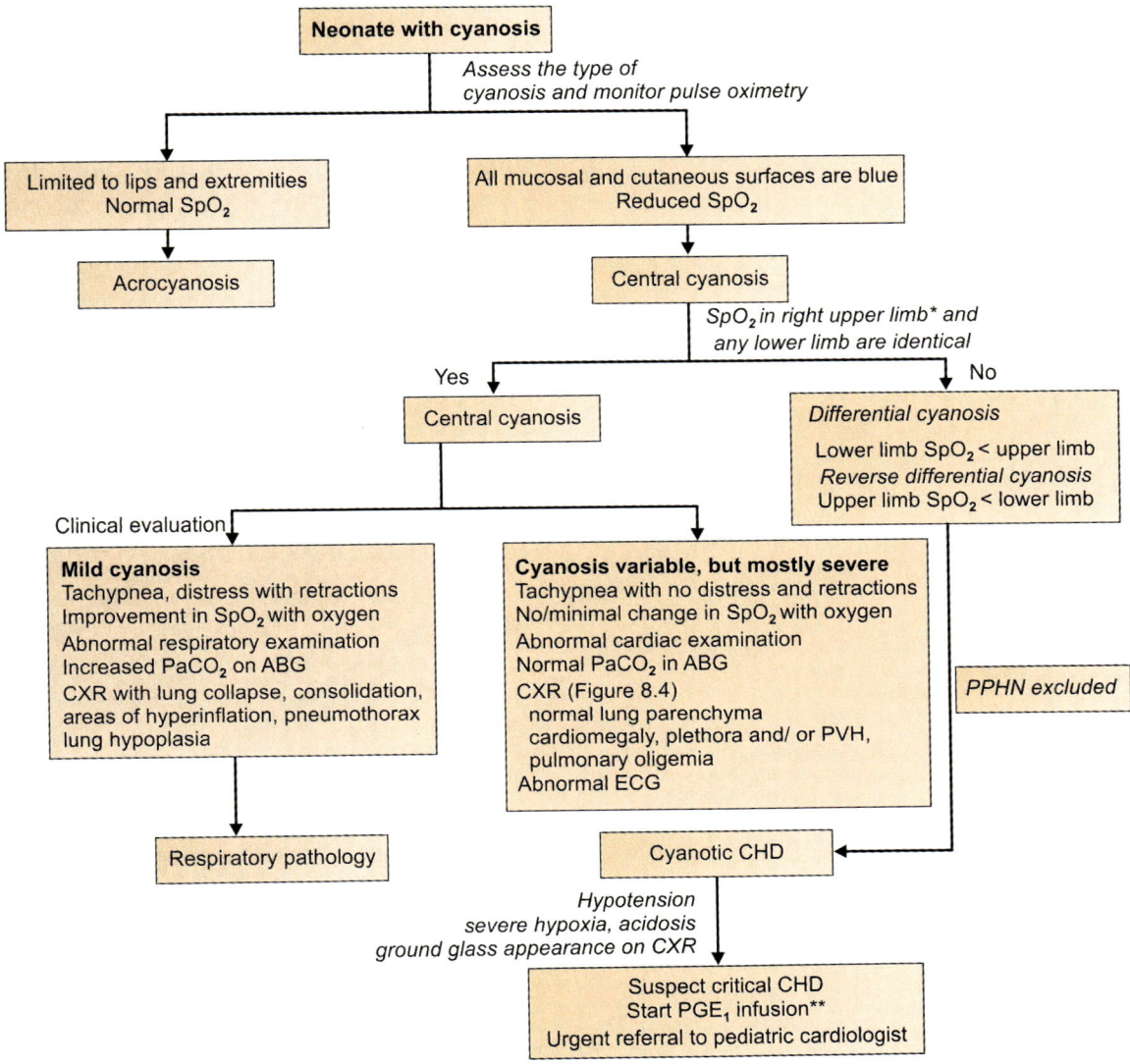

Figure 8.7 Algorithmic clinical approach to a neonate with cyanosis.

Large, non-restrictive VSD with PS (or pulmonary atresia) - TOF physiology

Any cardiac lesion with a large unrestrictive VSD and PS is included in a broad label of TOF physiology. Cyanosis in these children is proportionate to the severity of PS. There is no cardiomegaly and S_2 is single because P_2 is inaudible. An ejection systolic murmur (ESM) is audible at the base of the heart owing to turbulent blood flow across stenosed pulmonary valve. The intensity of ESM varies inversely to the severity of PS with only a faint murmur heard in patients with severe stenosis. In patients with pulmonary atresia, the outflow murmur is absent. The flow across VSD is not turbulent and does not produce any murmur. There is

no RVS_3 or S_4. An aortic ejection click may be audible in children with pulmonary atresia. CXR shows normal sized heart with oligemic lung fields. In addition, an upturned apex and concavity in the region of main pulmonary artery (pulmonary bay) gives it an appearance of Chinese boot (*Coeur en Sabot*). The aortic arch is right sided in approximately 25% cases (Figure 8.4D). ECG reveals RAD, RVH and early precordial transition (Figure 8.5).

Pulmonary stenosis (or atresia) with atrial septal defect

In these patients, right-to-left shunt occurs across an atrial septal defect (ASD) or patent foramen ovale (PFO). The PS is generally valvular and results in RVH

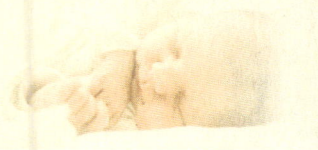

and left parasternal heave when stenosis is severe. The 'a' wave in jugular venous pulse (JVP) is prominent and in cases where tricuspid regurgitation (TR) develops, `v' wave also becomes prominent. The utility of assessment of jugular venous pressure (JVP) in neonates remains limited. P_2 is soft with wide, and variably split S_2 and RVS_4 may be audible. The classical finding is a prominent ESM at second left intercostal space. Unlike patients with TOF, the intensity of murmur is directly proportional to the degree of cyanosis. Once cardiac failure sets in, cardiomegaly occurs and murmur of tricuspid regurgitation (TR) appears. CXR shows cardiomegaly, right atrial (RA) enlargement and pulmonary oligemia. RAD and RVH is evident on ECG. The RV is hypoplastic in all patients with pulmonary atresia and in some patients with critical PS. The ECG in neonates with RV hypoplasia shows poor RV forces as evident by small R wave in lead V_1 and V_4R.

2. Increased Pulmonary Blood Flow with Pulmonary Artery Hypertension

Cardiac lesions in this subgroup represent conditions with PBF which is greater than the systemic blood flow. These neonates typically present with poor weight gain, tachypnea, tachycardia and cardiomegaly. Based on the pattern of blood flow, cardiac lesions in this group are further classified as follows:

Transposition of great arteries

These neonates have parallel systemic and pulmonary circulations instead of normal circulation in series. This peculiar arrangement of great arteries leads to deoxygenated blood circulating from vena cavae through RA and RV to the systemic circulation without getting oxygenated in the lungs. The oxygenated blood returning from pulmonary veins via left atrium (LA) and LV recirculates in pulmonary arteries without reaching body tissues. Instead, only a small amount of blood in these two parallel circulations mixes through ASD, VSD or PDA and allows some oxygenated blood to reach to the body. It is this intermixed blood that determines the oxygen saturation and in absence of a sizeable ASD, VSD or PDA, the child presents with severe hypoxia. VSD or PDA by allowing larger amount of blood to mix, improves the saturation markedly but at the cost of heart failure and PAH. ASD, on the other hand, allows mixing to occur with lower oxygen saturation.

These children tend to have a single and loud S_2. Cardiac murmur is absent in neonates without VSD or PDA. ECG is not useful in early neonatal period. CXR usually shows a narrow pedicle and cardiomegaly,

giving an appearance of 'egg-on-side' (Figure 8.4B). Narrow pedicle results from malposition of the great arteries, aorta lying anterior to the pulmonary artery with associated hypoplasia of thymus.

Admixture (intra-cardiac mixing) physiology

This group includes cardiac malformations that allow complete admixture of systemic and pulmonary venous blood. As a result, oxygen saturation in aorta and pulmonary artery is equal and is the hemodynamic hallmark of these lesions.

These neonates have cyanosis with features of increased PBF. If PS coexists, as in most of the patients with tricuspid atresia, the clinical presentation is like TOF physiology. CXR shows cardiomegaly and increased pulmonary vascularity. Absence of PS and increased PBF puts them at risk of rapid development of pulmonary vascular obstructive disease. These neonates should therefore be managed by early definitive surgical correction, as in patients with TAPVC or truncus arteriosus, or by pulmonary artery banding as the first step of palliation when correction is not possible.

3. Absence of Pulmonary Stenosis with Normal Pulmonary Artery Pressure

In this subgroup, neonates are minimally cyanosed and are usually asymptomatic. These cardiac lesions may escape detection till late in infancy or childhood. Nonetheless, some of these children are seriously ill in neonatal period. For example, a child with Ebstein's anomaly of tricuspid valve (TV), when symptomatic in neonatal period, is challenging to manage. The prognosis in such cases is poor even in the current era of intensive care and advanced neonatal cardiac surgeries. Severe tricuspid regurgitation impairs PBF and elevated pulmonary vascular resistance (PVR) in neonatal period further compromises PBF. The surgical options are reserved for severely symptomatic neonates and have limited success. Medical management remains the cornerstone and is aimed at supporting the neonate through the initial period of transition. The attempts should be made to reduce PVR by improving oxygenation and respiratory alkalosis and improve PBF with PGE_1 infusion. Associated pulmonary hypoplasia due to massive cardiomegaly *in utero* also contributes to poor clinical outcome and high mortality in these neonates. Another rare cardiac anomaly in this group includes anomalous drainage of systemic veins to LA. Normal cardiovascular assessment with cyanosis raises the suspicion but the confirmation is done with saline contrast echocardiography.

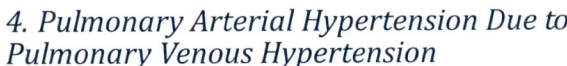

4. Pulmonary Arterial Hypertension Due to Pulmonary Venous Hypertension

This situation arises in patients with obstruction to pulmonary venous inflow as exemplified by HLHS, obstructed TAPVC and obstructive cor-triatriatum. The presentation is early in the neonatal period mostly with cyanosis, congestive heart failure and sometimes cardiogenic shock. Murmur and cardiomegaly are conspicuous by its absence. ECG characteristically shows RAD and RVH while CXR shows normal sized heart and severe PVH resulting in ground glass appearance of lungs. Majority of these cardiac malformations need urgent surgical intervention and therefore warrant prompt referral to a pediatric cardiology center.

Management of Neonates with Cyanotic CHD

Immediate Management

Medical management Medical management is the key to initial stabilization. Patients who are critically ill must be treated in consultation with pediatric cardiologist. Heart failure secondary to cyanotic CHD with increased PBF responds well to diuretic therapy. Beta blocker (intravenous metoprolol 0.1 mg/kg/dose 3–4 times/day or oral propranolol 1–4 mg/kg/day in 3–4 divided doses) is prescribed for children with reduced PBF, especially if the saturations are low or cyanotic spells are present. These drugs are well-tolerated in neonates and infants except when associated with congenital heart block, bradycardia, heart failure or shock. All children with cyanotic CHD should also receive iron supplementation to promote compensatory erythrocytosis.

There is no definite oxygen saturation or PaO_2 that defines adequate oxygenation in a child with cyanotic CHD. The emphasis must be placed on avoiding tissue hypoxia and metabolic acidosis. Cyanosis related to CHD is the result of intracardiac right-to-left shunt and there is only a slight improvement in oxygen saturation with administration of oxygen. Nonetheless, oxygen supplementation increases dissolved oxygen which is undoubtedly helpful for a child with severe hypoxia. Oxygen supplementation sometimes results in clinical worsening in a patient with increased PBF by causing pulmonary vasodilatation. Oxygen supplementation therefore must be restricted in neonates with severe hypoxia and should not be used routinely.

PGE_1 infusion Neonates with deep cyanosis, especially those with acidosis should be immediately started on PGE_1 infusion. Intravenous PGE_1 infusion, in a dose of 0.05–0.4 mcg/kg/min improves and maintains oxygen saturation. The infusion dose is guided by the degree of oxygen saturation. The availability of PGE_1 infusion has revolutionized the management of neonates with cyanotic CHD especially TGA. PGE_1 infusion is useful in almost all neonates with cyanotic CHD except when it is associated with severe PVH as seen in obstructed TAPVC, HLHS, mitral atresia with restrictive ASD and rarely in neonates with TGA with intact ventricular septum and restrictive ASD. The clinical worsening following PGE_1 infusion provides a useful clue regarding the existence of one of aforementioned malformations. Approximately 10–12% neonates receiving PGE_1 infusion develop side effects, most serious being apnea which is dose dependent and may need mechanical ventilation.

Percutaneous Intervention or Surgical Palliation

It is not uncommon to encounter a neonate in whom severe hypoxia or heart failure persists despite medical stabilization. These neonates require percutaneous intervention or surgical palliation for stabilization. A surgical aorto-pulmonary shunt such as Blalock-Taussig shunt or percutaneous PDA stenting improves saturation in patients with TOF physiology. Neonates with critical PS necessitate urgent percutaneous pulmonary valve balloon dilation (PVBD). Percutaneous balloon atrial septostomy improves saturation in neonates with TGA by enlarging pre-existing PFO or ASD. Patients with critical lesions such as obstructive TAPVC must be operated upon urgently.

Definitive Management

Surgery remains the definitive curative therapy for majority of cyanotic CHDs. All cyanotic CHDs are not amenable to corrective surgery and only palliative

Table 8.6 Definitive surgical management of common cyanotic CHDs	
Surgical correction	*Multistage surgical palliation***
Neonatal surgery or intervention	Single ventricle
TAPVC	DORV, Non-routable VSD
TGA	Tricuspid atresia, VSD
Critical PS or pulmonary atresia with IVS#	HLHS and mitral atresia
Surgery during infancy	
Truncus arteriosus	
Surgery during childhood	
TOF and TOF physiology*	
Single atrium	
Ebstein's anomaly	

#Percutaneous pulmonary valve balloon dilatation (PVBD)
*Severe hypoxia warrants Blalock Taussig shunt to improve saturation
**Absence of PS and resultant unrestricted PBF necessitates surgical PA banding during neonatal period or early infancy
CHD: congenital heart disease; DORV: double outlet right ventricle; HLHS: hypoplastic left heart syndrome; IVS: intact ventricular septum; PA: pulmonary artery; PS: pulmonary stenosis; TAPVC: total anomalous pulmonary venous connection; TGA: transposition of great arteries; TOF: tetralogy of Fallot; VSD: ventricular septal defect

surgery is possible in certain circumstances. Brief knowledge of surgical management for various cyanotic CHDs is important as it enables the pediatricians to decide the timing of referral and type of surgical intervention (Table 8.6). In addition, it is useful for preliminary counselling of parents.

SUMMARY

Cyanosis in a neonate, especially if not associated with respiratory distress, is diagnostic of cyanotic CHD. Although definitive management is based on accurate diagnosis, precise anatomic diagnosis at the bedside is not always possible. Identifying the hemodynamic subtype of CHD is far more important and useful for initial stabilization of the infant. The critical lesions, however, must be dealt urgently in consultation with a pediatric cardiologist.

Acknowledgement
Several Tables and Figures have been reproduced with permission from Gupta SK. Clinical approach to a neonate with cyanosis. *Indian J Pediatr* 2015, 82:1050–60.

BIBLIOGRAPHY

Allen HD, Driscoll DJ, Shaddy RE, Timothy FF (Ed). In: Moss and Adam's Heart disease in Infants, Children and Adolescents: including the Fetus and Young Adults. 8th edition, *Lippincott Williams and Wilkins*; 2012.

Cleveland RH. A radiologic update on medical diseases of the newborn chest. *Pediatr Radiol* 1995; 25:631–7.

Cloherty JP, Eichenwald EC, Stark AR (Ed). In: Manual of Neonatal Care. 6th edition, South Asian edition, 4th Indian reprint edition, *Wolters Kluwer Company*; 2009.

Ewer AK, Middletonn LJ, Furmston AT, Bhoyar A, Daniels JP, Thangaratinam S, Deeks JJ, Khan KS, PulseOx study group. Pulse oximetry screening for congenital heart defects in newborn infants (PulseOx): a test accuracy study. *Lancet* 2011; 378:785–94.

Ewer AK. Pulse oximetry screening for critical congenital heart defects in newborn infants: should it be routine? *Arch Dis Child Fetal Neonatal* 2014; 99:F93–F95.

Frank JE, Jacobe KM. Evaluation and management of heart murmurs in children. *Am Fam Physician* 2011; 84:793–800.

Fuloria M, Kreiter S. The newborn examination. Part I. *Am Fam Physician* 2002; 65:61–8.

Grifka RG. Cyanotic congenital heart disease with increased pulmonary blood flow. *Pediatr Clin North Am* 1999; 46:405–25.

Gupta SK, Saxena A. Approach to a cyanotic neonate. In: Essential Neonatology, NB Mathur (ed). *Noble Vision Medical Book Publishers, New Delhi.* pp 569–592.

Gupta SK. Clinical approach to a neonate with cyanosis. *Ind J Pediatr* 2015; 82:1050–60.

Hiremath G, Kamat D. Diagnostic considerations in infants and children with cyanosis. *Pediatric Annals* 2015; 44:76–80.

Jennis MS, Peabody JL. Pulse oximetry: an alternative method for the assessment of oxygenation in newborn infants. *Pediatrics* 1987; 79:524–8.

Koppel RI, Druschel CM, Carter T, Goldberg BE, Mehta PN, Talwar R, et al. Effectiveness of pulse oximetry screening for congenital heart disease in asymptomatic newborns. *Pediatrics* 2003; 111:451–5.

Lees MH. Cyanosis of the newborn infant. Recognition and clinical evaluation. *J Pediatr* 1970; 77:484–98.

Marino BS, Bird GL, Wernovsky G. Diagnosis and management of the newborn with suspected congenital heart disease. *Clin Perinatol* 2001; 28:91–136.

Newborn screening for CCHD. Answers and resources for primary care pediatricians. Available online at https://www.aap.org/en-us/advocacy-and-policy/aap-health initiatives/ PEHDIC/ pages/ Newborn- Screening-for-CCHD.aspx. Accessed on December 12, 2016.

Oliver TK Jr, Demis JA, Bates GD. Serial blood gas tensions and acid-base balance during the first hour of life in human infants. *Acta Paediatr* 1961; 50:346–60.

Rudolph AM. Oxygen uptake and delivery In: Congenital Diseases of the Heart, Rudolph AM (Ed), *Futura Armonk* 2001, p. 85.

Sasidharan P. An approach to diagnosis and management of cyanosis and tachypnea in term infants. *Pediatr Clin North Am* 2004; 51:999–1021.

Steinhorn RH. Evaluation and management of the cyanotic neonate. *Clin Pediatr Emerg Med* 2009; 9:169–75.

Tandon R. Bedside approach. In: The Diagnosis of Congenital Heart Disease. Tandon R (Ed). 2nd edition, New Delhi, Sitaram Bhartia Institute of Science and Research Publishers; 2011.

Thangaratinam S, Brown K, Zamora J, Khan KS, Ewer AK. Pulse oximetry screening for critical congenital heart defects in asymptomatic newborn babies: a systematic review and meta-analysis. *Lancet* 2012; 379:2459–64.

Wren C, Reinhardt Z, Khawaja K. Twenty-year trends in diagnosis of life-threatening neonatal cardiovascular malformations. *Arch Dis Child Fetal Neonatal* 2008; 92:33–35.

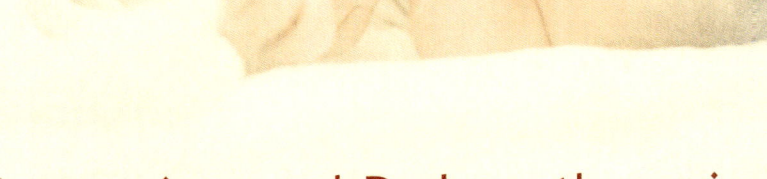

Anemia and Polycythemia

Swarna Rekha

ANEMIA

Anemia is a common hematological problem particularly in sick and preterm neonates. Anemia may be due to physiological reasons or as a consequence of blood loss, decreased production or increased destruction of red blood cells. It is important to recognise the presence of anemia, determine the etiology and treat appropriately. Acute anemia could be life-threatening and long-standing anemia can cause growth failure and may have some adverse implications for neuromotor development.

Definition

Anemia is defined as hematocrit value <45% in a term neonate. There is no single value definition in preterm neonates. In both term and preterm neonates, hemoglobin levels initially fall and then stabilise. The definition would therefore differ in term and preterm neonates and depends on the postnatal age.

Etiopathogenesis

In accordance with other age groups, anemia in neonates can occur due to blood loss, decreased production or increased destruction of RBCs. In addition there is an entity of physiologic anemia of infancy and anemia of prematurity. Pathologic causes of anemia include blood loss secondary to maternal, and fetal factors and neonatal disorders at birth or immediately after birth. The second most frequent cause of anemia is due to hemolysis, this could be immune mediated because of Rh or ABO incompatibility or non-immune as in G6PD deficiency, and spherocytosis. The bone marrow failure syndrome due to aplastic anemia and infiltrative disorders like leukemia can present with anemia in the neonatal period. Intrauterine and postnatal infections play an important role in development of anemia in neonates (Table 9.1).

Table 9.1 Causes of anemia
1. **Physiologic anemia of infancy**
2. **Anemia due to blood loss**
■ Fetomaternal hemorrhage
■ Twin-to-twin transfusion
■ Antepartum hemorrhage
■ Birth trauma
■ Umbilical cord bleeding
■ Pulmonary or intracranial hemorrhage
■ Excessive blood sampling
3. **Anemia due to decreased production of RBCs**
■ Parvovirus infection
■ Nutritional deficiencies
■ Diamond Blackfan syndrome
■ Fanconi's anemia
■ Leukemia
4. **Anemia due to increased destruction of RBCs**
■ Immune hemolysis (Rh, ABO)
■ Hemolytic anemias
i. Spherocytosis
ii. G6PD deficiency
iii. Thalassemias
■ Autoimmune hemolytic anemia

Approach to a Neonate with Anemia

The most common presentation of anemia is pallor. Before discussing approach to anemia it is important to recognize other causes of pallor in a neonate (Box 9.1).

BOX 9.1 Causes of pallor in a neonate
■ Anemia
■ Hypothermia
■ Hypoxia
■ Shock
■ Sepsis

History

- *Antenatal history*: Maternal infections, antepartum hemorrhage, and twin gestation
- *Mother's blood group*: Rh-negative, O-positive
- *Delivery details*: Mode of delivery, birth trauma, bleeding from umbilical cord
- *Gestation*: Preterm infants are likely to have anemia of prematurity
- *Family history of anemia, and neonatal jaundice*: G6PD deficiency, and spherocytosis
- *Age of onset*: Early onset is likely to be related to antepartum or birth events, late onset is most commonly due to anemia of prematurity
- History of blood sampling, sepsis, external or occult hemorrhage.

Physical Examination

- Severity of pallor
- *Jaundice*. In visceral or internal bleeding in a neonate, jaundice may be predominant finding compared to anemia
- *Site of bleeding*. Umbilical, and cephalhematoma, multiple subcutaneous hematomas, placenta with retroplacental clot
- Full anterior fontanel
- *Skin bleeds*. Ecchymosis and petichiae
- Dysmorphic features
- Hepatosplenomegaly
- Lymphadenopathy
- Cardiovascular compromise
  - Tachycardia
  - Tachypnea
  - Hepatomegaly due to cardiac failure
  - Increase in oxygen requirement.

Diagnostic Approach

It is important to determine the severity of anemia and decide regarding the need for blood transfusion. The next important thing is to determine the etiology. The algorithmic approach to anemia in a neonate is given in Figure 9.1. If there is history suggestive of bleeding the etiology is obvious. The second most common cause of anemia is hemolytic, blood group of mother and baby should be checked. Presence of blood group incompatibility or reticulocytosis and/or presence of jaundice are suggestive of hemolytic anemia. Bone marrow failure syndromes are less likely and should be confirmed by investigations (Box 9.2).

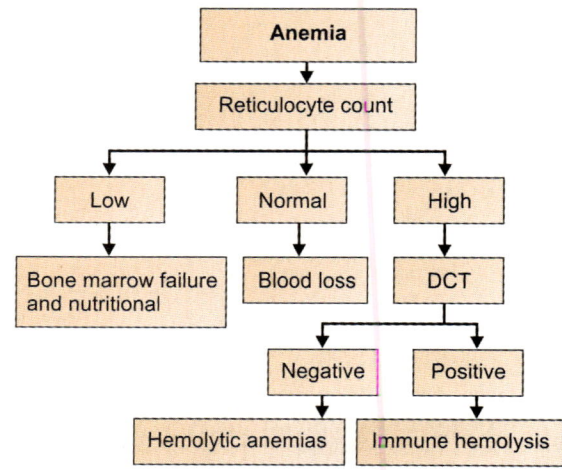

In blood loss, Hb/hematocrit should be checked every one hour to detect the drop.

Figure 9.1 Approach to anemia in a neonate

BOX 9.2 Basic investigations in a neonate with anemia

- Hemoglobin*
- Hematocrit (PCV)*
- Complete blood counts including platelets
- Reticulocyte count
- Peripheral smear
- Blood group (mother and baby)
- Direct Coombs' test (DCT)
- G6PD level
- Hemoglobin electrophoresis

*During acute bleeding, the fall in hemoglobin and hematocrit may take several hours.

Anemia of Prematurity

Anemia of prematurity should be suspected in the following situations:

- Anemia occurring in preterm neonates
- Presentation around 10 to 12 weeks of life (could be earlier in preterm neonates)
- There is no cause of anemia or hepatosplenomegaly
- Poor weight gain
- No history of bleeding or jaundice
- Physical examination is negative, except for pallor
- Investigations are noncontributory.

Etiopathogenesis

All neonates demonstrate a drop in hematocrit values due to various physiologic reasons in the first few weeks of life and this is known as physiologic anemia in term neonates and anemia of prematurity in preterm neonates. In sick neonates, hematocrit levels may drop further due to additional pathologic reasons. In term infants, hemoglobin levels may drop to 10 gm/dL by

Table 9.2 Hemoglobin levels in physiologic anemia		
Gestation/weight	Lowest Hb in gm/dL	Time when Hb is at its nadir
Term	10	10–12 weeks
1.0 to 1.5 Kg	8	6–8 weeks
<1 kg	7	6–8 weeks

Table 9.3 Transfusion guidelines for preterm neonates	
Restricted transfusion guidelines	Liberal transfusion guidelines
■ Hct <30% if infant requires moderate ventilator support (MAP >8 cm H$_2$O or FiO$_2$ >0.4) ■ Hct <25% for infants requiring minimal ventilator support (MAP, 8 cm H$_2$O or FiO$_2$ <0.4) ■ Hct <20 % if on supplemental oxygen ■ Hct <18% if asymptomatic (Retic should be <2%) ■ If blood loss >20% or >10% in a symptomatic baby	■ Hb <11 gm/dL or Hct <35% if on moderate ventilation ■ Hb <10 gm/dL or Hct <30% if on minimal ventilation ■ Hb <8 gm/dL if needing supplemental oxygen ■ Hb <7 gm/dL or Hct <20% if asymptomatic

Hb: hemoglobin, Hct: hematocrit, MAP: mean airway pressure, FiO$_2$: fraction of inspired oxygen, Rectic: reticulocyte count

about 10 to 12 weeks of life. In preterm neonates hemoglobin levels may drop to as low as 7 gm/dL.

The life span of RBCs in neonates is about 60 to 70 days and in preterm neonates it can be as low as 35 to 50 days compared to adult lifespan of 90 to 120 days. The timing and severity of physiologic anemia is shown in Table 9.2.

Treatment and Prevention of Anemia of Prematurity

Delayed Cord of Clamping

Numerous studies have shown that delayed cord clamping (30 to 120 seconds) is safe and beneficial to both preterm and term neonates. In preterm neonates, it reduces the need for transfusion, decreases incidence of necrotizing enterocolitis (NEC) and intracranial hemorrhage (ICH).

Iron Supplementation

All preterm neonates should be started on prophylactic iron supplementation at 2 to 4 weeks (elemental iron 1 mg/kg) till 1 year of age or atleast till iron fortified complementary or weaning foods are introduced.

Recombinant Erythropoietin

Low erythropoietin levels have been demonstrated in neonates with anemia of prematurity. Hence it is logical that administration of recombinant erythropoietin would decrease the need for blood transfusion. Studies have been equivocal and currently there is no definitive role of recombinant erythropoietin either for prophylaxis or treatment of anemia of prematurity. Studies have shown that it may decrease the number and volume of blood transfusions but does not eliminate the need for transfusion.

Blood Transfusion

There is no role for whole blood transfusion for treatment of anemia in neonates. Packed red cell transfusion is indicated if hemoglobin levels are low. The guidelines for transfusion are shown in Table 9.3. The basic philosophy is to avoid unnecessary transfusions because of several transfusion-related risks. The restricted guidelines are a little more stringent compared to the liberal guidelines. Special care should be taken in preterm neonates to prevent transmission of CMV by using irradiated blood whenever feasible.

Treatment of Anemia in Sick Preterm and Term Neonates

In a sick neonate, packed cell transfusion is given if hematocrit is 40 or less. The volume of transfusion is 10 to 15 mL/kg and there is no need to routinely administer furosemide. In neonates on IV fluids, the amount of transfused blood should be deducted from total volume of fluids.

Treatment of Specific Cause of Anemia

In immune hemolysis secondary to blood group incompatibility, exchange blood transfusion is done followed by top up transfusion. The underlying cause of anemia should be identified and appropriately treated (avoid certain medications in G6PD deficiency, administer IVIG in autoimmune hemolysis). Long term follow-up is needed in hemolytic anemias. If anemia is due to leukemia or red cell aplasia, specific treatment should be given.

Complications of Blood Transfusion

The common complications of blood transfusion in neonates are listed in Table 9.4. Blood transfusion may predispose preterm infant to develop necrotizing enterocolitis, bronchopulmonary dysplasia and retinopathy of prematurity.

Prognosis

Most neonates with anemia of prematurity do not need any treatment, other than appropriate iron

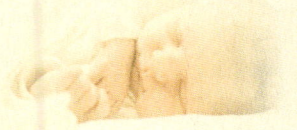

Table 9.4 Complications of blood transfusion in neonates
Immunologic
▪ Hemolytic reactions
▪ Febrile reactions
▪ GVHD
▪ TRALI
▪ T-antigen activation hemolysis
Metabolic
▪ Hypoglycemia
▪ Hypocalcemia
▪ Hyperkalemia
Infections
Cytomegalovirus, human immunodeficiency virus, Hepatisi B, C virus
Others
Necrotizing enterocolitis, retinopathy of prematurity, broncho-pulmonary dysplasia

*GVHD: Graft versus host disease, TRALI: Transfusion associated lung injury.

supplementation. The treatment of neonates with anemia due to pathologic causes depends on the severity and etiology of anemia. A neonate with immune hemolysis will recover completely whereas a neonate diagnosed to have spherocytosis will need long term follow-up and may need repeated blood transfusions.

POLYCYTHEMIA

Polycythemia is one of the common hematological problems occuring in neonates. The incidence of polycythemia varies between 1.8 to 2.2% in neonates born at sea level. The incidence may be as high as 15% in term SGA neonates. It can occur due to antenatal problems like intrauterine hypoxia or twin- to-twin transfusion or due to postnatal conditions such as delayed cord clamping or dehydration. The symptomatology is secondary to hyperviscosity which occurs as a result of polycythemia. Over the years there has been a change in the incidence and approach to managing this condition. The aim of treatment is to prevent immediate and long-term complications.

Definition

Polycythemia is defined as a venous hematocrit of more than 65% or venous hemoglobin concentration of more than 22.0 g/dL. However, the following physiologic facts need to be considered while diagnosing and treating polycythemia.

- *Timing of cord clamping.* Early (<30 seconds) *vs* late clamping (>120 seconds); late clamping may increase hematocrit levels by 10 to 30%.

- *Site of sampling.* The blood sample should always be collected from a large freely flowing blood vessel. Samples from small vessels or capillary samples will yield falsely elevated values. One study has shown that venous hematocrit of 65% would correlate with a capillary hematocrit of 70% and a central venous hematocrit of 63%.

- *Time of sampling.* Hematocrit will peak at 2 hours of age and then it slowly declines over next 6 to 12 hours. The upper limit of the normal hematocrit at the age of 2 hours has been reported to be 71% and at the age of 6 hours around 68%.

- *Method of testing.* Automated analysis (Coulter counter) yields lower values than those estimated after the spun.

Hyperviscosity

Hyperviscosity is defined as a viscosity greater than 14.6 cP at a shear rate of 11.5 per second. Polycythemia and hyperviscosity are often used synonymously, but they are different. Polycythemia refers to an increase in red blood cell mass, whereas hyperviscosity refers to the "thickness" or viscosity of blood. The relationship between hematocrit values and blood viscosity is linear till about 65% hematocrit, after this the viscosity increases exponentially. Since the clinical effects of polycythemia are secondary to hyperviscosity, it would be ideal to measure the viscosity. As measurement of hyperviscosity is rather difficult in clinical practice, diagnosis and treatment of polycythemia – hyperviscosity syndrome is usually based on hematocrit levels.

Pathophysiology

Higher red cell mass results in increased viscosity causing sluggish blood flow. There is an impairment of oxygenation and perfusion and formation of micro-thrombi. This can cause tissue hypoxia and acidosis. Increase in red cell mass leads to increased number of hemolyzing RBC's resulting in neonatal hyperbilirubinemia. Other metabolic effects include hypoglycemia and hypocalcemia. Polycythemia may cause renal vein thrombosis resulting in renal failure. Thrombosis in the cerebral vessels may cause cerebrovascular accident and seizures. It can also rarely cause cardiac failure and myocardial infarction.

Risk Factors

The predominant cause of polycythemia is chronic intrauterine hypoxia. The other causes include maternal diabetes mellitus. Therefore all small-for-gestational age, large-for-gestational age and postmature neonates are at risk for developing polycythemia. The secondary

Table 9.5 Causes and risk factors for polycythemia	
Primary causes	**Secondary causes**
■ Placental insufficiency	■ Delayed cord clamping
• Small-for-gestational age	■ Twin-to-twin transfusion
• Pre-eclampsia/eclampsia	■ Maternal-fetal transfusion
• Maternal heart disease	■ Perinatal asphyxia
• Maternal smoking	■ Dehydration
• Postmaturity	
■ Maternal diabetes mellitus	
■ Neonatal thyrotoxicosis	
■ Congenital adrenal hyperplasia	
■ Trisomy 13, 18, 21	
■ Beckwith-Wiedemann syndrome	

causes of polycythemia are related to timing of cord clamping, and twin-to-twin transfusion. A metaanalysis of early vs late cord clamping has shown that there is an increased risk of developing polycythemia in the late cord clamping group with a relative risk of 3.82; with 95% confidence interval. The leading primary and secondary causes of polycythemia are listed in Table 9.5.

Clinical Features

The salient clinical features of polycythemia are shown in Table 9.6. Most of the clinical features are secondary to hyperviscosity. Polycythemia can affect almost all organ systems. Nearly 50% of neonates with polycythemia may remain asymptomatic and are detected only during routine screening. Asymptomatic polycythemia is usually a benign condition and can resolve sponataneously. Occasionally, symptoms may be significant to require admission and treatment. The major concern is long-term sequelae which can be obvious or subtle like dyslexia.

Screening for Polycythemia

Almost 50% of neonates with polycythemia are asymptomatic, screening of the at-risk neonates is recommended to identify these neonates (Box 9.3). Though it is ideal to collect a venous sample preferably after 6 hours, for screening purposes a capillary sample from a prewarmed heel puncture can be collected. The recommended timing for screening are 2, 6, 12 and 24 hours. If the capillary hematocrit is 70% or more, this should be followed up by a venous sample to confirm the diagnosis of polycythemia.

Investigations

In neonates diagnosed to have polycythemia, other than serial monitoring for hemoglobin/hematocrit, the following investigations should be done. Investigations can be decided on the basis of symptoms.

■ Blood glucose
■ Serum calcium
■ Platelet count
■ X-ray chest if there is tachypnea
■ Abdominal X-ray if symptoms of NEC are present
■ Renal functions and ultrasound examination of abdomen if there is evidence of renal failure.

Table 9.6 Clinical features of polycythemia
Central nervous system
■ Lethargy
■ Poor feeding
■ Irritability
■ Jitteriness
■ Convulsions
■ Hypotonia
■ Neurodevelopmental sequelae
Respiratory
■ Tachypnea
■ Respiratory distress
Cardiovascular system
■ Cyanosis
■ Cardiac failure
Gastrointestinal
■ Vomiting
■ Necrotizing enterocolitis
Hematologic
■ Thrombosis
■ Thrombocytopenia
Renal
■ Renal vein thrombosis
■ Renal failure
Metabolic
■ Jaundice
■ Hypoglycemia
■ hypocalcemia
Others
■ Plethora
■ Priapism
■ Gangrene of toes

BOX 9.3 At risk neonates who require screening for polycythemia
■ Small-for-gestational age babies
■ Large-for-gestational age babies
■ Twins/multiple births
■ Infants of diabetic mothers
■ Trisomy 21

Management

Over the years there has been a change in the management of polycythemia. Earlier and effective feeding should be ensured to high-risk neonates to prevent dehydration and hemoconcentration. In the 80's and 90's there was a tendency to be aggressive in treating polycythemia, because of studies reporting significant long term sequelae. Currently the trend is to reserve the intervention only for symptomatic neonates or those with very high hematocrit values of more than 75%. Earlier colloids like plasma and albumin were used for exchange transfusion, current recommendation is to use normal saline. In the past, umbilical catheterization was done for exchange transfusion, now partial exchange transfusion is done through peripheral route.

The treatment of choice is peripheral partial exchange transfusion using normal saline. The indications for procedure include (i) symptomatic neonates with venous Hct >65% and (ii) asymptomatic neonates with venous Hct >75%. Neonates who are asymptomatic but have a venous Hct >70% should be monitored and one should consider increasing their fluid intake by 20 mL/kg per day. The protocol for management of polycythemia is shown in Figure 9.2.

Partial Exchange Transfusion

- The procedure must be done under aseptic precautions
- *Route*. Partial exchange transfusion can be done either through the umbilical vein or preferably through a peripheral artery and vein. The latter is the preferred method as there has been some reports of increased incidence of infection and NEC following umbilical cannulation and exchange through this route.

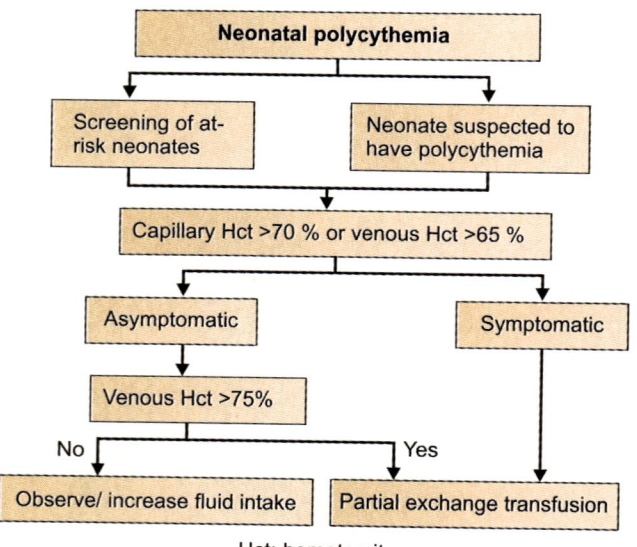

Figure 9.2 Algorithm for management of neonatal polycythemia.

- *Choice of fluid*. The current evidence shows that crystalloids are equally effective and hence the choice of fluid is normal saline. Earlier plasma and albumin were being used.
- *Method*. Once cannulation of a peripheral artery is done, small aliquots of blood are withdrawn (5 to 10 mL) from the artery and equal amount of saline is pushed through a vein.
- Volume of fluid to be exchanged is calculated as shown below:

> **Volume to be exchanged = observed HCT – desired HCT (55) × blood volume ÷ observed HCT**
> *Blood volume = 80 mL/kg in term neonates and 100 mL/kg in preterm neonates.*

Prognosis

Earlier studies have shown that symptomatic neonates if untreated may develop long-term sequelae. Current evidence suggests that asymptomatic neonates with lower hematocrit values are less likely to have sequelae even when managed by supportive measures. Neonatal polycythemia is mostly a benign condition and is often self-limiting and sequelae are unlikely if these infants are identified early and managed appropriately.

BIBLIOGRAPHY

Aher S, Malwatkar K, Kadam S. Neonatal anemia. *Semin Neonatal Fetal Med* 2008; 13:239–49.

Bell EF, Strauss RG, Widness JA. Randomised controlled trial of liberal vs restrictive guidelines for red cell transfusion in preterm infants. *J Pediatr* 2005; 115:1685–91.

Bishara N, Ohls RK. Current controversies in the management of anemia of prematurity. *Semin Perinatol* 2008; 33:29–34.

Black VD, Lubchenco LO, Koops BL, Foland RL, Powell DP. Neonatal hyperviscosity: randomized study of effect of partial plasma exchange transfusion on long-term outcome. *Pediatrics* 1985; 75:1048–53.

Colombatti R, Sainati L, Trevisanuto D. Anemia and transfusion in the neonate. *Semin Fetal Neonatal Med* 2016; 21(1):2–9.

de Waal KA, Baerts W, Offringa M, Systematic review of the optimal fluid for dilutional exchange transfusion in neonatal polycythemia. *Arch Dis Child Fetal Neonatal Ed* 2006; 91:F7–F10.

Demirel N, Aydin M, Zenciroglu A, Bas AY. Yarali N, Okumus N, Cinar G, Ipek MS. Neonatal thrombo-embolism: risk factors, clinical features and outcome. *Ann Trop Paediatr* 2009 Dec; 29(4):271–9.

Dempsey EM, Barrington K. Short and long term outcomes following partial exchange transfusion in the polycythemic newborn: a systematic review. *Arch Dis Child Fetal Neonatal Ed* 2006; 91:F2–F6.

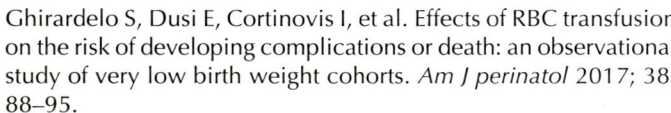

Ghirardelo S, Dusi E, Cortinovis I, et al. Effects of RBC transfusion on the risk of developing complications or death: an observational study of very low birth weight cohorts. *Am J perinatol* 2017; 38: 88–95.

Higgins RD, Patel RM, Josephson CD. Preoperative anemia and neonates. *JAMA Pediatr* 2016, 170(9):835–36.

Hopewell B, Steiner LA, Ehrenkranz RA, Bizzarro MJ, Gallagher PG. Partial exchange transfusion for polycythemia hyperviscosity syndrome. *Am J Perinatol* 2011; 28:557–64.

Hutton EK, Hassan ES. Late vs early clamping of the umbilical cord in full-term neonates: systematic review and meta-analysis of controlled trials. *JAMA* 2007; 297:1241–52.

Jeevasankar M, Agarwal R, Deorari AK, Paul VK. Management of polycythemia in neonates. *Indian J Pediatr* 2010; 77:1117–21.

Kripalani H, Whyte RK, Anderson C, et al. The premature infant in need of transfusion: A randomised control trial of restrictive vs liberal transfusion threshold for ELBW neonates. *J Pediatr* 2006; 149:301–7.

Kumar A, Ramji S. Effect of partial exchange transfusion in asymptomatic polycythemic LBW babies. *Indian Pediatr* 2004; 41:366–72.

Linderkamp O. Blood viscosity of the neonate. *Neo Reviews* 2004; 5:406.

McDonald SJ, Middleton P, Dowswell T, Morris PS. Effect of timing of umbilical cord clamping of term infants on maternal and neonatal outcomes. *Cochrane Database Syst Rev* 2013: CD004074.

Morag I, Strauss T, Lubin D, Eisen I, Kenet G, Kuint J. Restrictive management of neonatal polycythemia. *Am J Perinatol* 2011; 28:677.

Ohls RK. Evaluation and treatment of anemia in the neonate. In: Hematologic Problems of the Neonate. Christensen RD (Ed), *Philadelphia, WB Saunders* 2000 p 137–170.

Ozek E, Soll R, Schimmel MS. Partial exchange transfusion to prevent neurodevelopmental disability in infants with polycythemia. *Cochrane Database Syst Rev* 2010:CD005089.

Patil S, Saini SS, Kumar P, Shah R. Comparison of intra-procedural pain between a novel continuous arteriovenous exchange and conventional pull-push techniques of partial exchange transfusion in neonates: a randomized controlled trial. *J Perinatol* 2014; 34:693–97.

Ranjit T, Nesargi S, Rao PN, Sahoo JP, Ashok C, Chandrakala 3S, Bhat S. Effect of early versus delayed cord clamping on hematological status of preterm infants at 6 weeks of age. *Indian J Pediatr* 2015; 82:29–34.

Rossi CA, Prefumo F, Perinatal outcomes of twin anemia-polycythemia sequence: A systematic review. *J Obstet Gynaecol Can* 2014; 36:701–707.

Sarkar S, Rosenkrantz TS. Neonatal polycythemia and hyperviscosity. *Semin Fetal Neonat Med* 2008; 13:248–55.

Strauss RG, Anemia of prematurity: pathophysiology and treatment. *Blood Rev* 2010; 24:221–25.

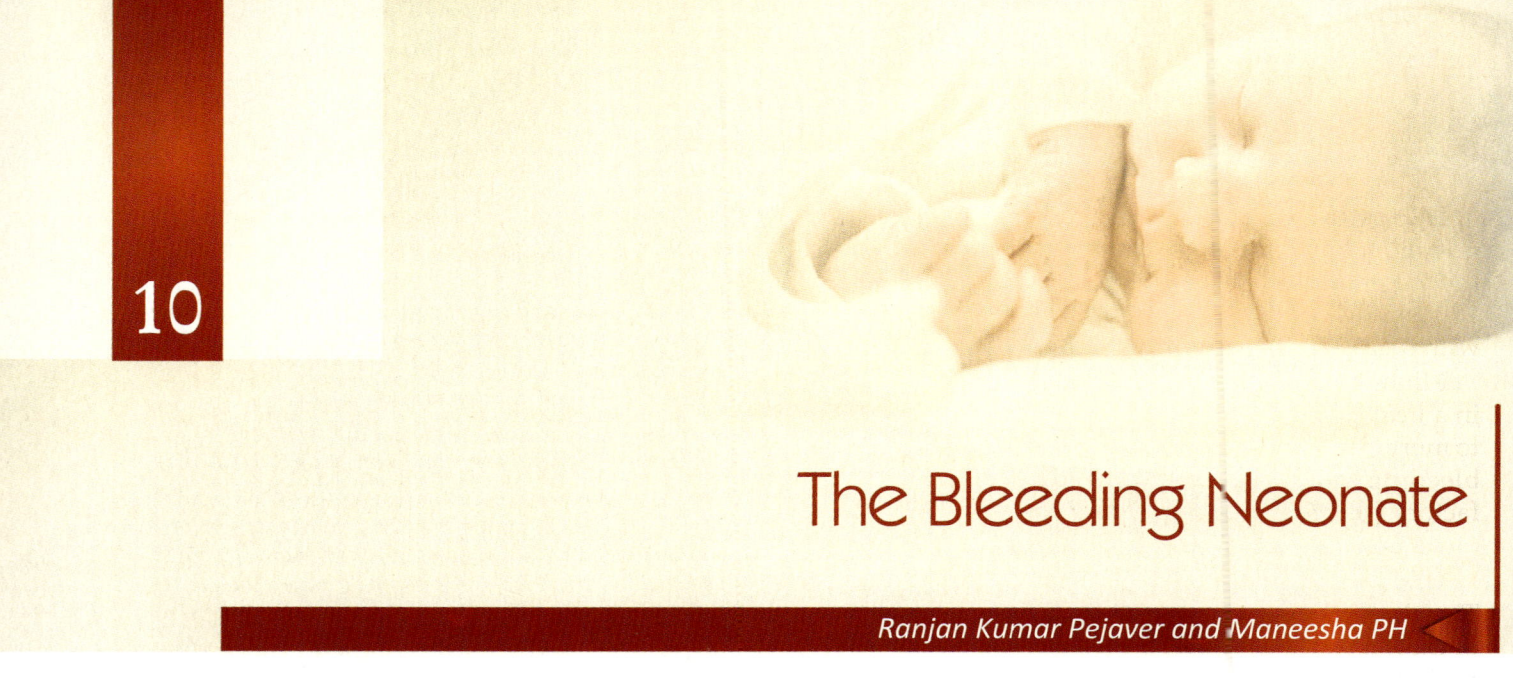

Ranjan Kumar Pejaver and Maneesha PH

The Bleeding Neonate

10

Bleeding in a newborn is a common problem encountered in clinical practice. The newborn baby's hemostatic mechanism is immature and does not develop fully until the age of 6 months. The liver is the site of synthesis of most of the coagulation proteins; the surfaces of platelets and endothelial cells are the predominant sites of protein activation. Plasma levels and functional abilities of most coagulation proteins are low at the time of birth and reach adult levels weeks to months after birth. With a blood volume of around 80–90 mL/kg, even small quantities of blood loss, can lead to hemodynamic instability and interfere with oxygen delivery.

Physiology of Coagulation Pathway

Hemostasis (coagulation) refers to the process in which bleeding is halted at the site of damaged and discontinued endothelium. This process is a dynamic interplay among the subendothelium, endothelium, circulating cells and proteins. The immediate response is confined to the area of injury so that pathologic thrombosis does not occur. The coagulation process is described in three phases; vascular, platelet and the plasma phase.

Vascular phase is mediated by release of local vasoactive agents and results in vasoconstriction at the site of injury. This results in reduced blood flow. The normal endothelial lining promotes fluidity of blood by secreting prostacyclin or prostaglandin 12 which inhibits platelet aggregation. Once endothelium is disrupted and subendothelium is exposed, and pro-coagulant proteins such as tissue factor, collagen, and von Willebrand factor (vWF) are released at the site of injury. Large multimeric proteins are activated and they coat the platelet receptor glycoprotein 1b. Platelets then bind to vWF forming a layer which is bound to the subendothelium in a process called platelet adhesion. Platelets are activated and release vasoactive and hemostatic substances including thromboxane A2, serotonin and adenosine diphosphate (ADP) leading to further vasoconstriction and platelet aggregation thus forming the platelet plug. During the plasma phase, initially tissue factor (TF) is released in the subendothelium. TF binds to and activates factor VII to form a TF-VIIa complex called extrinsic tenase. This binds to and activates factor X and converts prothrombin to thrombin. The thrombin burst takes place to form large amounts of thrombin. This leads to expression of Factor V on the platelet surface and activates it. Thrombin also leads to activation of Factor VIII by its release from vWF, and activates factor IX. Activated Factor VIII then binds to activated Factor IX to form the potent intrinsic tenase leading to activation of Factor X. This association of activated Factors X and V result in thrombin burst, leading to rapid generation of thrombin with formation of a fibrin clot. Thrombin activates Factor XIII and thrombin fibrinolysis inhibitor and renders the clot resistant to plaminogen activator mediated fibrinolysis.

Physiological Handicaps in Newborns

A number of physiological handicaps predispose neonates to develop bleeding manifestations.

1. Blood vessels are thin and fragile.
2. Most coagulation factors do not cross placenta.
3. Vitamin K dependent clotting Factors (II, VII, IX, X) are reduced.
4. Antithrombin III and plasminogen are low.
5. Platelets are functionally less active.

Hemostatic protein concentration is dependent on gestational age and postnatal age. They do not cross the placental barrier. Fetus starts synthesizing them by 10 weeks of gestation. Their concentration increases with increasing gestation and postnatal age.

Minor bleeding may not cause any clinical problem in a healthy neonate, but may contribute significantly to morbidity in the sick and premature infant. Neonatal bleeding can result from disorders of coagulation factors, platelets and vascular integrity.

Causes of Bleeding

The bleeding may rarely occur *in utero* (maternal intake of medications), or at birth and during early newborn period. The bleeding may occur as a consequence of derangements in the hemostatic system or secondary to anatomic defects, trauma or surgical procedure. The common causes of bleeding in a neonate are listed in Table 10.1.

Bleeding disorder may be present in multiple family members which points towards an inherited disorder. Bleeding may be confined to specific anatomic sites or may occur at multiple sites. The onset, severity and duration of bleeding may vary. All this information is important for the clinician to arrive at a correct diagnosis with minimal laboratory tests. History taking should be done meticulously, to identify predisposing factors.

Family history The family history of bleeding disorder or neonatal deaths should be asked. Drawing up a pedigree chart may indicate specific conditions like Hemophilia which is an X-linked recessively inherited disorder.

Maternal history Ask for history of pregnancy-induced hypertension which can result in thrombocytopenia in the newborn. The antihypertensive medications like methyldopa may cause neonatal thrombocytopenia albeit transient. History of diabetes mellitus in the mother is an important correlate of thrombosis. History suggestive of intrauterine infections may explain occurrence of anemia, thrombocytopenia and DIC in the newborn. Maternal ingestion of medications like antitubercular drugs, aspirin, anticonvulsants, may lead to thrombocytopenia in the neonate. History of connective tissue disorders like SLE can lead to neonatal thrombocytopenia.

Neonatal history A detailed history should be taken. Preterm infants are more prone to develop bleeding especially intracranial, pulmonary and DIC. Intrauterine growth restriction may occur as a result of intrauterine infections. History of birth trauma, and perinatal asphyxia should be elicited. Administration of vitamin K soon after birth should be confirmed or documented. History of bleeding from the cord or site of injury, points towards hereditary deficiency of coagulation factor.

Information regarding bleeding should include location, severity, and duration of bleeding. The site of bleeding may suggest the part of the hemostatic system affected. Mucocutaneous bleeding, and easy bruising are seen in neonates with disorders of primary hemostasis involving platelets and vWF. Patients with secondary hemostasis (coagulation factor deficiencies) manifest with deep tissue bleeding including joints, muscles and central nervous system. Generalized bleeding manifestations in a critically sick neonate are suggestive of sepsis, disseminated intravascular coagulopathy and hepatic disease. History of excessive bleeding after an hemostatic challenge like, minor surgery, trivial trauma and perinatal bleeding should be checked. Look for various maternal risk factors like maternal infection (including chorioamnionitis and viral infections), and prolonged rupture of membranes.

Table 10.1 Common causes of bleeding in neonates

Coagulation disorder

Well child
- Transient due to vitamin K deficiency
  - i. Physiologic
  - ii. Prematurity
  - iii. Total parenteral nutrition
  - iv. Broad spectrum antibiotics
- *Congenital disorders*
  - i. Hemophilia A
  - ii. Hemophilia B
  - iii. von Willebrand disease
  - iv. Afibrogenesis

Sick child
  - i. Sepsis with disseminated intravascular coagulation
  - ii. Necrotizing enterocolitis
  - iii. Liver disease

Platelet disorder
- Thrombocytopenia
- Thrombocytopathy
  - i. Bernard-Soulier syndrome
  - ii. Glanzmann thromboasthenia
  - iii. Wiscott–Aldrich syndrome
  - iv. Gray platelet syndrome

Medications (maternal and neonatal)

Antitubercular drugs, salicylates, anticonvulsants, antihypertensives, and warfarin

Maternal disorders

Pregnancy-induced hypertension, systemic lupus erythematosus

Physical Examination

Assess the vital parameters like heart rate, respirations, blood pressure and oxygen saturation. This will determine whether baby needs any urgent resuscitation in addition to planned management. It differentiates the baby into the two categories of well and sick neonate, which helps in determining the etiology through systematic work-up. Identify the type and site of bleeding, localized or generalized. Petechiae, purpura, eccchymosis are suggestive of thrombocytopenia. Cepahlhematoma and subarachnoid bleeding may occur in healthy infants and without any hemostatic disorder. However, large subaponeurotic and subdural bleeds may be associated with coagulation defects. Germinal matrix and intraventricular bleeds are associated with prematurity, vascular fragility and coagulation disorders.

It provides useful etiological guidelines to classify the bleeding neonate into a well or a sick baby (Table 10.2). Hepatosplenomegaly may point towards the possibility of intrauterine viral infections. Detailed examination should be conducted to look for other features of TORCH infections, syndromes associated with bleeding disorder and for any congenital defects.

Table 10.2 Etiology of bleeding on the basis of a well and sick baby	
Well baby	Sick baby
▪ Slipped cord ligature	▪ Sepsis
▪ Swallowed maternal blood	▪ Disseminated intravascular coagulation
▪ Vitamin K deficiency (HDN)	
▪ Localized vascular disorder	▪ Birth asphyxia
▪ Maternal drug intake	▪ Thrombosis
▪ Allo/Autoimmune thrombocytopenia	▪ Hypothermia
	▪ Metabolic acidosis
▪ Isolated congenital clotting factor deficiency	▪ Necrotizing enterocolitis

HDN: Hemorrhagic disease of the newborn

Work-up of a Bleeding Neonate

Laboratory evaluation The initial screening tests include complete blood count, prothrombin time, activated partial thromboplastin time and a screening

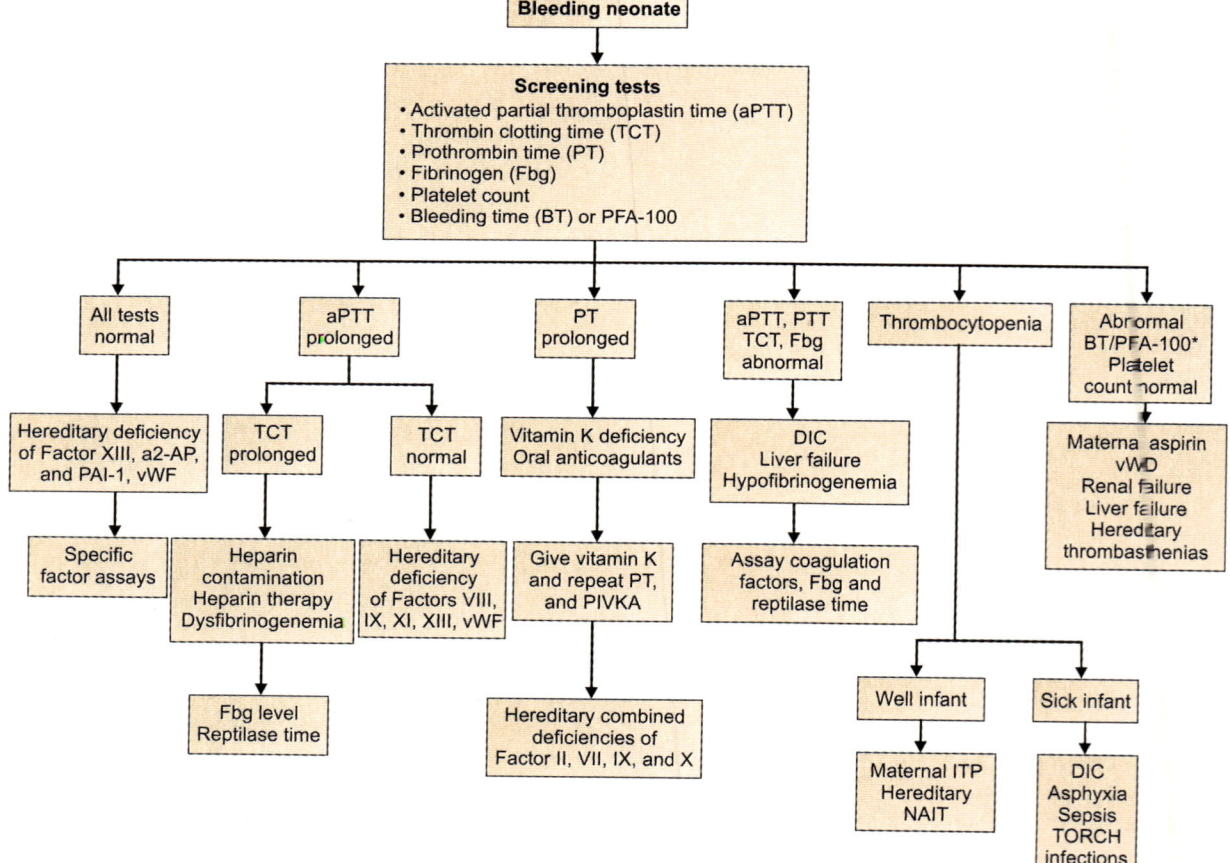

Abbreviations: PFA: Platelet function assay, PAI-1: Plasminogen activator inhibitor 1, a2-AP: Alpha 2 antiplasmin inhibitor, PIVKA: Protein induced by vitamin K deficiency or antagonists, NAIT: Neonatal alloimmune thrombocytopenia

Figure 10.1 Algorithm for laboratory investigations of a neonate with a bleeding disorder.

test for platelet functions with the help of platelet function analyzer (PFA). Assays of specific factors and more detailed examination of the platelet functions can be performed if indicated by the results of the screening tests. Screening tests may not be sensitive to identify several bleeding disorders including von Willebrand disease (vWD), factor XIII deficiency, plasminogen activator inhibition and alpha antiplasmin deficiencies. Abnormalities of certain screening tests like elevated PT, PTT and PFA may not necessarily mean presence of a pathologic process, as these tests are sensitive to handling, laboratory variations and are influenced by medications including herbal therapy. Algorithm for laboratory work-up of a neonate with a bleeding disorder is shown in Figure 10.1.

Laboratory Evaluation of Specific Disorders

The screening laboratory tests in sick and well neonates with a bleeding disorder are summarized in Table 10.3.

Platelet Disorders

Bleeding time It assesses the function of platelets and their interaction with vascular wall. The normal bleeding time varies between 4–8 minutes.

Platelet count The normal count varies between $1,50,000–4,00,000/mm^3$.

Platelet function analysis (PFA-100).

Platelet aggregation study ADP receptors, epinephrine, collagen, thromboplastin and restocetin parameters are assessed.

Coagulation Factor Deficiency

- *aPTT* It measures the initiation of clotting at the level of intrinsic Factors VII, IX, XI (normal 25–40 sec).
- *Prothrombin time (PT) and international normalized ratio (INR).* It measures the extrinsic clotting limb, i.e. Factors II, V, VII, X (normal 12–14 sec).

- *Thrombin time (TT)* It measures final step of clotting cascade (normal 11–15 sec). It is prolonged when there is deficiency of fibrinogen.
- *Fibrinogen level*
- *Fibrin degradation products* (FDPs) and D dimer assay level.
- *Peripheral smear* RBC morphology and number and size of platelets.

Management of a Bleeding Neonate

Immediate Management

The management should be directed to promote cardio-respiratory stability, which may require replacement of intravascular volume with 10 mL/kg normal saline bolus and other cardiorespiratory support measures. Following bleeding, when there is progressive fall in hematocrit, packed RBCs transfusion should be given. The underlying conditions like sepsis, hepatic failure and vitamin K deficiency should be treated. Vitamin K 1–2 mg should preferably be given through intravenous route.

Prevention of Vitamin K deficiency Bleeding (VKDB)

A single dose of intramuscular vitamin K (0.5 mg in preterm, 1.0 mg in term) after birth effectively prevents classic hemorrhagic disease of the newborn due to vitamin K deficiency. Oral vitamin K prophylaxis is also effective but it improves coagulation test results slowly over a period of 1–7 days.

Fresh frozen plasma (FFP) It has been traditionally used for a variety of indications, including volume replacement, treatment of disseminated intravascular coagulopathy (DIC), sepsis, bleeding due to vitamin K deficiency and inherited deficiency of coagulation factors.

Table 10.3 Screening laboratory tests in neonates with a bleeding disorder				
Health status	Platelets	PT/INR	aPTT	Bleeding disorder
Sick baby	↓	↑	↑	Disseminated intravascular coagulation
	↓	N	N	Infection, necrotizing enterocolitis, renal vein thrombosis
	N	↑	↑	Liver disease, heparin therapy
	N	N	N	Altered vascular integrity, extreme prematurity
Well baby	N	N	↑	Hemophilia
	↓	N	N	Immune thrombocytopenia, occult infection
	N	↑	↑	Hemorrhagic disease of the newborn
	N	N	N	Bleeding due to trauma, qualitative platelet abnormality, vascular fragility

aPTT: activated partial thromboplastin time, PT: prothrombin time, INR: international normalized ratio

Cryoprecipitate It is prepared from FFP by thawing at 2–4°C. Cryoprecipitate contains about 80 to 100 U of Factor VIII in 10–25 mL of plasma, 300 mg of fibrinogen and varying amounts of Factor XIII. It is stored at a temperature of –20°C or below. The specific indications for its use include congenital Factor VIII deficiency, congenital Factor XIII deficiency, afibrinogenemia and dysfibrinogenemia, and von Willebrand disease. The indications and benefits of various blood component therapy in a bleeding neonate are listed in Table 10.4.

Important Conditions Manifesting as Bleeding in a Neonate

Hemorrhagic Disease of the Newborn (HDN)

Vitamin K is essential for synthesis of coagulation Factors II (prothrombin), VII, IX and X by a process of carboxylation of glutamic acid in vitamin K-dependent proteins which helps in the process of coagulation. Blood PIVKA II (protein induced in vitamin K absence) is an excellent marker of vitamin K deficiency. The daily requirement of vitamin K is around 5 µg/d and an oral intake of about 10 µg/d is sufficient to provide for daily needs. Vitamin K exists in three forms. The naturally occurring vitamin K1 (Phylloquinone) is found in dietary sources like green leafy vegetables. Vitamin K2 (menaquinone) is indigenously produced in the gut by bacteroides fragilis and *E. coli.* Synthetic vitamin K3 (menadoine sodium bisulfite) is available as 10 mg/mL for parenteral administration.

Hemorrhagic disease of the newborn (HDN) is the commonest manifestation of vitamin K deficiency in infancy. Depending upon the age of onset, there are three types of hemorrhagic disease of the newborn.

1. Early HDN
The onset may be fetal or during first 24 hours of life. It is limited to babies of mothers receiving anticonvulsants, antitubercular drugs, coumarin derivatives, and salicylates during pregnancy. The site of bleeding is in the concealed cavities like cranium, thorax and abdomen.

2. Classic HDN
It has onset between 1–7 days of life and is usually limited to exclusively breastfed infants. The reported incidence varies between 0.25–0.5%. The common clinical manifestations include bleeding from umbilical stump and gastrointestinal tract. The bleeding is usually mild and can be managed by administration of vitamin K .

3. Late HDN
It has onset between 2–16 weeks of life. It is rare in formula fed infants and in infants who had received injectable vitamin K at birth. Intracranial bleeding is seen in over 50% cases of late HDN. It may occur following prolonged use of broad spectrum antibiotic therapy, chronic diarrhea and malabsorption, and cholestatic hepatitis.

Investigations

The blood sample should be collected before administration of vitamin K. Prothrombin time (PT) and plasma thromboplastin time (PTT) are prolonged because of low levels of Factors II, VII, XI, X. Blood PIVKA II (protein induced in vitamin K absence) levels as estimated by HPLC or ELISA are elevated.

Treatment

All neonates should receive single dose of vitamin K 0.5–1.0 mg IM at birth to prevent vitamin K deficiency bleeding (VKDB). It is credited to prevent both classic and late onset HDN. Oral administration of 2.0 mg (double the parentral dose) vitamin K is equally effective but there is no licensed preparation available in India.

Table 10.4 Blood components and products used in a bleeding neonate

Component/product	Content	Dose	Indications and outcome
Packed red blood cells (PRBc)	250–300 mL/unit	10–15 mL/kg	4 mL/kg increases Hb by 1.0 gm/dL
Platelet concentrate	5–7×10^7	1–2 units/ kg	Increases platelet count by 75,000/mm^3
Fresh frozen plasma (FFP)	1 unit/mL of clotting factor	10–15 mL/kg	Improvement in PT/PTT
Cryoprecipitate	Fibrinogen, Factor VII, vWF	15 mL/kg	Increases fibrinogen by 50–100 mg/dL
Exchange blood transfusion	All Factors and platelets	Double volume (160 mL/kg) exchange transfusion	Severe DIC; liver disease
Factor VIII concentrate	Factor VIII	25–50 U/kg	Hemophilia A
Intravenous immune globulins (IVIG)	All immune globulins	1–2 g/kg	Severe sepsis; thrombocytopenia due to transplacental gamma globulin antiplatelet antibodies

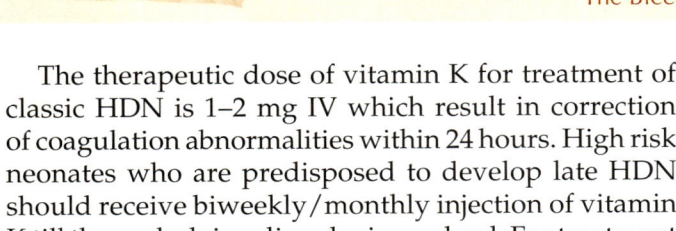

The therapeutic dose of vitamin K for treatment of classic HDN is 1–2 mg IV which result in correction of coagulation abnormalities within 24 hours. High risk neonates who are predisposed to develop late HDN should receive biweekly/monthly injection of vitamin K till the underlying disorder is resolved. For treatment of life-threatening hemorrhage, vitamin K should be followed by administration of fresh frozen plasma.

Disseminated Intravascular Coagulation (DIC)

DIC is defined as a systemic thrombo-hemorrhagic disorder seen in association with well-defined clinical situations and laboratory evidences of procoagulant and fibrinolytic activation, inhibitor consumption, biochemical and clinical evidences of endorgan damage or failure. Fibrinogen level is <100 mg/dL, with increased circulating fibrin degradation products (>100 µg/dL) and D-dimers (>0.5 mg/dL). The common underlying disorder is sepsis with multiorgan failure.

Treatment

Reversal of the underlying condition is paramount in achieving therapeutic success. The predisposing conditions like necrotizing enterocolitis, sepsis, and shock should be identified and appropriately managed. The important therapeutic interventions include volume resuscitation, correction of shock and coagulation abnormalities and ensuring urine output of at least 1 mL/kg per hour. Most infants require fresh frozen plasma and one unit of fresh platelet concentrate every 12–24 hours. The role of heparin is controversial.

Hemophilia

It is an X-linked recessive disorder; affecting males while females are carriers. The disease affects all racial groups and account for 90–95% of severe congenital coagulation deficiencies. Hemophilia A and B are inherited bleeding disorders caused by deficiencies of clotting Factor VIII (F VIII) and Factor IX (F IX), respectively.

Hemophilias may be missed in the newborn period. Excessive bleeding at the time of circumcision may provide earliest evidence of hemophilia. The bleeding manifestations are usually noticed when infant begins to crawl and walk leading to minor trauma and bruising. Clotting time is prolonged with reduced level of Factor VIII or Factor IX. In the newborns, Factor VIII may be elevated because of acute phase response elicited by the birth process while Factor IX is physiologically low in the newborn.

von Willebrand disease (vWD)

It is the commonest inherited bleeding disorder, with an estimated prevalence of 0.8–1.3%. It is inherited as an autosomal dominant disorder. Both superficial bleeding and intracranial hemorrhage have been reported in affected neonates. Type IIb vWD can be recognized during neonatal period because of presence of thrombocytopenia. Most other forms of vWD are masked by physiologically elevated levels of vWF and can be diagnosed in neonates by molecular analysis.

Neonatal Thrombocytopenia

Thrombocytopenia (platelet count <100,000/mm³) are seen in a quarter of sick neonates admited in the NICU. Thrombocytopenia is a useful marker of underlying disease and is an obvious risk factor for hemorrhage. Preterm neonates tend to have slightly lower mean platelet counts than term infants. Around 20% of neonates <28 weeks gestation develop severe thrombocytopenia. Transient thrombocytopenia may occur in healthy term infants while many sick neonates are likely to have low platelet counts.

The common causes of thrombocytopenia in neonates are listed in Table 10.5.

Table 10.5 Causes of thrombocytopenia in neonates
Secondary to maternal factors
■ Maternal autoimmune thrombocytopenia
■ Maternal diseases: Pre-eclampsia, lupus erythematosus, diabetes mellitus, hyperthyroidism
■ Maternal medications: Thiazides, sulfonamides, sedormid, quinine, quinidine
Congenital disorders
■ TAR (thrombocytopenia with absent radius) syndrome, Fanconi's anemia, congenital rubella syndrome, Trisomy 13 and 18, giant hemangioma (Kasabach-Merritt syndrome)
Poor production or functional defects
■ Congenital amegakaryocytic thrombocytopenia
■ Giant platelet syndrome
■ Alport syndrome
Increased platelet destruction
■ Infections (bacterial, viral, fungal, NEC)
■ Birth asphyxia and trauma
■ Disseminated intravascular coagulation
■ Thrombosis
■ Neonatal allo-immune thrombocytopenia (NAIT)
■ Congenital leukemia
Combined poor production and increased destruction
■ Rh-hemolytic disease of the newborn, hydrops fetalis, exchange blood transfusion
■ Intrauterine infections
■ Cyanotic heart disease
■ Polycythemia
■ Thrombosis
■ Wiskott-Aldrich syndrome

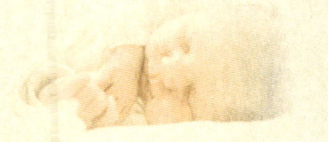

Early Thrombocytopenia

This is common in preterm infants following pregnancies complicated by placental insufficiency or fetal hypoxia (which may impair fetal/infant platelet production). These babies show a typical pattern of low/low-normal platelet counts at birth (100–200 × 10⁹/L), with levels falling to a nadir of 50–100 × 10⁹/L at 4–5 days. Counts generally return back to normal at 7–10 days. They usually have an associated transient neutropenia, increased number of nucleated RBCs and polycythemia. Clinically stable preterm infants following this pattern have a low risk of bleeding if platelet count remains above 50 × 10⁹/L. Other causes of early thrombocytopenia include neonatal alloimmune thrombocytopenia (NAITP), perinatal infections, maternal autoimmune diseases (ITP, SLE) and congenital disorders like thrombocytopenia with absent radius (TAR) and Wiskott-Aldrich syndrome.

Late Thrombocytopenia

Thrombocytopenia presenting in a neonate after the first 3 days of life is usually due to early-onset sepsis or NEC until proven otherwise. In such cases platelet count often drops rapidly to levels of 50 × 10⁹/L or below. These infants are at a significant risk of developing bleeding manifestations, while benefit of platelet transfusion is doubtful. The platelet count returns back to normal within 5–7 days when the underlying condition is treated by supportive and specific antimicrobial therapy. Other conditions in this group include intrauterine infections, late-onset sepsis, maternal ITP and SLE.

Immune Thrombocytopenias

Immune-mediated thrombocytopenia can be subdivided into three categories; transplacental crossing of the maternal antibodies directed against paternally inherited platelet antigen coated on fetal platelets (alloimmune thrombocytopenia), transplacental transfer of cross-reactive maternal autoimmune-derived antiplatelet antibodies (directed against both maternal and fetal platelets), and generation of autoreactive antiplatelet antibodies produced by the newborn (autoimmune thrombocytopenia).

Neonatal Allo-immune Thrombocytopenia (NAIT)

The fetomaternal alloimmune trombocytopenia, results from transplacental passage of maternal IgG alloantibodies directed against paternal antigens present on the fetal platelets, but lacking on maternal platelets. The mother will be healthy without any evidences of thrombocytopenia. Diagnosis is suspected when a healthy newborn born with an uneventful pregnancy and delivery, exhibits widespread petechiae or purpura at birth. The condition may manifest during first pregnancy in 50% cases. These infants are prone to develop fetal bleeding. Platelet antibodies are commonly present against HPA-1 or HPA-4.

Optimal treatment includes transfusion with platelet concentrates donated by the mother. In cases of severe thrombocytopenia or bleeding, random donor platelets may be used initially. High dose intravenous immune-globulins (IVIG), 400 mg/kg/day for 3 to 4 consecutive days, or 1 g/kg/day for 1 or 2 consecutive days, is effective in prolonging the survival of transfused platelets. All infants with NAIT should undergo cranial ultrasonography to rule out intracranial hemorrhage.

Autoimmune Thrombocytopenia

True autoimmune thrombocytopenia, in which a neonate generates antibodies against its own platelets, is rare in the newborn period. It is commonly associated with an underlying immune disorder. The bleeding manifestations are less severe and intracranial bleeding occurs in less than 1% cases. When immune-mediated maternal thrombocytopenia is associated, mother should receive corticosteroid therapy for 10–14 days.

SUMMARY

Bleeding in the newborn is often a serious event, which can present as a life-threatening emergency. The neonatologist should approach the problem in a systematic manner. Management should include strategies for prevention, measures to ensure hemodynamic stability, treatment of cause, and underlying problems, and replacement of coagulation factors. Counseling at all stages and proper follow-up is essential.

BIBLIOGRAPHY

Bakshi S., Deorari AK, Roy S, Paul VK, Singh M. Prevention of subclinical vitamin K deficiency based on PIVKA II levels: oral versus intramuscular route. *Indian pediatr* 1996, 33:1040.

BCHS Guidelines. The investigation and management of neonatal haemostasis and thrombosis. *Brit J Haematol* 2002, 119:295–309.

Buchanan GR. Coagulation disorders in the neonate. *Pediatr Clin North Am* 1986; 33:203–20.

Burrows RF, Kelton JG. Perinatal thrombocytopenia. *Clin Perinatol* 1995; 22:779–801.

Bussel JB, Sola-Visner M. Current approaches to the evaluation and management of the fetus and neonate with immune thrombocytopenia. *Obstet Gynecol Clin North Am* 2009; 33:457–66.

Homans A. Thrombocytopenia in the neonate. *Pediatr Clin North Am* 1996; 43:737–56.

McMillan DD, Wu J. Approach to the bleeding newborn. *Paediatr Child Health* 1998; 3(6):399–401.

Murray NA, Howarth U, McCloy MP, et al. Platelet transfusion in the management of severe thrombocytopenia in neonatal intensive care unit (NICU) patients. *Transfus Med* 2002; 12:35–41.

Murray NA, Roberts IAG. Neonatal transfusion practice. *Arch Dis Child FN* 2004; 89:101–107.

Pramanik AK. The bleeding neonate. In: Medical Emergencies in Children. Singh M (Ed.), revised 5th edition, *New Delhi, CBS Publishers & Distributors Pvt. Ltd.,* 2016, pp 306–336.

Puckett RM, Offringa M. Prophylactic vitamin K for vitamin K deficiency bleeding in neonates. *Cochrane Database Syst Rev* 2000(4):CD002776.

Roberts, IAG and Murray NA. Thrombocytopenia in the newborn. *Curr Opin Pediatr 2003; 15(1):17–23.*

Roberts IAG, Marray NA. Neonatal thrombocytopenia causes and management. *Arch Dis Child Ed* 2003, 88:F359–F364.

Sankar MJ, Chandrasekaran A, Paul VK. Vitamin K prophylaxis for prevention of vitamin K deficiency bleeding: a systematic review. *J Perinatol* 2016, May: 36 (suppl I):529–35.

Shearer MJ. Vitamin K deficiency bleeding (VKDB) in early infancy. *Blood Rev* 2009; 23:49–59.

Stanworth, SJ, Clarke, P, Watts, T, et al. Platelets Neonatal Transfusion Study Group. Prospective observational study outcomes in neonates with severe thrombocytopenia. *Pediatrics* 2009; 124:e826-e834.

The Diagnosis, Evaluation, and Management of von Willebrand Disease; NIH Publication No. 08-5832; December 2007.

Trotter L. Disseminated Intravascular coagulation in the neonatal period. *Newborn and Infant Nurs Rev* 2004; 4(4):176–80.

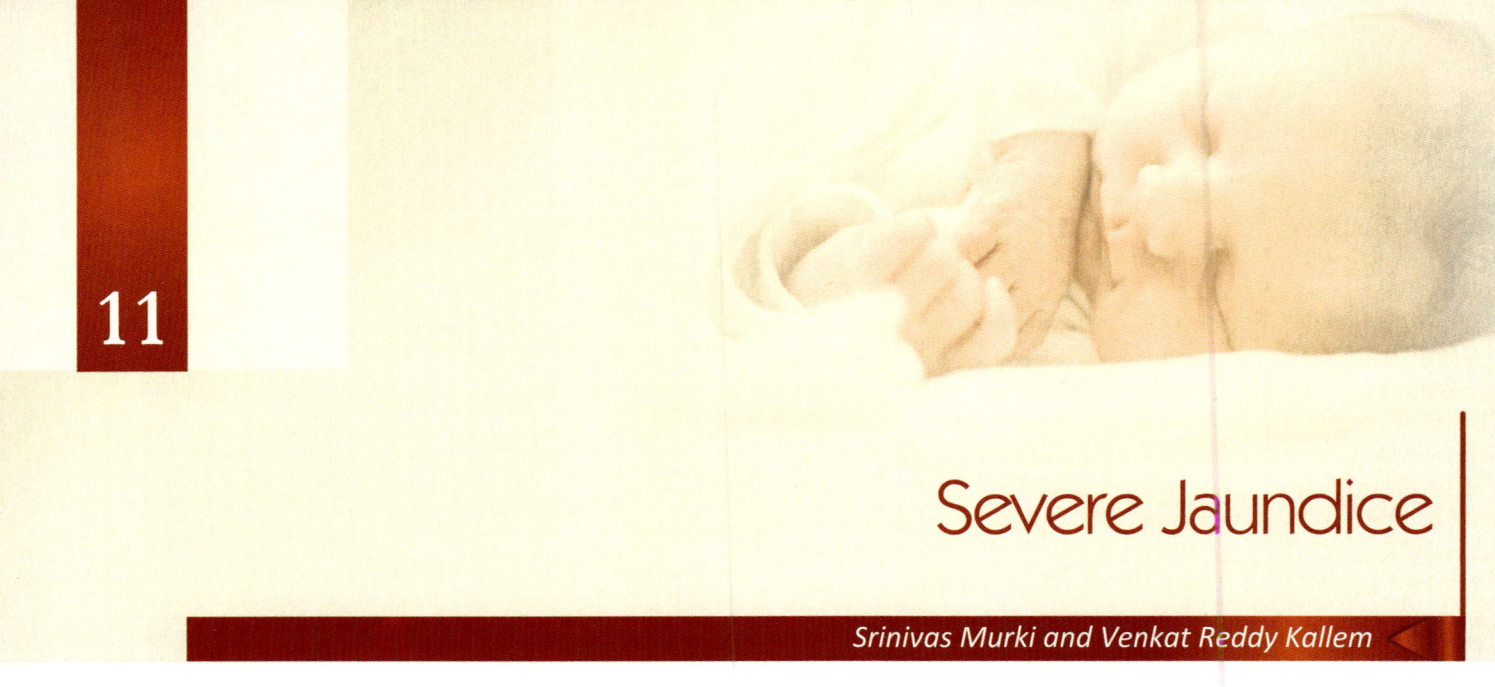

11

Severe Jaundice

Srinivas Murki and Venkat Reddy Kallem

Introduction

Severe neonatal jaundice or hyperbilirubinemia is considered as one of the medical emergencies during the newborn period and is associated with an increased risk of bilirubin induced neurologic dysfunction (BIND). Neonatal hyperbilirubinemia in infants with gestation greater than 35 weeks is defined as total serum or plasma bilirubin (TSB) >95th percentile on the hour specific nomogram and severe neonatal hyperbilirubinemia is defined as a TSB >25 mg/dL. The major complication of an elevated TSB (hyperbilirubinemia) is bilirubin-induced neurologic dysfunction (BIND), which occurs when circulating bilirubin crosses the blood-brain barrier and binds to brain tissue. Acute bilirubin encephalopathy (ABE) is the acute but reversible form of BIND, while kernicterus is the chronic and permanent neurologic sequelae of BIND. Advances in medical care with administration of Rh(D) immunoglobulins to Rh-negative mothers and introduction of effective phototherapy have resulted in reduction in the incidence of severe jaundice and need for exchange blood transfusions. Nevertheless, isolated cases of kernicterus continue to be reported. Population based data from developed countries is available to predict the risk of kernicterus on the basis of TSB concentrations (Box 11.1).

In a report from North India, out of 64 out-born newborns presenting with severe jaundice (TSB >24 mg/dL) in the first 72 hours of life, 28 (44%) had features of ABE. Almost all newborns with ABE developed some evidences of kernicterus at 6 months of age.

Assessment of Severity of Jaundice

Severity of jaundice is assessed based on the age of onset, intensity of skin discoloration, associated clinical signs of hemolysis, laboratory reports and clinical features of bilirubin induced neurologic dysfunction (BIND). The risk factors for development of ABE are listed in Box 11.2.

Severity of Yellow Discoloration of Skin

The clinical manifestations of hyperbilirubinemia occur due to deposition of bilirubin in the skin causing yellow

---

BOX 11.1 Risk of kernicterus in a term neonate based on total serum bilirubin

- TSB >20 and ≤25 mg/dL: Risk only in conjunction with a comorbid conditions
- TSB >25 but ≤30 mg/dL: 6 percent risk
- TSB >30 but ≤35 mg/dL: 14 to 25 percent risk
- TSB >35 mg/dL: Almost all infants will have signs of acute brain encephalopathy

TSB: Total serum bilirubin

BOX 11.2 Risk factors for development of acute bilirubin encephalopathy (ABE)

- Onset of jaundice within 24 hours of age with a rapid progression
- Jaundice affecting palms and soles
- Late preterms (35–37 weeks)
- Birth asphyxia
- Sepsis
- Integrity of blood-brain barrier
- Intrauterine growth restriction
- High bilirubin to albumin ratio (>3.5)
- High free bilirubin
- Hemolytic anemia
- Hypothermia
- Metabolic acidosis
- Hypoglycemia
- Administration of drugs blocking bilirubin binding sites

discoloration and/or occurrence of bilirubin induced neurological dysfunction (BIND). The yellow discoloration of skin is the time honored clinical sign of jaundice but it is not a reliable method to assess total serum bilirubin (TSB) concentration especially in infants with dark skin. The examination for jaundice should be performed with adequate natural sun light or under fluorescent daylight. Blanching of the skin with a finger reduces local skin perfusion and facilitates detection of jaundice. Jaundice usually progresses in a cephalo-caudal direction, appearing first on the face with a TSB levels of 4 to 8 mg/dL. The entire body, including palms and soles, appear yellow discolored when TSB exceeds 15 mg/dL. It is difficult to assess yellow discoloration of eyes due to physiologic photophobia in neonates but when scleral conjunctiva is visibly yellow, TSB is likely to be more than 15 mg/dL. If there is uncertainty regarding the presence or severity of jaundice, a TSB or a TcB (transcutaneous bilirubin) measurement should be performed. Other findings on physical examination that suggest an increased risk for hyper-bilirubinemia include pallor due to hemolytic anemia, enclosed hemorrhage (cephalhematoma, subgaleal bleed), bruising, and hepatosplenomegaly. The associated clinical signs of hemolysis like onset of jaundice within first 24 hours of life, anemia and hepato-splenomegaly are reliable correlates of severe jaundice with increased risk of BIND.

Pathological Jaundice

Jaundice due to physiological immaturity of neonates is seen in over 60% of term and 80% of a preterm babies. Jaundice should be closely watched to identify its onset, severity, features of BIND and its duration. A number of clinical and biochemical parameters are useful to identify pathological jaundice which may require photo-therapy and exchange blood transfusion (Box 11.3).

Neurologic Manifestations

Bilirubin is a useful anti-oxidant but a potential neuro-toxin. Term and late preterm (35–37 weeks) infants are at risk to develop BIND when TSB concentrations exceed 25 mg/dL. In general, at this threshold,

BOX 11.3 Clinical and biochemical parameters suggestive of pathological jaundice

- Onset of jaundice within 24 hours or after 72 hours of age.
- Distinct yellow staining of palms and soles with total serum bilirubin >15 mg/dL.
- Persistence of jaundice beyond 15 days of age.
- Jaundice with pallor, hepatosplenomegaly, and/or edema.
- Elevation of direct reacting serum bilirubin by >2.0 mg/dL (yellow colored urine and/or clay colored stool).
- Jaundice in association with clinical evidences of bilirubin-induced neurologic dysfunction (BIND).

unconjugated bilirubin, which is not bound to albumin (also referred to as "free" or unbound bilirubin), can enter the brain and cause cell death by apoptosis (programmed cell death) and/or necrosis. The exact mechanism for development of BIND remains uncertain. BIND is characterized by a spectrum of subtle neurologic findings and sequelae, which can adversely affect vision, hearing, gait, muscular rigidity, cognition, and language development. Acute bilirubin encephalopathy (ABE) may be reversible or result in permanent irreversible neurologic dysfunction (kernicterus). The brain regions which are most vulnerable to BIND include the basal ganglia and the brainstem nuclei concerned with oculomotor and auditory functions.

Acute bilirubin encephalopathy (ABE) typically progresses through three phases (Table 11.1). In the early phase, the clinical signs may be subtle. The infant is sleepy but arousable, and when aroused has mild to moderate hypotonia and a high-pitched cry. If no intervention is done, the intermediate phase evolves with progression of hyperbilirubinemia. The infant may be febrile, lethargic with a poor suck, or irritable and jittery. The cry is usually high pitched or shrill and the infant is difficult to console. Mild to moderate hypertonia develops, beginning with backward arching of the neck (retrocollis) and trunk (opisthotonos) especially when infant is disturbed. Immediate and emergent exchange blood transfusion at this stage may reduce the severity of BIND. The advanced phase is characterized by apnea, inability to feed, fever, seizures, and a semi-comatose state that may progress to coma.

Table 11.1 Bilirubin-induced neurological dysfunction (BIND) score

Features	Mild (score 1)	Moderate (score 2)	Severe (score 3)
Mental status	Sleepy and poor feeding	Lethargic and irritable	Semi coma and/or seizures
Muscle tone	Slight decrease	Hyper or hypotonia depending on the arousal state or mild nuchal/truncal arching	Markedly increased opisthotonos or decreased tone or increased bicycling movements
Character of cry	High pitched	Shrill	Inconsolable crying or absence of cry

Hypertonicity and rigidity presents as persistent retrocollis and opisthotonos with excessive bicycling movements or twitchings of the hands and feet. The cry is inconsolable, or may be weak or absent. Death usually occurs due to respiratory failure or intractable seizures.

Brainstem auditory evoked responses (BAER) can be evaluated to detect neurologic sequelae of hyper-bilirubinemia. Increased TSB correlates with prolonged brainstem conduction time. These abnormalities resolve as TSB values decline. Changes in BAER are associated with elevated unbound bilirubin levels. An abnormal BAER and normal otoacoustic emission (OAE) test suggest that severe hyperbilirubinemia may result in auditory neuropathy.

Identification of Etiology

Etiology of jaundice is evaluated from the history, course of jaundice, clinical examination and laboratory reports. Steps for evaluation of a jaundiced infant are summarized below.

Step 1 *Identification of features suggestive of hemolysis.*
The onset of jaundice within the first 24 hours of birth, and rapid progression of jaundice to cause yellow staining of trunk, palms and soles are suggestive of hemolysis.

Hemolytic anemia is characterized by pallor, splenomegaly, hematocrit <40% and reticulocyte count of more than 3%. Peripheral blood smear examination usually shows marked anisopoikilocytosis, spherocytosis, polychromasia and nucleated or fragile RBCs. In neonates with hemolysis, the severity of jaundice is out of proportion to the intensity of anemia.

Step 2 *Features suggestive of immune hemolysis*
There may be laboratory evidences of blood group incompatibility in the ABO (A, B or AB baby and O group mother) and Rh system (Rh-negative mother and Rh-positive baby). Mother's indirect Coombs test (ICT) is usually positive and infant's direct Coombs test (DCT) may be positive.

Step 3 *Infants with non-immune hemolysis*
The presence of cephalhematoma or subgaleal bleeds, or concealed internal hemorrhage may cause severe jaundice. Geographic origin of parents and rapidity of rise in bilirubin levels with mild or no clinical signs of hemolysis (G6PD deficiency) and family history of jaundice in previous siblings should be looked for. Family history of recurrent blood transfusions, jaundice, leg ulcers and splenectomy in the mother or father are suggestive of hereditary spherocytosis.

Step 4 *Non-hemolytic jaundice*
In an exclusively breastfed baby, persistence of jaundice beyond 2 weeks, slow progression of jaundice, absence of pallor, or any concealed hemorrhage and excessive weight loss are suggestive of breastfeeding jaundice. Poor feeding, lethargy, temperature instability, circum-oral grayish discoloration, cold peripheries, prolonged capillary refill time in the presence of severe jaundice are suggestive of sepsis. Infants with cretinism and cholestasis may have severe and prolonged jaundice.

Investigations

The jaundiced neonate should be investigated to assess the severity of jaundice (TSB), its likely etiology and to look for any evidences of bilirubin induced neurologic dysfunction (BIND). Transcutaneous bilirubin is a useful screening tool to asess the severity of jaundice but it is relatively less reliable at higher bilirubin levels. Total serum bilirubin level is the gold standard for assessing the severity of jaundice. There is no need to substract the direct bilirubin from the TSB unless the direct fraction exceeds 50% of the total serum bilirubin.

Blood group of the mother and the baby should be checked. Direct Coombs test (DCT) in the infant and indirect Coombs test (ICT) in the mother are useful to diagnose hemolytic disease of the newborn. Hematocrit of <40% is suggestive of anemia while a PCV >60% is suggestive of polycythemia.

Peripheral blood smear should be examined for anisopoikilocytosis, polychromasia, and nucleated RBCs. The presence of spherocytes, elliptocytes, and stomatocytes suggest RBC membrane defects. Reticulocyte count is elevated in hemolysis and blood loss. Sepsis screen and blood culture are done to exclude septicemia. Thyroid function tests are done to rule out cretinism as a cause of prolonged jaundice. G6PD screening is mandatory in endemic areas and whenever there is rapid rise in bilirubin level. When G6PD screening is done during acute hemolysis, it should be rechecked at the age of 3–4 months. Hypoalbuminemia, metabolic acidosis and hypoglycemia should be looked for because they increase the risk of bilirubin encephalopathy. BAER and MRI brain are useful to look for evidences of BIND.

Management

The decision regarding the time of intervention and its choice are based on total serum bilirubin level, gestation, birth weight, postnatal age of the infant, and presence of risk factors for ABE like isoimmune hemolytic disease, G6PD deficiency, asphyxia, temperature instability, sepsis, acidosis, hypoglycemia and hypo-albuminemia (serum albumin <3 g/dL).

Interventions Based on Risk Severity

Phototherapy is the initial intervention to reduce TSB. The cut-off values for phototherapy and exchange blood transfusion in healthy (without hemolysis) term and late preterm infants, with and without perinatal risk factors are shown in Table 11.2.

Phototherapy

Phototherapy remains the mainstay of treatment of neonatal hyperbilirubinemia. Indications for phototherapy are listed in Tables 11.2 and 11.3, and Figure 11.1. The

Table 11.2 Bilirubin cutoff values for intervention in healthy term and late preterm infants with and without risk factors

	Total serum bilirubin levels (mg/dL)						
	Phototherapy			Exchange Transfusion			
Age (hours)	24	48	≥72	24	48	72	>72
Term infants with no risk factors	>12	>15	>18	>19	>22	>24	>25
Term infants with risk factors	>10	>13	>15	>16.5	>19	>21	>21
Late preterm infants with no risk factors	>10	>13	>15	>16.5	>19	>21	>21
Late preterm infants with risk factors	>8	>11	>13.5	>15	>17	>18.5	>18.5

Term: ≥38 weeks, Late preterm: 35 to 37 weeks, Risk factors: Rh, ABO incompatibility, G6PD deficiency, asphyxia, sepsis, metabolic acidosis, hypoglycemia, low serum albumin.
Note: In newborns under intensive phototherapy, exchange transfusion is recommended if the TSB is not dropping below exchange threshold or if the newborn has signs of BIND

Table 11.3 Phototherapy and exchange transfusion cut-offs for preterm babies (<35 weeks)

Birth weight	Total serum bilirubin levels (mg/dL)			
	Healthy infant		Sick or high-risk infant	
	Phototherapy	Exchange transfusion	Phototherapy	Exchange transfusion
<1000 gm	5–7	11–13	4–6	10–12
1001–1500 gm	7–10	13–15	6–8	11–13
1501–2000 gm	10–12	15–18	8–10	13–15
2001–2500 gm	12–15	18–20	10–12	15–18

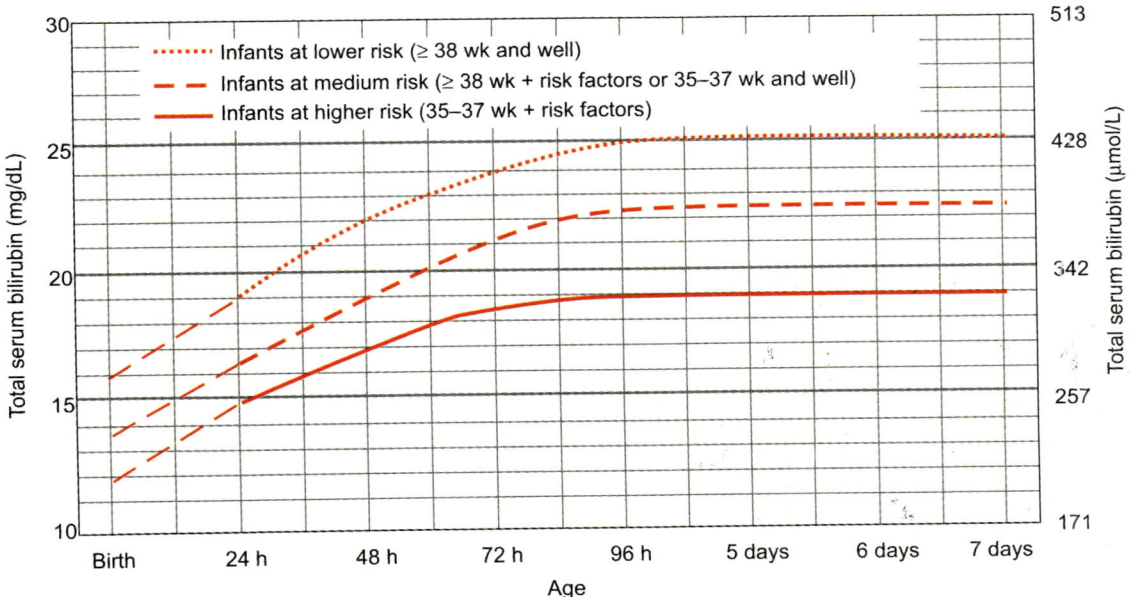

Figure 11.1 AAP nomogram for exchange transfusion in infants 35 or more weeks' gestation.

phototherapy units use a variety of light sources including fluorescent lamps of different colors and shapes, halogen bulbs, high intensity light emitting diodes (LED) and fiber-optic light sources. Compact fluorescent light (CFL) and LED phototherapy units are commonly used in our country. The light source should provide minimum of 15 mW/cm²/nm irradiance and ideally above 30 mW/cm²/nm to ensure effective phototherapy. Double surface or multiple sources of phototherapy are used if TSB is rising rapidly (> 0.5 mg/dL/hr), TSB is within 3 mg/dL of the threshold for exchange transfusion and/or TSB fails to respond to single surface PT in 6 hours.

Administration of Phototherapy

While under PT, the baby's eyes and genitals (male infants) should be covered without undue pressure on the face and nose by using PT goggles (Figure 11.2). Mother should be encouraged to remove the baby from under the lights, uncover the eyes and breastfeed every 2 to 3 hours.

The position of the baby should be changed every 2 hours or after each feed to expose maximum skin surface of the baby to PT. Temperature (every 4 hourly), body weight (once daily) and urine output (daily) of the baby should be monitored.

The light source should be as close to the baby as possible in order to increase the efficacy of PT. Monitor the progress of jaundice with frequent TSB measurements because TcB (transcutaneous bilirubin) and clinical assessment of jaundice becomes unreliable in an infant receiving phototherapy.

Efficacy of Phototherapy

The efficacy of PT depends on the type of light source, surface area of exposure, distance between the baby and light source, intensity of light, cause of jaundice and condition of the baby. The narrow spectral blue light is most effective for PT. Intensity of PT can be improved by using LED or CFL light. The higher the intensity of

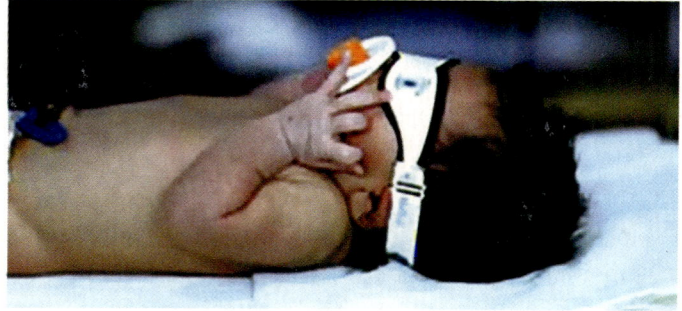

Figure 11.2 Phototherapy goggles.

irradiance, better is the efficacy. Intensity and efficacy of PT can also be increased by decreasing the distance between the lamps and the baby.

The surface area of skin exposed to PT can be increased by double or triple surface light sources, by using fiberoptic biliblanket along with CFL/LED, by frequently changing the position of the baby or by using reflectors. The efficacy of PT is improved of child is fed frequently to improve the status of hydration.

Stopping the Phototherapy

Phototherapy can be stopped once two TSB values, at least four hours apart, are 2 mg/dL below the PT cutoffs. Check for rebound rise in TSB after 8–12 hours in neonates with gestational age less than 35 weeks, birth weight of less than 2000 g, G6PD deficiency or hemolytic disease of the newborn.

Side Effects of Phototherapy

The common side effects of PT include impaired maternal infant bonding, skin rash, increased insensible water loss, passage of loose green stools and hypocalcemia. Hyperthermia, irritability and dehydration may occur. Infants having elevation of direct bilirubin due to parenchymal liver disease may develop peculiar bronze discoloration of skin.

Exchange Blood Transfusion

Indications for EBT are given in Tables 11.2, 11.3 and Figure 11.3. If TSB remains above the threshold for exchange transfusion after six hours of phototherapy, exchange blood transfusion is indicated. This approach reduces the number of infants requiring an invasive procedure of exchange blood transfusion, which is associated with significant morbidity and mortality. Exchange transfusion is reserved for symptomatic infants, with severe hyperbilirubinemia, who fail to respond to phototherapy. The type and cross-match of the infant's blood and placement of umbilical catheter are performed promptly, so that exchange transfusion can be started as quickly as possible. Urgent and intense phototherapy (referred to as crash cart phototherapy) is provided during the interim period needed to set-up the procedure. Infants who are likely to meet the criteria for exchange transfusion should be directly admitted or transferred to the neonatal or pediatric intensive care unit (NICU/PICU).

The bilirubin/albumin (B/A) ratio can be used as an additional parameter in determining the need for exchange transfusion. It should not be used alone, but in conjunction with TSB values. In term neonates, B/A

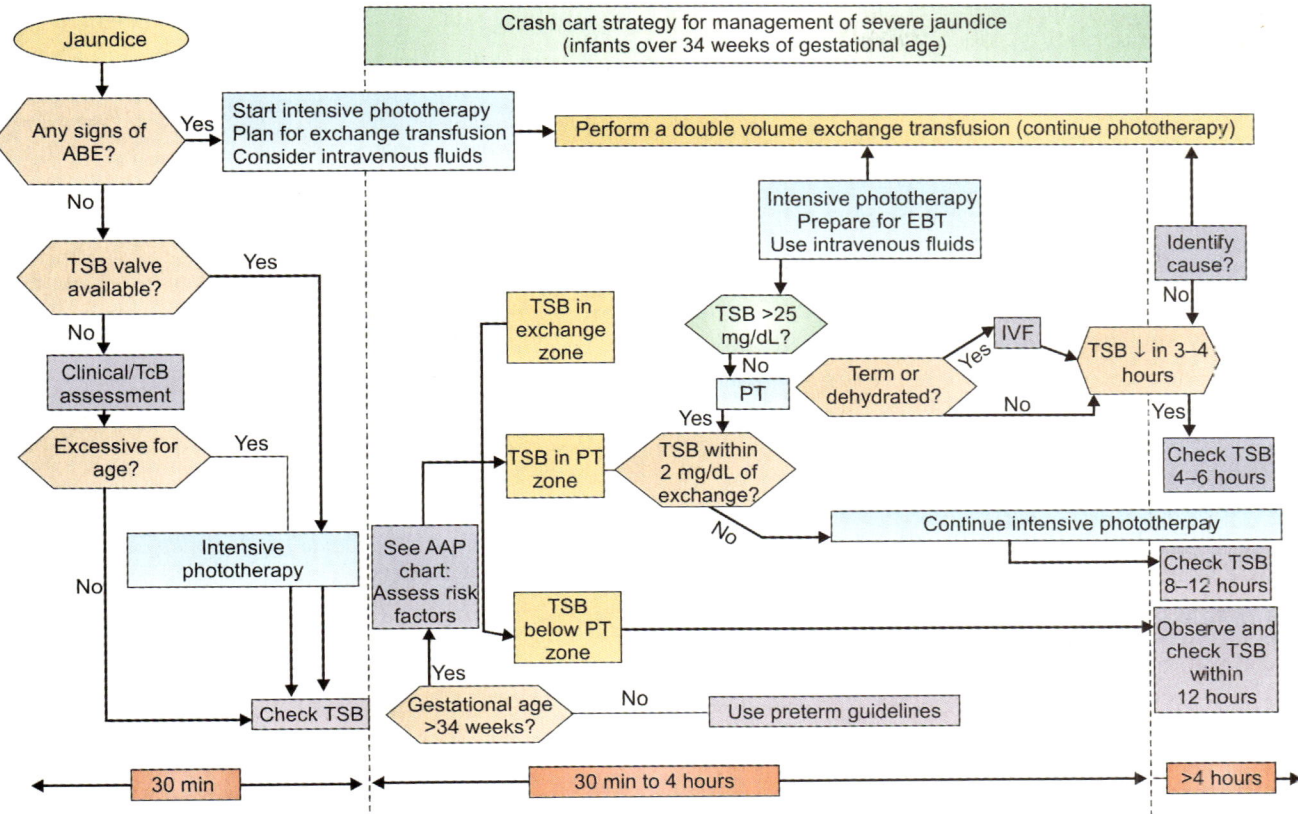

Figure 11.3 Algorithm for crash-cart management of neonatal jaundice as a pediatric emergency.

ABE: acute bilirubin encephalopathy; IVF: intravenous fluids; PT: phototherapy; TSB: total serum bilirubin; TcB: transcutaneous bilirubin; EBT: exchange blood transfusion.

ratio >7.0 (bilirubin mg/dL to albumin g/dL) indicate that all bilirubin binding sites on albumin are saturated. Any further increase in bilirubin would be associated with exponentially increasing levels of free bilirubin and increased risk of neurotoxicity. In preterm infants, additional confounding factors may affect the ability of albumin to bind bilirubin making it more challenging to predict their bilirubin binding capacity.

Exchange transfusion is indicated in infants with impending signs of acute bilirubin encephalopathy (ABE), such as significant lethargy, hypotonia, poor sucking, or high pitched cry, irrespective of the TSB level. The procedure for exchange transfusion should be set-up without any delay by arranging suitable matched irradiated fresh blood and by establishing vascular access for the procedure. Phototherapy should be provided in the interim period (Figure 11.1).

Preterm Infants below 35 Weeks of Gestation

There are no consensus guidelines for phototherapy or exchange blood transfusion in preterm infants. The proposed TSB cut-offs for phototherapy and exchange transfusion in preterm infants are arbitrary and clinical judgment should be exercised before making a decision (Table 11.3).

Indications of ET at Birth

In infants with Rh-hemolytic disease of the newborn, ET is planned at birth in following situations:

- Hydrops fetalis and hemolysis
- Cord hemoglobin <10 g/dL or hematocrit <30%
- Cord TSB > 5 mg/dL

Procedure of Exchange Blood Transfusion

The procedure of exchange blood transfusion (EBT) involves removal of the infant's blood having high bilirubin levels, antibody-coated red blood cells, partially hemolysed RBCs and simultaneous replacement with fresh donor blood providing fresh albumin with available binding sites for bilirubin.

Type of Blood

Depending upon the blood group of the mother and the infant, appropriate type of donor blood is ordered

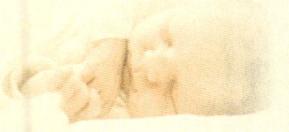

Table 11.4 Choice of blood for exchange transfusion		
Maternal blood group	*Infant blood group*	*Donor blood group*
O	O/A/B/AB	O
A/B/AB	O/A/B/AB	Infant blood group or O group
Rh negative	Rh positive/negative	Rh negative

(Table 11.4). Fresh donor blood (<5 days) is preferred to prevent the risk of hyperkalemia. The donor blood should be irradiated to deplete leucocytes to prevent graft versus host disease (GVHD). Before the procedure, the blood should be warmed to body temperature using either a water bath or by wrapping the container in a warm towel. Rapid rewarming by placing it under the radiant warmer, massaging between hands or placing under running hot water should be avoided to minimize hemolysis of the donor blood.

Blood Volume for ET

Assessment of infant's total circulating blood volume determines the efficacy of exchange blood transfusion. In a term neonate, the blood volume is around 80–90 mL/kg. The procedure of EBT that uses 80–90 mL/kg of donor blood is termed as single-volume exchange blood transfusion, and when 160–180 mL/kg blood is used for the procedure, it is termed as double-volume exchange blood transfusion. On the basis of the time constant of the procedure of exchange blood transfusion, single-volume exchange is credited to exchange 63% of the infant's blood while double-volume exchange achieves 86% exchange. However, because of tissue to intravascular dynamics, more bilirubin is removed from the infant than the actual volume of blood exchanged.

Single-catheter Pull Push Technique (Figure 11.4)

In this "central" technique, ET is usually performed through a catheter passed via the umbilical vein that has been placed in the inferior vena cava below its junction with the right atrium. The procedure is performed with continuous monitoring of vital signs and by placing the infant under the radiant warmer. Periumbilical area is cleaned as for a surgical procedure using betadine or chlorhexidine skin preparation. The operational area should be covered with sterile surgical drapes. A loose purse string should be placed around the base of the cord to ensure hemostasis after the procedure. Umbilical venous catheter size 5 or 8 Fr, prefilled with saline and attached to a 10-mL syringe, is gently inserted into the umbilical vein. The venous catheter is advanced into inferior vena cava below its junction with right atrium. The umbilical venous catheter

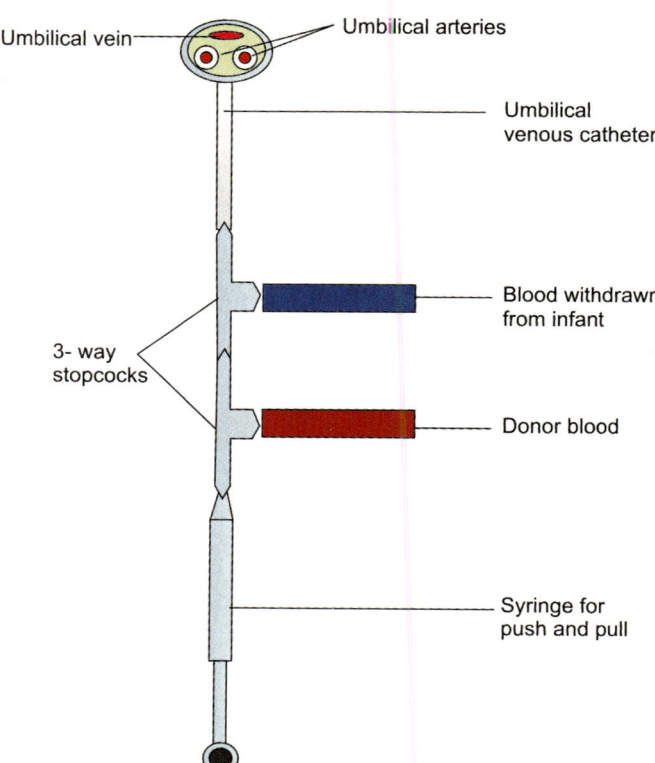

Figure 11.4 Schematic diagram for performing a single-catheter pull push exchange blood transfusion through the umbilical vein.

is connected to 2 three-way stopcocks or 1 four-way stopcock. The 4 channels of connection to the umbilical catheter include umbilical catheter, catheter draining the withdrawn blood, donor blood, and a saline prefilled syringe. All the connections should be prefilled with saline and they should never be left open to the atmosphere to prevent air embolism. The first aliquot of blood drawn from the neonate can be used for laboratory tests. During the procedure, the size of each aliquot should be approximately 5–8% of infant's estimated blood volume (smaller aliquots for smaller and sicker infants). In a term infant with a body weight appropriate for gestational age, usually 15 to 20 mL aliquots are withdrawn or infused at a rate of 5 mL/kg/min.

Double-catheter Pull Push Technique

In this technique, both umbilical vein and artery are catheterized. Blood is withdrawn from the umbilical artery and simultaneously equal volume of blood is replaced through the umbilical vein. Additional personnel are needed to operate each catheter and monitor their synchronization. Advantages include a timely completion of the procedure to achieve an iso-volumetric withdrawal and infusion.

Other Modalities of Management

Pharmacologic Agents

Pharmacologic agents including intravenous immune globulins (IVIG), phenobarbital, ursodeoxycholic acid (UDCA), and metalloporphyrins have been used to inhibit hemolysis, increase conjugation and excretion of bilirubin, increase bile flow, or inhibit the formation of bilirubin. However, among these modalities only IVIG is used for treatment Rh⁻ and ABO-hemolytic disease of the newborn.

Intravenous immune globulins

IVIG has been shown to reduce the need for exchange transfusion in infants with hemolytic disease caused by Rhesus (Rh) or ABO incompatibility. Several systematic reviews have shown that infants who received IVIG had lower rates of exchange blood transfusion. However, a meta-analysis of various studies concluded that the efficacy of IVIG is controversial. IVIG 0.5–1 g/kg is given intravenously over a period of two hours in infants with iso-immune hemolytic disease of the newborn if the total serum or plasma bilirubin is rising despite intensive phototherapy or is approaching within 2 or 3 mg/dL of the threshold for exchange transfusion. The dose of IVIG may be repeated after 12 hours if necessary. The exact mechanism of efficacy is uncertain, but IVIG is believed to inhibit hemolysis by blocking antibody receptors on the red blood cells.

Ursodeoxycholic acid

Ursodeoxycholic acid (UDCA) increases bile flow and helps to lower TSB levels. It is useful in the treatment of cholestatic jaundice. However, data are limited on the safety and overall efficacy of UDCA as adjunctive therapy.

Phenobarbital

Phenobarbital increases the conjugation and excretion of bilirubin and decreases postnatal TSB levels when given to pregnant women or infants. However, prenatal administration of phenobarbital is not very effective and may adversely affect the cognitive development and reproduction. Phenobarbital is not routinely used to treat indirect neonatal hyperbilirubinemia.

Metalloporphyrins

Synthetic metalloporphyrins such as tin mesoporphyrin (SnMP), reduce bilirubin production by competitive inhibition of hemeoxygenase. There is limited data on the safety and efficacy of SnMP and its use is controversial and not approved.

Hydration

It is important to maintain adequate hydration and urine output during phototherapy since urinary excretion of lumirubin is the principal mechanism by which phototherapy reduces TSB. During phototherapy the infant should continue to receive oral feeds from breast or with a spoon. Extra fluids @ 50 mL/kg either as additional spoon feeds or intravenous fluids, in neonates with severe jaundice (TSB >18 mg/dL) decreases the need for subsequent exchange transfusions. Intravenous hydration may be necessary to correct hypovolemia in infants with significant volume depletion because of inadequate oral intake.

Prognosis

The earliest evidences of asymptomatic bilirubin encephalopathy are seen on the MRI, auditory brainstem evoked responses, somato-sensory evoked responses and abnormalities on crying. In all newborns with a TSB >18 mg/dL or if there are signs of BIND, a BAER is best done at the time of discharge or at the age of one month. Auditory waves I, III, and IV-V complex are normally present in full-term neonates. Wave I originates from the auditory nerve, wave III the superior olive, and wave IV–V complex from the lateral meniscus and inferior colliculi. The latter three sites are classically involved in infants with kernicterus. Severe jaundice leads to loss of waves IV and V, with prolonged latency of the brainstem response. The changes represent aberrant brainstem functions, at both lower and upper brainstem levels. Although the auditory brainstem response is a specific reflection of auditory neural function, aberrant auditory brainstem responses are suggestive of widespread neural malfunction. Persistent abnormalities on the brainstem evoked response audiometry (BERA) at 3 and 9 months of age are indications of underlying hearing deficits and associated neurological handicaps (Figure 11.5).

Severe jaundice causes bilateral symmetrical hyper intense signals in the globus pallidus on both T1 and T2 weighted images on MRI of brain (Figure 11.6). High signal intensity is also seen in the hippocampus and thalamus. Following EBT, these MRI changes may disappear but persistence of abnormal signals on the MRI are suggestive of long-term neurological deficits.

Kernicterus or permanent sequelae of BIND develop during the first year of life. Infants with severe jaundice with acute bilirubin encephalopathy (ABE), cognitive functions are usually spared. The major features of kernicterus include choreoathetoid cerebral palsy, sensorineural hearing loss (SNHL) commonly

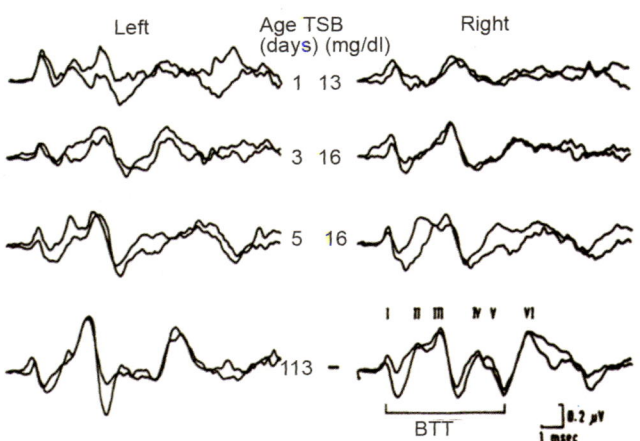

Figure 11.5 Serial BERA changes and bilirubin concentrations over a period of time.

Note: Serial auditory brainstem responses and bilirubin concentrations over a period of 16 weeks in a jaundiced infant. There is absence of waves IV–V and increasing amplitude and decreasing latency of wave III.

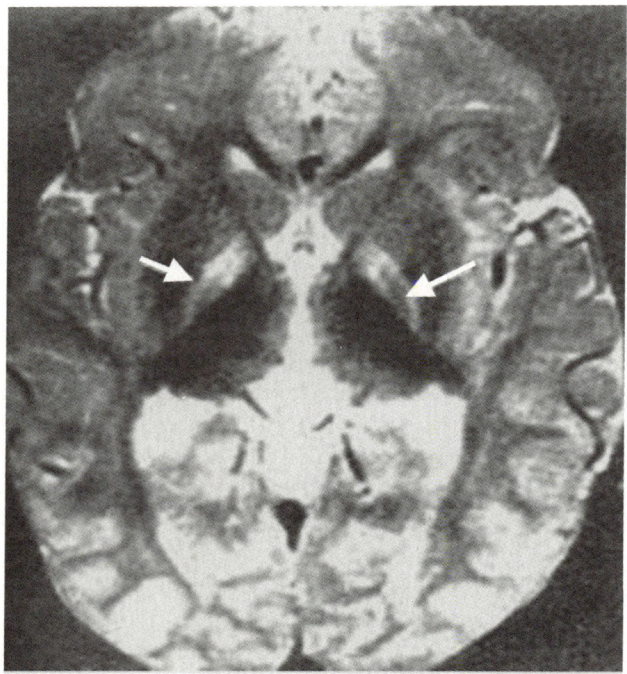

Figure 11.6 MRI picture showing bilirubin induced neurological damage. Note hyperintense signals in the globus pallidus (arrow mark).

manifesting as auditory neuropathy (abnormal BAER with normal OAE), gaze abnormalities, especially limitation of upward gaze and dysplasia of dental enamel.

Most infants who develop kernicterus, are likely to have manifested some or all of the findings associated with ABE in the neonatal period. However, there are case reports of infants who developed kernicterus with high TSB, but without any significant signs of ABE. The earliest manifestations of kernicterus include sunset sign, persistent atonic neck reflex (ATNR) and hearing deficits. In the first year, these infants feed poorly, develop high pitched cry, persistent and often obligatory atonic neck righting reflex. They are often hypotonic with increased deep tendon reflexes. Athetosis (involuntary, sinuous, writhing movements) may develop as early as 18 months but may be delayed as late as 8 to 9 years. Chorea and dystonia are the other abnormal movements which can occur in these children. Affected children may also have dysarthria, facial grimacing, drooling and difficulty in chewing or swallowing.

Hearing loss is generally most severe in high sound frequencies and is usually bilateral. The hearing deficit even when severe, may escape clinical detection for months or even longer and may be suspected on the basis of delayed acquisition of speech. Long term follow-up is required for infants with TSB levels >18 mg/dL, infants who underwent exchange blood transfusion, neonates with features suggestive of acute bilirubin encephalopathy and infants with presence of additional risk factors such as asphyxia, acidosis, hypoglycemia, sepsis and prematurity. Neurodevelopmental assessment should be continued till the age of 18 months to identify subtle features of kernicterus.

BIBLIOGRAPHY

American Academy of Pediatrics Subcommittee on Hyperbilirubinemia. Management of hyperbilirubinemia in the newborn infant 35 or more weeks of gestation. *Pediatrics* 2004 Jul; 114(1):297–316.

Balasubramanian K, Kumar P, Saini SS, Attri SV, Dutta S. Isotonic versus hypotonic fluid supplementation in term neonates with severe hyperbilirubinemia – a double-blind, randomized, controlled trial. *Acta Paediatr* 2012 Mar; 101(3):236–41.

Bhethanabhotla S, Thukral A, Sankar MJ, Agarwal R, Paul VK, Deorari AK. Effect of position of infant during phototherapy in management of hyperbilirubinemia in late preterm and term neonates: a randomized controlled trial. *J Perinatol* 2013 Oct; 33(10):795–9.

Bhutani VK, Johnson L. The jaundiced newborn in the emergency department: prevention of kernicterus. *Clin Ped Emerg Med* 2008, 9:149–59.

Bhutani VK, Johnson L. Kernicterus in late preterm infants cared for as term healthy infants. *Semin Perinatol* 2006, 30:89–97.

Bhutani VK, Stark AR, Lazzeroni LC, Poland R, Gourley GR, Kazmierczak S, et al. Predischarge screening for severe neonatal hyperbilirubinemia identifies infants who need phototherapy. *J Pediatr* 2013 Mar; 162(3):477–82.

Dennery PA. Metalloporphyrins for the treatment of neonatal jaundice. *Curr Opin Pediatr* 2005 Apr; 17(2):167–9.

Deorari AK, Singh M, Ahuja GK, Bisht MS, Verma A, Paul VK, et al. One year outcome of babies with severe neonatal hyper-bilirubinemia and reversible abnormality in brainstem auditory evoked responses. *Indian Pediatr* 1994 Aug; 31(8):915–21.

Gamaleldin R, Iskander I, Seoud I, Aboraya H, Aravkin A, Sampson PD, et al. Risk factors for neurotoxicity in newborns with severe neonatal hyperbilirubinemia. *Pediatrics* 2011 Oct; 128(4):e925–31.

Hansen TW. The role of phototherapy in the crash-cart approach to extreme neonatal jaundice. *Semin Perinatol* 2011 Jun; 35(3):171–4.

Kumar P, Murki S, Malik GK, Chawla D, Deorari AK, Karthik N, et al. Light emitting diodes versus compact fluorescent tubes for phototherapy in neonatal jaundice: a multicenter randomized controlled trial. *Indian Pediatr* 2010 Feb; 47(2):131–7.

Kumar R, Narang A, Kumar P, Garewal G. Phenobarbitone prophylaxis for neonatal jaundice in babies with birth weight 1000–1499 grams. *Indian Pediatr* 2002 Oct; 39(10):945–51.

Mehta S, Kumar P, Narang A. A randomized controlled trial of fluid supplementation in term neonates with severe hyperbilirubinemia. *J Pediatr* 2005 Dec; 147(6):781–5.

Murki S, Kumar P, Majumdar S, Marwaha N, Narang A. Risk factors for kernicterus in term babies with non-hemolytic jaundice. *Indian Pediatr* 2001 Jul; 38(7):757–62.

Murki S, Kumar P. Blood exchange transfusion for infants with severe neonatal hyperbilirubinemia. *Semin Perinatol* 2011 Jun; 35(3):175–84.

Rennie J, Burman-Roy S, Murphy MS. Guideline Development Group. Neonatal jaundice: Summary of NICE Guidelines. *BMJ* 2010; 340:c2409.

Sachdeva M, Murki S, Oleti TP, Kandraju H. Intermittent versus continuous phototherapy for the treatment of neonatal non-hemolytic moderate hyperbilirubinemia in infants more than 34 weeks of gestational age: a randomized controlled trial. *Eur J Pediatr* 2015 Feb; 174(2):177–81.

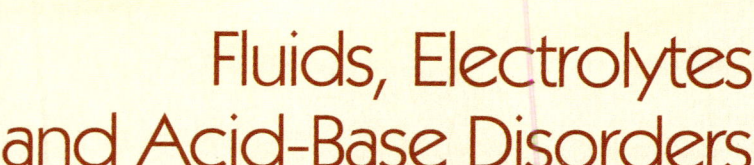

12

Fluids, Electrolytes and Acid-Base Disorders

FLUIDS AND ELECTROLYTES

The management of fluids and electrolytes plays a vital role in supportive care of high-risk neonates. The transition from fetal to neonatal life is associated with major changes in water and electrolyte homeostasis. Understanding the physiology of body fluids and transition from fetal to neonatal period would help in maintaining the normal fluid and electrolyte balance in sick newborn infants admitted in the neonatal intensive care unit (NICU).

Physiology

Fluids in the fetus and neonate is distributed among three main compartments; plasma, interstitial space and intracellular compartment. The amount of fluid in these compartments is based on gestational age, body weight, changes from the fetal to neonatal period, and during postnatal period.

At birth, the percentage of body weight represented by water is approximately 75% in term infants and 80% in premature infants. As gestational age increases, total body water and extracellular water decreases and intracellular fluid content increases (Figure 12.1).

Extracellular fluid decreases as the child grows, with a gradual rise in intracellular fluid. It is generally recognized that healthy term neonates lose on an average 5 to 10% of their body weight during the first week of life, with premature infants losing even more. It is important to recognize that in the first few days of life, physiologic weight loss in low birth weight infant represents isotonic contraction of body fluids.

Sodium Balance

Extracellular fluid (ECF) volume and plasma volume are determined by the total sodium content of the ECF.

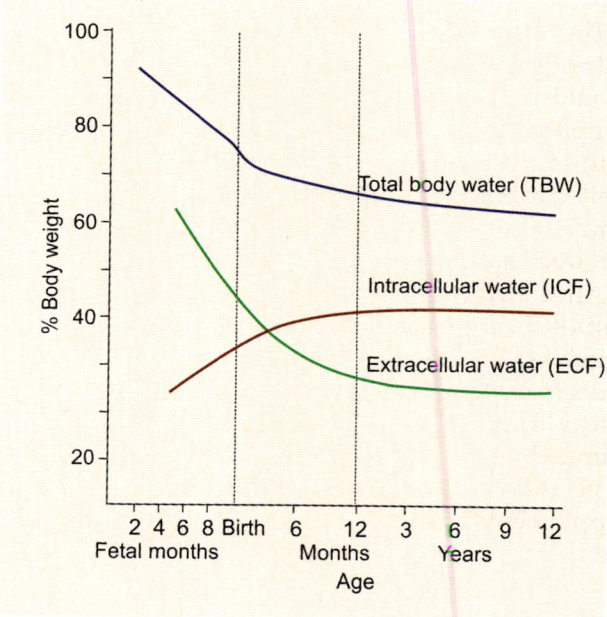

Figure 12.1 Changes in total body water with age.

Renal sodium handling plays a crucial role in maintaining sodium balance and protecting against volume depletion or overload. There are higher sodium losses from the renal tubules in immature babies resulting in hyponatremia. Table 12.1 shows the normal concentration of electrolytes in various body fluids.

Renal Function

The ability of immature kidneys in preterm neonates to compensate for changes in fluid and electrolytes is limited. Glomerular filtration rate in preterm infants is lower than term neonates. It increases with increasing gestational and postnatal age. Newborn infants have a decreased capacity to concentrate urine compared with

Table 12.1 Electrolyte composition of various body fluids

Fluid source	Sodium (mEq/L)	Potassium (mEq/L)	Chloride (mEq/L)
Stomach	20–80	5–20	100–150
Small intestine	100–140	5–15	90–120
Bile	120–140	5–15	90–120
Ileostomy	45–135	3–15	20–120

Table 12.2 Factors affecting insensible water loss

Factors that increase insensible water loss	■ Inversely related to gestational age and birth weight ■ Naked baby ■ Respiratory distress ■ Fever ■ Radiant warmer ■ Phototherapy ■ Activity ■ Skin defects: Omphalocele, gastroschisis ■ Non-humidified oxygen/environment
Steps to reduce insensible water loss	■ Antenatal steroids ■ Keep the baby covered and clothed ■ Effectively humidified incubators ■ Transparent plastic barriers to cover babies under radiant warmers ■ Applications of emollients on the skin ■ Covering skin defects ■ Using humidifiers in ventilators ■ Administration of humidified oxygen

adults. The concentrating capacity of an adult is 1500 mOsm/kg compared to 800 mOsm/kg in a term neonate and 600 mOsm/kg in preterm infants. The minimal water requirement to excrete a given solute load is greater in the preterm than a term infant. Hence in situations of fluid deficit, there is a limited tubular reabsorption of fluids, resulting in dehydration and hypernatremia especially in immature babies.

The discrepancy between the diluting capacity of kidneys in term and preterm infants (50 versus 70 mOsm/kg) is minimal. This may be slightly less compared to adults, but when a neonate is challenged with excessive administration of fluids, babies have limited capacity to handle fluids as compared to adults, which may be due to lower glomerular filtration rate and decreased reabsorption in distal tubules.

After birth there is a salt and water diuresis in the first 48–72 hours of life. Therefore, sodium supplementation is started after onset of initial diuresis, when there is decrease in serum sodium level or when baby has lost at least 5% of body weight. Preterm neonates have a limited tubular capacity to reabsorb sodium and hence have increased urinary losses. They need higher supplementation of sodium during the first month of life.

Fluid Losses

There is visible or obvious water loss from the kidneys and gastrointestinal system. Additional water loss occurs from the skin and respiratory tract, which is known as the insensible water loss. Transepidermal water loss (TEWL) contributes to 70% of insensible water loss and remaining 30% water loss occurs through the breath or respiratory tract. In neonates, efforts should be made to reduce insensible water losses instead of excessive administration of replacement fluids (Table 12.2).

Insensible Water Losses (IWL)

Insensible water loss is accorded major consideration in fluid and electrolyte therapy of extremely preterm neonates. Insensible water losses are higher in preterm infants due to thin immature skin and a large surface area to body weight ratio. The highest TEWL occurs during the first few days after birth. Each milliliter of water that evaporates from the skin is accompanied by a loss of 560 calories of heat, imposing a severe risk of development of hypothermia.

A high ambient humidity reduces TEWL and this effect is most pronounced in extremely low birth weight (ELBW) infants. TEWL represents a major component of the total water requirement in preterms compared to term infants and is highly variable. The infant has poor ability to modulate insensible water loss (IWL) which is calculated on the basis of urine output and weight changes.

IWL = Fluid intake – urine output + weight loss

or

IWL = Fluid intake – urine output – weight gain

Transitional Changes in Fluids and Electrolytes from Fetal to Neonatal Life

About 10% to 15% weight loss is common in preterm infants during the first postnatal week. The decrease in ECF volume is the result of a decrease in interstitial fluid (ISF) volume without any change in plasma volume. The magnitude of the contraction of the ECF space is inversely proportional to the gestational age.

Principles of Fluid and Electrolyte Therapy

Calculation of fluid and electrolyte requirements in the newborn is based on their maintenance needs, deficits, and ongoing losses. The critical factors that determine their fluid requirements include gestational age, renal function, ambient air temperature and humidity, nursing practices, clinical condition of the baby, ventilator dependence, presence of drainage tubes, and gastrointestinal losses.

Fluid Therapy

It is not possible to prescribe any uniform recommendation of maintenance fluids because their requirement is affected by a large number of factors. The maintenance fluid requirements in term neonates is given in Table 12.3. The initial fluids should be 10% dextrose to maintain glucose infusion rate of 4–6 mg/kg/min. Sodium and potassium are added after 48 hours of age. In preterm neonates, fluid requirements are higher as shown in Table 12.4.

Monitoring of Fluid and Electrolyte Status

A careful assessment of clinical indicators of volume status, including heart rate, blood pressure, skin turgor, capillary refill time, , and anterior fontanel is essential. The changes in body weight, serum electrolytes and renal functions should be closely monitored in sick neonates admitted in the NICU. Intravenous fluids should be *increased* in following situations:

a. Increased weight loss (>3%/day or a cumulative weight loss >20%)
b. Increased serum sodium (Na >145 mEq/dL)
c. Increased urine specific gravity>1.020 or urine osmolality >400 mOsm/L
d. Decreased urine output (<1 mL/kg/hr).

The intravenous fluids should be *restricted* in the presence of following situations:

a. Decreased weight loss (<1%/day or a cumulative weight loss <5%)
b. Decreased serum sodium in the presence of weight gain (Na <130 mEq/dL)
c. Decreased urine specific gravity <1.005 or urine osmolality <100 mOsm/L
d. Increased urine output (>3 mL/kg/hr).

Guidelines for Starting Electrolytes

Sodium and potassium should be added to the intravenous fluids after 48 hours, each in a dose of 2–3 mEq/kg/day. Calcium supplements are given in a dose of 4 mL/kg/day (40 mg/kg/day) of calcium gluconate during the first 3 days in certain high-risk situations like prematurity, infants of diabetic mothers and birth asphyxia. Dextrose infusion should be maintained at the rate of 4–6 mg/kg/min. In ELBW babies, it is preferable to use 5% dextrose solution to reduce the risk of hyperglycemia.

Replacement of Fluid Deficit

In infants with moderate (10%) to severe (15%) dehydration, fluid deficit is corrected gradually over 24 hours. If an infant is in shock, 10–20 mL/kg of normal saline is given immediately as a bolus followed by half correction of fluid deficit over 8 hours. The remaining fluid deficit is corrected over 16 hours. Assuming equal losses of fluids from the ECW and ICW, the replacement fluid after correction of shock, should consist of N/2 dextrose-saline (0.45% NS).

Maintenance Fluids

Maintenance sodium and chloride are usually not provided during the first 1 to 2 days of life due to

Table 12.3 Fluid requirement in term neonates

Day of life	Day 1	Day 2	Day 3	Day 4	Day 5	Day 6	Day 7 onwards
Volume (mL/kg)	60	75	90	105	120	135	150

Table 12.4 Fluid requirements in premature babies

Birth weight (g)	Insensible water loss (mL/kg/day)	Water requirements (mL/kg/day) by age		
		Day 1–2	Day 3–7	Day 8–30
<750	100–200	100–200	150–200	120–180
750–1000	60–70	80–150	100–150	120–180
1001–1500	30–65	60–100	80–150	120–180
>1500	15–30	60–80	100–150	120–180

relatively expanded state of blood volume of the newborn. Potassium is not provided in parenteral fluid until urinary flow has been established and normal renal function is ensured. After postnatal days 3 to 7, maintenance sodium and potassium are started in a dose of 2–3 mEq/kg/day.

Specific Clinical Conditions

Extreme Prematurity (Gestation <28 Weeks, Birth Weight <1000 g)

The insensible water losses may be very high in these babies resulting in higher needs for maintenance fluid requirements. The stratum corneum matures rapidly in 1–2 weeks and fluid requirements become comparable to larger infants by the end of the second week. Fluid requirement can be reduced by decreasing the IWL by covering the baby with plastic transparent barriers or double walled humidified incubators. The initial fluids on day one should be electrolyte free and should be prepared by using 5% dextrose solution to prevent risk of hyperglycemia.

Respiratory Distress Syndrome (RDS)

Fluid intake is restricted to reduce the risk of ductus arteriosus, necrotizing enterocolitis and bronchopulmonary dysplasia.

Perinatal Asphyxia and Brain Injury

Fluid restriction is recommended in the presence of hyponatremia. The intake should be restricted to two-thirds of maintenance fluids till serum sodium values return to normal. Once urine production increases by the third postnatal day, fluid intake may be gradually restored to normal levels.

Diarrhea

The principles of fluid therapy in diarrhea are the same as in older children. Due to limited renal concentrating capacity, newborn infants are more vulnerable to develop severe dehydration and shock. Water and electrolytes should be given to correct any existent deficits, meet maintenance requirements and replenish ongoing losses.

Phototherapy

Phototherapy is an additional source of radiant heat and may increase TEWL by as much as 30%. However, it is unnecessary to increase fluid intake routinely on starting phototherapy if steps have been taken to reduce insensible water loss.

COMMON ELECTROLYTE PROBLEMS

Sodium

The normal serum sodium level is 135–145 mEq/L. Marked fluctuations in sodium levels in preterm have been associated with poor neurological outcome.

Hyponatremia

It is defined as serum sodium level of less than 130 mEq/L. Severe hyponatremia (<125 mEq/L) may result in altered consciousness, apnea and convulsions. It may occur due to the inability to excrete water load, excessive sodium losses or inadequate intake of sodium (Table 12.5).

Treatment

The diagnosis and appropriate treatment of hyponatremia is controversial. At present there is no clear consensus regarding the best treatment for symptomatic hyponatremia. In hyponatremia of acute onset, urgent therapy is instituted while in a chronic case, it is necessary to treat the underlying cause.

Acute alterations in sodium concentration should be managed promptly by taking due care to avoid complications. Dilutional hyponatremia is managed by fluid restriction. When there is sudden fall of serum sodium below 120 mEq/L, consider administration of 3% saline solution to raise serum sodium level slowly up to maximum of 0.5 mEq/hr (up to 8–10 mEq/L in 24 hr) to avoid both cerebral edema and risk of myelinolysis. Hyperglycemia should be excluded before correcting hyponatremia. The algorithmic approach for management of hyponatremia is summarized in Figure 12.2.

Table 12.5 Causes of hyponatremia	
Increased free water load	▪ Increased maternal free water intake during labor ▪ Excess free water administration to the baby, e.g. improperly mixed formula ▪ Perinatal non-osmotic release of vasopressin, e.g. perinatal asphyxia, RDS, bilateral pneumothoraces, IVH and administration of drugs like morphine, barbiturate, carbamazepine
Decreased free water clearance	▪ Sick newborns and acute kidney failure (oliguria)
Negative sodium balance	▪ Inadequate sodium intake ▪ Excessive renal losses ▪ Preterms <28 week ▪ Tubulopathies like Bartter syndrome ▪ Disorders of aldosterone production or unresponsiveness such as congenital adrenal hyperplasia and pseudohypoaldosteronism

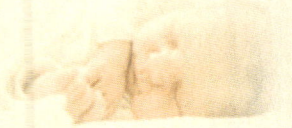

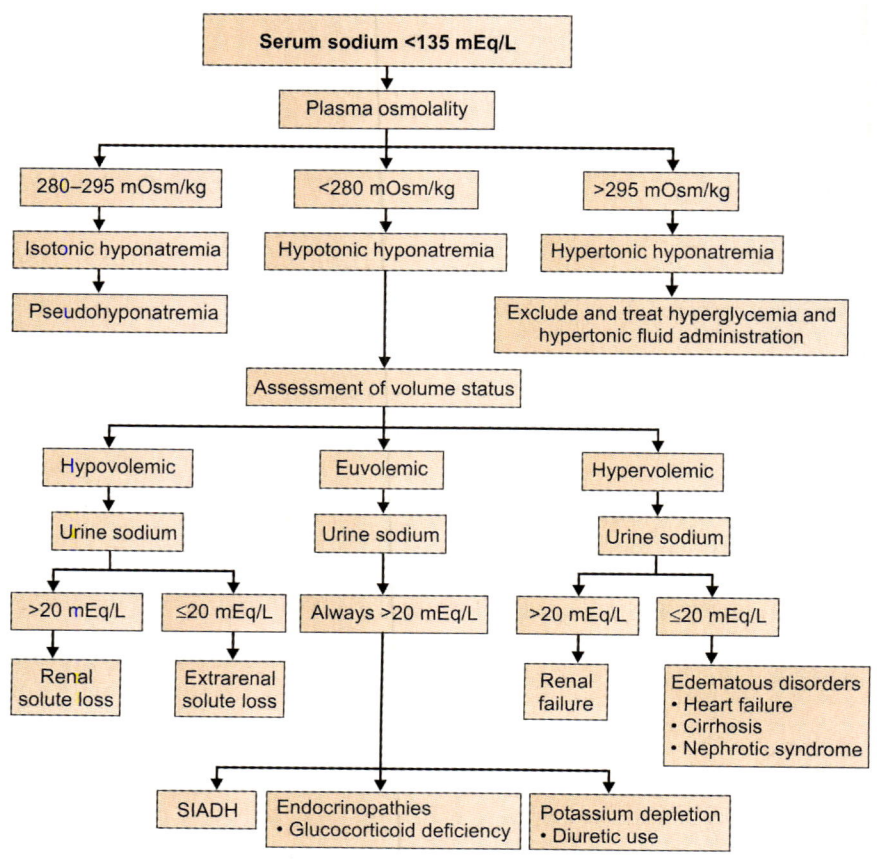

SIADH: syndrome of inappropriate antidiuretic hormone secretion.

Figure 12.2 Approach to a neonate with hyponatremia

Hypernatremia

It is defined as serum sodium level of more than 155 mEq/L. The common causes of hypernatremia in neonates are listed in Table 12.6. The symptoms vary depending upon the underlying etiology.

Table 12.6 Causes of hypernatremia

Hypovolemic hypernatremia
- Inadequate breast milk intake
- Diarrhea
- Radiant warmers
- Excessive sweating
- Osmotic diuresis

Euvolemic hypernatremia
- Decreased production of antidiuretic hormone
- Central diabetes insipidus, meningitis, or encephalitis

Decrease or absence of renal responsiveness
Nephrogenic diabetes insipidus, extreme immaturity, renal insult, and medications such as amphotericin, hydantoin, and aminoglycosides

Hypervolemic hypernatremia
- Improperly mixed formula
- Administration of sodium bicarbonate
- Administration of sodium chloride
- Primary hyperaldosteronism

Treatment

Treatment depends upon the underlying cause of the hypernatremia. The cornerstone of the management of hypernatremia is providing free water to correct the serum sodium level and associated volume depletion. Treatment of this condition is generally divided into two phases; the *emergency phase* where the intravascular volume is restored, by administration of 10 to 20 mL/kg of isotonic saline, and the *rehydration phase*, when the existent free water deficit and usual maintenance needs are administered during next 48 hours. Initial fluid resuscitation with 0.9% saline should be instituted followed by replacement and maintenance fluid therapy. A simple way of estimating the minimum amount of fluid necessary to correct the serum sodium is calculated by the following equation:

Free water deficit (mL) = 4 mL × lean body wt (kg) × (desired change in serum Na in mEq/L).

The amount of free water required to decrease serum sodium by 12 mEq/L over a 24-hour period when hypernatremia is *moderate* is calculated as follows:

Free water required = Body weight (kg) × 4 mL/kg × 12 mEq/L

The amount of free water required to decrease serum sodium by 12 mEq/L over a 24-hour period when hypernatremia is *severe* is calculated as follows:

Free water required = Body weight × 3 mL/kg × 12 mEq/L

The calculated deficit does not account for insensible losses or ongoing urinary or GI losses and maintenance fluids. The rate of correction of hypernatremia is largely dependent on the severity of hypernatremia and its etiology (Table 12.7). The correction should not exceed more than 10 mEq/L per day. In severe hypernatremia (>170 mEq/L) serum sodium should not be allowed to fall below 150 mEq/L in the first 48–72 hours.

One should be aware of the availability of various parenteral fluids and their electrolyte composition (Table 12.8). This will help in managing the fluid therapy appropriately.

POTASSIUM

Potassium is predominantly intracellular cation (98%) and only 2% is in extracellular space. Distribution of potassium in intracellular and extracellular compartment depends upon pH of the body compartments. Alkalosis causes influx of potassium in the cells and acidosis causes efflux from the cells resulting in hyperkalemia.

Hypokalemia

Hypokalemia is defined as serum potassium level less than 3.5 mEq/L. It can result in hypotonia, paralytic ileus, and cardiac arrhythmias. Areflexia, paralysis and death due to failure of respiratory muscles may be the presenting features of severe hypokalemia. The ECG changes include tachycardia, ST segment depression, flattened T waves, prominent U waves and prolonged QT interval. The common causes of hypokalemia are listed in Table 12.9.

Treatment

Treatment depends upon the underlying cause of hypokalemia. The drugs which are known to cause hypokalemia should be withdrawn. Intravenous correction is done by administration of potassium chloride. *Potassium should be administered only when urine flow is established.* The rate of correction should not exceed 0.5 mEq/kg/hour. Rapid administration of potassium chloride is not recommended, because it is associated with life-threatening cardiac dysfunction.

Table 12.7 Management of hypernatremia

Etiology	Treatment
Sodium and water loss	
■ Gastroenteritis	0.45 % dextrose-saline
Primary water loss	
■ Ineffective breast feeding	0.2 to 0.45% dextrose-saline
■ Nephrogenic diabetes insipidus	0.1 % saline in 2.5% dextrose water
Central diabetes insipidus	Desmopressin acetate
Sodium overload	5% dextrose in water Diuretics or dialysis may be needed

Table 12.8 Common intravenous fluids with their composition

IV fluid	Dextrose (g/L)	Sodium (mEq/L)	Potassium (mEq/L)	Chloride (mEq/L)	Lactate (mEq/L)	Calcium (mEq/L)	Osmolality (mOsm/L)
Normal saline (0.9%)	—	154	—	154	—	—	308
Ringer lactate	—	131	5	111	29	2	270
0.45 normal saline	—	77	—	77	—	—	154
5% dextrose	50	—	—	—	—	—	278
10% dextrose	100	—	—	—	—	—	556
Isolyte P	50	29	20	29	—	—	368
5% dextrose-saline (DNS)	50	154	—	154	—	—	585

Table 12.9 Causes of hypokalemia in neonates

GI losses	Diarrhea, vomiting, nasogastric and ileostomy drainage, GIT fistulae, and short gut syndrome
Renal losses	Alkalosis, renal tubular acidosis, tubulopathies, congenital adrenal hyperplasia, and diuretics
Decreased intake	Malnutrition, errors in administration of TPN
Intracellular shift	Insulin, alkalosis, beta adrenergic medications (Albuterol), hypokalemic periodic paralysis

Hyperkalemia

Hyperkalemia is defined as serum potassium level of more than 5.5 mEq/L. It may be asymptomatic or present with hypotonia, paralysis, and cardiac arrhythmias. The causes of hyperkalemia are summarized in Table 12.10. Severe hyperkalemia may cause tachyarrhythmia or bradyarrhythmia leading to cardiovascular collapse and death. ECG changes show tall T-waves, increased PR interval, QRS widening and slurring sine wave pattern due to ventricular fibrillations.

Treatment

Hyperkalemia is an emergency and needs urgent management as outlined in Table 12.11.

Table 12.10 Common causes of hyperkalemia

Decreased excretion	Acute renal failure, oliguria, adrenal insufficiency
Increased K+ release secondary to tissue destruction	Asphyxia, sepsis, IVH, hypothermia, trauma, cephalhematoma, intravascular or extravascular hemolysis, and major surgery
Miscellaneous conditions	Dehydration, use of old blood, accidental oral or IV administration of potassium

Table 12.11 Management protocol for hyperkalemia

Stabilization of conducting tissue	▪ Remove all sources of exogenous potassium. ▪ Calcium gluconate 2 mL/kg 1:1 diluted slowly IV under cardiac monitoring ▪ For refractory ventricular tachycardia, lidocaine/ bretylium should be considered
Ensuring intracellular shift of K+	▪ Sodium bicarbonate 7.5% solution 1–2 mEq/kg 1:1 diluted slowly IV (avoid in preterms) ▪ Glucose insulin drip @ 0.1 unit/kg regular insulin (max. 10 units) mixed with 2 mL/kg of 25% dextrose over 30 min. Repeat after 30–60 min if necessary. Salbutamol either as intravenous infusion or nebulization (2–5 mg in 2 doses 2 hr apart) in chronic renal failure
Enhanced excretion of K+	▪ Diuretic therapy by administration of furosemide 1 mg/kg ▪ Kayexalate (ion exchange resins) 1.0 g/kg orally or rectally ▪ Peritoneal dialysis or exchange blood transfusion

ACID-BASE DISORDERS

Introduction

Acid base management is essential for the care of sick newborns especially those born immature. Neonates have a limited ability to compensate for acid-base alterations and they are susceptible to significant morbidity and mortality because of acid-base imbalance. Arterial blood gas analysis reveals oxygenation status, adequacy of ventilation and acid-base status. Understanding and interpreting blood gases help in managing sick babies better and they should be correlated with the clinical picture.

Basic Physiology

The suffix "*emia*" refers to the state of *blood*, for example, acidemia is a condition of excessive blood acidity as indicated by pH. The suffix "*osis*" refers to a pathologic *process* in which acid or base is gained or lost from the body. Acidosis may not lead to acidemia, depending on the patient's ability to compensate. The terms acidosis and alkalosis refer to the processes that alter the acid-base status of the infant.

An acid is a substance that dissociates to produce H^+ while a base neutralizes or accepts H^+ ions. In blood gas measurement, the pH and $PaCO_2$ levels are measured by machine, while HCO_3^- level and base excess or deficit are calculated values. The core body temperature of the infant is fed into the blood gas machine which measures all parameters at 37°C. It is desirable to have values of pH, $PaCO_2$ and PaO_2 corrected for infant's temperature. Base excess refers to excessive base in relation to total buffer base, the normal buffer base is about 48 mmol/L. If buffer base is 40 mmol/L, it means buffer base is reduced by 8 mmol/L or base excess (BE) is –8 (also called as **base deficit**). In case buffer base is 60 mmol/L, it means buffer base has increaed by 12 mmol/L or base excess is +12.

Anion Gap

Measurement of anion gap gives a clue to the cause of metabolic acidosis. Anion gap is the difference between the unmeasured anions and cations. This is calculated as a difference between the measured cations and anions as follows:

Anion gap = Serum $(Na^+ + K^+) - (Cl^- + HCO_3^-)$

When acidosis is associated with normal anion gap, it suggests loss of bicarbonate or rapid dilution of ECF. Chloride is proportionately increased in these conditions because of loss of HCO_3^- through gastrointestinal tract or kidneys. The anion gap is increased when there is accumulation of a strong acid in the system in conditions with lactic acidosis, ketonemia, renal failure and excessive salt therapy (Ringer lactate and acetate).

Oxygen Saturation

It is expressed as amount of oxygen that is actually combined with hemoglobin (Hb) divided by the total amount of oxygen that can be combined with Hb (percent saturation of Hb). Pulse oximetry is convenient and useful for monitoring trends in oxygenation. The curve may shift to right due to low pH, high $PaCO_2$, high temperature, high 2–3 diphosphoglycerate (DPG) and adult hemoglobin which has less affinity for oxygen resulting in more delivery of oxygen to the peripheral tissues (Figure 12.3). The shift of the oxygen-dissociation curve to the left would result in tissue hypoxia due to higher affinity of oxygen to bind with the hemoglobin.

The plasma HCO_3^- is a commonly used parameter for interpretation of acid base status and is easily calculated from $PaCO_2$ and pH using Henderson - Hasselbalch equation. The standard plasma bicarbonate is obtained after the blood has been equilibrated at 37°C with a $PaCO_2$ of 40 mmHg. It overcomes the changes in HCO_3^- due to respiratory causes and reflects a non-respiratory acid-base change. The machine calculates the pH, PCO_2 and PO_2 from the sample while other parameters are derived from the Henderson-Hasselbach equation. The Siggaard Anderson nomogram can be used to derive values of HCO_3^- and base excess on the basis of pH and $PaCO_2$ values measured by the blood gas machine (Figure 12.4).

The normal range of ABG values in neonates include pH 7.35–7.45, PaO_2 50–70 mmHg, $PaCO_2$ 35–45 mmHg, HCO_3^- 20–24 mEq/L and base excess ±5.

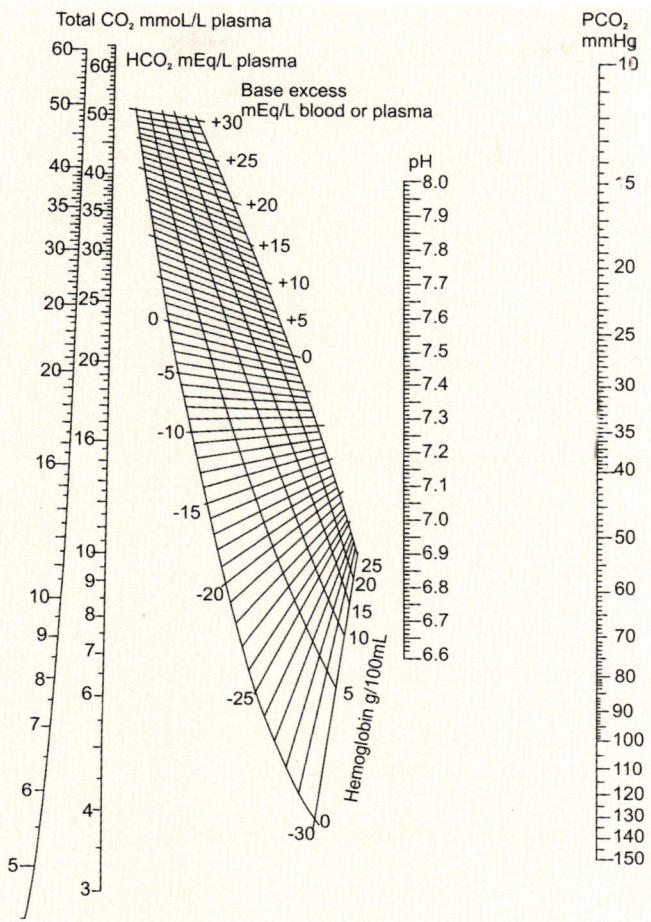

Figure 12.4 Siggaard Anderson nomogram

Buffer Systems

The acid-base balance is regulated by a combination of the respiratory, buffer, and renal systems. Buffer system resists change in pH when acid or alkali is added, due to their capacity to absorb or release H^+. The three main buffer systems in the body include bicarbonate, phosphate and protein systems. The protein and phosphate buffer systems are intracellular and act as 'sinks' for extracellular H^+ which are exchanged with intracellular potassium (K^+) and sodium ions (Na^+). The bicarbonate buffer system is extracellular and consists of a mixture of carbonic acid (H_2CO_3) and sodium bicarbonate ($NaHCO_3$). Carbonic acid is a weak acid and readily dissociates to give CO_2, which is transported in dissolved form to the lungs for excretion, as shown below:

$$H^+ + HCO_3^- \leftrightarrow H_2CO_3 \leftrightarrow H_2O + CO_2$$

Buffers are most potent when there is equal amount of H^+ and HCO_3^- in solution. The buffer systems are useful to serve as the primary mechanism for maintaining acid-base balance in the newborn.

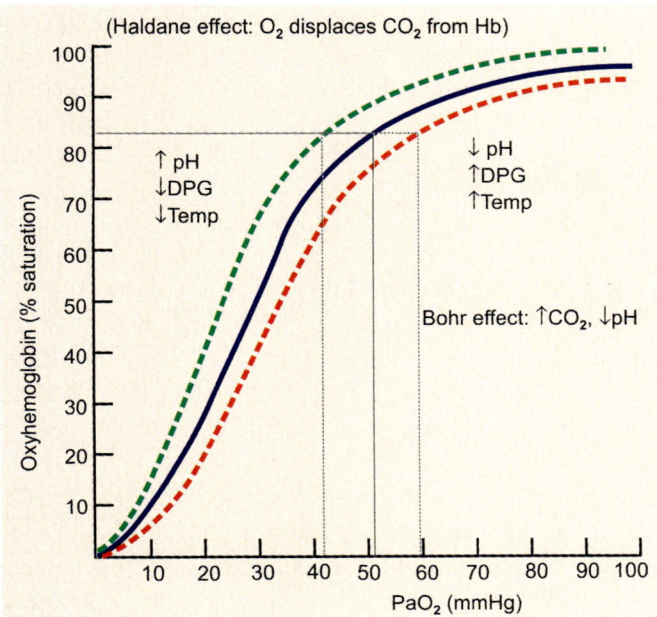

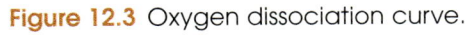

DPG: 2-3 diphosphoglycerate, Temp: core body temperature

Figure 12.3 Oxygen dissociation curve.

Respiratory Regulation

The respiratory system operates within minutes to hours as part of the acute response to acidosis. This system modifies pH by balancing production of H^+ with ventilatory clearance of carbon dioxide. The H^+ ions directly stimulate chemoreceptors in the respiratory center of the brainstem, producing an increase in respiratory rate with washout of CO_2 and carbonic acid. Acidosis may not lead to acidemia, depending on the patient's ability to compensate. Premature infants are often not able to compensate for metabolic acidosis and respiratory alkalosis by alterations in ventilation.

Rules of Compensation

Compensation is a response to the primary disorder, attempting to bring the pH to as close as possible to normal pH. Full compensation is generally not achieved, and blood gases that appear to have fully compensated for the primary problem are most likely to display a mixed picture, rather than complete correction. The acid-base balance is maintained closely by complex interactions between the respiratory system and the kidneys (Table 12.12).

Steps in Interpretation of Blood Gases

1. Is acidosis or alkalosis present?
2. Is the imbalance respiratory ($PaCO_2$) or metabolic (HCO_3^-) in origin?
3. Is any compensation present?
4. What is PaO_2?
5. Identify possible cause of the acid-base imbalance
6. What is the rational management for the imbalance?

The correlates for various types of acid-base disorders are shown in Figure 12.5.

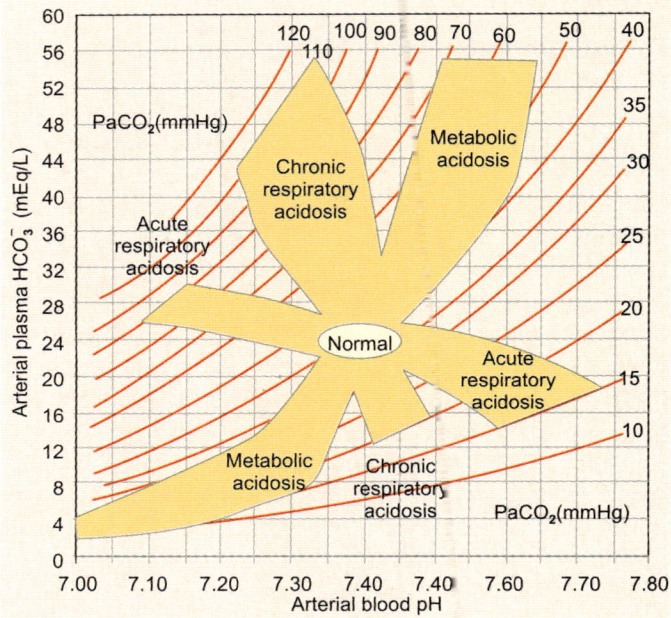

Figure 12.5 Map of acid and base disorders.

Acid-base Disorders

Acid-base disorders are classified according to their cause whether they are metabolic or respiratory. Metabolic acidosis occurs as a result of accumulation of increased amounts of nonvolatile acid or decreased amounts of HCO_3^- in the ECF. Metabolic alkalosis occurs as a consequence of increased amounts of HCO_3^- in the ECF. Respiratory acidosis is usually caused by hypoventilation and decreased excretion of volatile acid (CO_2), whereas respiratory alkalosis is caused by hyperventilation and increased excretion of volatile acid (CO_2).

Metabolic Acidosis

Metabolic acidosis is a common problem, particularly in critically ill newborns. It occurs when drop in pH is caused by accumulation of acid other than H_2CO_3, resulting in loss of available HCO_3^-, or by the direct loss of HCO_3^- from body fluids. Patients who have metabolic acidosis are divided into those with an elevated anion gap and those with a normal anion gap (Table 12.13).

The morbidity and mortality of metabolic acidosis depend on the underlying pathologic process, the severity of the acidosis, and the responsiveness of the disorder to clinical management. Correction of the underlying cause is the most important therapeutic measure in the management of metabolic acidosis. Bicarbonate administration should be reserved for severe acidosis,

Table 12.12 The compensatory attempts on the part of the body to maintain acid-base balance			
Simple disorders	pH	$PaCO_2$	HCO_3^-
Metabolic acidosis	↓	↓	↓
Metabolic alkalosis	↑	↑	↑
Respiratory acidosis	↓	↑	↑
Respiratory alkalosis	↑	↓	↓
In simple disorders, CO_2 and HCO_3^- move in same direction.			
Mixed disorders			
Acidosis	↓	↑	↓
Alkalosis	↑	↓	↑
In mixed disorders, CO_2 and HCO_3^- move in opposite direction.			

Table 12.13 Causes of metabolic acidosis

Increased anion gap	1. Lactic acidosis: Asphyxia, sepsis, hypothermia 2. Inborn errors of metabolism: Organic acidemias, primary lactate acidosis 3. Others: Renal failure, late metabolic acidosis
Normal anion gap	1. Renal losses: Prematurity, renal tubular acidosis 2. GI losses: Diarrhea, ileostomy 3. Others: Administration of carbonic anhydrase inhibitor, excessive administration of chloride

especially when cardiac output is compromised. The dose of bicarbonate is calculated as follows:

Dose of bicarbonate (mEq) = Base deficit (mEq/L) × Body weight (kg) × 0.6

(0.6 being volume distribution factor for bicarbonate).

Most clinicians use half of the calculated dose for initial therapy to avoid overcorrection. The subsequent doses depend upon periodic testing of ABG values and clinical status of the neonate.

Respiratory Acidosis

Respiratory acidosis occurs when an increase in $PaCO_2$ develops secondary to impairment in alveolar ventilation that result in an arterial pH of less than 7.35. Primary respiratory acidosis is a common problem in newborns, and important causes include hyaline membrane disease, pneumonia owing to infection or aspiration, patent ductus arteriosus with pulmonary edema, chronic lung disease, pleural effusion, pneumothorax, and pulmonary hypoplasia.

Management of respiratory acidosis is directed toward improving the alveolar ventilation and treating the underlying disorder. *There is no role of administration of sodium bicarbonate.*

Metabolic Alkalosis

Metabolic alkalosis is characterized by a primary increase in the extracellular HCO_3^- concentration sufficient to raise the arterial pH above 7.45. In the newborn, metabolic alkalosis occurs when there is a loss of H^+, gain of HCO_3^-, or depletion of the extracellular volume with the loss of more chloride than HCO_3^-. Chloride loss may occur due to chloride losing diarrhea, Bartter's syndrome, chloride loss through skin in infants with cystic fibrosis.

The common causes of of metabolic alkalosis in the newborn period include continuous nasogastric aspiration, persistent vomiting, and diuretic treatment. One of the commonly encountered clinical scenario of chronic metabolic alkalosis is a form of mixed acid-base disorder in a preterm infant with chronic lung disease on long-term diuretic treatment.

Respiratory Alkalosis

When a primary decrease in $PaCO_2$ results in an increase in the arterial pH beyond 7.45, it is suggestive of respiratory alkalosis. The primary cause of respiratory alkalosis is hyperventilation, which may occur due to fever, sepsis, retained fetal lung fluid, aspiration pneumonia, and central nervous system disorders. In the neonatal intensive care unit, the most common cause of respiratory alkalosis is iatrogenic as a consequence of hyperventilation of the intubated newborn. There is an association between hypocapnia and the development of periventricular leucomalacia; hence it is important to avoid hyperventilation, low CO_2 and respiratory alkalosis in neonates.

BIBLIOGRAPHY

Baumgart S, Costarino AT. Water and electrolyte metabolism of the micropremie. *Clin Perinatol* 2000, 27:131–46.

Bhatia J. Fluid and electrolyte management in the very low birth weight neonate. *J Perinatol* 2006; 26:S19–S21.

Brewer ED. Disorders of acid-base balance. *Pediatr Clin North Am* 1990; 37:430.

Chawla D, Agarwal R, Deorari AK, and Paul VK. Fluid and electrolyte management in term and preterm neonates. *Indian Pediatr* 2008; 75(3):255–60.

Hartnoll G. Basic principles and practical steps in management of fluid balance in newborn. *Semin Neonatol* 2003; 8:307.

Horacio JA, Nicholas EM. Hypernatremia. *New Engl J Med* 342(20); May 18, 2000: 1493–99.

Jin Xiong Lian. Interpreting and using arterial blood gas analysis. *Nursing Crit Care* 2010, 5 (3): 26–36.

Lakhwani S, Shanker V, Gathwala G, Waswani ND. Acid base disorders in critically ill neonates. *Indian J Crit Care Med* 2010 Apr-Jun; 14 (2):65–69.

Lorenz J. Fluid and electrolyte therapy in the very low birthweight neonate. *Neo Reviews* 2008; 9;e102–e108.

Modi N. Management of fluid balance in the very immature neonate. *Arch Dis Child Fetal Neonatal Ed* 2004; 89:F108–F111.

Quigley R, Baum M. Neonatal acid base balance and disturbances. *Semin Perinatol* 2004, Apr 28 (2): 97–102.

13

Shock

B. Vishnu Bhat and Nishad Plakkal

Background

Shock is commonly encountered in critically sick neonates, and preterm infants are at an increased risk. More than a one-third of very low birth weight (VLBW) neonates receive volume expanders or inotropes. Majority of neonates under 28 weeks of gestation are treated for hypotension during their hospital stay. The diagnosis and management of shock in neonates pose special challenge in neonates compared to older children. Older children and adults have pulmonary and systemic circulations which are connected in series. On the other hand, newborn infants are transitioning from a fetal circulation, where the right and left ventricles operate independently as a parallel circulation. Fetal shunts may continue to operate well into the neonatal period, particularly in small and sick newborns. These features limit the value of blood pressure, which is the most relied-upon clinical measurement in the management of neonatal shock. Neonates are also inherently more susceptible to circulatory failure. The immature myocardium of the neonate is structurally and functionally different from that of the older child, and has only a limited capacity to increase stroke volume. In addition, neonates have a higher hematocrit, a predominance of fetal hemoglobin, and a higher cardiac index, all of which can affect tissue oxygen delivery and cardiac output. Neonates, especially if preterm, are more susceptible to develop infection and hypoxia.

The problem of shock in neonates is often viewed in the context of an ancient Indian story when six blind men touched different parts of the elephant and developed different perceptions about the elephant. The lack of universally agreed criteria to diagnose neonatal shock reflects gaps in knowledge regarding the pathophysiology of shock. There is paucity of data from randomized controlled trials in its management, and lack of evidence about the long-term effects of various management strategies. Shock is commonly treated with fluid boluses, inotropes and vasoconstrictors, but using the wrong therapy could be life-threatening. For example, administration of fluid boluses in the presence of myocardial dysfunction without hypovolemia is likely to aggravate cardiac failure. It is desirable to tailor the therapy in accordance with the underlying pathophysiology, while we await robust data from on going trials.

This chapter attempts to revisit the physiology of fetal, transitional and neonatal circulation, and summarizes the state of the art strategies in the management of shock in neonates

Transition from Fetal to Neonatal Circulation

In the fetus, blood is oxygenated in the placental circulation, which has a low vascular resistance. The stream of oxygenated blood returning through the umbilical vein, the ductus venosus and into the right atrium is redirected into the left atrium by the Eustachian valve. This ensures that the left ventricular output, which flows to the brain, has better oxygenation. Most of the right ventricular output is shunted to the lower part of the body through the ductus arteriosus because of high pulmonary vascular resistance. Thus, the systemic circulation is effectively supported by both ventricles operating in parallel. In the normal course, after delivery, elimination of the placental circulation and closure of the fetal shunts result in two distinct circulations connected in series; a low-resistance pulmonary circulation and a high-resistance systemic circulation. This transition from the fetal to the neonatal circulation may be delayed by infection, prematurity, intrauterine growth restriction, asphyxia and congenital heart disease, among other causes.

Pathophysiology of Shock

The delivery of oxygen and nutrients to tissues is dependent on adequate blood flow. Shock is characterized by inadequate delivery of oxygen to tissues, which leads to anerobic metabolism. The etiology of shock in neonates can be diverse; some important causes are summarized in Table 13.1. Whatever the etiology, understanding the pathophysiology is key to successful management of these infants. Hypovolemia (leading to decreased preload), vasodilation or increased systemic vascular resistance (increased afterload), poor cardiac contractility, and arrhythmias are some of the common mechanisms of circulatory failure in neonates. Unfortunately, the common clinical signs of shock, i.e. tachycardia, decreased blood pressure (BP), prolonged capillary refill, cold (or less commonly warm) extremities and oliguria are not always reliable to identify the physiologic derangements.

Cardiogenic Shock

Although the myocardium of neonates is immature, cardiac dysfunction is not always the primary cause of circulatory failure. The neonates with perinatal asphyxia, shock and sepsis often develop secondary to myocardial dysfunction. Asphyxia can directly injure the myocardium, as evidenced by ECG changes or elevated levels of myocardial markers such as troponin T, troponin I or CK-MB. Decrease in stroke volume, ejection fraction and left ventricular output are commonly observed on echocardiography in asphyxiated infants. Myocardial dysfunction is also common in preterm infants following PDA ligation.

Table 13.1 Common causes of shock in neonates

Cardiogenic shock
- Perinatal asphyxia
- Septic shock
- Hypertrophic cardiomyopathy (infants of diabetic mothers)
- Arrhythmias (supraventricular tachycardia, atrial flutter)
- Congenital complete heart block
- Structural congenital heart disease

Vasodilation
- Septic shock
- Necrotizing enterocolitis
- Relative adrenal insufficiency

Hypovolemia
- Fetomaternal or twin-to-twin hemorrhage
- Cord rupture
- Vasa previa
- Congenital adrenal hyperplasia
- Subgaleal or other causes of obvious or occult hemorrhage
- Gastrointestinal diseases

Infants with septic shock often present with low cardiac output and peripheral vasoconstriction. However, hemodynamic changes in shock are complicated and more variable in neonates. Myocardial dysfunction can be a significant component of circulatory failure in neonates with septic shock, especially in those presenting later in the course of the disease.

Infants of diabetic mother may have hypertrophic cardiomyopathy, typically presenting with features of congestive heart failure. Although self-limited in the long-term, this condition is important to consider and recognize early in the neonatal period, because the obstruction can be severe and the usual treatments for congestive heart failure, including diuretics and digoxin, can worsen the cardiac output. Other cardiomyopathies and myocarditis can cause shock, albeit less commonly.

Shock due to arrhythmias can be readily reversed if the disorder is recognized and treated promptly. Supraventricular tachycardia and atrial flutter are common tachyarrythmias in the neonates. Complete heart block can result in shock due to decreased cardiac output. Critical congenital heart disease often presents with circulatory failure and shock in the neonatal period.

Vasodilation

Preterm infants are particularly prone to develop shock as a result of vasodilation. In conditions associated with systemic inflammation, such as sepsis or necrotizing enterocolitis (NEC), circulating cytokines mediate excessive vasodilation. Bacterial endotoxins and tumor necrosis factor alpha (TNF-α) can also induce the production of inducible NO synthase (iNOS) in the vascular endothelium, increasing local levels of nitric oxide (NO). The paracrine effects of NO result in vasodilation mediated by cyclic guanosine monophosphate (cGMP). Cardiac output is normal or increased in most neonates with early septic shock, but the findings may depend on the time of presentation and the type of the organism causing sepsis. Relative adrenal insufficiency is common in preterm neonates. While it is accepted that the hypothalamic-pituitary-adrenal axis is immature in preterm infants, it is not clear what cut-offs for cortisol values should be used to diagnose adrenal insufficiency.

Hypovolemia

Unlike older children, hypovolemia is not a common cause of shock in neonates. But fetomaternal transfusion, twin-to-twin transfusion, vasa previa, cord rupture, placental abruption, and large subgaleal or liver hematomas can all lead to hypovolemic shock. Excessive fluid loss due to polyuria or transepidermal water loss or capillary leak in the third space due to NEC or sepsis can also result in hypovolemia. In developing and underdeveloped countries, it is not uncommon to see neonates presenting with diarrhea and dehydration, especially if they are not exclusively breastfed. Salt-wasting forms of congenital adrenal hyperplasia often present with vomiting, dehydration, hyperkalemia and shock in the neonatal period. This is often the presenting feature in male infants with severe enzyme deficiency which may be missed because of normal looking external genitalia. In female infants ambiguous genitalia often provide useful clinical lead for early diagnosis. While 21-hydroxylase deficiency is more common, 11-hydroxylase deficiency can also present in the neonatal period. Although not due to hypovolemia, a decrease in venous return and hence preload can lead to shock in infants with tension pneumothorax or cardiac tamponade.

Hemodynamic Monitoring

Intra-arterial BP measurement is traditionally considered as the "gold standard", but it is invasive and not universally available in most NICUs. Smaller catheter size, improper calibration and the presence of bubbles or clots in the tubing can affect the accuracy of measured values. Although BP measurements are commonly used to diagnose shock and guide therapy, many questions and dilemmas remain. It is not uncommon that invasive and noninvasive methods of BP measurements may give significantly different values in the same infant. Which blood pressure should we target, systolic, diastolic or MAP? Is blood pressure a better guide to therapy than superior vena cava (SVC) flow or other proxies for cerebral blood flow or oxygenation? Are existing normative values appropriate for our population given that India has a high incidence of small-for-gestational age (SGA) and growth restricted infants? Does the use of specific BP targets improve long-term neurologic outcome in preterm or VLBW infants?

From a purely physical perspective, the key determinant of blood flow to any tissue depends upon the driving pressure (which is the blood pressure minus the venous pressure) and the vascular resistance in the tissue. Thus, one expects the systemic blood flow to be directly dependent on the blood pressure and inversely dependent on the systemic vascular resistance (SVR). However, blood pressure itself is not an independent variable and depends on the cardiac output and the SVR. The presence of a patent ductus arteriosus (PDA)

and several other factors which influence SVR further complicate this picture. As a result, there is poor correlation between the blood pressure and the systemic (especially cerebral) blood flow, especially in preterm infants. The association between hypotension and the development of germinal matrix hemorrhage, intraventricular hemorrhage (GM-IVH) or white matter injury is not consistent. In view of the ease of measuring BP (unlike SVR, cardiac output or cerebral blood flow) and the preponderance of data linking low blood pressure to poor outcome, BP measurements continue to be an important parameter in the management of shock.

In 1992, a Joint Working Group of the British Association of Perinatal Medicine (BAPM) and the Research Unit of the Royal College of Physicians suggested that in the immediate postnatal period, mean BP should be maintained at or above the gestational age of the infant in weeks. Although based on expert opinion and not on any data, this recommendation remains popular, and is easy to use at the bedside. However, it does not take into consideration the rapid rise in blood pressure over the first 5 days of life, and a slower increase during subsequent two weeks. These changes in blood pressure occur even in the most preterm infants. Zubrow's charts provide mean and 95% confidence intervals for systolic and diastolic BP (but not mean BP) obtained by oscillometry on the first day of life for various gestations and birth weights, and also for up to 46 weeks of corrected age.

More recently, normative BP measurements for non-ventilated stable preterm (28–36 weeks) neonates were reported by Kent et al. Like Zubrow, they also used an oscillometric method, but in a more homogenous group of infants, and reported the mean arterial blood pressure (MAP) in addition to the systolic (SBP) and diastolic (DBP) blood pressures. MAP is calculated by the equations: (2 × diastolic + systolic) ÷ 3. Their results suggested that a mean BP of 1–2 mmHg above the gestation in weeks in the first few days of life fell within the 10–90th centiles, providing some justification for the BAPM recommendations mentioned vide supra. Preterm infants have BPs similar to that of term infants after 2 weeks of life. When compared to appropriate-for-age infants, small-for-gestational age infants have relatively lower blood pressures.

In practice, it is a good idea to remember that measurements with the oscillometric technique for non-invasive blood pressure (NIBP) can be significantly different from invasive measurements. In extremely low birth weight (ELBW) infants, NIBP measurements tend to overestimate systolic, diastolic and mean BP when compared to intra-arterial measurements.

Given the limitations of clinical assessment and BP measurements, clinicians increasingly rely on point-of-care ultrasound (clinician performed cardiac ultrasound; CPCU) to individualize hemodynamic assessment and treatment of shock in neonates. In CPCU, a focused assessment is used to guide clinical decision-making regarding the choice of volume expanders, inotropes, vasoconstrictors, etc. and to monitor response to therapy. Measurements of left or right ventricular outputs may over estimate the systemic blood flow in neonates due to shunting through the PDA or at the atrial level. Use of superior vena cava (SVC) flow, 80% of which represents cerebral venous return, is considered a better indicator of cerebral blood flow. The use of near-infrared spectroscopy (NIRS) to assess cerebral oxygenation and guide therapy can be considered experimental at this stage. Future neonatologists will have to master the art of integrating clinical findings and BP with cardiac ultrasound findings to identify the specific pathophysiology and offer individualized, rational therapy to neonates in shock.

Management

General Measures

Prevention and treatment of hypothermia and hypoglycemia are important components of care for any sick newborn, including those with shock. Once the airway is secured and ventilation is established, treatment of shock should be initiated promptly. Most neonates with shock requiring significant inotropic support will require mechanical ventilation. In view of recent evidence indicating higher mortality and increased risk of necrotizing enterocolitis with low oxygen saturation targets, SpO$_2$ should be maintained between 90–95% in preterm infants, especially below 28 weeks. Antibiotics should be started and continued until infection is ruled out.

Volume Expanders

The common practice of resuscitating neonates in shock with volume expanders has very little evidence to support it. While volume expansion is beneficial in an hypovolemic infant, increasing the preload may worsen cardiac function in infants with myocardial dysfunction. Hence it appears prudent to limit fluid boluses to 10–20 mL/kg, especially in the preterm infants whose immature myocardium is more sensitive to preload, unless there is definitive evidence of hypovolemia.

Apart from normal saline, other crystalloids or colloids are sometimes used for volume expansion. There is no evidence that colloids are superior to crystalloids in treating neonatal shock. Two small studies suggested that dopamine was better than fluid boluses for correcting low BP in preterm, hypotensive infants. A Cochrane Systematic Review in 2004 concluded that there was insufficient evidence to determine whether infants with cardiovascular compromise benefit from volume expansion.

Inotropes and Vasoactive Drugs

Dopamine is one of the most commonly used inotropes, and is an endogenous catecholamine. It has been shown to raise the blood pressure better than albumin or dobutamine in hypotensive infants. Whether this translates into better outcomes is not clear. Dopamine causes systemic and pulmonary vasoconstriction at higher doses, resulting in increased cardiac afterload. Although urine output improves with low-dose dopamine, there is no effect on serum creatinine or clinical outcomes. Given the variability of adrenergic receptor expression in preterm infants, it is better to start with a low dose (2–5 µg/kg/minute) and gradually increase to 20 µg/kg/minute if shock persists. Dopamine is arrhythmogenic, and there is a risk of extravasation injury. Dopamine has endocrine effects, and can cause transient hypopituitarism as well as reduced thyroid hormones in infants and children; long-term consequences are not known.

Dobutamine, on the other hand, is synthetic and does not have endocrine effects. It is inotropic, and can cause some vasodilation. This makes it useful when there is myocardial dysfunction, especially if the SVR is elevated. There is some evidence that dobutamine is better than dopamine in increasing systemic blood flow in preterm neonates with low systemic flow. While dopamine is more effective in treating hypotension than dobutamine, a Cochrane review found no differences in mortality, periventricular leukomalacia or severe intraventricular hemorrhage. The usual dose of dobutamine is 5–20 µg/kg/minute. Arrhythmias can also occur with dobutamine.

Epinephrine is commonly used when shock is refractory to dopamine and dobutamine. At low doses, β-adrenergic effects result in a net fall in SVR with positive inotropic and chronotropic effects. Peripheral and renal vasoconstriction are more common with doses above 0.3 µg/kg/minute. The usual dosage range is 0.05 to 1 µg/kg/minute, although higher doses have been used. High doses of epinephrine should be used cautiously as it can cause intense vasoconstriction, and tends to worsen lactic acidosis.

Hydrocortisone is used when shock is resistant to infusions of one or more catecholamines. As an alternative to dopamine for treatment of hypotension, it is equally effective in VLBW infants. It is logical to consider its early use in the VLBW neonates who are at an increased risk of relative adrenal insufficiency. Hydrocortisone acts by increasing adrenergic receptor

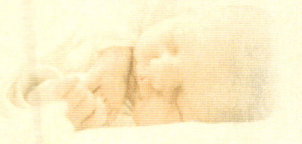

density and enhancing vascular sensitivity to catecholamines. Hyperglycemia is a common short-term side effect. Concurrent use of hydrocortisone with indomethacin is best avoided, given the risk of spontaneous intestinal perforation. The use of short-course hydrocortisone is not associated with neuro-sensory or cognitive impairment, unlike dexamethasone.

Vasopressin is a potent vasoconstrictor and acts through V1 receptors. It may be more useful in vaso-dilatory shock, and has been used in catecholamine-resistant septic shock. It may overcome alpha-receptor down-regulation in septic shock because it acts through different receptors.

Milrinone is a phosphodiesterase-III inhibitor and has cAMP-mediated positive inotropic effects without significant chronotropy. In addition, it causes systemic and pulmonary vasodilation. This profile is beneficial in the setting of myocardial dysfunction with increased SVR or persistent pulmonary hypertension (PPHN). Milrinone has been shown to be useful in the management of post-PDA ligation circulatory failure in neonates. Improved oxygenation and hemodynamics in neonates with PPHN has also been reported. Systemic vasodilation can result in hypotension after administration of milrinone; this may require volume expansion.

Norepinephrine has potent vasoconstrictive effects, acting through α-adrenergic receptors. Although effective in raising the blood pressure, higher doses can result in hypoperfusion of vital organs and increased myocardial work due to the higher afterload. Levosimendan is a newer inodilator more commonly used in the setting of heart failure in adults; its use in

neonates is currently anecdotal. The various drugs used in the management of shock in neonates are summarized in Table 13.2.

Monitoring Therapeutic Response

No single therapeutic endpoint can reliably assess the response to the treatment of shock. Clinical assessment is based on monitoring of vital signs, physical examination and urine output. This is often reinforced with blood gas analysis and serum lactate measurements. Blood pressure is the most commonly tracked therapeutic endpoint.

While invasive monitoring allows for accurate measurement of BP, CVP and central venous oxygen saturation is increasingly used, the benefits have to be weighed against the risk of infection, thrombosis and other complications. Mixed or central venous oxygenation ($ScvO_2$) targeting can be problematic in the neonate because of the presence of fetal hemoglobin. The blood lactate level of more than twice the normal is indicative of inadequate tissue oxygenation. Lactate levels can be followed to monitor the response to therapy.

CPCU can be used at the bedside to monitor response to treatment. An SVC flow of more than 40 mL/kg/minute is targeted to ensure adequate cerebral blood flow. Low SVC flows are associated with intraventricular hemorrhage and neurodevelopmental delay. Measurement of ventricular contractility and shunt across the PDA are other useful parameters. Long-term benefits of CPCU-guided therapy are unknown. When CPCU is not available, an algorithmic approach is useful to manage a neonate with shock (Figure 13.1).

Table 13.2 Drugs used in the treatment of shock			
Drug	*Mechanism of action*	*Usual dosage*	*Comments*
Crystalloids (commonly normal saline)	Volume expansion	10–20 mL/kg	Consider higher volume in hypovolemia, term infants, older children
Dopamine	Inotropic, chronotropic, vaso-constrictor (higher doses). Dopamine, α and β receptors. Endogenous neurotransmitter has endocrine effects	2–20 μg/kg/min	Naturally occurring inexpensive; commonly used. Vasodilator to kidneys, intestines, coronaries. More effective than dobutamine for raising BP. There are concerns regarding its endocrine effects
Dobutamine	Predominantly β-agonist. Inotropic and chronotropic. Very little vasoconstriction (α effect); can cause some peripheral vasodilation	5–20 μg/kg/min	Synthetic; does not increase vascular resistance. Shown to increase superior vena cava flow (more than dopamine). Less effective for raising BP. No endocrine effects
Milrinone	Phosphodiesterase-III inhibitor. Inodilator (inotropic and vasodilator), lusitropic (improves diastolic relaxation of myocardium)	50 μg/kg loading followed by 0.25–1 μg/kg/min	Relatively expensive. Systemic and pulmonary vasodilator (risk of hypotension that usually responds to fluid boluses). Useful in the setting of post-PDA ligation, circulatory failure and in PPHN. Limited experience in neonatal shock

(Contd...)

Table 13.2 Drugs used in the treatment of shock (*Contd...*)

Drug	Mechanism of action	Usual dosage	Comments
Levosimendan	Calcium sensitizer; K-ATP channel opener and inodilator	6 to 12 µg/kg loading dose over 10 minutes followed by 0.05–2.0 µg /kg/min	Increases cardiac contractility without corresponding increase in oxygen requirement. Coronary and peripheral vasodilator; anti-stunning effect on myocardium. No neonatal trials; most studies in adults with heart failure
Adrenaline	α and β adrenergic receptor agonist	0.1–1 µg/kg/min	Inexpensive; reduces systemic and pulmonary vascular resistance in lower doses due to β effects; vasoconstriction with higher doses
Noradrenaline	α and β adrenergic receptor agonist	0.05–1 µg/kg/min	Predominant α effect. Vasoconstrictor. Increases afterload and myocardial work.
Vasopressin	Acts through V1 receptors	0.0002 to 0.004 units/kg/min (higher doses for shock). 0.0002–0.0004 units/kg/min for PPHN	More commonly used for septic shock in older children. Anecdotal experience in PPHN (low dose) in neonates. Terlipressin is analogue with longer half-life
Hydrocortisone	Increased sensitivity to catecholamines; cytokine suppression (glucocorticoid effect). Sodium retention (mineralocorticoid)	2–4 mg/kg/day	Consider early administration in very preterm infants; check pre-treatment cortisol level when possible. Risk of GI perforation is higher when used concurrently with NSAIDs for closure of PDA

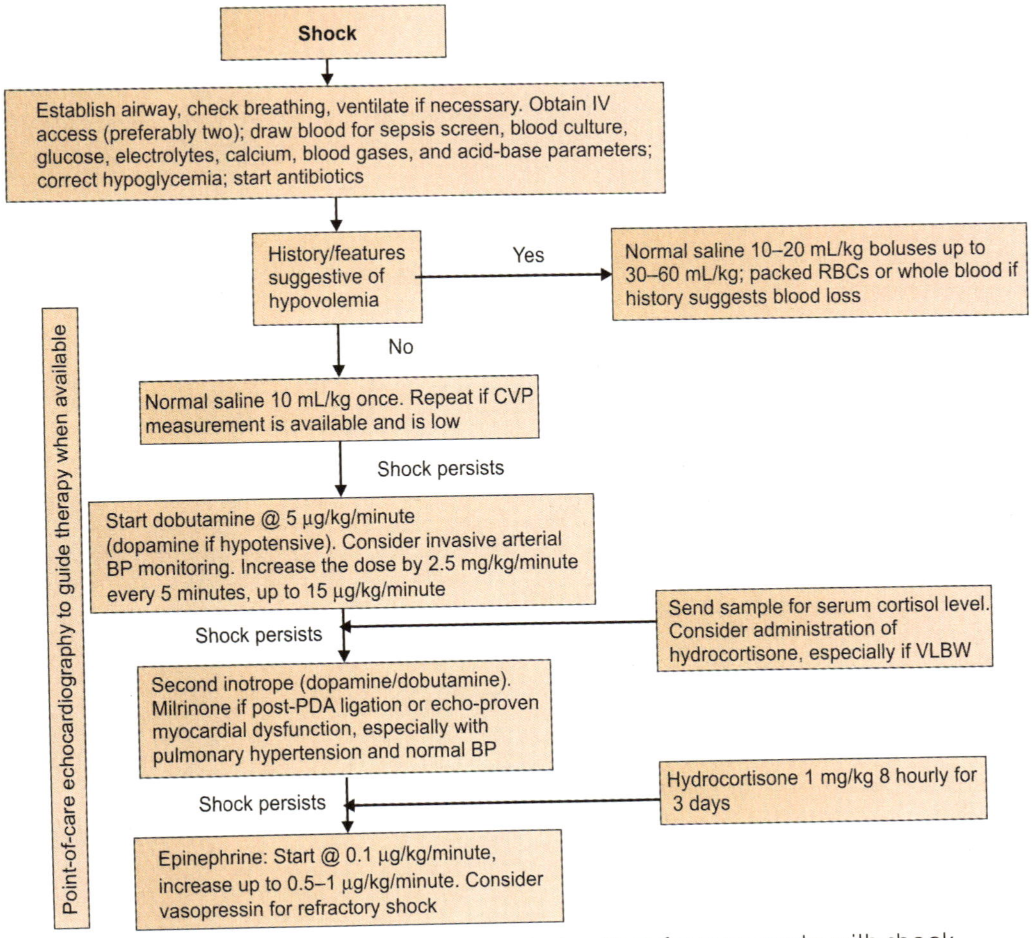

Figure 13.1 Suggested management algorithm for a neonate with shock.

The use of near infrared spectroscopy (NIRS) to measure regional cerebral tissue oxygenation and guide therapy is attractive in theory because it is noninvasive and can provide a continuous measurement of what appears to be a clinically relevant end-point. However, normative values have not been established, and there is wide variability in readings between patients and between devices from different manufacturers. At this stage, the use of NIRS to guide the treatment of shock should be considered as experimental.

Early Goal-directed Therapy

Early goal-directed therapy (EGDT) involves the use of defined resuscitation end points in initial management of septic shock, and is endorsed by the Surviving Sepsis campaign. Maintaining CVP and maximizing mixed or central venous oxygen saturation are key features of EGDT. This demands invasive monitoring. EGDT for septic shock has not been studied in neonates. The role of EGDT in adults and older children is being questioned because two large trials in 2014 did not show any benefit when compared to 'conventional care'.

SUMMARY

Early detection and prompt treatment of shock can reduce mortality and improve neurologic outcome. The goal of therapy is to maintain perfusion and oxygen delivery to tissues. Volume expanders must be used cautiously in the absence of hypovolemia. An algorithmic therapeutic approach is recommended. Clinician performed cardiac ultrasound can be used to guide fluid and inotrope therapy and monitor response, but trained personnel and equipment are not always available, and long-term benefits are unknown. Future research should be directed at long-term survival and neurodevelopmental outcomes following various management strategies.

BIBLIOGRAPHY

Brierley J, Carcillo JA, Choong K, et al. Clinical practice parameters for hemodynamic support of pediatric and neonatal septic shock: 2007 update from the American College of Critical Care Medicine. *Crit Care Med* 2009; 37:666–88.

Cheung PY, Barrington KJ, Pearson RJ, et al. Systemic, pulmonary and mesenteric perfusion and oxygenation effects of dopamine and epinephrine. *Am J Respir Crit Care Med* 1997; 155:32–7.

Dellinger RP, Levy MM, Rhodes A, et al. Surviving sepsis campaign: international guidelines for management of severe sepsis and septic shock 2012. *Crit Care Med* 2013; 41:580–637.

Evans N. Which inotrope for which baby? *Arch Dis Child Fetal Neonatal Ed* 2006; 91:F213–F20.

Femitha P, Bhat BV. Early neonatal outcome in late preterms. *Indian J Pediatr* 2012; 79:1019–24.

Friedrich JO, Adhikari N, Herridge MS, Beyene J. Meta-analysis: low-dose dopamine increases urine output but does not prevent renal dysfunction or death. *Ann Intern Med* 2005; 142:510–24.

Gill AB, Weindling AM. Echocardiographic assessment of cardiac function in shocked very low birthweight infants. *Arch Dis Child* 1993; 68:17–21.

Jain A, Sahni M, El-Khuffash A, et al. Use of targeted neonatal echocardiography to prevent postoperative cardiorespiratory instability after patent ductus arteriosus ligation. *J Pediatr* 2012; 160:584–9.

Kluckow M, Evans N. Relationship between blood pressure and cardiac output in preterm infants requiring mechanical ventilation. *J Pediatr* 1996; 129:506–12.

Kluckow M, Evans N. Superior vena cava flow in newborn infants: a novel marker of systemic blood flow. *Arch Dis Child Fetal Neonatal Ed* 2000; 82:F182–F7.

Kluckow M. Use of ultrasound in the haemodynamic assessment of the sick neonate. *Arch Dis Child Fetal Neonatal Ed* 2014; 99:F332–F7.

Lechner E, Hofer A, Leitner-Peneder G, et al. Levosimendan versus milrinone in neonates and infants after corrective open-heart surgery: a pilot study. *Pediatr Crit Care Med* 2012; 13:542–8.

Noori S, Friedlich PS, Seri I. Pathophysiology of shock in the fetus and neonate. In: Fetal and Neonatal Physiology. Polin RA, Fox WW, Abman SH, eds. 4th ed. Philadelphia: *Elsevier Saunders* 2011; pp 853–63.

Nuntnarumit P, Yang W, Bada-Ellzey HS. Blood pressure measurements in the newborn. *Clin Perinatol* 1999; 26:981–96.

Osborn DA, Evans N. Early volume expansion for prevention of morbidity and mortality in very preterm infants. *Cochrane Database Syst Rev* 2004:CD002055.

Osborn DA, Evans N. Early volume expansion versus inotrope for prevention of morbidity and mortality in very preterm infants. *Cochrane Database Syst Rev* 2001:CD002056.

Peake SL, Delaney A, Bailey M, et al. Goal-directed resuscitation for patients with early septic shock. *N Engl J Med* 2014; 371:1496–506.

Peltoniemi O, Kari MA, Heinonen K, et al. Pretreatment cortisol values may predict responses to hydrocortisone administration for the prevention of bronchopulmonary dysplasia in high-risk infants. *J Pediatr* 2005; 146:632–7.

Saugstad OD, Aune D. Optimal oxygenation of extremely low birth weight infants: a meta-analysis and systematic review of the oxygen saturation target studies. *Neonatology* 2014; 105:55–63.

Subhedar NV, Shaw NJ. Dopamine versus dobutamine for hypotensive preterm infants. *Cochrane Database Syst Rev* 2003:CD001242.

Tibby S, Hatherill M, Marsh M, Murdoch I. Clinicians' abilities to estimate cardiac index in ventilated children and infants. *Arch Dis Child* 1997; 77:516–8.

Van den Berghe G, de Zegher F, Lauwers P. Dopamine suppresses pituitary function in infants and children. *Crit Care Med* 1994; 22:1747–53.

Wright IM, Goodall SR. Blood pressure and blood volume in preterm infants. *Arch Dis Child Fetal Neonatal Ed* 1994; 70: F230–F31.

14

Respiratory Emergencies

Shalabh Garg and Sunil Sinha

Respiratory disorders are one of the most common causes of serious illness in newborns which require immediate treatment. Optimal management of these conditions require good understanding of the etiology, pathogenesis and rationale for treatment strategies. These disorders may present at birth, soon after birth or during the later neonatal period. The normal establishment of regular and effective breathing requires transition from intrauterine to extrauterine life which involves a number of processes including conversion of the fluid filled lungs into an organ distended with air to support effective gaseous exchange. This results in establishment of 'adult' type circulation leading to reduced pulmonary vascular resistance. An effective breathing at birth also requires integrity of respiratory center in the brain, breathing apparatus (airways, lungs, respiratory muscles) and cardiovascular system. Therefore, any supportive care provided in the immediate newborn period must be based on an understanding of the pathophysiology of these homeostatic mechanisms.

Respiratory Physiology

1. Oxygen Transport

Oxygen is essential for the production of adenosine triphosphate (ATP), which is responsible for storage and release of energy. Severe hypoxemia greatly reduces the production of ATP and the resultant anerobic metabolism produces lactic acid. Lactic acid accumulation significantly contributes to the development of metabolic acidosis.

2. Carbon Dioxide Transport

Carbon dioxide may be transported dissolved in the blood, but is mainly present as bicarbonate ions (HCO_3^-).

Carbon dioxide is produced as a by-product of cellular respiration and is liberated into the blood. It diffuses through the alveoli to be excreted in the expired air. The CO_2 content of the blood is referred to as the partial pressure of CO_2 or $PaCO_2$.

3. Acid-base Balance

In the presence of the enzyme carbonic anhydrase, carbon dioxide dissolved in plasma forms carbonic acid, which in turn dissociates to H^+ and HCO_3^- ions. As a result of this dissociation, carbonic acid can be indirectly excreted through the lungs. Lactic acid must be excreted through the kidneys which occurs more slowly to prevent rapid pH changes. Disturbance of the acid-base balance can produce either acidosis or alkalosis, which may be due to metabolic or respiratory causes. The acid-base status of the infant can be derived from the blood gases. Table 14.1 provides a normal biochemical indices for arterial blood gases in term and preterm infants.

Apart from establishment of normal gaseous exchange, the act of breathing also requires the development and maturation of the various components of the 'breathing apparatus'. This is made up of the conducting system (airways) and a gas exchange organ (the lung). The respiratory movements of the chest wall

Table 14.1 Normal values of arterial blood gases and acid-base parameters

Parameter	Preterm neonate	Term neonate
pH	7.25–7.4	7.32–7.4
PaO_2 (kPa)	6–12	7–10
$PaCO_2$ (kPa)	5–8	4.5–6
Bicarbonate	16–24	18–24
Base excess	–4 to +4	–2 to +2

*1kPa = 7.5 mmHg

are further supported by intercostal muscles and diaphragm (muscles of respiration). The effective functioning of the respiratory system also requires normal functioning of respiratory centers in the brain as well as good cardiac function with a change over from fetal to adult type of circulation. The causes of respiratory failure in newborns are listed in the Table 14.2.

Assessment of Respiratory Status

This is done on the basis of information obtained on detailed perinatal/neonatal history, clinical observations, blood gases (arterial or capillary), chest X-rays, pulmonary function tests and 3D echocardiography.

The collective information obtained from these investigations provide useful data regarding the likely cause, underlying respiratory status and severity of the disease process but each of them when used individually may have poor specificity.

Table 14.2 Causes of respiratory failure depending upon the site of the respiratory system involved

Site of disease	Causes
Brain	▪ Neonatal encephalopathy ▪ Apnea of prematurity ▪ Intracranial hemorrhage
Lungs	▪ RDS ▪ Pneumonia ▪ Pulmonary hemorrhage ▪ Pneumothorax and pneumomediastinum ▪ Pulmonary hypoplasia ▪ Aspiration (meconium, blood, milk) ▪ Diaphragmatic hernia ▪ Congenital cystic adenomatoid malformation ▪ Lobar emphysema
Airways	▪ Laryngomalacia ▪ Tracheomalacia ▪ Subglottic stenosis ▪ Atresia (choanal, tracheal agenesis) Esophageal atresia with TEF ▪ Pierre Robin sequence
Muscles of breathing	▪ Congenital myopathy ▪ Werdnig-Hoffmann syndrome ▪ Spinal cord lesions ▪ Myasthenia gravis
Miscellaneous conditions	▪ Persistent pulmonary hypertension ▪ Congenital heart defects ▪ Tetanus neonatorum ▪ Hydrops fetalis

RDS: respiratory distress syndrome; TEF: tracheo-esophageal fistula.

Table 14.3 Salient changes in blood gases in respiratory and metabolic acidosis or alkalosis

Acid-base disorder	pH	Bicarbonate	PaCO₂
Respiratory acidosis	↓	↑	↑
Respiratory alkalosis	↑	↓	↓
Metabolic acidosis	↓	↓	↓
Metabolic alkalosis	↑	↑	↑
Mixed acidosis	↓	↓	↑
Mixed alkalosis	↑	↑	↓

The *clinical assessment* requires detailed obstetric history and baby's condition at birth. The physical signs associated with respiratory distress include increased respiratory rate, subcostal and intercostal retractions, nasal flaring, grunting and cyanosis.

The *blood gas analysis* gives information regarding the status of oxygenation and whether infant is having respiratory or metabolic acidosis, or alkalosis (Table 14.3).

Chest radiograph is an integral part of diagnostic evaluation. Other imaging modalities including CT and MRI are useful in selected cases.

Pulmonary mechanic testing or pulmonary graphics have now become available at bedside and can be used to provide important information about the lung volume and airflow. This in turn can be used to calculate *compliance* (elasticity of the lung), *resistance* (to the gas flow during inspiration and expiration) and work of breathing. This can also be used to assess the progress of the disease and response to any therapeutic intervention. *Cardiac assessment* is also an important aspect of assessment and management of a baby with respiratory symptoms and signs. This requires clinical examination of cardiovascular system but if facilities are available, a bedside echocardiography provides useful information about the cardiac functions (filling, contractility, systemic and pulmonary circulation) as well as presence of any structural abnormality.

Treatment of Respiratory Failure

Mainstay of treatment of babies with respiratory failure is to provide artificial respiratory support but affected babies may also have multisystem failure and they require additional supportive care. The strategies to provide artificial respiratory support are listed below:

▪ Oxygen therapy
▪ Noninvasive forms of mechanical respiratory support
▪ Assisted ventilation through mechanical ventilators

The aim of the oxygen therapy is to achieve optimal oxygenation without causing oxygen toxicity and therefore babies on oxygen therapy require close monitoring. The commonly used indices of oxygenation are alveolar-arterial oxygen pressure difference, oxygenation index and arterial to alveolar oxygen tension ratio (a/A ratio). Newer equipment have also now become available which monitor and adjust oxygen administration using automated control systems to maintain arterial oxygen level within optimal range. But this device is not yet universally available.

Depending on the degree of respiratory insufficiency, some babies will require assisted mechanical ventilation. Although life saving, this is an invasive procedure and may cause damage to the lungs. Therefore, the operators using the mechanical ventilators should have special skills to understand how the ventilators work and how to make adjustments in the settings to get maximum benefit with minimal harm. Goals of mechanical ventilation, irrespective of the ventilatory device or mode of ventilation, are listed below.

- Achieve adequate pulmonary gas exchange
- Reduce work of breathing
- Overcome alveolar atelectasis
- Avoid ventilator-induced lung injury
- Maximise patient's comfort

The factors which affect oxygenation include fraction of inspired oxygen (FiO_2) and mean airway pressure (MAP) which is determined by positive end-expiratory pressure (PEEP), peak inspiratory pressure (PIP), inspiratory time and gas flow rate. Increase in respiratory rate has minimal effect on oxygenation. The CO_2 removal is determined by minute volume (MV) which is equal to tidal volume (TV) multiplied by inspiratory rate. The tidal volume is dependent on distending pressure which is equal to difference between PIP and baseline PEEP.

Recently, there has been increasing interest in use of noninvasive modes of respiratory support which include continuous positive airway pressure (CPAP), high flow nasal cannula (HFNC) and noninvasive intermittent positive pressure ventilation (NIPPV). They all seem to work and there is no current compelling evidence that one method is superior to the other. They have been used successfully as an initial treatment for mild to moderate respiratory failure or as a continuing respiratory support to babies who have been extubated after a period of mechanical ventilation. The use of these forms of noninvasive respiratory support has increased in recent past because they are gentler modalities and cause less damage to the lungs. However, this has not been proven conclusively by long term respiratory or neurological outcomes of several scientific trials. Whatever method is chosen, the operators should understand the basis of their action and limitations of the therapeutic modality in order to get the best results.

COMMON LIFE-THREATENING RESPIRATORY DISORDERS

As mentioned in the anatomy and physiology of respiratory system, the specific etiology may present with characteristic or nonspecific symptoms but if not treated early it will ultimately lead to respiratory failure. The investigations and management depend upon the site and nature of disease process. In the following section, some common neonatal respiratory emergencies are described starting from pathologies arising in central nervous system and then going on to describe problems with airways, chest wall and the lungs.

Apnea and Bradycardia

These signs can be present either at birth or later in the course of neonatal illness. The apnea that occurs subsequently is most commonly due to 'Apnea of Prematurity'. Sometimes the non-respiratory causes can also lead to apnea especially in preterm babies with neonatal sepsis, anemia, gastroesophageal reflux, electrolyte or metabolic imbalance or seizures.

The apnea and bradycardia due to perinatal hypoxia manifests as an emergency at birth. Most term babies establish spontaneous breathing soon after birth unless compromised or depressed by perinatal hypoxic ischemic injury, maternal drugs or general anesthesia. The babies who remain apneic or bradycardiac even after providing basic life support, generally have central nervous system involvement.

Congenital Central Hypoventilation Syndrome (CCHS)

It is a well-recognised but ill understood cause (Ondine's curse) of apnea. In most cases it will become apparent soon after birth when the baby starts to hypoventilate while falling asleep. In this condition, the responses of autonomic nervous system to hypoxia or hypercarbia are impaired which manifests as 'fast and deep' breathing in normal infants. There is loss of automatic control of breathing during sleep which is preserved while awake. The genetic basis for this condition has been described as mutation in homeobox gene. The milder cases may be diagnosed late in infancy or childhood. Some workers believe that this could be the basis of some of the cases of Sudden Infant Death Syndrome (SIDS). The management mostly involves in providing mechanical ventilation on a long-term basis especially during the nights. Although most cases are congenital in nature but acquired cases are reported in children and adults mainly due to ischemic insults leading on to central infarcts especially of ventrolateral medulla.

In cases of traumatic instrumental deliveries (especially the rotational forceps), high spinal cord injuries should be suspected as a cause for apnea and bradycardia. In these cases, the central respiratory center is intact and infant exhibits signs of distress and makes efforts to breathe but is unable to do so due to complete diaphragmatic paralysis. These cases also require long-term mechanical ventilation. The long-term prognosis is generally poor and most of these infants die in the early neonatal period.

Neonatal Emergencies Related to Upper Airways

Choanal atresia This is an acute respiratory emergency that presents at birth with obstructive apnea and cyanosis as soon as the baby stops crying. The neonates are obligatory nose breathers during first few weeks of their life and any obstruction in the mouth (during breast or bottle-feeding) causes intense respiratory distress and cyanosis. It is caused by either a bony or membranous (or more commonly both) obstruction of the posterior nasal passages. Clinically, the diagnosis is confirmed by inability to pass nasogastric tube through the nasal passage. The other tests that can be done to confirm the diagnosis are endoscopy or CT scan. It is mostly unilateral (60–75%) in which case no immediate surgical intervention is required but rare cases of bilateral choanal atresia of bony nature will invariably need surgical correction during the neonatal period. Bilateral choanal atresia is associated with other genetic abnormalities in 75% of the cases including CHARGE association, Crouzen's and Treacher Collins syndromes. Until the surgery is performed, the condition is managed by insertion of an oral (special nipple with a large hole) or oropharyngeal airway. If these are not available or do not provide any relief, mechanical ventilation is provided.

The other *airway anomalies* that can present as respiratory emergency in newborn babies are *Pierre Robin sequence* (severe micro and/or retrognathia), severe macroglossia (Beckwith-Wiedemann syndrome or sometimes with Trisomy 21) or tracheo-esophageal fistula (TEF). They are either related to obstruction of the airway due to abnormal upper airway anatomy or due to aspiration as in tracheo-esophageal fistula. In TEF, there may be history of polyhydramnios and the baby may present with copious frothy mucus secretions

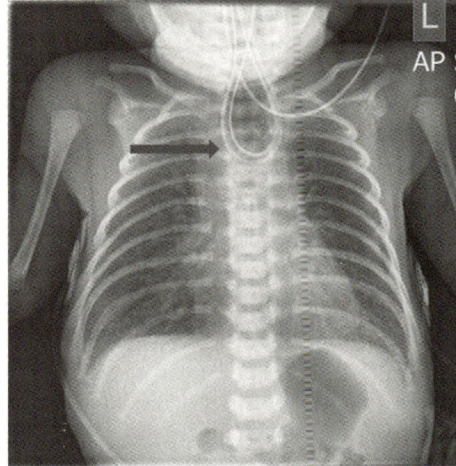

Figure 14.1 Esophageal atresia with tracheo-esophageal fistula. The curled up nasogastric tube is suggestive of esophageal atresia while presence of stomach bubble indicates the presence of fistula.

from oral or nasal orifices. The baby may develop symptoms of choking and cough that worsen with any attempts on feeding. The diagnosis is confirmed by finding a curled up stiff rubber catheter in the upper pouch of esophagus on chest X-ray (Figure 14.1). After stabilization and identification of associated malformations, these infants should be transferred to the surgical unit for surgical correction as early as possible.

At times, trachea may be partially or completely obstructed by thick particulate meconium, mucus or blood which demands effective endotracheal suctioning to achieve successful resuscitation. One of the worst nightmares of any neonatologist is complete *congenital tracheal agenesis* and total inability to ventilate or oxygenate the baby at birth. This condition is rare and should be suspected in a baby where endotracheal intubation is not successful despite adequate technique and attempts by a senior neonatologist. Immediate ENT intervention for tracheostomy may be lifesaving in these infants.

Some of the cases of congenital stridor (vocal cord palsy, subglottic hemangioma or tumor, external airway compression by abnormal blood vessel) may present as upper airway obstruction. These infants need services and expertise of ENT colleagues for their work-up and management.

Pulmonary Air Leaks

Pulmonary air leaks are a group of disorders that are caused by collection of air outside the lungs. These include pneumothorax (air in pleural space), pneumo-mediastinum (mediastinal air) and pneumopericardium (air in the pericardial sac). If there is significant leak, any of these can lead on to sudden cardio-respiratory collapse. Sometimes these leaks can be seen in interstitial lung spaces (pulmonary interstitial emphysema).

Pneumothorax Pneumothorax is the most common air leak syndrome in newborns. One of the main risk factor for development of pneumothorax is provision of positive-pressure ventilation (invasive or noninvasive) for respiratory failure in preterm and term babies. The incidence of pneumothorax has reduced significantly with widespread use of antenatal steroids, surfactant therapy as well as gentler ventilation strategies. In term vigorous babies, sometimes providing continuous positive airway pressure (CPAP) may cause pneumothorax. Spontaneous pneumothorax occurs in 1% of babies born by vaginal deliveries and 1.5% of those born by cesarean section.

Pneumothorax should always be suspected and ruled out in a baby on ventilator who deteriorates suddenly, for example, desaturating, needing increased oxygen, dropping blood pressure, and worsening of blood gases. This is mostly a clinical diagnosis but sometimes the diagnosis is made incidentally on chest radiograph (Figure 14.2). If not treated promptly, a simple pneumothorax can develop into a tension pneumothorax which is life-threatening emergency and needs immediate decompression. As mentioned above, diagnosis is mainly clinical with reduced air entry on one side (beware of bilateral pneumothoraces in which air entry may not be different on two sides), hyper-expanded chest on normal side, reduced chest wall movements or positive transillumination on affected side. Transillumnation can be false negative (especially in bigger babies) if the ambience is not dark or the pneumothorax is small.

The condition is treated with urgent needle thoracocentesis followed by chest drain insertion if required. Needle thoracocentesis is performed in second intercostal space in the midclavicular line. The chest drain is placed in the 4th or 5th intercostal space in anterior or midaxillary line. The two methods of chest drain insertion are traditional Trocar-cannula approach or more recently Seldinger technique using a pigtail catheter (Figure 14.3). Our experience of using the Seldinger technique is quite encouraging allowing us to put chest drains without any blunt or surgical dissection. There is no need to apply any sutures and there are less chances of accidental dislodgement. Some neonatologists use needle thoracocentesis without inserting any chest drain. Although a recent Cochrane review showed inconclusive results while comparing needle thoracocentesis and chest drains for pneumothoraces in neonates.

Sometimes babies are born with congenital pleural effusion due to fetal hydrops or as an isolated pleural effusion. One of the most common causes of neonatal pleural effusions is *chylothorax*. Chyle is a non-inflammatory fluid composed mainly of fat, cholesterol, electrolytes, proteins, glucose, and abundant lymphocytes. This can occur due to the several pathologies that cause obstruction to the lymphatic drainage, for example, lymphangiectasia, pulmonary venous obstruction, absence or atresia of thoracic duct but also in some congenital heart diseases. Depending upon the size of the effusion as well as the gestation at which the effusion developed, it may be associated with pulmonary hypoplasia or poor lung expansion at birth. This may necessitate immediate drainage of pleural fluid in the delivery suite to achieve stable respiratory status. This can be done by large bore cannula attached

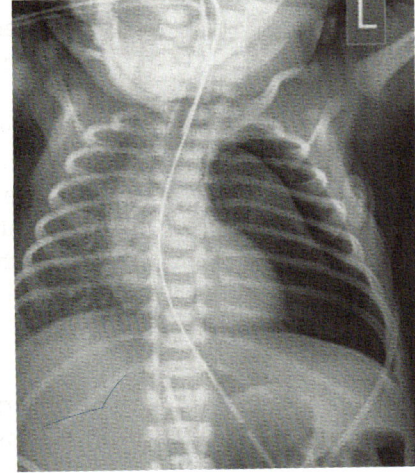

Figure 14.2 Chest radiograph showing left sided pneumothorax in a preterm baby on mechanical ventilator.

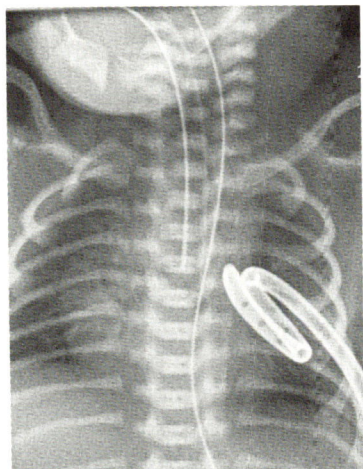

Figure 14.3 Pigtail chest drain *in situ* inserted by Seldinger technique.

to three way tap which can be closed after drainage of the fluid while leaving the cannula *in situ* until the definitive chest drain is placed after transfering the baby to the neonatal intensive care unit. In some cases, the pleural effusion accumulates rapidly during antenatal period and chest drains are placed *in utero*.

Respiratory Distress Syndrome (RDS)

Respiratory distress is a nonspecific combination of signs and symptoms (tachypnea, nasal flaring, chest recessions, grunting, wheezing, stridor, cyanosis) that leads on to increased work of breathing. On the other hand, Respiratory Distress Syndrome (RDS) is a name given to a specific clinical condition that is mostly (but not always) seen in preterm infants. This is also sometimes referred to as idiopathic respiratory distress syndrome or hyaline membrane disease. This condition mainly occurs due to lack of the endogenous production or deactivation of surfactant in the alveoli of the premature lungs. Multiple clinical trials have been performed to understand the pathophysiology of RDS and the role of surfactant in its occurrence and management. Once a major cause of neonatal mortality until mid-20th century, currently RDS remains an important cause of respiratory morbidity that demands admission to neonatal unit, surfactant administration as well as positive pressure respiratory support. The mortality due to RDS has gradually decreased over last 50–60 years with the use of different treatment modalities most importantly being antenatal steroids, mechanical ventilation (noninvasive and invasive) and and administration of synthetic surfactant.

Incidence

RDS is one of the most common causes of post-delivery respiratory disease in preterm babies. Although the absolute diagnosis can only be made by quantitative analysis of surfactant deficiency or by histology, none of which are feasible in routine clinical practice. Hence most of the studies quoting the incidence of RDS are mainly based on clinical and radiological parameters in a preterm baby. The incidence of RDS is inversely proportional to the gestational age as illustrated in Figure 14.4.

Pathophysiology

The main correlate of RDS is a decrease in production of surfactant because of prematurity. Type 2 pneumocytes in the alveoli are mainly responsible for the surfactant production that starts at about 20–22 weeks of gestation; but it is not until late in pregnancy when it is sufficient and mature enough to work effectively. The surfactant is chemically composed mainly of phospholipids (70–80%) and proteins. In addition to

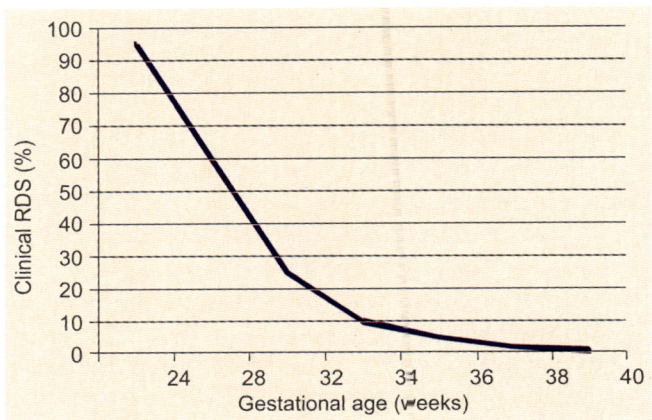

Figure 14.4 Incidence of clinical RDS in relation to gestational age.

gestational age, the surfactant production/activity is also dependent upon several other factors such as body temperature, acidosis, perfusion, meconium, sepsis and other inflammatory triggers like oxygen and ventilator induced baro/volutrauma. Histologically, diffuse atelectasis with only few dilated alveoli is evident along with an eosinophilic membrane lining the alveolar ducts and terminal bronchioles.

The physiological function of surfactant in the alveoli is to reduce the surface tension at the alveolar surface and prevent alveolar collapse at the end of expiration. The surfactant deficiency leads to collapse of alveoli across both the lungs and difficulty in maintaining functional residual capacity. As per the Laplace law ($P = 2T/r$, where P is the pressure; T the surface tension and r is the radius), the pressure needed to inflate collapsed alveoli will be much higher if the surface tension is high.

Clinical Features

The clinical presentation of RDS in preterm babies include features of respiratory distress (tachypnea, grunting, chest recessions, increased oxygen requirement, hypoxia and hypercarbia) along with characteristic radiographic changes including fine reticulo-granular pattern described as 'ground glass appearance'. The clinical symptoms can be mild to start with but may progress to severe distress if no treatment is given and can lead on to respiratory failure. In the current era of antenatal steroids and postnatal surfactant use, the typical radiological changes may not be evident and the chest X-ray may even be normal. The presence of air-bronchogram or in severe cases with almost complete collapse, the lung fields will show complete 'white out' (Figure 14.5). The clinical severity of RDS may gradually increase over first 2–3 days of life before resolving phase begins.

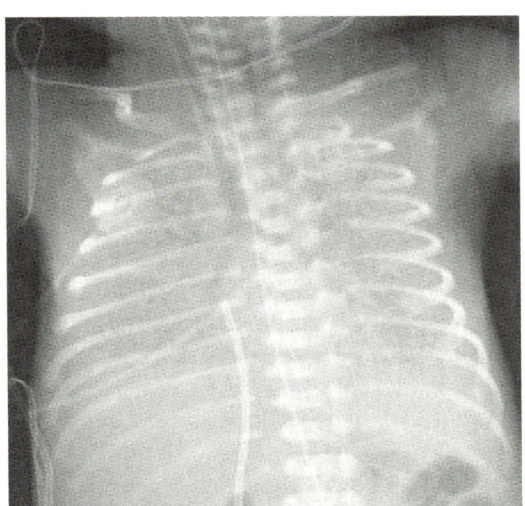

Figure 14.5 Chest radiograph showing 'white out' lung fields in a case of severe RDS.

Prevention and Treatment

Significant advancements have been made in the management of RDS over last few decades. Once a disease of high mortality, most preterm babies now survive this disease especially in developed countries where several modalities of respiratory support are readily available. Preventive measures mainly include administration of antenatal steroids (betamethasone 12 mg 1M every 24 hr for 2 doses or dexamethasone 6 mg 1M every 12 hr for 4 doses) to the women who develop preterm onset of labor (<34 weeks) or where the preterm delivery is anticipated for other maternal or fetal reasons.

The mainstay of treatment is surfactant replacement therapy and provision of artificial respiratory support (noninvasive or invasive). The surfactant is most commonly administered through endotracheal tube into the bronchi and to the lungs. It can be used as prophylactic therapy (in most infants born less than 28 weeks gestation) where the baby is intubated after birth and surfactant is given before the RDS manifests. In more mature babies (generally above 28 weeks gestation), noninvasive respiratory support in the form of continuous positive airway pressure (CPAP) is currently the modality of choice. In these cases, rescue surfactant therapy is used if the respiratory disease is progressing with evolving respiratory failure needing mechanical ventilation. Since its first use, a variety of surfactants (natural or synthetic) have been used. Most natural surfactants are derived from bovine or porcine lungs. The newer regimens of surfactant administration and dosage schedules are being tried in different units and individual units should consider devising their own guidelines or policies depending upon current scientific evidence and clinical experience of the unit. The need for respiratory support and overall management should be guided by cardio-respiratory monitoring (clinical, blood gases and radiological), acid-base balance and need for administration of antibiotics to treat super added infection. The rest of the management remains supportive. Despite the advancements in the treatment, the clinicians need to be aware of potential complications including pulmonary interstitial emphysema (PIE), pneumothorax, bronchopulmonary dysplasia, and retinopathy of prematurity.

Persistent Fetal Circulation or Persistent Pulmonary Hypertension of Newborn (PPHN)

This condition is caused by failure of systemic and pulmonary circulation to switch from the fetal to 'normal' postnatal or adult type of circulation. In the antenatal period, the pulmonary pressures are high as the lungs do not participate in fetal oxygenation. This physiology needs to change after the delivery when lungs are functional. In certain pathological conditions causing hypoxemia, the pulmonary pressures remain high and lead of to right- to-left shunt through foramen ovale or ductus arteriosus. This manifests clinically as refractory hypoxemia, poor perfusion and ultimately leading to severe respiratory failure. The conditions that can cause delayed adaptation to postnatal life and development of PPHN include neonatal sepsis, congenital pneumonia, severe surfactant deficient lung disease, meconium aspiration syndrome, congenital diaphragmatic hernia or pulmonary hypoplasia. At the bedside, it can be diagnosed by pre-ductal to post-ductal oxygen saturation difference of ≥15%. If echocardiography is available, the features like significant tricuspid regurgitation, supra-systemic pulmonary pressure and right-to-left shunt at ductus arteriosus are suggestive of PPHN after excluding congenital cyanotic heart disease.

The treatment includes providing adequate ventilatory support to achieve normal oxygenation. It is important to maintain normothermia, normal acid-base indices as well as good systemic blood pressure. If the conventional ventilation fails to achieve normal oxygenation, rescue high frequency oscillatory ventilation (HFOV) is used. Inhaled nitric oxide (iNO) therapy is beneficial in reducing the pulmonary pressure and improving oxygenation in these cases. In poor resource setting where HFOV or nitric oxide is not available, sildenafil or prostacyclin can be tried to reduce the pulmonary pressures. In developed countries, term babies who are not responding to HFOV and nitric oxide and if the oxygenation index (OI) remain more than 30–40 {OI = Mean airway pressure (cm of H_2O) × FiO_2 (%) ÷ post ductal partial pressure of arterial oxygen (mmHg)}, they are considered suitable for extra corporeal membrane oxygenation (ECMO).

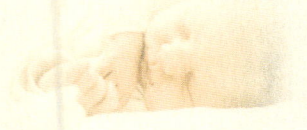

Meconium Aspiration Syndrome (MAS)

Meconium staining of amniotic fluid (MSAF) is present in about 13% deliveries and is an indication of some degree of fetal distress. The meconium staining of liquor may be normal in breech deliveries. This should not be confused with MAS which occurs in only about 5% cases of all babies with MSAF. It most commonly presents in babies born at term and very rarely in preterm babies. Most babies born through meconium will not need any resuscitation but still it is important that a person (obstetric or neonatal) competent in initiating newborn resuscitation is present at the time of delivery to assess the baby and take appropriate actions if needed. It is no longer recommended to aspirate meconium from the nose and mouth of the infant when the head is just delivered. There is no need to do any tracheal or oropharyngeal suction if the baby is crying and vigorous at birth. When faced with a floppy, apneic infant born through thick particulate meconium, it is recommended to inspect the oropharynx and suck any meconium or particulate matter. Tracheal intubation should not be routine in the presence of meconium and should only be performed for suspected tracheal obstruction. Most babies who aspirate meconium do so *in utero* due to gasping response to intrapartum distress or hypoxia which migrates down to smaller airways once the respiration is established.

The clinical features of MAS vary from mild respiratory distress needing oxygen and some pressure support to significant respiratory failure needing mechanical ventilation.

The various pathological mechanisms that cause respiratory distress in MAS are listed below.

- Mechanical obstruction of the airways causing alveolar collapse. In some areas this may cause 'ball-valve' effect and result in hyperinflation and risk of pulmonary air leaks.
- Chemical pneumonitis due to irritant effects of meconium.
- Secondary inactivation of endogenous surfactant.
- Marked V/Q mismatch leading to right-to-left shunting and development of PPHN.
- In some case secondary bacterial infection supervenes.

Diagnosis is made by passage of thick meconium stained liquor at delivery, clinical features as well as radiological appearances of heterogenous diffuse patchy opacities in bilateral lung fields. There may be presence of pneumothorax or pneumomediastinum. Sometimes blood or amniotic fluid aspiration can also mimic the clinical features of meconium aspiration syndrome in the absence of meconium staining of liquor

although the treatment essentially remains the same. If the cardiorespiratory status is not optimised promptly, the mild respiratory distress may worsen leading to development of PPHN over few hours. The treatment is the same as with any other cause of respiratory distress and involves positive-pressure ventilation support to maintain optimal ventilation and oxygenation, exogenous surfactant, antibiotics, and maintenance of fluid and acid-base balance. In severe cases, high frequency oscillatory ventilation and inhaled nitric oxide therapy are required. When these measures fail, the infant is referred for extracorporeal membrane oxygenation (ECMO) treatment which is available in few advanced centers and may involve long distance road or air ambulance transfer. The mortality rate without ECMO can be as high as 80% but in established centers, the success rate of ECMO in meconium aspiration syndrome is quite promising (80 to 100% survival) with good long-term outcome.

Congenital Diaphragmatic Hernia (CDH)

CDH is an important cause of neonatal respiratory emergency that needs prompt diagnosis and specific management to prevent mortality. In developed countries, where the antenatal anomaly scanning is universal, such cases are identified early in the pregnancy and the delivery is planned at a specialized center. Antenatal counselling involving multi-disciplinary team plays a vital role in overall management of these cases. However, a number of these cases may remain undiagnosed and present as a respiratory emergency soon after birth. A high degree of clinical suspicion is required in a baby who needs unexpectedly disproportionate degree of resuscitative measures, especially if a baby is becoming worse on bag and mask resuscitation.

Diaphragmatic hernia occurs mostly on the left side (90%) and the clinical features depend upon the size and duration of the defect as well as upon the amount of herniated intestine and other organs. This often leads to development of variable degree of pulmonary hypoplasia on the ipsilateral side which determines the severity of clinical features and likely outcome.

The infant generally presents with significant respiratory distress at birth or later. These infants may have scaphoid abdomen and hyperinflated hemithorax. On auscultation, one may hear the bowel sounds with decreased breath sounds on the herinated side. *In the suspected cases, bag and mask ventilation must be avoided.* A nasogastric tube should be passed soon after birth to avoid gastric and intestinal distension which will further compromise oxygenation. The diagnosis is

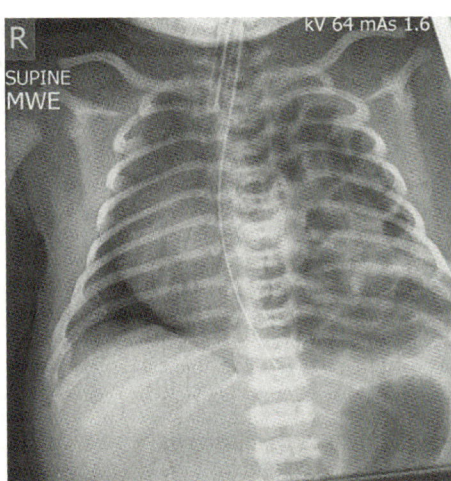

Figure 14.6 Chest radiograph showing left sided congenital diaphragmatic hernia.

confirmed by chest radiograph (Figure 14.6) which will show stomach and small bowel in the thoracic cavity.

The management strategy involves respiratory support and prevention of development of PPHN. This include prompt ventilator support (conventional and may be upgraded to HFOV at an early stage), keeping infant settled (sedation and or paralysis) and optimisation of cardiovascular status by using inotropic support. Most neonatologists also use surfactant. The aim is to achieve pre-ductal saturations above 85% and this may necessitate use of inhaled nitric oxide if PPHN has set in. A gentle ventilation strategy should be adopted to avoid barotrauma and development of pneumothorax.

The previous approach of early surgical correction is no longer advocated. The intra and post-operative mortality is significantly reduced if the newborn is allowed to be stabilised for first few days and the PPHN is resolved. ECMO treatment is also used and has improved survival in cases with severe PPHN before the surgical repair is undertaken. In Europe, a CDH Euro Consortium was established that has published recommendations for standardised postnatal management of patients with CDH. Some specialized centers in USA and Europe have performed fetal surgeries to promote development of hypoplastic lung by tracheal occlusion surgery but the results are not very encouraging at this stage and the procedure carries high-risk of complications. The best predictor of survival is the oxygenation index at 24 hours regardless of the antenatal intervention.

Pulmonary Hypoplasia

The lung development *in-utero* is dependent upon adequate amniotic fluid as well as fetal breathing movements. Keeping in mind these development needs, the following conditions can cause pulmonary hypoplasia:

- Oligohydramnios/anhydramnios due to prolonged preterm rupture of membranes, renal agenesis or urethral obstruction.
- Inadequate fetal breathing efforts due to neuro-muscular disorders.
- Poor lung expansion because of diaphragmatic hernia, pleural effusion, arthrogryposis multiplex congenita, and thoracic masses.

The baby develops severe respiratory distress soon after birth and has significant ventilator needs. The babies develop marked hypoxia and hypercarbia and may quickly progress to develop significant PPHN. The lungs are very stiff and prone to develop pneumothoraces. A significant number of babies with severe pulmonary hypoplasia die in immediate or early neonatal period.

Management involves specific ventilation strategies including early promotion to high frequency oscillatory ventilation and drainage of pneumothorax as well as cardiovascular support.

Pulmonary Hemorrhage

This is one of the important respiratory emergencies that occur more commonly in preterm babies and term infants with intrauterine growth retardation. The typical scenario is an extremely preterm baby on ventilator with a stable clinical condition and infant suddenly starts to pour blood stained fluid or fresh blood through the endotracheal tube. This is immediately followed by worsening of the ventilator status and circulatory collapse and metabolic acidosis. The incidence is inversely related to the gestational age and is thought to be caused by mechanical ventilation for management of respiratory distress syndrome (RDS). These babies are likely to have significant patent ductus arteriosus (PDA) leading on to development of hemorrhagic pulmonary edema. The treatment involves the following steps:

- Maintaining adequate respiratory status by providing appropriate ventilatory support such as increasing PIP, high PEEP to provide stenting effect or HFOV.
- Cardiovascular resuscitation by intravenous infusion of fresh frozen plasma, packed red blood cells or normal saline. Inotropic support is mostly required.
- Correction of any bleeding diathesis by giving vitamin K, cryoprecipitate or platelet transfusion.
- Medical or surgical treatment of PDA once the baby is stable and has an echo confirmation of a hemodynamically significant PDA.

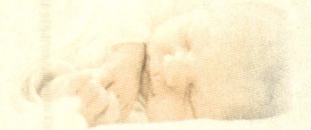

BIBLIOGRAPHY

Ali K, Bendapudi P, Polubothu S, Andradi G, Ofuya M, Peacock J, Hickey A, Davenport M, Nicolaides K, Greenough A. Congenital diaphragmatic hernia: influence of fetoscopic tracheal occlusion on outcomes and predictors of survival. *Eur J Pediatr* 2016 Aug; 175(8):1071–6.

Bahrami KR, Van Meurs KP. ECMO for neonatal respiratory failure. *Semin Perinatol* 2005 Feb; 29(1):15–23.

Bruschettini M, Romantsik O, Ramenghi LA, Zappettini S, O'Donnell CP, Calevo MG. Needle aspiration versus intercostal tube drainage for pneumothorax in the newborn. *Cochrane Database Syst Rev* 2016 Jan 11; (1):CD011724.

Donn SM and Sinha SK (Eds). *Manual of Neonatal Respiratory Care.* 4th ed. *Springer Publications,* 2016.

Engle WA. American Academy of Pediatrics Committee on Fetus and Newborn. Surfactant replacement therapy for respiratory distress in the preterm and term neonate. *Pediatrics.* 2008; 12: 419–32.

Gelfand SL, Fanaroff JM, Walsh MC. Meconium stained fluid: approach to mother and the baby. *Pediatr Clin North Am* 2004; 51:655–67.

Halliday HL. Recent clinical trials of surfactant treatment of neonate. *Biol Neonate* 2006; 30:296–304.

MacKinnon JA, Perlman M, Kirpalani H, Rehan V, Sauve R, Kovacs L. Spinal cord injury at birth: diagnostic and prognostic data in twenty-two patients. *J Pediatr* 1993 Mar; 122(3):431–7.

Martin, RJ, Fanaroff, AA, Walsh, MC (Eds). Neonatal-Perinatal Medicine. 10th ed. *Elsevier Publications,* 2015, pp 1113–1146.

Murki S, Deorari AK, Vidyasagar D. Use of CPAP and surfactant therapy in newborns with respiratory distress syndrome. *Indian J Pediatr* 2014; 81(5):481–88.

Pedroso JL, Baiense RF, Scalzaretto AP, Neto PB, Teixeira de Gois AF, Ferraz ME. Ondine's curse after brainstem infarction. *Neurol India* 2009 Apr; 57:206–7.

Pfister RH, Soll RF. Initial respiratory support of preterm infants. The role of CPAP, INSURE methods and non-invasive ventilation. *Clin Perinatol* 2012; 39:459–81.

Sinha S, Miall L and Jardine L (Eds). Essential Neonatal Medicine. 5th ed. *Wiley Blackwell Publications,* 2012, pp 145–187.

Snoek KG, Reiss IK, Greenough A, Capolupo I, Urlesberger B, Wessel L, Storme L, Deprest J, Schaible T, van Heijst A, Tibboel D; CDH EURO Consortium. Standardized postnatal management of infants with congenital diaphragmatic hernia in Europe: The CDH EURO Consortium Consensus - 2015 Update. *Neonatology* 2016; 110(1):66–74.

Sweet DG, Carnielli V, Greisein G et al. European Consensus Guidelines on the Management of Neonatal Respiratory Distress Syndrome in Preterm Infant 2010 update. *Neonatology* 2010; 91:402–17.

Weese-Mayer DE, Berry-Kravis EM, Ceccherini I et al. An official ATS clinical policy statement: congenital central hypoventilation syndrome: genetic basis, diagnosis, and management. *Am J Respir Crit Care Med* 2010 Mar 15; 181:626–44.

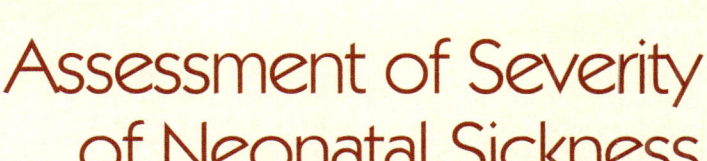

15

Assessment of Severity of Neonatal Sickness

Piyush Shah and Sanjay Wazir

Introduction

Every newborn must undergo a clinical assessment soon after birth, which guides newborn resuscitation in the delivery room. The assessment helps the attending pediatrician to provide a triage of care to the neonate in the special care unit or high dependency neonatal intensive care unit (NICU). During NICU care, the baby is constantly observed, monitored and assessed to either escalate or de-escalate treatment options. The assessment of a sick newborn helps not only in planning care of the baby but is useful to prognosticate the outcome. Every neonate must have successful transition from dependent fetal life to independent neonatal existence with effective breathing (ventilation and oxygenation), ability to maintain body temperature, tolerate and metabolize enteral feeds and excrete waste products.

The ability of a newborn to achieve the above independent physiological needs is inversely proportional to the gestational age and birth weight. The time honored Apgar score for assessment of a neonate at birth was proposed by Virginia Apgar in 1952.

Apgar Score

Apgar score can be remembered by the acronyn, **A**ppearance, **G**rimace, **A**ctivity and **R**espiration (Table 15.1). It remained a popular tool for assessment of a neonate at birth and make decisions for resuscitation of baby who is faced with a difficult transition from a dependent fetal life to independent breathing and effective circulation after birth. It is no longer used to make decisions for resuscitation but Apgar score at 5 minutes or later is useful to prognosticate the outcome of an asphyxiated newborn. The decision for resuscitation is now based on a single criterian whether a baby is

breathing or apneic at birth because all other criteria of Apgar score or wellbeing of the baby are dependent on whether a baby is having effective independent breathing or not. However, when Apgar score at 5-minute or later is 3 or less, despite resuscitation efforts, the infant is at risk to develop hypoxic ischemic encephalopathy (HIE) and neuromotor disability later in life. When Apgar score is low at 1-minute, it should be assessed every 5-minute till the score is 7 or more. In view of the limitation of clinical assessment of heart rate, it is recommended to assess the oxygen status and heart rate of an asphyxiated neonate with the help of a pulse oximeter. According to International Liaison Committee on Resuscitation (ILCOR) guidelines 2015, if there is no heartbeat at 10 minutes or later, the attempts at resuscitation may he abandoned because these infants are likely to die or develop severe neuromotor disability on survival. However, because of the availability of therapeutic hypothermia, these guidelines may need to be revised when more data is available.

Table 15.1 Apgar scoring system			
		Score	
Criteria	0	1	2
▪ Breathing	Absent	Slow, gasping	Crying
▪ Heart rate/min	Absent	Up to 100	More than 100
▪ Muscle tone	Flaccid	In-between	Fully flexed
▪ Reflex response*	Nil	Grimace	Cough, sneeze, cry
▪ Color	Blue or pale	Peripheral cyanosis	Pink

*By inserting a catheter in the nostrils or tactile stimulation

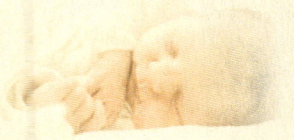

Breathing

Effective breathing is essential for ventilation and oxygenation. The minute ventilation depends upon tidal volume × respiratory rate. Tidal volume is decreased in various conditions with decreased compliance, e.g. surfactant deficiency, pneumonia, aspiration, pulmonary hypoplasia, etc. In order to compensate for decrease in tidal volume, the newborn breathes faster to maintain the oxygenation. In a term neonate, the resting respiratory rate varies between 40–60/min and there is no grunt or retractions.

Respiratory distress is diagnosed if 2 or more of the following signs are present; namely tachypnea (RR >60/min), grunt and increased work of breathing (subcostal, intercostal, suprasternal retractions, flaring of *alae nasi*).

Respiratory failure is defined as ineffective ventilation or oxygenation or both. It is characterised by increasing respiratory distress with low arterial oxygen saturations on pulse oximetry ($SpO_2 \leq 93\%$), low partial pressure of oxygen on the arterial blood gas ($PaO_2 \leq 60$ mmHg) and/or high partial pressure of carbon dioxide ($PaCO_2 \geq 45$ mmHg) with respiratory acidosis (pH ≤ 7.2). It may lead to apnea with cyanosis and non-responsiveness.

Clinical Scores to Assess the Severity of Respiratory Distress

A number of scores are available to assess the severity of respiratory distress (Table 15.2 and Figure 15.1).

Table 15.2 Modified Downes score

Criteria	Score		
	0	*1*	*2*
Respiratory rate (breaths/min)	<60	60–80	>80
Cyanosis	None	In room air	In 40% oxygen
Retractions	None	Mild	Moderate-severe
Grunting	None	Audible with stethoscope	Audible without stethoscope
Air entry	Good	Decreased	Barely audible

Source: Downes JJ, Vidyasagar D, Boggs TE, Morrow GM. *Clin Pediatr* 1970; 9:325–31.

When score is worsening, blood gases should be analyzed and timely decision made to provid CPAP or assisted ventilation.

Oxygen Saturation (SpO_2, SaO_2)

Pulse oximetry is a simple noninvasive method to assess arterial oxygen saturation. It also provides reliable estimate of heart rate. It should be recorded from right arm (pre-ductal). SpO_2 of $\leq 90\%$ in room air or $\leq 93\%$ when receiving oxygen through head box is suggestive of hypoxia. It is desirable to make early diagnosis of congenital malformations, aspiration syndromes and bronchopneumonia. The presence of reduced lung volume due to atelectasis and white out reticular granular pattern are suggestive of idiopathic RDS.

	Retractions of upper chest	Retractions of lower chest	Xiphoid retractions	Flaring of nostrils	Expiratory grunt
Grade 0	Synchronized	No retractions	None	None	None
Grade 1	Lag on inspiration	Just visible	Just visible	Minimal	With stethoscope
Grade 2	See-saw movements	Marked	Marked	Marked	Naked ear

Source: Silverman WA, Anderson DH. *Pediatrics* 1956; 171(1):1–10.

Figure 15.1 Silverman–Anderson score.

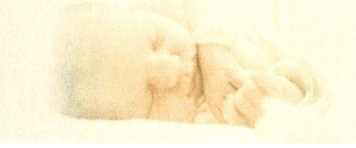

Respiratory acidosis on ABGs is diagnosed on the basis of pH ≤7.2, $PaCO_2$ ≥45 mm of Hg and worsening oxygenation with PaO_2 < 60 mmHg on supplemental oxygen.

Cardiovascular Status

Heart rate (HR) Heart rate of 100–160/min in a term and 120–180/min in a preterm is considered normal. In a resting or sleep state, HR may fall to as low as 80/min in term and 100/min in preterm neonates. Tachycardia may occur due to hyperthermia, handling, pain, septicemia, anemia and shock. Bradycardia may occur due to hypoxia and congenital heart block.

Blood pressure Both invasive intra-arterial and non-invasive oscillometric BP monitoring is used in the NICU. The noninvasive method is unreliable in critically sick infants with severe hypotension and shock. The BP norms are based on gestational age or birth weight and postnatal age of the infant. The diagnosis of hypotension is made when systolic BP is ≤30 mmHg, mean BP less than the gestational age in weeks, or a low BP value associated with clinical evidences of end organ perfusion failure (decreased urine output, poor peripheral perfusion, and/or lactic acidosis).

Cardiac output It is calculated by multiplying HR with stroke volume. The delivery of oxygen to the tissues depends upon cardiac ouput and content of oxygen in arterial blood.

Capillary refill time (CRT) CRT is useful to assess peripheral perfusion in the newborn. It is checked over the upper sternum and is less than 2 sec in a healthy term infant. In stable VLBW babies, CRT may be 3 sec or more. It is a crude marker of peripheral perfusion. The prolonged CRT may be associated with marked differences between core and peripheral body temperature.

Serum lactate It is a useful indirect marker of cellular oxygen delivery. Elevated levels of serum lactate of >4 mmol/L, has been shown to correlate with low superior vena cava (SVC) flow in preterm infants. This suggests decreased blood flow to brain because of decreased end organ perfusion. A single value of serum lactate is unreliable but elevated values of lactate on serial measurements are suggestive of compromised circulation and adverse outcome.

Arterial oxygen saturation (SpO$_2$) The use of SpO_2 measurement after 24 hours of life is increasingly used to screen a neonate for duct dependent congenital cardiac defect (Figure 15.2). The point-of-care echocardiography is done when an infant fails SpO_2 screen.

Functional echocardiography Doppler studies to measure blood flow and myocardial contractibility, are being increasingly used to guide hemodynamic management of sick neonates in NICU. The point-of-care functional echocardiography requires expertise and resources which may not be readily available.

Near infrared spectroscopy (NIRS) NIRS is a useful modality to measure end organ perfusion. It is increasingly being validated for use in preterm neonates. It uses the technique of calculating blood flow based on changes in oxygenation over time or the difference between oxygenated and deoxygenated hemoglobin. Both cerebral blood flow and splanchnic circulation can be checked to assess blood flow and adequacy of circulation.

Based on the aforementioned observations, no single cardiovascular vital finding can assist in precise prognostication of a sick neonate. There is a need to use multiple vital parameters (tachycardia, low mean BP, rising serum lactate levels) along with evidences of poor end organ perfusion (decreased urine output, delayed CRT, hypothermia, increasing difference between core and peripheral temperatures, altered sensorium) to assess the cardiovascular status of the baby.

Body Temperature

Hypothermia is an important contributor to both morbidity and mortality in newborns. WHO defines hypothermia as core body temperature below normal range (36.5°C–37.5°C) and is further classified as mild (36.0°C–36.5°C), moderate (32°C–35.9°C), and severe (<32°C) hypothermia (Figure 15.3). The likelihood of development of hypothermia in a newborn is inversely related to birth weight and gestational age of the infant. Both, extreme preterm (≤28 weeks) and/or extreme low birth weight (ELBW, ≤1000 gm), infants are vulnerable to develop hypothermia.

The severity of hypothermia is directly associated with morbidity and mortality. The clinical manifestations of hypothermia include cold trunk and extremities to touch, acrocyanosis, skin mottling, bradycardia, apnea, decreased activity, poor feeding and poor weight gain. The comorbidities secondary to hypothermia include metabolic acidosis, hypoxia, hypoglycemia, pulmonary vasoconstriction and thermal shock with DIC, and multi-organ failure.

Hyperthermia (temperature >37.5°C), is also associated with adverse outcome. Hyperthermia may occur due to raised environmental temperature in summer or due to life-threatening disorders like sepsis (often causes hypothermia in a preterm infant), meningitis,

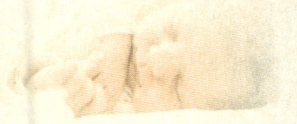

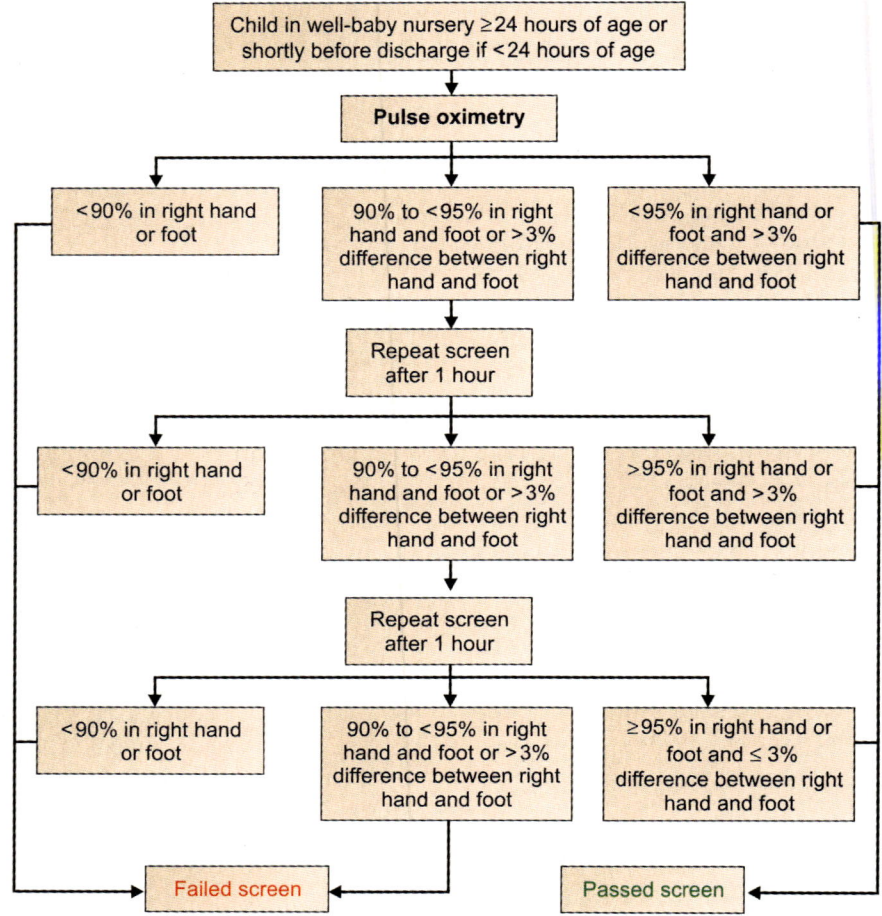

Figure 15.2 Screening for congenital heart disease.

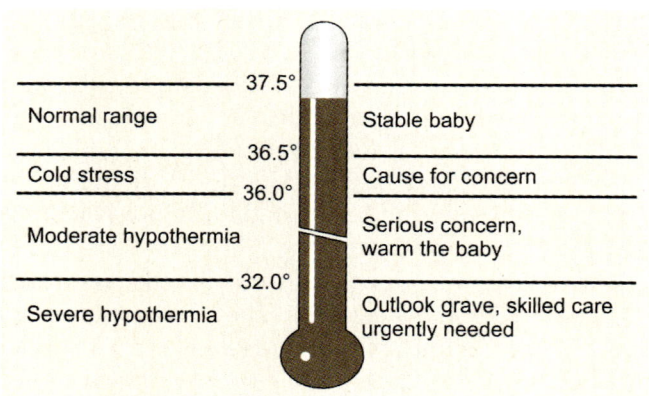

Figure 15.3 WHO classification of hypothermia in the newborn.

dehydration, and malnutrition. Hyperthermia in NICU is likely to be due to iatrogenic causes, dislodgement of skin probe of servo control system or high set up of ambient temperature on manual control mode of overhead warmer. Other causes of accidental hyperthermia in ELBW neonates include intraventricular hemorrhage and burns due to electrocution.

Central Nervous System

Healthy term neonate has a flexed posture with increased muscle tone, and normal automatic reflexes (Moro's, rooting, sucking, plantar reflex). They have long hours of sleep, wake up and are alert for short periods. The tone, primitive reflexes, and posture are inversely related to the gestational age. Preterm infants are hypotonic, with extended posture and poor reflexes. Therefore, lethargy, poor feeding, hypotonia, depressed neonatal reflexes which are inappropriate for the gestation are suggestive of a sick newborn. Similarly, a full or tense anterior fontanel, abnormal movements, hypertonia, opisthotonos, apnea, poor sucking or a change in sucking behavior is associated with poor outcome.

In literature, various scoring systems are available to assess the neurologic status of the baby (Tables 15.3, 15.4 and 15.5). They have been originally developed to assess infants with hypoxic-ischemic encephalopathy (HIE) but can be used assess prognosis of encephalopathy due to any cause.

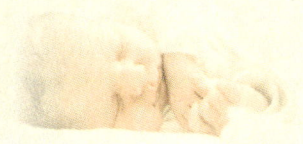

Table 15.3 Levene scoring for hypoxic ischemic encephalopathy

Feature	Mild	Moderate	Severe
Consciousness	Irritable	Lethargic	Comatose
Tone	Hypotonia	Marked hypotonia	Severe hypotonia
Seizures	None	Common	Persistent
Sucking/respiration	Poor suck	Unable to suck	No spontaneous breathing

Source: Levene MI. The asphyxiated newborn infant. In: Levene MI, Lilford RJ. Fetal and Neonatal Neurology and Neurosurgery. *Edinburgh; Churchill Livingstone*, 1995, pp 405–26.

Table 15.4 Sarnat scoring system for various stages of hypoxic ischemic encephalopathy

Feature	Stage 1	Stage 2	Stage 3
Consciousness	Hyper-alert	Lethargic	Stupor or coma
Muscle tone	Normal	Hypotonia	Flaccidity
Tendon reflexes	Normal/increased	Increased	Depressed/absent
Seizures	None	Present, focal or multifocal	Uncommon except decerebration
Sucking	Active	Weak	Absent
Moro	Exaggerated	Incomplete	Absent
Grasping	Normal/exaggerated	Exaggerated	Absent
Pupils	Dilated, reactive	Small, reactive	Variable, fixed
Occulocephalic reflex (Doll's eyes)	Normal	Over-reactive	Reduced/ absent

Source: Sarnat HB, Sarnat MS. Neontal encephalopathy following fetal distress, *Arch Neurol* 1976; 33(10):696–705.

Table 15.5 Thompson scoring system for hypoxic ischemic encephalopathy

Sign	Score			
	0	1	2	3
Tone	Normal	Increased tone	Hypotonia	Flaccid
Consciousness	Normal	Over-alert, stare	Lethargic	Comatose
Seizures	None	Infrequent, <3 per day	Frequent, >3 per day	None
Posture	Normal	Fisting, cycling	Distal flexion	Decerebrate
Moro	Normal	Partial	Absent	—
Grasp	Normal	Poor	Absent	—
Suck	Normal	Poor	Absent ± bites	—
Respiration	Normal	Hyperventilation	Apnea	—
Anterior fontanel	Normal	Full, not tense	Tense	—

Source: Thompson CM, Puterman AS, Linley LL, et al. The value of a scoring system for hypoxic ischemic encephalopathy in predicting neurodevelopmental outcome. *Acta Paediatr* 1997; 86(7):757–61.

Conventional EEG (cEEG) and amplitude integrated EEG (aEEG)

The conventional EEG (cEEG), is a gold standard for evaluating neurological activity, and is used as a valuable tool in early prediction of the neurodevelopmental outcome of neonates following brain injuries. cEEG receives electrocortical signals through at least nine electrodes attached to the scalp (maximum of 40 electrodes). The electrical activity is inversely proportional to the gestation, preterm infants having lower electrocortical signals and longer periods of brain inactivity than term healthy infants. cEEG recording for a duration of 45–60 mins usually provides the snapshot picture of the current electrical activity of the brain.

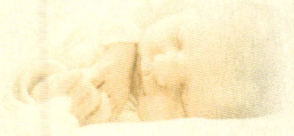

Amplitude-integrated EEG (aEEG), in contrast to cEEG, measures continuous electrocortical activity of the brain. It is recorded with a single- or double-channel EEG that uses 3–5 electrodes affixed to the scalp. It continuously captures the general background pattern of the brain activity in real time for an extended period. aEEG correlates with cEEG for monitoring background activity of the brain of a healthy and neurologically compromised neonates. It is reliable and sensitive for diagnosing neonatal seizures. However, aEEG tracings may not be sensitive enough to pick-up certain focal, low-amplitude and very short seizure episodes. In general, aEEG is being increasingly used for early detection of abnormal brain activity and provides guidelines for performing more definitive cEEG and detailed neurologic examination.

Biochemical Parameters

Glucose Hypoglycemia is diagnosed in neonates when serum glucose level is <40 mg/dL. The presence of hypoglycemia at admission is associated with increased morbidity and mortality in neonates.

Bilirubin levels Hyperbilirubinemia in the newborn is physiologically related to immature liver function during first week of life. The high levels of unconjugated bilirubin are associated with increased risk of bilirubin induced neuronal damage (BIND) causing kernicterus. The risk of BIND is inversely proportional to the maturity of blood brain barrier, thus lower gestation and higher levels of bilirubin in early life are likely to cause BIND. The assessment of severity of BIND is summarized in Tabe 15.6. The common causes for excessive rise of bilirubin include increased hemolysis of red blood cells (Rh or ABO incompatibility, G-6-PD deficiency), sepsis, and prematurity. The guidelines for management of neonatal hyperbilirubinemia are discussed in detail in Chapter 11.

Table 15.6 Bilirubin-induced neurologic dysfunction (BIND) score

Clinical features	Mild (score 1)	Moderate (score 2)	Severe (score 3)
Mental status	Sleepy and poor feeding	Lethargic and irritable	Semi coma and/or seizures
Muscle tone	Slight decrease	Hyper/hypotonia	Opisthotonos/decreased tone/increased bicycling movements
Character of cry	High pitched	Shrill	Inconsolable

Source: Johnson L, Bhutani VK. The clinical syndrome of bilirubin-induced neurologic dysfunction. *Semin Perinatol* 2011; 35(3):101–113.

Gastric Aspirate

The volume and quality of gastric residuals in an enterally fed neonate is useful to assess the tolerability of oral feeds. The volume of gastric residuals can be measured before administration of nasogastric feed in preterm infants. The presence of abdominal distension, excessive pre-feed gastric residuals (>50% of the last feed volume) and bilious or blood stained gastric aspirate are suggestive of feed intolerance due to dysmotlity of gut in a sick neonate. The common causes of feed intolerance and abdominal distension include ELBW babies or a sick baby having electrolyte imbalance, sepsis, necrotizing enterocolitis, shock and intestinal obstruction. When gastric aspirate is bilious green even after repositioning the nasogastric tube, surgical cause of intestinal obstruction should be ruled out.

SCORING SYSTEMS

Scoring systems are increasingly being used by clinicians and researchers to assess a sick neonate. They are useful to assess the prognosis and outcome when a neonate is critically sick. The scoring systems use appropriately weighted demographic, physiological, biochemical and clinical data to calculate a score to quantify the risk of morbidity and mortality in NICU babies.

The extremely low gestational age (ELGA) or birth weight (ELBW) babies are likely to have poor outcome, for example birth weight <500 g or gestational age <23 week is often used as a reason for a considered decision to deny intensive care. The clinical scores are usually derived from observations collected over a period of hours or days, and then collectively used to predict the outcome. The scoring system is useful to assess and compare the outcome of sick neonates in various neonatal intensive care units. The utility of clinical score for assessment of an individual baby is less useful, and only serves as a quality control or a research tool. The commonly used clinical scores such as CRIB, CRIB II, SNAP, BERLIN, etc. as summarized in Table 15.7. The variables amongst different scores are extensive and rather cumbersome. They serve as a useful research tool to compare a large number of interventions to improve the outcome of sick neonates. However, for an individual baby, simple score like TOPS score [temperature at admission, oxygenation (SpO$_2$), perfusion and blood sugar] have been used and found to have similar predictive value compared to complex scoring system like CRIB II. Some of these scores are used to assess the risk of transport of sick neonates.

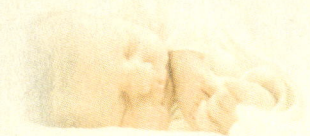

Table 15.7 The available scoring systems for objective assessment of sick neonates

CRIB I
Birth weight
Gestation
Congenital malformation
Maximum base deficit in first 12 h
Minimum appropriate FiO_2 in first 12 h
Maximum appropriate FiO_2 in first 12 h

CRIB II
Birth weight by gestation
Maximum base deficit in first 12 h
Sex
Admission temperature

BERLIN score
Birth weight
Grade of RDS
Apgar score at 5 min
Artificial ventilation
Base excess at admission

NICHD score
Birth weight
Small-for-gestational age
Race
Sex
Apgar score at 1 min

NMPI
Gestational age
Birth weight
Cardiac arrest
PaO_2/FiO_2 ratio
Major congenital malformations
Sepsis
Base excess

SINKIN 12 hour
Birth weight
Gestational age
Apgar score at 5 min
Peak inspiratory pressure at 12 h

NBRS
Blood pH
Hypoglycemia
Intraventricular hemorrhage
Periventricular leucomalacia
Seizures
Infection
Need for mechanical ventilation

SNAP-I
Blood pressure
Heart rate
Respiratory rate
Temperature
PaO_2
PaO_2/FiO_2 ratio
$PaCO_2$
Oxygenation index
Packed cell volume
White blood cell count
Immature to total white blood cell ratio
Absolute neutrophil count
Platelet count
Blood urea nitrogen
Creatinine
Urine output
Indirect bilirubin
Direct bilirubin
Sodium
Potassium
Calcium (ionised)
Calcium (total)
Glucose
Serum bicarbonate
Serum pH
Seizure
Apnea
Stool guaiac

SNAP-II
SNAP **plus**
Mean blood pressure
Lowest temperature
PaO_2/FiO_2 ratio
Serum pH
Multiple seizures
Urine output

SNAP-PE I
SNAP score **plus**
Birth weight
Apgar score <7 at 5 min
Small-for-gestational age

SNAP-PE II
SNAP II score **plus**
Birth weight ≤749 g
Apgar score <7 at 5 min

NTISS
Supplemental oxygen
Surfactant administration
Tracheostomy placement
CPAP administration
Endotracheal intubation
Mechanical ventilation
Mechanical ventilation with paralysis
High frequency ventilation
Extracorporeal membrane oxygenation
Indomethacin administration
Volume expansion
Vasopressor administration
Pacemaker on standby
Pacemaker used
Cardiopulmonary resuscitation
Antibiotics
Diuretics (enteral)
Steroids (postnatal)
Anticonvulsants
Aminophylline
Other unscheduled medications
Diuretics (parenteral)
Treatment of metabolic acidosis
Potassium binding resin
Frequent vital signs
Cardiorespiratory monitoring
Phlebotomy
Thermoregulated environment
Noninvasive oxygen monitoring
Arterial pressure monitoring
CVP monitoring
Urinary catheter
Quantitative intake and output
Gavage feeding
Intravenous fat emulsion
Intravenous amino acid solution
Phototherapy
Insulin administration
Potassium infusion
Transfusion
Intravenous γ-globulin
Red blood cell transfusion
Partial volume exchange transfusion
Pericardial tube

CRIB: clinical risk index for babies; FiO_2: fractional inspired concentration of oxygen; NICHD: national institute of child health and human development. NBRS: neurobiological risk score; NMPI: neonatal mortality prognosis index; NTISS: neonatal therapeutic intervention scoring system; PO_2: partial pressure of oxygen; RDS: respiratory distress syndrome; SNAP: score for neonatal acute physiology; SNAP-PE: score for neonatal acute physiology-perinatal extension.

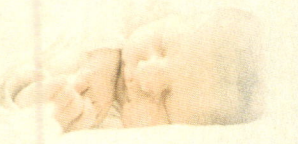

CONCLUSION

The assessment of severity of disease process in a sick newborn requires a constellation of a number of clinical and laboratory parameters. The individual or a single parameter per se is not reliable to judge the severity of disease process. Also, the disease process is dynamic in nature and therefore, a continuum of assessment is mandatory for better prognostication and management strategies compared to one time or isolated assessment.

BIBLIOGRAPHY

Broughton SJ, Berry A, Jacobe S, Cheeseman P, Tarnow-Mordi WO. The mortality index for neonatal transportation score: A new mortality prediction model for retrieved neonates. *Pediatrics* 2004; 114(4):e424–31.

Dammann O, Shah B, Naples M, et al. Interinstitutional variations in prediction of death by SNAP-II and SNAPPE-II among extremely preterm infants. *Pediatrics* 2009, 124(5):e1001–1006.

Dawnes JJ, Vidyasagar D, Boggs TR, Morrow GM. Respiratory distress syndrome of newborn infants: 1. New clinical scoring system (RDS score) with acid-base and blood gas correlations. *Clin Pediatr* 1970 Jun, 9(5):325–31.

Dorling JS, Field DJ, Manktelow B. Neonatal disease severity scoring systems. *Arch Dis Child Fetal Neonatal Ed* 2005; 90:F11–F16.

Gagliardi L, Cavazza A, Brunelli A, Battaglioli M, et al. Assessing mortality risk in very low birth weight infants: a comparison of CRIB, CRIB-II and SNAPPE-II. *Arch Dis Child Fetal Neonatal Ed* 2004; 89:F419–F422.

Maier RF, Rey M, Metz BC, Obladen M. Comparison of mortality risk: a score for very low birth weight infants. *Arch Dis Child Fetal Neonatal Ed* 1997, 76:F146–F150.

Mathur NB, Arora D. Role of TOPS (a simplified assessment of neonatal acute physiology) in predicting mortality in transported neonates. *Acta Paediatr* 2007, 96(2):172–75.

Parry G, Tucker J, Tarnow-Mordi W. CRIB II: an update of the clinical risk index for babies score. *Lancet* 2003; 361:1789–91.

Richardson DK, Corcoran JD, Eseobar GJ, Lee SK. SNAP-II and SNAPPE-II: simplified newborn illness severity and mortality risk scores. *J Pediatr* 2001; 138(1):92–100.

Richardson DK, Gray JE, McCormic MC, Workman K, Goldmann DA. Score for neonatal acute physiology: a physiologic severity index for neonatal intensive care. *Pediatrics* 1993; 91(3);617–23.

Shannon M, Groer M, Keller G, Ashmeade T. A systematic review: The utility of revised version of the score for neonatal acute physiology among critically ill neonates. *J Perinat Neonatal Nurs* 2015 Oct–Dec, 29(4):315–44.

Silverman WA, Anderson DH. A controlled clinical trial of effects of water and mist or obstructive respiratory signs, death rate and necropsy findings among premature infants. *Pediatrics* 1956,17(1):1–10.

The International Neonatal Network. The CRIB (clinical risk index for babies) score: a tool for assessing initial neonatal risk and comparing performance of neonatal intensive care units. *Lancet* 1993; 342:193–98.

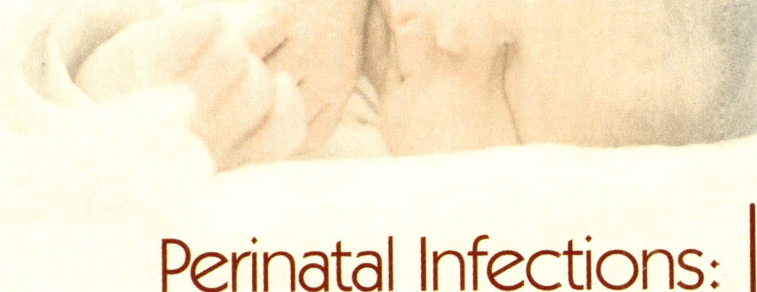

16

Perinatal Infections: Bacterial and Spirochetal

Suja Mariam and Praveen Kumar

BACTERIAL INFECTIONS

Bacterial infections are a major indication for admission to neonatal emergency and intensive care units. They contribute to nearly one-third of neonatal mortality worldwide. In India, sepsis contributes up to 52% of neonatal deaths in community and 36% of deaths in hospitalized newborns. With advances in technology, more and more preterm newborns are surviving initial neonatal period, they have a prolonged stay in the NICU and succumb to hospital acquired infections subsequently.

Neonatal sepsis is a diagnostic and therapeutic challenge. It is crucial to accurately determine without delay whether a symptomatic baby is infected or not because neonatal sepsis carries high case fatality rate. The disease can progress rapidly in 'apparently well appearing' newborns, more so in preterm neonates.

Definitions

Neonatal sepsis is defined as the presence of genera- lized systemic features of sepsis associated with pure growth of bacteria from one or more sites which are known as sterile. Box 16.1 shows the criteria for diagnosing systemic inflammatory response syndrome (SIRS).

Probable sepsis The clinical and laboratory findings are consistent with bacterial infection but blood culture is sterile or contaminant.

Severe sepsis Sepsis associated with cardiovascular dys- function (hypoperfusion abnormalities or hypotension) or acute respiratory distress syndrome or dysfunction of 2 or more of other organ systems. Manifestations of hypoperfusion include but are not limited to prolonged capillary refill time, borderline blood pressure, lactic acidosis, oliguria or an acute alteration in sensorium.

BOX 16.1 Systemic inflammatory response syndrome (SIRS)

The presence of at least two of the following four criteria, one of which must be abnormal temperature or leukocyte count.

- Core temperature of >101.3°F (38.5°C) or <96.8°F (36°C) and/ or leukocyte count elevated or depressed for age or >20% immature to total neutrophil ratio or C-reactive protein >10 mg/dL.
- Tachycardia, defined as a mean heart rate >cut-off in the absence of medications or painful stimuli; or otherwise unexplained persistent elevation of heart rate 20% above baseline over a 0.5- to 4-hr time period.
- Bradycardia, defined as a mean heart rate < cut-off for age in the absence of external vagal stimulus, beta blocker drugs, or congenital heart disease; or otherwise unexplained persistent depression of heart rate 20% below baseline over a 0.5-hr time period.
- Mean respiratory rate > 60 per minute or mechanical ventila- tion for an acute process not related to underlying surfactant deficiency or neuromuscular disease or administration of general anesthesia.

Septic shock Sepsis-induced hypotension despite fluid resuscitation.

Multi-organ dysfunction syndrome Presence of altered functions of several body organs in an acutely ill septic neonate so that homeostasis cannot be maintained without intervention.

Classification

Neonatal sepsis is classified into early-onset and late- onset sepsis on the basis of age at onset of symptoms. Early-onset sepsis (EOS) is defined as any evidence of infection presenting before 48–72 hours of life. However, the median time of presentation is about 6 hours and a large proportion of symptoms are present within first 2 hours of life. In EOS, the neonate acquire the bacteria from mother (vertical transmission). Late- onset sepsis (LOS) refers to an infection which is acquired after 48–72 hours of life. The infection is acquired after birth either during resuscitation or subsequently from personnel, patients and fomites either from community or hospital environment.

In developing countries, due to poor aseptic practices in the delivery room, health care associated infections (HAIs) may be acquired early and can manifest within 24 to 72 hours of age. The classical late-onset HAIs most commonly present within first week of hospital stay in India when maximum interventions take place, unlike in the developed countries, where they manifest after 2 to 4 weeks of NICU stay.

Incidence

The incidence of hospital-acquired neonatal sepsis in our country as per National Neonatal-Perinatal Database (NNPD) in the year 2002–03 was 30 per 1000 live births in contrast to developed countries where incidence of neonatal sepsis is less than 1 per 1000 live births. EOS contributed to 67% of infections in NNPD data while in a recent study from Delhi, 83 % of infections had an onset within 72 hours of age.

With improved obstetric care and use of intrapartum antibiotics, the incidence of early onset neonatal sepsis is decreasing. However, it still contributes to a major proportion of neonates who receive antibiotics. The diagnosis of EOS may be missed or delayed due to lack of clear cut risk factors or correlates and poor predictive value of laboratory tests in the first few days of life. The actual community based incidence and burden of early onset/perinatal sepsis is likely to be under reported from developing countries in view of home deliveries, lack of availability of diagnostic tests, and poor reporting system.

Pathogenesis

Bacteria can reach the fetus from mother to the neonate or from environment through multiple routes.

- A maternal bloodstream infection can cause placental invasion and placentitis leading to fetal bloodstream infection.
- Maternal bloodstream infection may cause invasion of amniotic fluid which is swallowed by fetus causing pneumonitis.
- Direct invasion of the amniotic fluid may occur by procedures like amniocentesis or intrauterine transfusion.
- Bacteria colonizing maternal genital tract can reach the fetus through following routes:
  a. Ascending infection through intact membranes.
  b. Ascending infection through ruptured membranes.

c. Infection of neonate while passing through birth canal during delivery.

The incidence of amniotic fluid invasion in women with term pregnancy is <1% while it increases to 32% in women with preterm labor with intact membranes , and up to 75% in women with preterm premature rupture of membranes (pPROM).

There are many factors which predispose a neonate, who has been colonized with pathogenic bacteria either from maternal or hospital environment, to develop serious infection. One of the most important risk factors is immaturity of immune system of the neonate. There is no transplacental transfer of IgM antibodies which can protect against *Enterobacteriaceae*. The preterm neonates do not get the full quota of IgG from mother which gets maximally transferred after 32 weeks of gestation and infants do not produce sufficient quantities of IgG antibodies until 3 months of life. Moreover, complement system protein levels and phagocytic capacity of neutrophils is greatly reduced in neonates as compared to an adult.

Risk Factors for Perinatal Bacterial Infections

The maternal risk factors associated with an increased risk of perinatal bacterial infection are listed below.

- Prolonged labor >24 hours
- Prolonged rupture of membranes >18 hours
- Foul smelling liquor
- Clinical or subclinical chorioamnionitis
- Single unclean/>3 sterile vaginal examinations
- Maternal urinary tract infection
- Preterm or very low birth weight infants
- Male infants

The probability of an infant born to a woman with clinical chorioamnionitis or foul smelling liquor, to develop EOS is very high. However, the risk of EOS in infants born with other risk factors is relatively low. Therefore, presence of 3 or more aforementioned risk factors is considered to have a high probability for occurrence of EOS in the newborn. Scoring systems taking into account the differential risks associated with different factors have also been derived to predict the risk of EOS among asymptomatic neonates born at <35 weeks gestation (Box 16.2).

Bacteriology

The bacteriology of EOS has both temporal and geographic differences. In developed countries, in early 20th century, Gram-negative bacilli were the most common organisms causing EOS. After 1960s, Group B streptococcus (GBS) became the most common organism in developed countries. At present GBS and

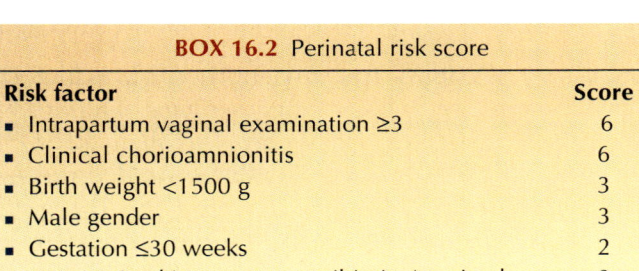

BOX 16.2 Perinatal risk score

Risk factor	Score
▪ Intrapartum vaginal examination ≥3	6
▪ Clinical chorioamnionitis	6
▪ Birth weight <1500 g	3
▪ Male gender	3
▪ Gestation ≤30 weeks	2
▪ Not received intrapartum antibiotics/received antibiotics <4 hours prior to delivery	2

▪ Neonates with a score of ≤7 should be empirically started on antibiotics. A blood culture must be sent prior to initiation of antibiotics. However, lumbar puncture need not be done in asymptomatic neonates unless blood culture is positive. Neonates with a risk score of 0–6 should be carefully monitored for features of sepsis atleast for 72 hours.

▪ Neonates with extreme risk factors like (a) very prolonged rupture of membranes (≤72 hours), (b) very prolonged labor (≥24 hours), (c) foul smelling liquor, (d) unclean per vaginal examinations, (e) maternal septicemia or other systemic infections, must be started on empirical antibiotics, irrespective of the score.

E. coli contribute to more than 70% of EOS in developed countries. Late-onset sepsis in developed countries is most commonly due to coagulase negative staphylococci (CONS), *E. coli* and Candida spp.

In developing countries like India, Gram-negative bacteria like *K. pneumoniae* and *E. coli* contribute to the major burden of EOS. The National Neonatal-Perinatal Database (NNPD) project reported 1248 isolates from 18 hospitals in 2002–03. The most common organisms were *K. pneumoniae*, *Staphylococcus aureus* and *E. coli* (Figure 16.1). There was no difference between intramural and extramural babies. Over the years, multi-drug resistant Acinetobacter especially *Acinetobacter baumanii* has emerged as the most important organism in overcrowded hospitals receiving a large number of outborn referrals and walk-in deliveries. In a recent study from three Delhi hospitals, of the 1005 isolates, Acinetobacter spp (22%), Klebsiella spp (17%) and *E. coli* (14%) were the major organisms with multi-drug resistance. *Acinetobacter baumanii* is not only notorious because of high drug resistance rates but it also frequently leads to meningitis and ventriculitis. It has also been documented that in our country, there is no significant difference in the bacteriology of early-onset and late-onset sepsis.

Staphylococcus aureus, which used to be very common, has decreased in incidence over the years with better implementation of hand hygiene practices. However, coagulase negative *Staphylococcus aureus* (CONS), which is a common inhabitant of skin and mucus membranes, has emerged as an important pathogen in the intensive care unit, especially in very low birth weight infants.

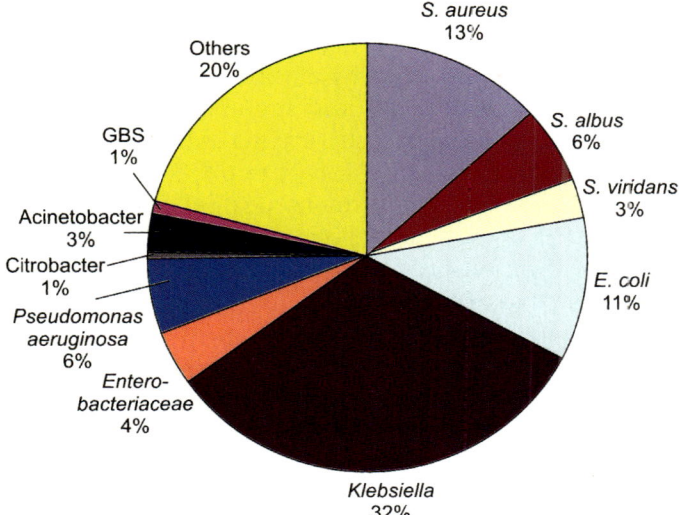

A. Bacteriology in intramural neonates

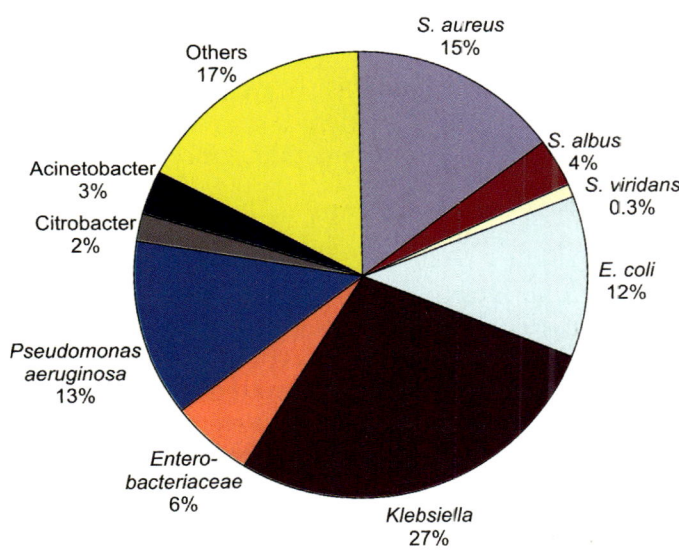

B. Bacteriology in extramural neonates

Figure 16.1 Organisms causing sepsis in newborn (*Source:* NNPD 2002-2003).

In the recent Delhi study, CONS and *Staphylococcus aureus* contributed to 15% and 12% of isolates respectively. Among these isolates, 61% and 38% were methicillin resistent respectively.

Clinical Features

The neonate responds to sepsis in a stereotyped manner as in case of other perinatal disorders. Therefore, the symptoms and signs are widely variable and non-specific. EOS typically presents with respiratory symptoms and signs which may progress to involve other organ systems. In hospitalized preterm infants, the common symptoms of LOS include lethargy/hypotonia, tachycardia or bradycardia, fever, abdominal distension, increased or altered gastric aspirates, chest, retractions, grunting, hypotension/prolonged capillary refill time, apnea, abnormal skin color, increased ventilator requirements and metabolic acidosis. In isolation, no single symptom or sign has high sensitivity or specificity. A combination of multiple features are more reliable to make a diagnosis. Sclerema, shock, features of disseminated intravascular coagulation (DIC), and pulmonary hemorrhage are late signs and are suggestive of severe sepsis.

In view of the widely varied non-specific features and frequent occurrence of sepsis, possibility of sepsis must be considered whenever there is clinical deterioration of a neonate, while alternative possibilities are being considered.

In the community setting, WHO Young Infant Study Group identified seven signs (history of difficulty in feeding, convulsions, body movements or arousal only when stimulated, respiratory rate of 60 breaths per minute or more, severe chest retractions, temperature of 37·5°C or more, or below 35·5°C) which have a reasonable sensitivity and specificity for predicting serious bacterial illness in infants less than 2 months of age.

Laboratory Investigations

Blood Culture

The gold standard for diagnosing septicemia in a symptomatic neonate is isolation of pathogenic bacteria from blood. Conventional blood culture systems are being replaced by semi-automated or automated systems like BACTEC. These systems detect CO_2 production by bacteria to diagnose growth. The advantage of these techniques include significantly shorter time to positivity and higher isolation rates as compared to conventional methods. Most positive cultures show bacterial growth within a maximum period of 24 to 48 hours. Single blood culture with 1.0 mL of blood is sufficient when special pediatric bottles are used. Inoculation of 0.5 mL of blood has been shown to be insufficient as low birth weight babies can be symptomatic even when CFU(colony forming unit) is less than 4/mL. The ideal method to draw blood for culture is through a fresh venipuncture. A freshly placed umbilical artery catheter is the next best alternative. Umbilical venous and other peripheral vascular catheters are not suitable for collecting blood sample for culture.

The major limitation of blood cultures is that it can take 24–72 hours to detect growth, identify the organism and do antibiotic sensitivity testing. Inadequate volume of inoculum, prior antibiotic exposure and improper collection technique can give both false negative as well as false-positive results.

Other Culture Studies

Urine culture Urinary tract infection in EOS is almost always secondary to bacteremic seeding. Therefore, urine culture is not required as part of work up for EOS. However, neonates 7 days or older should undergo urine culture as part of work up for LOS. The gold standard technique for collecting urine for culture is suprapubic aspiration. A freshly placed urethral catheter can be used as an alternative. Routine urine microscopy is not reliable in neonates.

Body surface culture There is no role of skin surface cultures from axilla, umbilicus or other body surfaces for diagnosis of sepsis.

Tracheal aspirate Routine tracheal aspirates have no role in the diagnosis of pneumonia. A semi-quantitative culture may be of some value if sample is collected from a freshly placed endotracheal tube.

Sepsis Screen

The inherent delay in getting blood culture report and frequent false negative results have led to a search for rapid diagnostic tests for neonatal sepsis. An ideal rapid diagnostic test should have high sensitivity and specificity, high positive and low negative likelihood ratio, 24 × 7 round-the-clock availability and short turn around time. No single test satisfies all of these criteria. The interpretation of all hematological and biochemical parameters is complicated by the wide normal ranges, especially in first 72 hours of life and the influence of perinatal events on hematological indices. The commonly used screening tests in clinical practice are described below:

i. *WBC count and neutrophil indices* Neonates with sepsis typically respond with lowering of WBC counts and increase in proportion of immature neutrophils. Total leucocyte counts and differential counts, though done frequently, often yield little because of the wide normal ranges. Neutrophil indices like absolute neutrophil count, absolute band cell count and immature to total neutrophil ratio (I/T ratio) have proved useful in ruling out rather than ruling in the diagnosis of sepsis. Amongst these, I/T ratio has best sensitivity and maximum negative predictive value. The interpretation of neutrophil counts should be based on nomograms. Recently, revised reference parameters have been published by Henry et al based on a very large database and they reiterate a very wide normal ranges and need for caution in their interpretation.

ii. *C-reactive protein (CRP)* CRP is an acute phase reactant secreted by liver in response to stimulation by interleukin-6. It starts rising 6 to 8 hours after an infection but peak concentrations are reached only after 24 to 48 hours. For this reason, sensitivity of CRP in first 8–12 hours is as low as 66%. After 24 hours, 2 sequential CRP values 8–12 hours apart, have a sensitivity of 99.7%. CRP levels are estimated reliably by immuno-turbidimetric and latex enhanced immuno-nephelometric assays. Varying cut-offs have been used in different studies. Using a cut-off of more than 10.0 mg/L is useful to reduce false positives due to non-infective conditions. Qualitative latex agglutination tests are often used at bedside but have high false-positive rates and several quality control issues.

Two normal CRP values 24 hours apart have been shown to have a negative predictive value of 99.7% and a negative likelihood ratio of 0.15 for proven neonatal sepsis. This can be used to discontinue antibiotics if the infant is well and culture is sterile.

iii. *Procalcitonin* Procalcitonin is a propeptide of calcitonin and is secreted by monocytes and hepatocytes. It increases within 2 hours of onset of infection and reaches peak values within 12 hours. The half-life in peripheral blood is about 24 hours. Instead of single absolute cut-off, age based nomograms should be used. Cheisa et al have published reference ranges for preterm as well as term infants. The normal value in first 48–72 hours can reach as high as 10 µg/L. In general, procalcitonin is more likely to be increased in bacterial rather than viral infections and is more sensitive and specific than CRP. However, it is much more expensive and is not widely available.

iv. Other biomarkers like interleukin-6, interleukin-8, tumor necrosis factor-α, INF-γ, sICAM and CD markers like CD 64 have been studied and shown to have variable sensitivity and specificity. They have not been able to fulfill the criteria for a reliable rapid diagnostic test and are currently used as research tools.

Sepsis Screen Panels

Because no single test has been shown to have adequate sensitivity as well as specificity, it has been suggested that a combination of 3 to 5 tests should be used to improve its sensitivity and specificity. These have included a combination of CRP, WBC indices and other hematologic tests like micro-ESR. Two sepsis screens performed 24 hours apart have been shown to have high sensitivity and negative predictive value. Box 16.3

BOX 16.3 Key points regarding sepsis screen

- Sepsis screen is useful to 'rule out' but not to 'rule in' sepsis. For example, a negative screen has high negative predictive value , especially if two screens are done 12–24 hr apart. A positive screen simply means you are unable to rule out sepsis and one should treat until proven otherwise (i.e. based on cultures and clinical course).
- Sepsis screen does not include blood culture, X-ray chest or CSF examination because these are definitive tests.
- In early-onset infection, sepsis screen has a limited role because it takes several hours for the acute phase reactants to rise and they may also rise in response to various perinatal events.
- Sepsis screen is done in any of the following three situations:
  1. There is clinical ambiguity, i.e. you are not sure whether to give antibiotics or not, e.g. mild abdominal distension with milky aspirate, but otherwise baby looks well. In this situation, if screen is negative, you should withhold antibiotics; if sepsis screen is positive, it is desirable to give antibiotics.
  2. On the other hand, if in your clinical judgment, you feel that antibiotics have to be started, e.g. very sick baby with shock, screen serves no purpose, one should take a blood culture and start antibiotics.
  3. In a situation where you feel antibiotics need not be started, e.g. one episode of apnea in a preterm baby on day 3 and baby is otherwise well; sepsis screen will not serve any purpose.
- In other words, if the sepsis screen is likely to change your decision about administration of antibiotics , do it; otherwise there is no need to waste resources and time.

---

summarizes certain practical points for effective utilization of sepsis screen.

Newer Diagnostic Methods

Molecular techniques have emerged as promising tools for diagnosis of neonatal bacterial infections.

Polymerase chain reaction (PCR) PCR extracts bacterial DNA from blood and identifies species specific genes by sequencing. Real-time PCR (RT-PCR or qPCR) can also provide information regarding bacterial load. Compared to blood culture, PCR has higher sensitivity, shorter turnaround time (as short as 30 minutes) and requires a small blood volume. The disadvantage is that the PCR is directed against a specific pathogen only. A multiplex PCR technique targeting multiple gene sequences of all possible etiological organisms is likely to be more useful. It is now available commercially, but is very expensive.

DNA microarray This is another recent technique which can give information regarding nature of bacteria, their load, virulence and host immune responses.

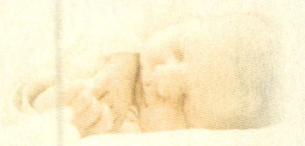

Other Supportive Investigations

Additional or adjunctive investigations are done to assess homeostasis of the infant and identify associated complications to improve management and outcome.

- *X-ray chest* It should be done in all cases especially when there is respiratory distress or need for oxygen requirement.
- *Platelet count and coagulation profile* There is high incidence of thrombocytopenia and DIC in neonatal sepsis. The counts and coagulogram should be monitored for therapeutic implications in the presence of bleeding tendency, especially in preterm infants.
- Electrolytes and renal function tests are mandatory.
- Arterial blood gases and acid-base status should be checked in all cases.

Lumbar Puncture

In septicemic neonates, the incidence of meningitis may be as high as 23%. The symptoms and signs of meningitis in neonates are nonspecific and at times the CNS symptoms may be totally absent. Irritability, seizures and full or bulging anterior fontanel may be seen in 60%, 20–50% and 25% of cases respectively. Therefore, lumbar puncture must be done in all symptomatic neonates being treated for probable sepsis, with the exception of preterm neonates presenting only with respiratory distress at birth and having no risk factors for sepsis. The incidence of meningitis is much higher in LOS. About 38% of newborns with meningitis are likely to have sterile blood cultures.

CSF culture and Gram stain are gold standards for diagnosis of meningitis. CSF sugar, protein and WBC counts are useful for a presumptive diagnosis of bacterial meningitis if culture is sterile. However, the range of normal values of CSF leukocytes, sugar and protein varies according to gestation, birth weight and chronological age, and there is a considerable overlap of these parameters between neonates with and without meningitis. In 1.0 to 10% of neonates with proven bacterial meningitis, CSF sugar, protein and cell count may be absolutely normal. Based on recent data, the currently suggested cut-offs of CSF parameters for presumptive diagnosis of meningitis are shown in Table 16.1.

There is no need to estimate concurrent blood glucose as CSF to blood glucose ratios are not useful in neonates. Correction of CSF WBC count for presence of RBCs in traumatic lumbar puncture, does not improve the diagnostic accuracy and can result in loss of sensitivity with only a slight gain in specificity. Therefore, CSF should be sent only for culture when CSF is blood stained. CSF glucose is the main variable with a high specificity in diagnosing meningitis. But delay in processing the CSF sample can supuriously decrease CSF glucose values.

Treatment

Interventions to Prevent Early-onset Sepsis in Infants Born to Mothers with Risk Factors

The only intervention that has proven beneficial is treatment of mother with antibiotics once there is evidence of infection or premature rupture of membranes. A recent Cochrane Systematic Review showed statistically significant reduction in chorioamnionitis [average risk ratio (RR) 0.66, 95% confidence interval (CI) 0.46 to 0.96], number of babies born within 48 hours [average RR 0.71, 95% CI 0.58 to 0.87] and after 7 days [average RR 0.79, 95% CI 0.71 to 0.89]. There was reduction in neonatal infection [RR 0.67, 95% CI 0.52 to 0.85], need for surfactant [RR 0.83, 95% CI 0.72 to 0.96], oxygen therapy [RR 0.88, 95% CI 0.81 to 0.96], and

---

Table 16.1 Guidelines for empirical treatment of meningitis based on CSF parameters

Cut-off values to diagnose meningitis	Among neonates with suspected sepsis	Among neonates with culture proven sepsis
	Preterm babies WBC >25/mm^3 and protein >170 mg/dL OR WBC >100/mm^3 OR Glucose <25 mg/dL	**Preterm babies** WBC >10/mm^3 OR Glucose <25 mg/dL OR Protein >170 mg/dL
	Term babies WBC >21/mm^3 OR Glucose <20 mg/dL	**Term babies** WBC >8/mm^3 OR Glucose <20 mg/dL OR Protein >120 mg/dL

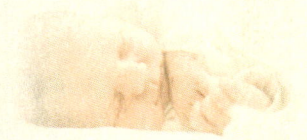

abnormal cerebral ultrasound scan prior to discharge from hospital [RR 0.81, 95% CI 0.68 to 0.98].

There is no role for maternal prophylactic antibiotics in preterm onset of labor, meconium stained amniotic fluid and pPROM in infants > 34 weeks.

Treatment of Sepsis in Newborn

Antibiotics The mainstay of treatment is early administration of appropriate antibiotics in the right dose, through intravenous route and for the right duration. The first dose should be administered within one hour of clinical diagnosis.

Choice of antibiotics The choice of antibiotics depends upon prevalent bacteria, their sensitivity patterns, presence of meningitis and comorbidities. Each hospital or geographic area should review their culture results of past year and have a clear written antibiotic policy based on their data. The isolates and their sensitivity profile should be reviewed periodically. In the absence of such information, the policy should be decided based on best available data from the region. The first line antibiotics should be able to cover at least 70% of the prevalent bacteria. In general, the empirical first line therapy needs to cover both Gram-negative as well as Gram-positive organisms till culture results are available when targeted therapy can be given.

Although ampicillin and gentamicin are used and recommended as first line antibiotics in the developed world by WHO and recently announced National Treatment Guidelines, one should confirm from available local data whether the organisms are sensitive

to this combination. The NNPD data had shown less than 30% antibiotic sensitivity to this combination and currently most hospitals report even lower figures. Cephalosporin use is best restricted to neonates with CNS involvement as widespread use of cephalosporins is associated with increased incidence of necrotizing enterocolitis, fungal infections and increased mortality.

Duration of antibiotic therapy The duration of antibiotic therapy depends upon culture results and clinical course. Table 16.2 shows the suggested duration of therapy in different clinical scenarios.

Adjunctive Therapies for Neonatal Sepsis

Current evidence does not support routine use of any of the following adjunctive therapies.

Intravenous immunoglobulins Systematic reviews of treatment with IgG based immunoglobulins have not shown improvement in mortality in neonatal sepsis. In a small number of infants enrolled in trials using IgM enriched immunoglobulin, there was a benefit in in improving survival but the numbers were too small to provide concrete evidence.

G-CSF, GM-CSF Administration of granulocyte colony stimulating factor (G-CSF) and granulocyte-monocyte colony stimulating factor (GM-CSF) has not shown any reduction in 14 day mortality. In the sub-group of neonates with absolute neutrophil count $<1.7 \times 10^3/dL$, a reduction in mortality was seen with G-CSF but the numbers were too small for a confident estimate.

Table 16.2 Duration of antibiotic therapy based on various clinical scenarios	
Clinical scenario	**Duration of therapy**
No clinical features but risk factors are present (e.g. chorioamnionitis, unclean vaginal examinations)	Stop antibiotics when culture is reported as sterile after 48 hours
Clinical features are suggestive of sepsis, screen negative, culture sterile, no clinical evidences of meningitis	Stop antibiotics once alternative diagnosis is made/signs resolve and culture is sterile
Clinical features probably due to sepsis, screen positive, cultures sterile, and no evidences of meningitis	If clinical features completely resolve; stop antibiotics once culture is sterile after 48 hours. In case signs persist and an alternative diagnosis is not available, give antibiotics for 5–7 days or repeat sepsis screen
Blood culture positive sepsis	10–14 days for Gram-negative organisms
	7 days for coagulase negative staphylococci
	14 days for *Staphylococcus aureus*
CSF culture positive meningitis	21 days for Gram-negative; 14 days for Gram-positive organisms
Complicated meningitis, e.g. ventriculitis, brain abscess	6 to 8 weeks depending upon response
Probable meningitis (culture –ve)	Determine the duration of antibiotic therapy based on blood culture positivity and overall clinical picture
Bone and joint infections	6 weeks depending on response
Urinary tract infection	7–14 days

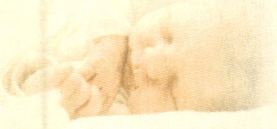

Granulocyte transfusions Granulocyte transfusions did not show any reduction in 14 day mortality.

Exchange blood transfusion Studies from India have shown some benefits in hematological and immunological parameters and survival following exchange transfusion. However, it is a risky procedure especially in the setting of septicemia. Correct timing of the procedure during the course of sepsis is difficult to decide. Exchange transfusion with relatively fresh blood may be considered in infants not responding or worsening on adequate supportive and appropriate antibiotic treatment, provided the general condition of the baby permits the procedure.

Supportive Treatment

Early and comprehensive supportive care is a must for better outcome. Failure of various organ systems should be anticipated and prospective monitoring should be done to provide timely respiratory and hemodynamic support.

- Infants with respiratory distress and hypoxemia should be givn oxygen, CPAP or mechanical ventilation as indicated.
- Monitor and maintain blood pressure and peripheral perfusion. Inotropes and vasoactive agents should be started without any delay. Adrenaline is the inotrope of choice for septic shock in the newborn.
- Prevent and correct hypoglycemia. Maintain blood glucose in euglycemic range.
- When infant is hemodynamically stable, start enteral nutrition as per tolerance.
- Transfuse blood products as required.

Special Conditions

Meningitis

Meningitis in the newborn is a dreaded complication because of high risk of neurodevelopmental sequelae and mortality. The incidence of culture proven meningitis in cases of suspected sepsis in infants less than 3 months age varies between 4.7 and 7.9%. Meningitis in neonates may be insidious in onset and it is difficult to distinguish it from sepsis alone. Rarely a neonate may develop localizing features of meningitis like seizures and bulging anterior fontanel and timely lumbar puncture should be done when indicated. Lumbar puncture can be deferred when the neonate is hemodynamically unstable and has serious bleeding diathesis.

In addition to antibiotic sensitivity profile of commonly isolated microbes of a NICU, the other major factors that determine the choice of antibiotics is the

Table 16.3	Complications of meningitis
Complications	**Clinical/laboratory features**
Brain abscess	Seizures, focal neurological signs, persistent leucocytosis/leucopenia
Hydrocephalus	Rapidly increasing head size, widened sutures, sun setting sign, increased frequency of apnea, and seizures
SIADH	Abnormal weight gain, oliguria, hyponatremia, seizures, depressed sensorium if hyponatremia is not treated
Cerebral venous thrombosis	Sudden alteration in sensorium, features of raised ICP, full or bulging anterior fontanel
Cerebral infarct	Focal neurological signs

SIADH; syndrome of inappropriate diuretic hormone

degree of CSF penetration of the drug. Usually CSF sterilization occurs with 3 days in case of Gram-ve bacteria and 24–48 hours in case of Gram +ve bacteria. It may be prudent to repeat a CSF analysis in neonates not showing adequate clinical recovery or having positive CSF culture, especially in a case of multi-drug resistant organism. The complications of bacterial meningitis in a neonate are mentioned in Table 16.3.

Bone and Joint Infections

Bone and joint infections in neonates usually occur following septicemia, secondary to heel pricks or venipuncture or occasionally secondary to pPROM in mother. Though *S. aureus* is reported as the most commonly isolated organism, the bacterial profile mimics that of microbial spectrum causing sepsis. Therefore, in Indian scenario, Gram-negative bacteria like *Klebsiella* and *E. coli* are equally common. The presentation can be insidious with localized inflammatory swelling or with features of systemic infection. Bone radiographs are first line investigation but their sensitivity can be as low as 75%. The destructive changes in bone may be delayed till 7–14 days. Ultrasound can detect abnormalities at an early stage, but traditional findings of osteomyelitis may not be seen. MRI has sensitivity of 95% and specificity of 97%. Technetium-99m scan has also high sensitivity (90–95%) and can detect osteomyelitis as early as 24 to 48 hours after the onset of infection. Initial empiric antibiotic therapy should include cover for staphylococci and Gram-negative organisms. Antibiotic therapy is given for 4–6 weeks based on response and resolution of local signs.

Long-term Sequelae

Perinatal bacterial infections are associated with a number of long-term sequelae including bronchopulmonary

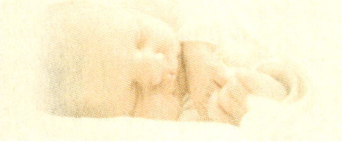

dysplasia, periventricular leukomalacia and risk of neuromotor developmental delay. The risk of hearing loss and neurodevelopmental delay is higher in the presence of meningitis and other CNS complications.

SPIROCHETAL INFECTIONS

The term "spirochetes" refers to a group of flagellated bacteria which includes Treponema, Leptospira and Borrelia, but only syphilis caused by *Treponema pallidum* is discussed in this chapter.

Introduction

Syphilis is caused by the spirochete *T.pallidum*, a macro-aerophilic Gram-negative flagellated bacteria with humans as the sole natural host. Untreated primary or secondary syphilis infection can cause catastrophic fetal outcomes during second or third trimesters of pregnancy. There has been a worldwide decrease in the incidence of congenital syphilis over the years. A clinician may suspect congenital syphilis in a neonate on the basis of clinical features or may be faced with an asymptomatic neonate born to a mother with syphilis.

Maternal Syphilis

Syphilis in the pregnant woman can cause recurrent abortions, stillbirths and preterm labor. The prevalence of syphilis in pregnant women has decreased from 3% to <0.5% in India in the past decade. Most mothers infected with syphilis are asymptomatic. All pregnant women should be tested by a non-treponemal antibody test for syphilis during their first antenatal visit preferably before 16 weeks of gestation (Table 16.4). If tested positive, one should confirm the diagnosis with a treponemal antibody test. For high-risk population, even when the first titer is negative, a repeat titer should

---

> ### Table 16.4 Laboratory diagnosis of syphilis
>
> *T. pallidum* cannot be cultured rapidly and requires special dark field microscopy for identification. Presumptive diagnosis can be made by either one of the treponemal or non-treponemal tests.
>
> **Non-treponemal antibody tests**
> - Venereal Diseases Research laboratory (VDRL) test
> - Rapid plasma reagin (RPR) test
>
> They are rapid, less specific, and easy to perform. Their titers usually correlate with the disease severity and they become negative after successful treatment.
>
> **Treponemal antibody tests**
> - MHA-TP: Microhemagglutination test for *T. pallidum*
> - TPHA: *T. pallidum* hemagglutination test

---

be checked at 28–32 weeks of gestation and prior to delivery. Contemporary evaluation of fetus includes detailed ultrasonography to identify stigmata of *in-utero* transmission. The most commonly reported sonographic markers of fetal syphilis include hepatomegaly, placentomegaly, polyhydramnios, ascites, intrauterine growth restriction and other signs of hydrops fetalis.

Fetal Transmission

Transplacental transmission of *T. pallidum* can occur any time during pregnancy though it is less likely before 4th month of pregnancy because of protective effect of Langerhan's cell layer of placenta. This cell layer atrophies by 6th month of pregnancy after which treponemes in maternal circulation can pass through placenta into the fetus. The fetal manifestations of syphilis occur only after 18th week of gestation. The risk of transmission is greatest if mother is in the early infectious stage of disease (primary, secondary or early latent phase). Excluding stillbirths and abortions, vertical transmission rate of syphilis in case of untreated mothers is around 66%. The transmission is maximum for primary and secondary syphilis (60–100%) and it decreases in early latent phase (40%) and late latent phase (8%). Syphilis can also affect the fetus during subsequent pregnancies.

Congenital Syphilis

Congenital syphilis is a multisystem disorder that can cause profound neurological or skeletal abnormalities in newborn. The disease in almost entirely preventable by early treatment of mother before or during pregnancy.

Clinical Features

About two-thirds of the neonates born with congenital syphilis are asymptomatic at birth. The clinical manifestations are arbitrarily divided into early and late stages:

- *Early stages* Neonates are symptomatic at birth. The most common features include nasal discharge (snuffles or hemorrhagic rhinorrhea), skin rash, jaundice and hepatosplenomegaly. The skin rash can be vesiculobullous or maculopapular, often with desquamation, over palms and soles. Other types of skin lesions like erythematous targetoid, scaly or pustular rash can be seen. There may be associated pneumonitis and lymphadenopathy.
- *Late stages* The late manifestations of syphilis can appear anytime after 2 years of age. These include Hutchinson's triad, i.e. notched central incisors, sensorineural hearing loss and interstitial keratitis.

- *Other features* They include facial defects in the form of saddle nose, Clutton's joints (symmetrically enlarged painless joints) most commonly involving the knees due to synovitis, mulberry molars due to poorly formed molar cusps, palatal perforation, rhagades, (fissures, cracks or fine scars at the angles of nose and mouth), lymphadenopathy, radiological signs of dactylitis, osteochondritis and periosteitis. There is localized bilateral metaphyseal destruction of the medial proximal tibia (Wimberger sign). CNS manifestations include seizures, hydrocephalus and cranial nerve palsies. Eye involvement can present as optic atrophy, chorioretinitis, uveitis and corneal scarring.

- *Sensorineural hearing loss* Children present with sudden bilateral and profound hearing loss without associated vestibular symptoms. The overall incidence of hearing loss due to congenital syphilis is 38%. Therefore, hearing screening should be done at initial diagnosis and at 24–30 months. If treatment of congenital syphilis was incomplete, hearing should be checked annually.

Approach to an Infant Born to a Mother with Syphilis

The following investigations should be performed:

i. Quantitative non-treponemal serologic test (RPR or VDRL) on neonatal blood. Umbilical cord blood is not a preferred sample.

ii. Clinical examination of the neonate for features of congenital syphilis.

iii. Pathologic examination of placenta and umbilical cord (use of specific fluorescent anti-treponemal antibody staining if possible).

iv. If newborn has clinical features of congenital syphilis and mother's serology is unknown or not tested, do a non-treponemal antibody test on the mother for confirming the diagnosis.

The approach to evaluation and treatment of congenital syphilis is summarized in Table 16.5.

Diagnosis of Neurosyphilis

- Infants with reactive CSF VDRL
- CSF leukocytosis ($\geq$25 WBC per mm^3) and elevated protein content ($\geq$150 mg/dL in full term and $\geq$170 mg/dL in preterm infants)

In centers where complete work up is not possible and referral to a higher center is not feasible, complete treatment for 10 days should be given, presuming that the neonate is having neurosyphilis.

Table 16.5 Management of congenital syphilis

Scenario 1

Infants with an abnormal physical examination that is consistent with congenital syphilis

Evaluation

- CBC and differential WBC and platelet count
- Do blood VDRL
- CSF analysis for VDRL, cell count, and protein
- Other tests as clinically indicated (long-bone radiographs, chest radiograph, liver function tests, cranial USG, ophthalmologic examination, and auditory brainstem response)

Treatment Aqueous crystalline penicillin G 100,000–150,000 units/kg/d, administered as 50,000 units/kg/dose IV every 12 h during the first 7 d of life and every 8 h thereafter for a total of 10 d (3 weeks if CNS involvement is suspected) or procaine penicillin G 50,000 units/kg/dose IM in a single daily dose for 10 d. If more than one day of therapy is missed, the entire course should be restarted.

Scenario 2

Infants with a normal physical examination and VDRL titer same or less than fourfold of the maternal titer, and have any one of the following features:

1. Mother was not treated, inadequately treated, or has no documentation of having received treatment
2. Mother was treated with non-penicillin regimen
3. Mother received treatment for less than 4 weeks before delivery

Evaluation

- CBC and differential blood count and platelet count
- CSF analysis for VDRL, cell count, and protein
- Long-bone radiographs

Treatment Crystalline penicillin G (see dose above), or procaine penicillin G (*see dose above*) or benzathine penicillin G 50,000 units/kg/dose IM in a single dose (use this schedule only if evaluation is normal and follow-up is certain)

Scenario 3

Infants who have a normal physical examination and VDRL titer same or less than fourfold of the maternal titer and

1. Mother was treated during pregnancy, treatment was appropriate for the stage of infection, and treatment was administered >4 weeks before delivery; and
2. Mother has no evidence of reinfection or relapse

Evaluation No evaluation is required.

Treatment Benzathine penicillin G (see dose above). No treatment is required if mother was treated adequately before pregnancy and VDRL was non-reactive during pregnancy

Infection Control

Baby is no longer infectious after 24 hours of penicillin therapy. There is thus no need to isolate the baby after 24 hours of penicillin therapy.

Follow-up

- In sero-reactive babies, follow-up VDRL should be checked every 2–3 months until the test becomes non-reactive or the titer decreases by fourfold. VDRL should normally decline by 3 months and should be non-reactive by 6 months of age if adequately treated. If VDRL titers are stable or increase after age 6–12 months, the child should be retreated with a 10-day course of parenteral penicillin G.

- Infants whose initial CSF evaluations are abnormal, should undergo a repeat LP every 6 months until the results are normal. A reactive CSF VDRL test or abnormal CSF indices that cannot be attributed to any other ongoing illness, require re-treatment for possible neurosyphilis.

BIBLIOGRAPHY

Aradhya AS, Sundaram V, Kumar P, Ganapathy SM, Jain A, Rawat A. Double volume exchange transfusion in severe neonatal sepsis. *Indian J Pediatr* 2016; 83(2):107–13.

Chiesa C, Natale F, Pascone R, Osborn JF, Pacifico L, Bonci E, De Curtis M. C-reactive protein and procalcitonin: reference intervals for preterm and term newborns during the early neonatal period. *Clin Chim Acta* 2011; 412(11–12):1053–9.

Clinical signs that predict severe illness in children under age 2 months: a multicentre study. *Lancet* 2008; 371(9607):135–42.

Dutta S, Reddy R, Sheikh S, Kalra J, Ray P, Narang A. Intrapartum antibiotics and risk factors for early onset sepsis. *Arch Dis Child Fetal Neonatal Ed* 2010; 95(2):F99–F103.

Goldstein BG, Randolph A. International pediatric sepsis consensus conference: Definitions for sepsis and organ dysfunction in pediatrics. *Pediatr Crit Care Med* 2005; 6(1):2–8.

Henry E, Christensen RD. Reference intervals in neonatal hematology. *Clin Perinatol* 2015; 42(3):483–97.

Investigators of the Delhi Neonatal Infection Study (DeNIS) Group. Characterisation and antimicrobial resistance of sepsis pathogens in neonates born in tertiary care centers in Delhi, India: a cohort study. *Lancet Glob Health* 2016; 4(10):e752–e60.

Lawn JE, Zupan J. The Lancet Neonatal Survival Steering Team. 4 million neonatal deaths: when? where? why? *Lancet* 2005; 365:891–900.

National Neonatal Perinatal Database Report 2002–03. Available at url: www.nnfi.org Accessed on January 20, 2017.

Sexually Transmitted Diseases Guidelines: Congenital syphilis. Center for Disease Control and Prevention, USA. Available at url: http://cdc.gov accessed January 20, 2015.

Stocker M, Fontana M, El Helou S, Wegscheider K, Berger TM. Use of procalcitonin-guided decision-making to shorten antibiotic therapy in suspected neonatal early-onset sepsis: prospective randomized intervention trial. *Neonatology* 2010; 97(2):165–74.

Tarnow-Mordi W, Dutta S. Adjunctive immunologic interventions in neonatal sepsis. *Clinic Perinatol* 2010; 37:481–99.

Walker GJ, Walker DG. Congenital syphilis: a continuing but neglected problem. *Semin Fetal Neonatal Med* 2007; 12(3):198–206.

Wijesooriya NS, Rochat RW, Kamb ML, Turlapati P, Temmerman M, Broutet N, et al. Global burden of maternal and congenital syphilis in 2008 and 2012: A health systems modelling study. *Lancet Global Health* 2016; 4(8):e525–e33.

17

Perinatal Infections: Viral, Fungal and Parasitic

Arvind Shenoi

Introduction

Infection in the neonate is one of the commonest medical emergencies. Neonates being immunocompromised are prone to develop infections some of which may be non-bacterial like viral, fungal and parasitic. Bacterial infections are common, amenable to treatment with antibiotics, and multiple tests are available to diagnose them early, and monitor response to therapy. Of late viral, fungal and parasitic infections are being increasingly recognized in neonates. The clinical signs often mimic bacterial disease and hence there is often a delay in the diagnosis as well as therapy. The clinician must have a high degree of suspicion and should be aware of the possibility of a non-bacterial infection, especially when the tests for bacterial infection are negative or alternatively when the neonate does not improve in spite of adequate antibiotic therapy. The therapeutic options for viral infections are also evolving, although currently limited to few viruses. Fungal and parasitic infections have definite therapeutic options but the diagnosis is often delayed.

When to suspect a non-bacterial infection?

Viral infections are transmitted vertically from mother to neonate, or horizontally from health care workers or family members. The suspicion for viral infection should arise if the mother has fever, rash or flu like symptoms in pregnancy; or alternatively a health care worker or family member has some of these symptoms. Viral infections often present in syndromic manner like encephalitis (Herpesvirus), hepato-splenomegaly (Rubella, CMV), respiratory distress (RSV), etc. However, there is considerable overlap, rubella and CMV can present as encephalitis or as hepatosplenomegaly with development of conjugated jaundice. There is increasing incidence of dengue fever and chikunguniya in neonates due to endemicity of these infections. Viral infections should be suspected when there is suggestive history or tests for bacterial infection are negative.

Parasitsic infections like toxoplasmosis are transmitted vertically and are suspected when the neonate has stigmata of intrauterine infection like chorio-retinitis, hydrocephalus or intracranial calcification. Malaria is a common parasitic infection in our country and Africa, which affects the maternal and neonatal outcome. History of malaria in the mother should alert the clinician about the possibility of congenital malaria.

Fungal infections can present as surface colonization or invasive fungal infections. The distinction is fairly easy when fungus is isolated from the blood, CSF and body tissues. Isolation of fungus from urine is difficult to interpret due to colonization of skin of genitals and perineum with candida. In our country, fungal colonization and surface infection such as oral thrush are common in term newborns, while invasive fungal infections are more common in extremely preterm neonates requiring intensive care. The risk factors for fungal infections in the newborn include prolonged antibiotic therapy (especially third generation cephalosporins, or carbapenem), prolonged parenteral nutrition, presence of central venous catheter, assisted ventilation, use of H_2 receptor blockers and abdominal surgery. Vaginal and breast nipple candidiasis in the mother is a risk factor for oral thrush in the newborn. Bottle feeding is also a recognized risk factor for oral thrush in the neonates.

Diagnosis

Diagnosis of viral infections is often based on clinical features with positive serology. Viral cultures are not widely available. Polymerase chain reaction (PCR) based detection of viral DNA or RNA is available in some advanced centers but is expensive. Fungal infections are diagnosed by culture methods. Rapid diagnosis by identification of fungal hyphae in urine, or CSF with India ink preparation are available for some fungal infections.

VIRAL INFECTIONS

Rubella

Maternal rubella infection in pregnancy may lead to fetal embryopathy called congenital rubella syndrome, abortion or fetal death. Congenital rubella syndrome (CRS) is a social emergency as the child is likely to have a constellation of congenital anomalies like cataract, PDA, peripheral pulmonary artery stenosis, and microcephaly. The risk of CRS is as high as 85% when rubella occurs during first trimester of pregnancy and progressively fall when disease occurs late in pregnancy. The disease can be mild or manifest with hepatosplenomegaly, thrombocytopenia, interstitial pneumonitis, dermal erythropoiesis and growth restriction. Many of these children manifest neurological problems like sensorineural hearing loss, autism and mental retardation on follow-up. A number of CRS cases are reported from our country making a strong case for universal rubella vaccination in our country.

Diagnosis is made on the basis of a characteristic clinical spectrum of CRS and a positive rubella specific IgM antibodies. However, false-negative and false-positive serology tests are known to occur. The diagnosis can also be suspected by elevated or increasing titers of rubella specific IgG antibodies. The virus can be cultured from throat or nasal swab, or alternatively rubella virus RNA can be detected by polymerase chain reaction (PCR).

The treatment is essentially symptomatic under the guidance of multiple specialists. The baby must be isolated from other neonates, children and pregnant women as the infant with CRS may shed virus for as long as one year.

Human Immunodeficiency Virus Infection (HIV)

HIV infection in the newborn is rarely symptomatic. However, the prevention of vertical transmission of infection starts with screening of pregnant women, counseling for safe sexual practices, anti-retroviral therapy, birth planning and infant feeding options; post-partum therapy for the mother and baby, and early diagnosis of the infection in the infant as per the NACO guidelines.

Cytomegalovirus (CMV) Infection

Both congenital and acquired CMV infection can occur in the newborn. Congenital CMV infection can occur transplacentally if the mother has viremia in pregnancy, or if the baby is delivered vaginally through infected secretions. Acquired CMV can occur through blood transfusion, or by ingestion of infected breast milk. Congenital CMV is frequently asymptomatic with only about 10% of the neonates manifesting features of intrauterine growth restriction, hepatosplenomegaly, conjugated jaundice, thrombocytopenia, microcephaly, intracranial periventricular calcifications and retinitis. Sensorineural hearing loss commonly occurs in infants with congenital CMV, incidence of about 50% in symptomatic neonates and 15% among asymptomatic neonates.

In preterm neonates CMV infection may be transmitted through breast milk and blood transfusion. It causes a "viral sepsis" like syndrome, interstitial pneumonia, hepatitis, or thrombocytopenia. The condition is after confused with bacterial sepsis and chronic lung disease which is known to affect preterm infants.

Diagnosis of congenital CMV is difficult. Isolation of the virus from blood or cerebrospinal fluid by viral culture is diagnostic but may require more than 28 days. Detection of viral DNA by PCR on a blood spot confirms congenital CMV but absence does not rule out the disease. A strongly positive IgM antibody titer before 2 weeks of age in association with chorio-retinitis or intracranial calcification is diagnostic. However, the elevation of IgM antibodies alone has low specificity, and do not distinguish between congenital and postnatal infection occurring after 2–4 weeks of age.

Antiviral therapy is indicated for neonates with symptomatic CMV. Asymptomatic congenital CMV does not qualify for anti-viral treatment. Oral valganciclovir 16 mg/kg/ dose given twice daily for 6 months has been shown to improve auditory and neuro-developmental outcome at 2 years of age in infants with symptomatic congenital CMV if treatment is started within one month of life. Neonates who cannot be given oral therapy, ganciclovir 6 mg/kg/dose every 12 hour as an infusion over 2 hours can be given till the neonate is able to tolerate oral therapy. Therapy of preterm infants with hepatitis, pneumonitis and thrombocytopenia should start with intravenous ganciclovir till the symptoms and signs have resolved. However, the long-term outcome of this therapy has not been reported.

The transmission of CMV through blood transfusion can be prevented by filtering the blood with leucocyte filters. Freezing red cells in glycerol and removal of the

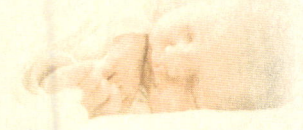

buffy coat are the other methods to prevent transmission of CMV through blood transfusion. Donor human milk can be pasteurized or frozen to decrease the risk of transmission of CMV.

Herpes Simplex Virus (HSV)

There are two strains of Herpes simplex virus, HSV-1 and HSV-2. They are enveloped double stranded DNA viruses. Transmission occurs at birth during passage through the maternal genital tract or by virtue of ascending infection with intact or ruptured amniotic membranes. The risk of transmission is as high as 25–60% when primary infection occurs just before delivery, while risk is minimal when reactivation of HSV infection occurs during early pregnancy. Rarely postnatal transmission through contact with oral secretions or hands of the caregiver has been documented.

Herpes simplex virus infection in the neonate can present in three different ways. Disseminated herpes infection can present with involvement of liver, lungs and brain in about 25% of the cases. Localised meningo-encephalitis may occur with or without skin involvement in about 30% of cases. Nearly 67% of neonates with disseminated or CNS disease may have skin lesions, but not necessarily at the time of onset of symptoms. Skin, eyes and mouth (SEM) disease can occur in 45% of cases. Nearly 80% cases of SEM disease have skin vesicles and the remaining 20% may have involvement of eyes or oral mucosa. It is difficult to suspect herpes in the absence of skin lesions. Herpes infection should be suspected in a neonate with sepsis syndrome with negative bacterial cultures, severe liver dysfunction or disseminated intravascular coagulation. Asymptomatic HSV infection is uncommon in neonates. The disease manifests in the first 2 weeks of life in the disseminated and SEM format, while CNS involvement occurs during 2nd and 3rd week of life.

Diagnosis of HSV infection is made by PCR of the viral DNA in the CSF, blood or from the vesicular fluid. Culture of the virus from the skin or mouth lesions can be done but is not available in most centers. The ELISA test for HSV IgM or IgG is not useful as the median time for sero-conversion is 21 days.

HSV infection is treated with intravenous acyclovir 20 mg/kg/dose every 8 hourly for 14 days for SEM disease or 21 days in case of CNS or disseminated disease. It is recommended that the CSF PCR should be repeated at the end of 21 days of therapy and if positive the parenteral acyclovir therapy continued for 7 more days. Thereafter, oral suppressive therapy is continued by administration of acyclovir in a dose of 300 mg/m^2/dose 3 times in a day for a period of 6 months, by monthly adjustments of dose. This is believed to improve the neuro-developmental outcome of survivors, as well as prevent skin recurrences. Eye involvement should be treated with topical 1% trifluridine, 0.1% iododeoxyuridine, or 0.15% ganciclovir, along with parenteral therapy.

The baby born to a woman with suspected or proven genital herpes should be observed closely for clinical signs of HSV. Surface cultures from conjunctiva, mouth, nasopharynx and rectum are taken for PCR study, as well as blood is sent for PCR. If these are negative, the baby is discharged after educating the family about the signs and symptoms of neonatal HSV infection. If the blood or surface PCR is positive, the baby is started on intravenous acyclovir therapy after collecting CSF sample for HSV PCR and blood sample for alanine transaminase. During follow-up, whenever a baby develops signs of possible HSV disease, CSF samples are collected and parenteral acyclovir therapy is started.

In a mother with genital herpes, baby should be delivered by cesarean section within 4 hours of rupture of membranes. Antenatal acyclovir therapy is not uniformly beneficial though it reduces the risk of recurrence of genital herpes during subsequent pregnancies.

Varicella Virus (Chickenpox)

Maternal chickenpox infection during pregnancy can cause severe illness in the mother, fetus (congenital varicella syndrome) or neonate (neonatal varicella). Perinatal chickenpox has a high perinatal mortality especially if the neonate develops varicella pneumonitis. Women who develop chickenpox in pregnancy need careful counseling and follow-up. It is essential to screen the fetus for congenital varicella syndrome by antenatal ultrasound examination. The features of congenital varicella syndrome include scarring of skin, hypoplasia of limbs and CNS abnormalities (microcephaly, cortical atrophy), and ocular abnormalities (micro-ophthalmia and chorioretinitis). The diagnosis is essentially clinical. All women should be protected against chickenpox by administration of varicella vaccine before marriage. VZIG (varicella zoster immune globulin) can be given to pregnant women who have been exposed to varicella in pregnancy to prevent congenital varicella syndrome. Maternal herpes zoster during pregnancy does not seem to cause congenital varicella syndrome.

Maternal varicella in the peri-partum period can affect the neonate. The infection is mild if adequate amounts of maternal antibodies have been transmitted to the baby, but the neonatal disease is likely to be severe if a high viral load has been transferred to the baby with no or low amounts of varicella antibodies. The highest morbidity occurs if the mother develops the rash 7 days prior to the delivery or within 2 days after the delivery. VZIG is recommended for this group of neonates in a dose of 62.5 units (1/2 vial) for neonates weighing less than 2 kg and 125 units (1 vial) for neonates weighing 2 kg or more. If the neonate develops chickenpox in spite of receiving VZIG or if VZIG was not given, intravenous acyclovir therapy is recommended. Acyclovir 20 mg/kg/dose is given 8 hourly orally for 7–10 days.

Dengue Virus

Dengue is an illness caused by infection with one of the 4 related RNA viruses of the genus Flavivirus. The incubation period in humans is 3 to 14 days. Perinatal dengue in the newborn has been described in our country when mother develops the infection around the time of birth. Disease may occur postnatally through the bite of infected *Aedes aegyptie* mosquitoes. As in older children, the neonate presents with thrombocytopenia, pleural effusion, ascites and shock. The disease is characterized by hemodynamic instability and capillary leak. Diagnosis is confirmed by detection of the dengue non-structural protein antigen (NS1) in the baby. Management strategies include aggressive fluid and vasopressor therapy, with supportive intensive care including ventilator support. The challenge is to recognize the illness when the disease in the mother has been mild, because dengue fever may present like neonatal sepsis.

Chikungunya

Neonatal chikungunya infection has been reported from our country and Reunion Island in the Indian Ocean. The disease is transmitted vertically if the mother has viremia around the time of delivery. It presents with fever, swelling and pain in joints including dactylitis, erythematous maculo-papular generalized rash, which lasts for 3–4 days. The baby may develop diffuse hyperpigmentation of skin which lasts for a few weeks. Rare instances of neonatal encephalitis have been reported with perinatal chikungunya virus infection. Treatment is supportive and symptomatic.

Hepatitis B Virus (HBV)

In-utero transmission of Hepatitis B is about 2% and mostly occurs during labor and delivery. About 90% of the neonates who acquire the disease perinatally go on to develop chronic Hepatitis B infection if the mother is both HBsAg and HBeAg positive and 5–20% if she is HBsAg positive but HBeAg negative. The vertical transmission of HBV from mother to her offspring can be prevented by screening of pregnant women followed by active and passive immunization. The symptoms and signs of neonatal HBV infection are mild, but rarely fulminant hepatic failure has been reported in perinatally acquired hepatitis B disease in the newborn. The diagnosis is made by detecting elevated levels of HbsAg, HbeAg and HBV DNA. The treatment of acute hepatitis B is supportive and the baby needs follow-up for detection of chronic carrier state and HBV reactivation disease.

In neonates weighing more than 2 kg at birth, Hepatitis B vaccine (HBV) and Hepatitis B immunoglobulin (HBIG) are administered at 2 different sites within 12 hours of birth, followed by 2nd and 3rd doses of the vaccine at 1–2 months and 6 months. In neonates weighing less than 2 kg at birth, HBIG and HBV are given as described above followed by 3 additional doses of vaccine at 1, 2–3, and 6 months. It is recommended to check the anti-HBs antibodies and HBsAg titer at 9–18 months on follow-up.

Enterovirus Infection

The group of enteroviruses includes polioviruses, Coxsackie, Parechoviruses, Echoviruses and Enterovirus 71. Vertical transmission from mother to child may occur including horizontal transmission from siblings to the neonate. In general, the horizontal transmission tends to be milder while vertical transmission from the mother can be life-threatening. The infection may range from asymptomatic to life-threatening myocarditis (Coxsackie B), hepatitis (Echovirus), meningitis or sepsis like picture (Enteroviruses), encephalitis and white matter injury (Parechovirus, Herpesvirus, CMV, Rubella, Chikungunya). Generally the mother has a viral illness around the time of delivery. Diagnosis is made by PCR but the cost of the test is often prohibitive and hence most viral infections go undiagnosed in our country. Treatment is supportive and symptomatic.

Parvovirus B19 Infection

Maternal infection with Parvovirus B19 during pregnancy may cause spontaneous abortion, some anomalies, but chiefly causes a temporary suppression of erythropoiesis in the fetus, resulting in hydrops fetalis. Fetal myocarditis due to the virus has also been documented. Treatment with intrauterine transfusion has been tried. The infant is treated with blood transfusion and multiparacentesis but the outcome is guided.

Respiratory Syncytial Virus (RSV), Rhinovirus, and Influenza Virus Infections

RSV, Rhinovirus or Influenza infections may be transmitted to the neonate by hospital staff or family

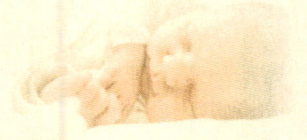

members. They present with apnea, tachypnea, increased oxygen or ventilator requirement, and feeding difficulties. Treatment is essentially supportive. A Cochrane review on use of nebulized ribavirin (20 mg/mL in a dose of 190 µg/L of nebulized gas for 12–18 hours a day) in RSV infection had shown only marginal therapeutic benefit. Monoclonal antibody palivizumab (15 mg/kg IM once a month) has been tried as a preventive measure against RSV infection. Currently its utility and cost-effectiveness are questioned.

Influenza infections of the neonates have been described during the pandemics of classical as well as H1N1 viral infections. Neonates present with respiratory symptoms like cough, fever and nasal congestion. Preterm neonates present with increased requirement of supplemental oxygen, or even respiratory failure requiring ventilation. Oseltamivir has been used to treat H1N1 infection in neonates in a dose of 1 mg/kg every 12 hourly for 5 days. It is recommended to prevent influenza infection in the nursery by immunization of mothers and health personnel. No vaccine is available for Rhinovirus and RSV infections.

PARASITIC INFECTIONS

Toxoplasmosis

Toxoplasmosis is a zoonotic infection caused by a coccidian parasite *Toxoplasma gondii*. Cats are the only known definitive hosts. Unsporulated oocysts are shed in the cat's feces. Humans become infected by consuming food or water contaminated with cat feces. Infection can also occur by eating undercooked meat of animals harboring tissue cysts. Maternal infection with the parasite causes fetal infection. The risk is lowest in the first trimester (14%), increasing to 29% and 59% in the second and third trimesters respectively. The severity of the disease falls with increasing gestation. Fetal infection results in classic triad of chorioretinitis, punctate intracranial calcification, and hydrocephalus. Additional clinical manifestations include skin rash, hepatosplenomegaly, and conjugated jaundice. Diagnosis is based on identification of *T. gondii* specific IgM and IgA antibodies. Detection of nucleic acid in CSF by PCR techniques is diagnostic. Pyrimethamine (loading dose of 1 mg/kg/dose every 12 hourly for 2 days; 1 mg/kg/day from day 3 to 6 months; and subsequently 1 mg/kg/day 3 times a week is given till one year) along with sulfadiazine 50 mg/kg 12 hourly for one year. Folinic acid 10 mg 3 times weekly is given for the entire period of therapy. Some authorities recommend adjunctive prednisone therapy 0.5 mg/kg every 12 hourly when there is high CSF protein or severe chorio-retinitis.

Malaria

Four species of malarial parasites that cause disease in humans include *Plasmodium vivax, P. falciparum, P. malariae* and *P. ovale*. Malaria can occur in the newborn when these parasites are transmitted transplacentally, or through blood transfusion, or mosquito bite postnatally. Congenital malaria is defined as demonstration of the parasite on peripheral smear within 7 days of birth. Many case reports of malarial infection with *P. vivax* and *P. falciparum* in neonates are available from our country. Fever, anemia, jaundice, hepatosplenomegaly and thrombocytopenia are the presenting features. Treatment consists of administration of chloroquine base 25 mg/kg total dose over 3 days; reports are available for use of quinine intravenous, and oral mefloquine and artesunate in individual cases. Simultaneously, maternal treatment as per WHO guidelines should be given. Prevention of malaria during pregnancy with antimalarials or insecticide treated bed nets has been shown to reduce the incidence of severe antenatal anemia, parasitemia and perinatal mortality.

FUNGAL INFECTIONS

Candida infections

Candida infection may present at birth or soon afterwards as dermal infection or as systemic candidiasis in ELBW babies receiving parenteral nutrition and life support measures in the NICU. It is characterized by respiratory distress, hepatosplenomegaly, and a 40% risk of mortality. Candida dermatitis on the other hand is a disease of term infants presenting as a diaper rash and is amenable to topical anti-fungal therapy. Oral thrush has been described in term and preterm infants with or without prolonged antibiotic therapy. Bottle-fed infants are more susceptible to it compared to breastfed neonates. When oral thrush does occur in a breastfed neonate, it may be associated with candida infection of the maternal nipples which can interfere with breastfeeding.

Systemic candida infection or candidemia occurs in ELBW infant receiving intensive care, total parenteral nutrition, broad spectrum antibiotics and H_2 blockers. It can present with all the signs of sepsis including shock, circulatory failure and disseminated abscesses. Multi-organ involvement is common with meningitis, chorioretinitis, brain abscess, endocarditis, nephritis, and hepatitis. Renal candida infection can present as parenchymal candidiasis, fungal ball in the pelvis, or candida urinary tract infection. Endophthalmitis with blindness may occur in 3% cases. Intestinal candidiasis has been described and it may cause spontaneous intestinal perforation and has a high mortality. It mimics NEC but there is no pneumatosis intestinalis and it is potentially treatable with systemic antifungals. Candida meningitis and brain abscess occur in 10–15% and 4% of candidemic patients respectively. Lumbar puncture along with culture for fungus is essential as the cell count may be low along with low glucose. Candida endocarditis is associated in 5% of infants with candidemia. Diagnosis is made by fungal culture of the blood and CSF. Molecular methods like PCR are now available in our country which give the diagnosis within 24 hours but their cost is prohibitive.

Treatment of candida infections is based on whether there is blood-borne candidemia or mucocutaneous candidiasis. Candidemia or invasive fungal infections require systemic antifungal medications and the removal of all indwelling catheters. Rarely surgical resection may be required if systemic fungal therapy fails as in case of a urinary fungal ball or fungal endocarditis. Mucocutaneous candidiasis requires topical therapy in term neonates, unless it is widespread or disseminated.

A variety of systemic antifungals are available and they include polyenes (amphotericin B), triazoles (fluconazole), nucleoside analogues (flucytosine) and echinocandins (caspofungin). Amphotericin B is the most commonly used antifungal agent and is active against all candida species except C. lusitaniae. Conventional amphotericin B is well-tolerated though nephrotoxicity can occur. It is given in a dose of 0.5–1.5 mg/kg/day intravenously. The duration of therapy for disseminated and CNS candidiasis is a total cumulative dose of 25–30 mg/kg over 4–6 weeks, and for catheter associated fungemia, it is 10–15 mg/kg 14–21 days. Fluconazole is a triazole antifungal agent which inhibits fungal cytochrome P450. It is given in a dose of 12 mg/kg/day while some authorities recommend an intial loading dose of 25 mg/kg/day. It has a better safety profile than amphotericin B. The only drawback is risk of emergence of fluconazole resistance in C. krusei, C. glabrata and C. parasilosis. Flucytosine is a nucleoside analogue of cytosine and inhibits DNA synthesis. It is active against all species of candida except C. krusei. The recommended dose is 25–100 mg/kg orally once daily. It should never be given as monotherapy because of the rapid development of resistance. It has been used in combination therapy for CNS and renal candidiasis. Echinocandins prevent the formation of glucan polymers which are essential for integrity of fungal cell walls. Echinocandins include caspofungin, anidulafungin and micafungin. Available studies suggest they are well-tolerated in neonates. However, further data on their safety and efficacy in neonates are needed before they are recommended for routine use. Oral and mucocutaneous candidiasis can be treated with miconazole gel or oral fluconazole 3 mg/kg/day for 7 days.

Prophylaxis of Fungal Infections

Prophylactic systemic antifungal therapy with fluconazole reduces the incidence of colonization and invasive fungal infection in very low birth weight infants, but does not influence mortality. Oral nystatin or miconazole gel has been associated with lower risk of invasive fungal infection but without any reduction in mortality. The general consensus is to use fluconazole intravenously in ELBW infants who are at high risk of fungal sepsis in a dose of 3–6 mg/kg/day. Some centers use this protocol 2–3 times a week.

Measures to reduce the risk of fungal infections include delivery by cesarean section for high-risk infants, avoidance of unnecessary endotracheal intubation, minimal duration of antibiotic therapy, minimum use of central catheters, TPN, H_2 blockers and postnatal corticosteroids. Some trials using bovine lactoferrin with or without *Lactobacillus rhamnoses* (probiotic) showed a lesser rate of invasive fungal disease. This needs further confirmation with larger trials.

Aspergillus, Pichia, and Zygomycosis

Neonatal Aspergillosis has been reported in the preterm and term infants. The cutaneous disease is more common in the preterm and invasive disease in the full term. *Pichia anomala* is sacchromycetes fungus found in the soil and has been reported to cause fungemia in premature neonates. The Zygomycetes (Rhizopus, Mucor, and Absidia) are found in the soil and are known to cause fungemia in preterm newborn. These fungal infections are also treated with amphotericin B.

Perinatal Infections and Cerebral Palsy

Infections transmitted from the mother or acquired in the neonatal period are known to cause cerebral palsy through cytokine induced white matter brain injury and systemic inflammatory response syndrome. In addition, perinatal infections are a recognized risk factor for preterm birth, placental insufficiency and perinatal asphyxia which are independent risk factors for development of cerebral palsy. The survivors of neonatal viral, fungal and parasitic infections are at high-risk of developing cerebral palsy and must be followed closely for neuromotor development during infancy.

Conclusion

Viral, parasitic and fungal infections do occur in neonates, though they are relatively less common than

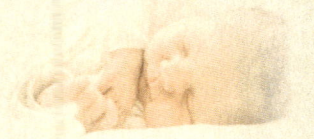

the bacterial infections. History of viral infection in the mother provides an important clue to the diagnosis of a viral infection in the neonate. Viral infections present in a syndromic pattern with features of encephalitis, respiratory distress and hepatosplenomegaly. Treatment is supportive except in the case of herpes simplex, CMV and varicella viruses. Parasitic infections have been reported in the newborn and should be suspected if there is maternal history. Treatment for malaria and toxoplasmosis is well-defined. Fungal infections occur in ELBW and sick babies expoed to high-risk factors. Treatment consists of anti-fungal therapy in the form of antifungal drugs like polyenes (amphotericin B), triazoles (fluconazole), nucleoside analogues (flucytosine), or echinocandins. Prophylaxis in the form of oral or systemic fluconazole has been shown to be beneficial in high-risk groups. The long-term outcome in perinatal infections is guarded with all survivors being at high-risk to develop cerebral palsy.

BIBLIOGRAPHY

Ascher SB, SmithPB, Watt K, et al. Antifungal therapy and outcomes in infants with invasive candida infections. *Pediatr Infect Dis J* 2012; 31:439.

Austin N, Cleminson J, Darlow BA, McGuire W. Prophylactic oral/topical non-absorbed antifungal agents to prevent invasive fungal infection in very low birth weight infants. *Cochrane Database Syst Rev* 2015; CD003478.

Baley JE, Kliegman RM, Fanaroff AA. Disseminated fungal infections in the very low birth weight infants; clinical manifestations and epidemiology. *Pediatrics* 1984; 73:144–52.

Benjamin DK Jr, Poole C, Steinbach WJ, Rowen JL, Walsh TJ. Neonatal candidemia and end organ damage: a critical appraisal of the literature using meta-analytic techniques. *Pediatrics* 2003; 112:634–40.

Cherry JD, Krogstad P. Enterovirus and parechovirus infections. In: Infectious Diseases of the Fetus and Newborn Infant, Remington JS, Klein JO, Wilson CB, Nizet V, Maldonado Y (Eds). *Philadelphia: Elseiver,* 7th Ed. 2011. pp. 759–799.

Cleminson J, Austin N, McGuire W. Prophylactic systemic antifungal agents to prevent mortality and morbidity in very low birth weight infants. *Cochrane Database Syst Rev* 2015; CD003850.

Department of AIDS control; Govt. of India, Ministry of health and family welfare. Updated Guidelines for Prevention of Parent to Child Transmission (PPTCT) of HIV using multidrug anti-retroviral regimen in India 2013.

Desai M, ter Kuile FO, Nostern F, McGready R, Asamoa K, Brabin B, Newman RD. Epidemiology and burden of malaria in pregnancy. *Lancet Infect Dis* 2007; 7:93–104.

Dewan P, Gupta P. Burden of congenital rubella syndrome in India; a systematic review. *Indian Pediatr* 2012; 49:377–99.

Gandhoke I, Aggarwal R, Lal S, Khare S. Congenital CMV infection in symptomatic infants in Delhi and surrounding areas. *Indian J Pediatr* 2006; 73:1095–97.

Giorgio E, Oronzo MAD, Iozza I et a . Parvovirus B19 during pregnancy: a review. *J Prenat Med* 2010; 4:63–66.

Giri S, Kindo AJ. A review of Candida species causing blood stream infection. *Indian J Med Microbiol* 2012; 30:270–78.

Hermansen MC, Hermansen MG. Perinatal infections and cerebral palsy. *Clin Perinatol* 2006; 33:315–33.

Hollier LM, Wendel GD. Third trimester antiviral prophylaxis for preventing maternal genital herpes simplex (HSV) recurrences and neonatal infection. *Cochrane Database Syst Rev* 2008; Issue 1. Art. No.:CD004946.doi:10.1002/14651358.CD004946.pub2

Hsieh E, Smith BP, Benjamin DK Jr. Neonatal fungal infections: when to treat? *Early Hum Dev* 2012; 88(2):S6-S10. Doi:10.106/S0378-3782(12)70004-X.

Jain A, Chaturvedi UC. Dengue in infants: an overview. *FEMS Immunol Med Microbiol* 2010; 59:119–30.

Jones CA, Walker KS, Badawi N. Antiviral agents for treatment of herpes simplex virus infection in neonates. *Cochrane Database Syst Rev* 2009; Issue 3. Art No: CD004206. Doi: 10.1002/14651858.CD004206.pub2

Kimberlin DW, Lin CY, Jacobs RF, et al. Natural history of neonatal herpes simplex virus infection in the acyclovir era. *Pediatrics* 2001; 108:223–29.

Leick-Courtois C, Hays S, Perpoint T, et al. Influenza A H1N1 in neonatal intensive care unit: analysis and lessons. *Arch Pediatr* 2011; 18:1069–75.

Manicklal S, Emery VC, Lazzarotto T, Bopanna SB, Gupta RK. The "silent" global burden of congenital cytomegalovirus. *Clin Microbiol Rev* 2013; 26:86–102.

Manzoni P, Mostert M, Jacqz-Aigrain E, Farina D. The use of fluconazole in neonatal intensive care units. *Arch Dis Child* 2009; 94:983.

Miller E, Cradock-Watson JE, Pollock TM. Consequences of confirmed maternal rubella at successive stages of pregnancy. *Lancet* 1982; 2:781–84.

Parikh TB, Nanavati RN, Patnakar CV, Rao SFN, Bisure K, Udani RH, Mehta P. Fluconazole prophylaxis against fungal colonization and invasive fungal infection in very low birth weight infants. *Indian Pediatr* 2007; 44:830–37.

Passi GR, Khan YZ, Chitnis DS. Chikungunya infection in neonates. *Indian Pediatr* 2008; 45:240–41.

Remington JS, McLeod R, Wilson CB, Desmonts G. Toxoplasmosis. In: Infectious Diseases of the Fetus and Newborn Infant, Remington JS, Klein JO, Wilson CB, Nizet V, Maldorado Y. *Philadelphia, Elseiver,* 7th edn 2011. pp 918–1041.

Shrim A, Koren G, Yudin MH, Farine D. Maternal Fetal Medicine Committee. Management of varicella infection (chickenpox) in pregnancy. *J Obstet Gynaecol Can* 2012; 34:287–92.

Singh J, Soni D, Mishra D, Singh HP, Bijesh S. Placental and neonatal outcome in maternal malaria. *Indian Pediatr* 2014; 51:285–88.

Ventre K, Randolph A. Ribavarin for respiratory syncytial virus infection of the lower respiratory tract in infants and young children. *Cochrane Database Syst Rev* 2000; Issue 5. Art no: CD000181. Doi10.1002/14551858.CD000181. pub 4

Weese-Mayer DE, Fondriest DW, Brouilette FT, Shulman ST. Risk factors associated with candidemia in the neonatal intensive care unit: a case control study. *Pediatr Infect Dis J* 1987; 6:190–96.

18

Neonatal Meningitis

Ashok Kumar and Sriparna Basu

Introduction

Meningitis is an important cause of mortality and long-term neurodevelopmental sequelae in neonates. Meningitis is more common in neonatal age group than at any other period of life. Majority of the cases of neonatal meningitis are bacterial in origin; viruses, fungi and other uncommon pathogens account for a smaller number of cases. The causative organisms of bacterial meningitis in neonates vary with the gestational age, postnatal age, place of delivery (home or hospital) and geographic location. Confirming the diagnosis of meningitis is often difficult in newborns, especially in preterm babies, as the clinical signs are nonspecific, there is a wide variation in the cerebrospinal fluid (CSF) cell count and protein levels even in healthy newborns, and CSF culture positivity is often compromised by antepartum or postnatal antibiotic exposure. Moreover, meningitis may occur in infants without bacteremia and with normal CSF parameters. High index of suspicion along with early treatment with appropriate antibiotics and good supportive measures are essential to optimize outcome.

Definition

Neonatal meningitis is defined as the inflammation of the meninges, subarachnoid space, and brain vasculature resulting from infection during the first 28 days of life. Neonatal sepsis and meningitis share similar risk factors, pathogens, and clinical manifestations. Approximately 15% of neonates with sepsis have concomitant meningitis. The incidence of neonatal meningitis is approximately one-fourth to one-tenth of neonatal sepsis. Meningitis is more frequent in newborns presenting with late-onset sepsis than in early-onset sepsis.

Etiology

The etiology of neonatal bacterial meningitis differs between developed and developing countries. In developed countries, *Group B streptococcus* (GBS) is the most common cause of bacterial meningitis, accounting for 50% of all cases. *Escherichia coli* (*E. coli*) accounts for another 20%. Other organisms include *Listeria monocytogenes*, other Gram-negative enteric bacteria and *Enterococci*.

In developing countries, *Klebsiella pneumoniae, E. coli* and *Staphylococcus aureus* are predominant pathogens responsible for meningitis. Unlike western countries, GBS is rare in our set up. Other causative organisms are *Acinetobacter*, Coagulase-negative *Staphylococci* (CONS), *Enterobacter, Enterococci, Citrobacter, S. agalatae, S. Epidermidis, Serratia,* and *Salmonella* species are important pathogens responsible for nosocomial infection in newborns, especially in very low birth weight (VLBW) infants.

Among non-bacterial pathogens, Herpes simplex virus (HSV) is the most common cause of neonatal viral meningitis. Rarely, enteroviruses especially Parechovirus-3 may cause neonatal meningitis. Congenital infections such as cytomegalovirus, toxoplasma, rubella, lymphocytic choriomeningitis virus, varicella zoster and human immunodeficiency virus infection can also cause neonatal meningitis. Recently with increased survival of VLBW infants, fungal meningitis, especially caused by *Candida* spp. has emerged as an important problem in high-risk neonates.

Incidence

The incidence of neonatal bacterial meningitis ranges from 0.25 to 1 per 1000 live births in developed countries. The incidence is higher in developing countries and ranges from 0.8 to 6.1 per 1000 live births. The true incidence may be underestimated in resource-poor settings due to lack of diagnostic facilities. The incidence of HSV meningitis is estimated to be 0.02–0.5 cases per 1000 live births and the reported frequency of fungal meningitis among VLBW infants is around 1.6%.

Risk Factors

Risk factors for neonatal meningitis are listed in Box 18.1. Early-onset infections reflect vertical transmission from maternal genital tract flora to fetus/newborn. Late-onset infections are horizontally acquired in the hospital or at community level.

Pathogenesis

The most common mechanism for the development of neonatal meningitis is primary bloodstream infection followed by secondary hematogenous spread to the CNS. In early onset sepsis, organisms present in the maternal genitourinary tract ascend through the vagina, and infect the amniotic fluid through disruptions in the amniotic membranes causing fetal infection. *Listeria monocytogenes* can be directly transmitted transplacentally. Organisms can also colonize neonatal skin and mucosa during passage through the birth canal. In late onset sepsis, organisms are acquired from the colonized mother, caregivers, hospital staff and fomites due to poor hand hygiene, failure of maintenance of asepsis during invasive procedures and cross infection from other septic neonates.

Clinical Features

Clinical diagnosis of neonatal meningitis is often difficult and requires a high index of suspicion as the early symptoms and signs are similar to those of neonatal sepsis without meningitis. In addition to non-specific features of sepsis, the clinical pointers to development of meningitis include high pitched inconsolable crying, fever, vomiting, marked lethargy, seizures and bulging anterior fontanel.

Symptoms

The most commonly encountered clinical symptoms are listed below.

- Temperature instability (hypothermia or hyperthermia)
- Irritability or lethargy
- Altered sensorium
- Poor feeding/or intolerance of feeds
- Vomiting
- Paralytic ileus
- Staring look
- Mottled skin
- High pitched inconsolable crying
- Seizures
- Respiratory distress or apnea
- Vasomotor instability
- Disseminated intravascular coagulation

Signs

Examination may reveal a full or bulging non-pulsatile anterior fontanel which is present in approximately 25% of cases. Hypo- or hypertonia may be present. Signs of meningeal irritation are generally absent. Nuchal rigidity is present in approximately 15% of neonates and is a late finding.

Diagnosis

Diagnosis of neonatal bacterial meningitis is based on both clinical manifestations and laboratory findings including CSF examination.

Lumbar Puncture (LP)

CSF examination is essential to establish the diagnosis of bacterial meningitis and to identify the causative organism and antibiotic susceptibility. There is a long-standing debate on the need to perform LP in septic newborns; whether it should be done in all cases, or only in those with a strong clinical suspicion of meningitis. Performing LP in all septic neonates will expose many of them without meningitis to this hazardous procedure. On the other hand, performing LP in a very selective population may miss cases of meningitis, as clinical manifestations may be minimal or subtle. It is generally agreed that LP should be done in all cases of late-onset sepsis (>3 days) to rule out

---

BOX 18.1 Risk factors for neonatal meningitis

- Low birth weight (LBW) and prematurity
- Prolonged rupture of membranes (>18 h)
- Maternal chorioamnionitis
- Intrapartum fever (>38°C)
- Male sex
- Invasive procedures
- Failure of breastfeeding
- Indwelling intravascular catheters
- Prolonged stay in NICU
- Prolonged mechanical ventilation
- Long duration of total parenteral nutrition
- Documented maternal GBS colonization
- Overuse of broad spectrum antibiotics in the NICU
- Poor hand hygiene
- Unhygienic infant care practices in the community

Abbreviation: GBS: Group B streptococci

meningitis. In neonates with early-onset sepsis (<3 days), LP is indicated only when blood culture is positive or there are definite signs of meningitis such as seizures, full fontanel, or meningeal signs. The other viewpoint is that LP should be done in all symptomatic newborns evaluated for sepsis, regardless of the time of presentation. An LP should be done ideally before starting antibiotics. However, a critically sick newborn may not tolerate the procedure and in such cases antibiotics should be started in meningitic doses after taking blood culture and LP is deferred until the neonate becomes clinically stable, generally after 24 to 48 hours. LP should also be deferred in the presence of uncorrected coagulopathy.

Culture and sensitivity CSF culture is the gold standard for diagnosis of meningitis, though prior antibiotic administration may decrease the yield of CSF culture. Antibiotic susceptibility of the isolates help in choosing or modifying the antibiotic therapy for best therapeutic dividends.

Gram stain Gram stain is a rapid, inexpensive, and easy method for diagnosis of bacterial meningitis. Gram stains of CSF may provide useful information, even if CSF culture is not available. Its positivity rates depend on concentration of bacteria in the CSF. A positive Gram stain test result may guide in selection of appropriate antibiotic agents and duration of therapy.

CSF cell count, protein and glucose Evaluation of leukocyte count, glucose, and protein levels in the CSF may help in the diagnosis of neonatal meningitis. Characteristic CSF findings for acute bacterial meningitis are polymorphonuclear pleocytosis, hypoglycorrhachia, and increased protein concentrations.

Interpretation of CSF findings in newborns can be very challenging. Reference values for CSF cell count, protein and glucose are highly variable in neonates depending upon their gestational age, chronologic age, and birth weight. Moreover, there is considerable overlap between CSF parameters in neonates with and without meningitis and similar CSF findings can be demonstrated for neonates with other conditions such as intraventricular hemorrhage. The normal values of CSF white blood cell (WBC) count, protein and glucose levels are shown in Table 18.1.

In general, a CSF WBC count of >20/µL and/or neutrophil count of >6/µL is suggestive of bacterial meningitis in neonates. CSF leucocyte count is higher in neonates with Gram-negative meningitis than in Gram-positive meningitis. CSF protein and glucose values are highly variable. A CSF protein of >150 mg/dL in preterm and >100 mg/dL in term infants and a CSF glucose concentration <30 mg/dL in a term infant or <20 mg/dL in a preterm infant are considered to be consistent with bacterial meningitis. CSF to serum glucose ratio is less helpful in sick newborns as their serum glucose may be elevated due to stress or parenteral glucose infusion. It should be remembered that neonatal bacterial meningitis may occasionally occur in the absence of CSF pleocytosis and with normal CSF protein and glucose levels.

Traumatic LP is a common problem in newborns due to small intervertebral space. CSF cell count is difficult to interpret in traumatic LP. Various formulae have been devised but they are of not much practical help. CSF protein increases by 1 mg/dL for every 1000 RBCs. The level of glucose is not altered in traumatic CSF and a low CSF glucose should be considered an important finding. The traumatic sample must be sent for culture which may grow organisms.

Ancillary tests Non-culture tests, such as latex agglutination, polymerase chain reaction, loop-mediated isothermal amplification method, microarray or microchip, and immune-chromatography of CSF

Table 18.1 CSF cytology and biochemistry in normal neonates				
	Preterm		Term	
	≤7 days	>7 days	≤7 days	>7 days
WBC count/µL				
Median (IQR)	3 (1–7)	3 (1–4)	3 (1–6)	2 (1–4)
95th percentile	18	12	23	32
Protein (mg/dL)				
Median (IQR)	116 (93–138)	93 (69–122)	78 (60–100)	57 (42–77)
95th percentile	213	203	137	158
Glucose (mg/dL)				
Median (IQR)	53 (43–65)	47 (40–58)	50 (44–56)	52 (45–64)
5th percentile	10	13	26	17

IQR; Interquartile range

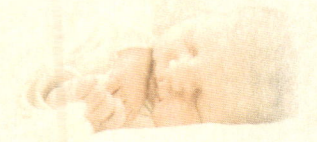

may be considered for neonates who need earlier identification of pathogens, have previously received antibiotics, or had a history of intraventricular hemorrhage. A number of CSF biomarkers such as tumor necrosis factor-α, interleukin (IL) 1β, IL-6, IL-8, IL-12, and IL-17 have been examined for differentiating bacterial meningitis from viral meningitis and non-infectious encephalopathy. The results are encouraging but with a wide range of sensitivities and specificities. Measurement of CSF procalcitonin on admission is useful, and a normal C-reactive protein (CRP) level has a high negative predictive value for bacterial meningitis. Significantly higher lipocalin-2 levels in CSF are documented in neonates with confirmed acute bacterial meningitis compared to those with acute viral meningitis. Other suggested biomarkers include neutrophil gelatinase-associated lipocalin, soluble triggering receptor expression on myeloid cells, heparin-binding protein, S100B, and brain-derived neurotrophic factor.

Repeating the LP The need for a repeat LP during treatment in an infant with bacterial meningitis is debatable. Some authors recommend repeating an LP routinely in all neonates at 48 hours of initiating antibiotics to document sterilization of CSF, whereas others suggest repeating an LP only if clinical condition has not shown significant improvement by 48–72 hours after beginning therapy. In general CSF becomes sterile in 2 days in Gram-positive meningitis and 3 days in Gram-negative meningitis. There is no need to repeat LP at the end of therapy to document cure unless the course is complicated.

Sepsis screen and blood culture Sepsis screen including peripheral WBC counts and CRP are poor predictors of neonatal meningitis. Blood cultures are positive in 40–60% of cases and among infants with positive blood cultures, up to 30% may have a concurrent positive CSF culture. In infants with confirmed meningitis, 15–38% may have a negative blood culture. In rare cases, the blood and CSF cultures can be discordant. Therefore, when only infants with confirmed bacteremia are evaluated for meningitis, we may miss the diagnosis of meningitis in some neonates. Hospitalized neonates, especially VLBW infants receiving broad spectrum antibiotics are at risk of fungal infection. Therefore in these cases blood sample should be sent for fungal culture in addition to bacterial culture during evaluation of late-onset sepsis, especially beyond one week of age.

Neuroimaging

Neuroimaging is indicated to identify the potential complications of neonatal meningitis, to extend the duration of antibiotic therapy if necessary, and to determine the prognosis.

Cranial ultrasonography (CUS) CUS is done early in the course of infection to assess ventricular size and identify the presence of ventriculitis, intraventricular hemorrhage, echogenic sulci, abnormal parenchymal echogenicities, and extracerebral fluid collections.

Magnetic resonance imaging (MRI) MRI can be done 48 to 72 hours before the anticipated end of therapy to detect the degree of cerebral edema, obstruction to CSF flow, infarction, abscess, and subdural fluid collections. Later on, contrast-enhanced MRI can be done to detect areas of infarct, encephalomalacia, degree of cerebral cortical and white matter atrophy and hydrocephalus.

Management

Management of neonatal meningitis includes meticulous clinical as well as laboratory monitoring, supportive care, prompt and optimal use of appropriate antibiotics.

Monitoring

Clinical Monitor temperature, respiratory rate, heart rate, color, oxygen saturation, capillary refill time/blood pressure, urine output, daily body weight and weekly head circumference.

Laboratory

- *Biochemical* Blood glucose, serum electrolytes, renal function tests, C-reactive protein, arterial blood gases
- *Hematological* Complete blood counts, and coagulation profile
- *Radiological* Cranial ultrasound.

Supportive Management

1. Provision of thermoneutral environment to ensure normal core temperature (36.5–37.5°C).
2. Gentle care should be provided by minimal handling with reduced environmental stimuli because of excessive light and sound. Painful procedures should be minimized and clustered together with appropriate pain relief.
3. Patent airway should be ensured with positioning and suction of secretions.
4. Oxygenation should be guided by pulse oximetry, respiratory support should be provided in the form of oxygen by hood/nasal prongs, CPAP or mechanical ventilation as per need.
5. Secure intravenous line should be established to provide fluids, antibiotics and parenteral nutrition. Blood culture sample should be collected before starting antibiotics. Normal maintenance fluids as appropriate for postnatal age should be given. There is no need to restrict daily fluid intake unless there

is abnormal weight gain or edema or decreased urine output. Enteral nutrition should be started with expressed breast milk once the infant is hemodynamically stable and seizure free.

6. In infants with prolonged capillary refill time or shock, saline should be infused at the rate of 10 mL/kg over 20–30 minutes, followed by vasopressors (dopamine or dobutamine).

7. If bedside dextrostix shows blood glucose level <40 mg/dL, 10% dextrose 2 mL/kg stat should be given followed by a glucose infusion with an infusion rate of 6–8 mg/kg/min.

8. Vitamin K 1.0 mg should be administered IV if not received earlier or there is active bleeding from any site.

9. If the neonate develops seizures, metabolic abnormalities in the form of hypoglycemia (blood glucose level <40 mg/dL) and hypocalcemia (ionized calcium <1 mmol/L) should be ruled out and managed appropriately. If seizures persist even after correction of hypoglycemia and hypocalcemia, injection phenobarbitone (20 mg/kg infused over 20 minutes) should be given intravenously. Newer antiepileptic agent levetiracetam can be tried as the first line agent in neonates with seizures.

Antibiotic Therapy

The management of neonatal meningitis is based on early and optimal intravenous administration of appropriate antibiotics. There are no randomized controlled trials on the choice of antibiotics in neonatal meningitis for rational antibiotic therapy. In the absence of high quality evidence, antibiotic therapy should be guided by the sensitivity pattern of prevalent microbial flora of the NICU. Therefore, every neonatal unit should have a strict policy to obtain blood cultures in suspected cases of sepsis before starting antibiotics and maintain records meticulously. The availability of culture profile and their antibiotic sensitivity pattern is critical for appropriate choice of antibiotics. The biggest concern for the choice of antibiotics is the growing resistance to commonly used antibiotics. Most Gram-negative bacilli are resistant to β-lactam antibiotics (penicillin, ampicillin) with increasingly growing resistance to cephalosporins and aminoglycosides. Empirical antibiotic therapy should cover common causative pathogens and should achieve adequate bactericidal activity in the CSF without toxicity. For infants <60 days of age, WHO recommends initial antibiotic therapy with a penicillin and an aminoglycoside (e.g. gentamicin). Though CSF penetration of penicillins is generally poor but when the meninges are inflamed, adequate concentrations can be achieved for susceptible organisms by more frequent and higher doses without

any risk of toxicity. In current practice most experts treat early-onset neonatal meningitis (<72 hours) with ampicillin and a third generation cephalosporin (cefotaxime, ceftazidime). For late-onset meningitis (>72 hours), it is recommended to use vancomycin and a third generation cephalosporin as first line empirical therapy. Third generation cephalosporins are preferred over aminoglycosides as they demonstrate good CSF penetration, have excellent activity against Gram-negative pathogens, and have minimal toxicity. Unlike cefotaxime, ceftazidime has potent anti-pseudomonal activity. Ceftriaxone should not be used in newborns as it may displace bilirubin from albumin and thus potentiate the risk of bilirubin neurotoxicity. Some experts advocate a combination of ampicillin, gentamicin and cefotaxime for treatment of neonatal meningitis. However, there is no evidence to show that this combination is superior to ampicillin and cefotaxime alone.

Empirical upgradation must be done if the expected clinical improvement with the first line of antibiotics does not occur in 48–72 hours. Vancomycin and meropenem may be considered empirically as the second line antibiotics for early-onset meningitis. For late-onset meningitis with inadequate response to first-line antibiotics, replace cefotaxime with meropenem and continue with vancomycin. Antibiotics are modified once CSF culture reports are available. In Gram-negative meningitis, cefepime or polymixin B or ciprofloxacin may be used in selected cases showing resistance to commonly used antibiotics. For nosocomial infections, vancomycin and meropenem is a reasonable empirical choice. Fungal meningitis should be considered in neonates (especially VLBW babies) who have prolonged hospital stay and are exposed to broad spectrum antibiotics. Intravenous fluconazole may be started on empirical basis as the first line antifungal agent after sending blood and CSF culture for fungal growth and antifungal susceptibility. Antifungal agent may be modified after receipt of culture and sensitivity report. Liposomal amphotericin B may be considered as the second line antifungal agent if the neonate does not show any improvement on fluconazole.

Duration of antibiotics In general, antibiotics are continued for 2 weeks after sterilization of CSF or for 2 weeks of total duration of Gram-positive meningitis and 3 weeks for Gram-negative meningitis. Longer treatment courses are recommended for infants with meningitis with delayed clinical improvement after beginning of therapy or with complications such as brain abscess, ventriculitis, or brain infarction. Doses of commonly used antibiotics for treatment of neonatal meningitis are given in Table 18.2.

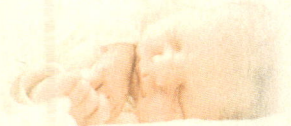

Table 18.2 Doses of antibiotics in neonatal meningitis

Antibiotic	Weight	Postnatal age	Dose/kg	Dosing frequency
Amphotericin – B (Liposomal)	All weights	All ages	5–7 mg	24 h
Amikacin	<1,000 g	≤14 days	15 mg	48 h
	<1,000 g	>14 days	15 mg	24–48 h
	1,000–2,000 g	≤7 days	15 mg	48 h
	1,000–2,000 g	>7 days	15 mg	24–48 h
	>2,000 g	≤7 days	15 mg	24 h
	>2,000 g	>7 days	15 mg	12–24 h
Ampicillin	All weights	≤7 days	50–100 mg	8 h
	All weights	>7 days	50–75 mg	6 h
Cefepime	<1,000 g	≤14 days	30–50 mg	12 h
	<1,000 g	>14 days	50 mg	8–12 h
	1,000–2,000 g	≤7 days	30–50 mg	12 h
	1,000–2,000 g	>7 days	50 mg	8–12 h
	>2,000 g	All ages	50 mg	8–12 h
Cefotaxime	<1,000 g	≤14 days	50 mg	12 h
	<1,000 g	≤14 days	50 mg	12 h
	1,000–2,000 g	≤7 days	50 mg	12 h
	1,000–2,000 g	>7 days	50 mg	8–12 h
	>2,000 g	≤7 days	50 mg	12 h
	>2,000 g	>7 days	50 mg	6–8 h
Ceftazidime	<1,000 g	≤14 days	50 mg	12 h
	<1,000 g	>14 days	50 mg	8–12 h
	1,000–2,000 g	≤7 days	50 mg	12 h
	1,000–2,000 g	>7 days	50 mg	8–12 h
	>2,000 g	≤7 days	50 mg	12 h
	>2,000 g	>7 days	50 mg	8 h
Ciprofloxacin	All weights	All ages	10 mg	12 h
Fluconazole	All weights	All ages	12 mg	24 h
Gentamicin	<1,000 g	≤14 days	5 mg	48 h
	<1,000 g	>14 days	4–5 mg	24–48 h
	1,000–2,000 g	≤7 days	5 mg	48 h
	1,000–2,000 g	>7 days	4–5 mg	24–48 h
	>2,000 g	≤7 days	4 mg	24 h
	>2,000 g	>7 days	4 mg	12–24 h
Meropenem	<1,000 g	≤14 days	20 mg	12 h
	<1,000 g	>14 days	20 mg	8 h
	1,000–2,000 g	≤7 days	20 mg	12 h
	1,000–2,000 g	>7 days	20 mg	8 h
	>2,000 g	All	20 mg	8 h
Piperacillin-tazobactam	<1,000 g	≤14 days	100 mg	12 h
	<1,000 g	>14 days	100 mg	8 h
	≥1,000 g	≤7 days	100 mg	12 h
	≥1,000 g	>7 days	100 mg	8 h
Vancomycin	<1,200 g	All ages	15 mg	24 h
	1,200–2,000 g	<7 days	10–15 mg	12–18 h
	1,200–2,000 g	≤7 days	10–15 mg	8–12 h
	>2,000 g	<7 days	10–15 mg	8–12 h
	>2,000 g	≤7 days	10–15 mg	6–8 h
Polymixin-B	All weights	All ages	40,000 U/kg/day	8 h

Adjunctive Therapy

Several adjunctive therapies have been explored, including the use of intraventricular antibiotics, intravenous immunoglobulins, and granulocyte or granulocyte macrophage colony stimulating factor. At present, none of the proposed adjunctive therapies are found to be useful in routine practice.

Based on current evidence, use of steroids is not recommended for treatment of neonatal meningitis. Similarly, intravenous immunoglobulins do not appear to improve the outcome of meningitis and are not recommended.

As aminoglycosides have poor penetration into CSF, intraventricular instillation of gentamicin was thought to achieve higher CSF concentrations than intravenous route alone. However, it has been documented that intraventricular use of gentamicin resulted in 3-fold increased relative risk for mortality compared to the standard treatment alone in Gram-negative meningitis and ventriculitis.

Neurologic Complications of Neonatal Meningitis and their Management

Neurologic complications of neonatal meningitis can be divided into acute and chronic.

Acute Complications

Acute complications include cerebral edema, increased intracranial pressure (ICP), ventriculitis, cerebritis, hydrocephalus, brain abscess, cerebral infarction, and subdural effusion or empyema.

Ventriculitis It is defined as inflammation of lining of the ventricles, usually occurring in association with obstruction to CSF flow. It is a common complication of neonatal bacterial meningitis occurring in approximately 20% of cases. There are no definite clinical signs but it should be suspected when the neonate fails to respond clinically and bacteriologically in spite of appropriate and optimal use of antimicrobial therapy.

Diagnosis is made by neuroimaging. The findings suggestive of ventriculitis on cranial ultrasound include intraventricular strands attached to ventricular surface, echogenic ependyma, and dilated ventricles. Enhancement of the lining of the ventricles is seen on MRI.

Aspiration of ventricular fluid is indicated for infants who have ventriculitis with an obstruction to the flow of CSF. Culture and sensitivity of ventricular fluid should be performed as infection may persist for a longer period. The duration of antimicrobial therapy should extend as long as six to eight weeks to sterilize the ventricular CSF. Pediatric neurosurgical consultation should be taken.

Hydrocephalus The overall incidence of hydrocephalus is around 24% of infants with neonatal bacterial meningitis. Higher incidence is observed in cases of Gram-negative infections, especially with K1 *E. coli* infection (30–44%) and in those who succumbed to the illness (56%). The clinical features of hydrocephalus include signs of increased intracranial pressure as evidenced by bulging non-pulsatile anterior fontanel, sun-setting sign, bradycardia, hypertension, and respiratory depression. Increase in head circumference (HC) is a late feature.

Diagnosis of hydrocephalus is made by CUS. Management is done in consultation with pediatric neurosurgeon. Neonates with rapidly progressive hydrocephalus require urgent surgical intervention, either with a CSF shunt or endoscopic third ventriculostomy. Patients showing signs of impending herniation and critically sick neonates may require placement of a temporary external ventricular drain. Other options include diuretics such as furosemide and acetazolamide to decrease CSF production and serial lumbar punctures, though these are less effective and can be used for short periods in slowly progressive hydrocephalus.

Brain abscess Brain abscess may occur in approximately 13% cases of neonatal bacterial meningitis. It is more common with Gram-negative infections and in meningitis caused by *Citrobacter koseri, Serratia marcescens, Proteus mirabilis, Enterobacter sakazakii (Cronobacter)* and extended-spectrum beta-lactamase producing *Klebsiella pneumoniae*. Clinical features may be subtle and include vomiting, bulging fontanel, hydrocephalus, decreased limb movements, focal seizures, and leukocytosis. The abscess generally develops in the second week of illness. In neonates with bacterial meningitis, development of brain abscess should be suspected if the neonate develops seizures, prominent focal cerebral signs, or shows poor clinical response to antibiotic therapy.

LP may show marked CSF pleocytosis, with a predominance of mononuclear cells, increased protein and decreased CSF glucose concentration. Marked clinical deterioration with further increase in CSF pleocytosis and protein can occur if the abscess ruptures into the lateral ventricle or subarachnoid space.

The diagnosis of brain abscess is made by neuroimaging studies. CUS can demonstrate an echogenic rim with a hypoechogenic center, but differentiation between hemorrhagic necrosis and abscess is difficult. MRI is preferred and shows variably circumscribed areas of decreased attenuation and contrast enhancement of the rim. The surrounding edema may occur due to cerebritis. Serial brain imaging at weekly or bi-weekly intervals should be performed to monitor the evolution and outcome of abscess.

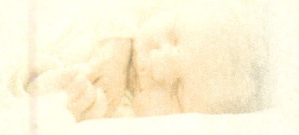

Management is done in consultation with a pediatric neurosurgeon for the need for surgical intervention in the form of needle aspiration or excision. The minimum duration of treatment for brain abscess complicating Gram-negative meningitis is 4 weeks. At times, the duration of antibiotic therapy may need to be extended to six to eight weeks depending on the clinical and radiographic response. The development of a brain abscess is associated with poor outcome in the form of increased mortality or development of neurologic sequelae such as seizures and developmental delay.

Infarction Arterial ischemic stroke and cerebral sinovenous thrombosis may complicate 30–50% cases of fatal neonatal meningitis. Infarction usually develops early in the course of the disease, most commonly within the first week. Clinical manifestations include focal seizures and limb paresis. There is no specific treatment.

Subdural effusion Clinically significant subdural effusion is uncommon in neonates with bacterial meningitis, though it can develop in neonates with Gram-negative meningitis. Clinical findings are often subtle or absent including bulging fontanel, signs of raised ICP and hydrocephaly. Most subdural effusions resolve spontaneously. Aspiration is indicated in suspected cases of subdural empyema, development of focal neurologic findings, and/or evidence of increased ICP.

Chronic Complications

Chronic complications of neonatal bacterial meningitis include hydrocephalus, cystic encephalomalacia with porencephaly and cerebral cortical and white matter atrophy. The clinical manifestations of these complications include developmental delay, cerebral palsy, seizure disorder, hearing loss and cortical blindness.

Outcome

In developed countries, mortality from neonatal meningitis has dropped from nearly 50% in the 1970s to approximately 10% in 2000s, but morbidity remains substantial. About 20–58% of survivors are known to have serious neurological sequelae, moderate to severe sensorineural hearing loss being most common. Other complications include intellectual impairment, visual impairment, epilepsy, neuromotor disability and hydrocephalus. Approximately 20% survivors develop severe disability and 35% have mild to moderate disability. Poor outcome is more common in Gram-negative infection and very low birth weight neonates.

Follow-up

Long-term multidisciplinary follow-up of survivors of neonatal meningitis should be done by a team of neonatologist/pediatrician, pediatric neurologist, occupational therapist, ophthalmologist, audiologist and radiologist. Regular monitoring of growth, neuro-motor development, hearing, vision, and other morbidities should be done. Hearing should be evaluated by evoked response audiometry within four to six weeks of completion of therapy. Survivors of neonatal meningitis are at risk for developmental delay and should be provided with early intervention physiotherapy.

Predictors of Poor Prognosis

The presence of the following factors predict increased risk of mortality and high-risk of neurologic sequelae:

- LBW and prematurity.
- Delayed diagnosis for more than 24 hours after the onset of symptoms.
- Leukopenia and neutropenia.
- Meningitis caused by Gram-negative bacteria.
- Focal neurological deficits, hypertonicity and dysphagia.
- Seizures occurring more than 72 hours after onset of symptoms.
- Requirement for mechanical ventilatory support or inotropes.
- Low voltage EEG.
- Delayed sterilization of the CSF.
- Presence of thrombi, abscess and encephalomalacia on neuroimaging.

Key Messages

- Neonatal meningitis is an important cause of neonatal mortality and survivors are at high-risk for neurologic damage and lifelong sequelae.
- Clinical signs are often subtle and a high index of clinical suspicion is necessary for early diagnosis and institution of therapy.
- CSF culture is the gold standard for diagnosis of neonatal meningitis.
- While blood cultures and CSF parameters (WBC count and biochemical parameters) may be helpful in cases where the diagnosis is uncertain, bacterial meningitis may occur in infants without bacteremia and with normal CSF parameters.
- On clinical suspicion of neonatal meningitis, appropriate broad spectrum antimicrobial therapy with adequate CSF penetration should be initiated as soon as possible. In Indian set-up, a combination

of ampicillin and cefotaxime is used for early-onset meningitis and vancomycin and cefotaxime for late-onset meningitis. Empirical antimicrobial therapy should be changed accordingly as soon as the causative organism and its antimicrobial susceptibility pattern is known. Duration of antibiotic therapy varies from 14–21 days, depending on the nature of causative organism.

- Regular neuroimaging is important to detect neurological complications at their earliest.
- Long-term multidisciplinary follow-up for survivors of neonatal meningitis is necessary to detect developmental delay and hearing loss.

BIBLIOGRAPHY

Barichello T, Fagundes GD, Generoso JS, Elias SG, Simões LR, Teixeira AL. Pathophysiology of neonatal acute bacterial meningitis. *J Med Microbiol* 2013; 62(12):1781–9.

Furyk JS, Swann O, Molyneux. Systematic review: neonatal meningitis in the developing world. *Trop Med Int Health* 2011; 16(6):672–9.

Garges HP, Moody MA, Cotten CM, Smith PB, Tiffany KF, Lenfestey R, Li JS, Fowler VG Jr, Benjamin DK Jr. Neonatal meningitis: what is the correlation among cerebrospinal fluid cultures, blood cultures, and cerebrospinal fluid parameters? *Pediatrics* 2006; 117(4):1094–100.

Greenberg RG, Benjamin DK Jr, Cohen-Wolkowiez M, et al. Repeat lumbar punctures in infants with meningitis in the neonatal intensive care unit. *J Perinatol* 2011; 31(6):425–9.

Khalessi N, Afsharkhas L. Neonatal Meningitis: Risk factors, causes and neurologic complications. *Iran J Child Neurol* 2014; 8(4):46–50.

Klinger G, Chin CN, Beyene J, et al. Predicting the outcome of neonatal bacterial meningitis. *Pediatrics* 2000; 106(3):477–82.

Ku LC, Boggess KA, Cohen-Wolkowiez M. Bacterial meningitis in infants. *Clin Perinatol* 2015; 42(1):29–45.

Ogunlesi TA, Odigwe CC, Oladapo OT. Adjuvant corticosteroids for reducing death in neonatal bacterial meningitis. *Cochrane Database Syst Rev* 2015; (11):CD010435.

Shah SS, Ohlsson A, Shah VS. Intraventricular antibiotics for bacterial meningitis in neonates. *Cochrane Database Syst Rev* 2012; (7):CD004496.

Srinivasan L, Shah SS, Padula MA, Abbasi S, McGowan KL, Harris MC. Cerebrospinal fluid reference ranges in term and preterm infants in the neonatal intensive care unit. *J Pediatr* 2012; 161(4): 729–34.

Zaidi AK, Thaver D, Ali SA, Khan TA. Pathogens associated with sepsis in newborns and young infants in developing countries. *Pediatr Infect Dis* 2009; 28 (Suppl. 1):S10–S18.

19

Neonatal Encephalopathy

Ashok Kumar and Sriparna Basu

Introduction

Neonatal encephalopathy is a heterogeneous disorder of varied etiology characterized by signs of neurologic dysfunction in newborn infants. Neonatal encephalopathy may lead to adverse consequences such as death, cerebral palsy, epilepsy and other significant neuro-cognitive, developmental and behavioral sequelae. Clinically it manifests as an abnormal level of consciousness, seizures, tone and reflex abnormalities, unexplained apnea and feeding difficulties. Correct diagnosis and prompt therapy can improve the outcome of neonatal encephalopathy in many cases.

Definition

As per the American College of Obstetricians and Gynecologists' Summary Statement (2014), neonatal encephalopathy is a clinically defined syndrome characterized by disturbed central nervous system (CNS) function in the earliest days of life in an infant born at or beyond 35 weeks of gestation. Encephalopathy is manifested by a subnormal level of consciousness or seizures, and often accompanied by difficulty in initiating and maintaining respirations at birth with depression of tone and reflexes.

This definition of neonatal encephalopathy refers to CNS dysfunction in term and late preterm infants only, encephalopathy of preterm infants has not been included. Other definitions which are also commonly used to describe neonatal encephalopathy include persistence of two or more symptoms of encephalopathy lasting for more than 24 hours or low 5-minute Apgar score. However, these definitions are less specific and often affected by maternal conditions or prematurity.

Incidence

The incidence of neonatal encephalopathy ranges from 2–9/1000 term births depending on the definition used. As per a study in US (2010), the estimated incidence of neonatal encephalopathy is 3.0/1000 live births (95% CI 2.7–3.3). No Indian data is available.

Etiology and Pathology

Neonatal encephalopathy is multifactorial in origin. The most common antecedent of neonatal encephalopathy is hypoxia-ischemia, but, it is only one of the many possible contributors to neonatal encephalopathy. Other insults potentially responsible for neonatal encephalopathy include infection/inflammation, metabolic, traumatic, cerebral malformations, genetic, and toxic causes, either alone or in combination.

Pathological changes in brain often encountered in neonatal encephalopathy include bilateral abnormalities in basal ganglia, thalami, cortex, or white matter, and focal infarction. In neonates presenting with seizures, acute ischemic or hemorrhagic strokes are also likely to be present.

Risk Factors

The nature of risk factors for neonatal encephalopathy varies depending on the time of CNS insult. Approximately 69% cases of neonatal encephalopathy are known to be associated with antepartum adverse events, 25% are associated with both antepartum and intrapartum risk factors, 4% have evidence of only intrapartum risk factor. No identified risk factors are found in 2% even after detailed investigations. The details of antepartum and intrapartum risk factors are summarized in Table 19.1. Among the antepartum risk factors, intrauterine growth restriction (IUGR) has

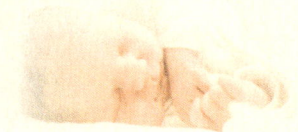
Table 19.1 Risk factors for neonatal encephalopathy

Antepartum

- *Maternal* Poor socio-economic status, chorioamnionitis, family history of seizures or neurologic disorder, thyroid disease, assisted reproductive technique
- *Placental* Severe pre-eclampsia, post-dated pregnancy, placental abnormalities such as placental thrombosis, infection, and compromised utero-placental flow
- *Fetal* Intrauterine growth restriction

Intrapartum

- Persistent occipito-posterior position
- Shoulder dystocia
- Emergency cesarean section, failed forceps or vacuum extraction
- Perinatal hypoxia-ischemia
- Acute intrapartum or sentinel events like uterine rupture, placental abruption, cord prolapse, tight nuchal cord, maternal shock/death
- Inflammatory events like maternal fever, sepsis, and prolonged rupture of membranes

Metabolic and genetic abnormalities

- *Disorders of amino acid metabolism* Maple syrup urine disease, phenylketonuria, nonketotic hyperglycinemia
- *Hyperammonemia* Urea cycle defects
- Neonatal hypoglycemia
- Organic acidemias
- Mitochondrial disorders
- Severe peroxisomal disorders like Zellweger syndrome
- Sulfite oxidase deficiency and molybdenum cofactor deficiency
- *Genetic disorders* Prader-Willi syndrome, chromosomal abnormalities

Others

- Brain anomalies
- Perinatal infection
- Sinovenous thrombosis
- *Intracranial hemorrhage* Idiopathic, related to birth trauma, congenital vascular malformation, coagulation disorder and thrombocytopenia
- Perinatal stroke
  - i. *Maternal* Prothrombotic disorders, addiction to narcotics, barbiturates, alcohol, tricyclic antidepressants, and serotonin reuptake inhibitors
  - ii. *Placental* Pre-eclampsia, chorioamnionitis and placental vasculopathy
  - iii. *Neonatal* Prothrombotic disorders, congenital heart disease, meningitis, and systemic infection

strongest association with neonatal encephalopathy. The common intrapartum events, placental abruption or uterine rupture is associated with a four-fold increased risk of neonatal encephalopathy. Other commonly recognized underlying disorders responsible for neonatal encephalopathy include perinatal stroke, perinatal infection, CNS malformations, intracranial hemorrhage, infarction and metabolic disorders.

Clinical Presentation

In the delivery room, the neonate is likely to have a weak or absent cry, requires resuscitation and has low Apgar score. Subsequent presentation include an abnormal state of consciousness ranging from hyperalert, irritable, lethargic or obtunded state, diminished spontaneous movements, respiratory or feeding difficulties, poor tone, abnormal posturing, absent primitive reflexes, or seizure activity.

Depending on the severity, neonatal encephalopathy is classified as mild, moderate, or severe as per following criteria.

- *Mild.* Hyperalert, hyperexcitable, normal muscle tone, no seizures.
- *Moderate.* Lethargy, hypotonia, decreased movements, and seizures
- *Severe.* Stuporose, flaccid, and absent primitive reflexes, seizures are uncommon but evident on EEG.

The signs and events suggestive of an acute peripartum or intrapartum adverse events are listed below:

Apgar score <5 at 5 and 10 minutes Low Apgar scores at 5 minutes and 10 minutes suggest perinatal hypoxia-ischemia. If the Apgar score at 5 minutes is ≥7, peripartum hypoxia-ischemia is reasonably ruled out as a cause of neonatal encephalopathy.

Fetal umbilical artery acidemia Fetal umbilical artery pH < 7.0, or base deficit ≥12 mmol/L, or both, increases the probability that neonatal encephalopathy is secondary to perinatal hypoxia-ischemia. If the cord arterial pH levels are above 7.20, intrapartum hypoxia is unlikely. However, the presence of metabolic acidemia does not indicate the time of the onset of an hypoxic-ischemic insult.

Presence of multisystem organ failure Multisystem organ failure including injury to renal and hepatic parenchyma, hematologic abnormalities, cardiac dysfunction, metabolic derangements, and gastrointestinal injury, or a combination of all these indicate hypoxia-ischemia as the cause of neonatal encephalopathy. *It should be remembered that in neonatal encephalopathy secondary to hypoxia-ischemia, the severity of brain injury does not always correlate with the degree of injury and dysfunction of other organ systems.*

Neuroimaging evidences of acute brain injury Normal neuroimaging findings after initial 24 hours of life reasonably rules out hypoxia-ischemia as a cause of neonatal encephalopathy.

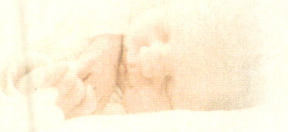

Diagnosis

The diagnosis of neonatal encephalopathy is based on the presence of clinical as well as laboratory evidences of potential etiology.

Clinical

History Details of maternal and family history should be recorded, including history of medical and obstetric disorders, prior pregnancy loss, maternal infection, thromboembolic disorders and maternal drug abuse. Details of obstetric antecedents, intrapartum factors including fetal growth, antenatal fetal monitoring and details of delivery should be noted. Assess condition of the baby at birth, Apgar score at 5 minutes and details of resuscitation provided. The onset of seizures within 36 hours of life is highly suggestive hypoxia-ischemia. A gross and histological examination of the placenta and umbilical cord may provide evidences of a possible cause, such as a placental vascular lesion or infection, or an umbilical cord thrombosis.

Clinical examination The neonate should be examined thoroughly for level of consciousness, muscle tone, movements of limbs and primitive reflexes. The presence of IUGR, oliguria, cardiomyopathy, or abnormal liver function tests may suggest a global hypoxic-ischemic event. Metabolic derangements, unusual odors, dysmorphic features, and congenital anomalies are useful correlates of an inborn error of metabolism (IEM) or genetic disorder. Blood samples should be drawn to determine umbilical artery cord pH and base deficit. Toxic and metabolic screening should be carried out in suspected cases.

Neuroimaging

Various neuroimaging modalities have been used to evaluate infants with neonatal encephalopathy, including cranial ultrasonography (CUS), computed tomography (CT), magnetic resonance imaging (MRI) and magnetic resonance spectroscopy (MRS).

Cranial MRI MRI is the best neuroimaging modality to define the nature and extent of cerebral injury in neonatal encephalopathy. It is a useful modality to predict later neurodevelopmental status. However, the facilities for transporting, monitoring, and supporting sick babies for MRI are not readily available in most set ups in India.

A cranial MRI is recommended to establish the presence and pattern of CNS injury, and to predict neurologic outcome for infants with neonatal encephalopathy. It is a reliable modality to detect cortical and white matter injury, deep grey matter lesions, arterial infarction, hemorrhage, developmental malformations of brain, and other underlying causes of neonatal encephalopathy. Deep gray matter lesions involving the bilateral basal ganglia and thalami are particularly common findings on brain MRI in encephalopathic term infants with a recognized preceding sentinel hypoxic-ischemic event such as placental abruption, uterine rupture, or umbilical cord prolapse. Brainstem injury is also common in these circumstances. The characteristics of brain injury considered to be typical of hypoxia-ischemia in term and late preterm infants are summarized below.

A. Injury to the deep gray nuclei especially in the region of lateral thalami and posterior putamin are indicative of acute total asphyxia.

B. Parasagittal injury of the cerebral cortex and subcortical white matter in the arterial watershed distribution, is suggestive of mild hypoxia or prolonged ischemia.

In contrast, presence of focal arterial infarcts, venous infarction, isolated intraparenchymal or intraventricular hemorrhage and porencephaly on MRI of brain suggest metabolic encephalopathies rather than peripartum hypoxia-ischemia as a cause of neonatal encephalopathy. Developmental brain malformations can also be identified as the underlying cause for neonatal encephalopathy. In addition to conventional MRI, MRS and diffusion-weighted imaging (DWI) techniques can provide useful information.

Neuroimaging provides useful information regarding the type and timing of brain injury. Normal MRI or MRS, obtained after the first 24 hours of life rules out significant peripartum or intrapartum hypoxic–ischemic brain injury as a significant factor causing neonatal encephalopathy. *It is important to remember that the full extent of cerebral injury may not be evident on MRI until after the first week of life.* Early MRI obtained between 24 to 96 hours of life is useful for the delineation of the timing of perinatal cerebral injury, but an MRI undertaken between 7 and 21 days of life (optimally at 10 days of life) is most useful to delineate the full extent of cerebral injury.

Cranial USG CUS has the advantage of being non-invasive and easily available at point-of-care. It has a high sensitivity and specificity for diagnosis of intraventricular hemorrhage and assessing ventricular size. It may also detect severe parasagittal white matter damage and obvious cystic lesions, but it is not reliable to image the outer limits of the cerebral cortex, and it is not a sensitive tool to identify milder white matter abnormalities that can be detected by cranial MRI.

CUS can also be used to detect cerebral edema which is characterized by increased echogenicity causing obliteration of sulci and fissures, blurring of other anatomical landmarks, decreased arterial pulsations, and compression of the cerebral ventricles. After a few days following hypoxic-ischemic injury, areas of echodensity corresponding to the regions of necrosis may be evident. However, differentiation of early echodensities as areas of infarction or hemorrhage is not always possible by CUS.

Cranial CT Cranial CT is more sensitive than CUS for diagnosing intracranial hemorrhage. Gray matter can be distinguished from white matter easily and cerebral edema is denoted by decreased attenuation of white matter in cranial CT. Other easily identified findings include cerebral atrophy, abnormal ventricular size, and severe white matter lesions. However, as the white matter in a term newborn brain has high water content, milder degrees of edema and white matter injury may sometimes be missed on cranial CT. *Moreover, CT should preferably be avoided in a newborn because of the hazards of high radiation exposure.*

Electroencephalography

An electroencephalogram (EEG) can identify subclinical seizures and help to distinguish neonatal seizures from other non-epileptic phenomena. Although, EEG is not helpful to determine the cause of neonatal encephalopathy, it can provide evidence for the presence and severity of encephalopathy, as well as prognostic information. Amplitude integrated EEG (aEEG) using a continuous, single- or dual-channel bedside recording of background cerebral electrical activity, is a useful modality as the seizure activity can be interpreted easily.

Metabolic Screening

If IEM is suspected, specific testing for acidemia, ammonia, lactate and pyruvate, serum amino acids, and urine organic acids along with tandem mass spectroscopy (TMS) should be obtained to rule out a metabolic cause of neonatal encephalopathy. The investigations should be done after introduction of enteral feeds and when baby is symptomatic.

Management

Prevention

Prompt identification and management of potentially modifiable risk factors which can prevent or lessen the severity of neonatal encephalopathy, are listed below.

- Early identification and adequate treatment of pre-pregnancy medical disorder in the mother.
- Proper antenatal care with regular fetal monitoring.
- Early recognition and management of pregnancy-induced disorders.
- Timely management of labor and delivery.
- Skilled resuscitation at birth.
- Good immediate postnatal care in the NICU.

Treatment

Major goals of immediate treatment include maintenance of physiological homeostasis and treatment of ongoing brain injury. The management is tailored to the specific etiology of neonatal encephalopathy. The broad principles of management are summarized below.

1. *Therapeutic hypothermia* It is the treatment of choice for perinatal asphyxia with moderate to severe hypoxic ischemic encephalopathy wherein intervention is started within first six hours of age along with provision of effective supportive management in late preterm and term neonates. In neonates with non-asphyxial encephalopathy, ensure normothermia (36.5–37.5°C).
2. Gentle handling with avoidance of various environmental stimuli.
3. Monitoring of vital signs including pulse oximetry.
4. Arterial blood gas analysis, serum calcium, magnesium, glucose, and electrolytes. These parameters should be assessed early and repeated as needed to maintain normal metabolic status and normoglycemia.
5. Respiratory support by providing oxygen inhalation, continuous positive airway pressure (CPAP) or mechanical ventilation. Maintenance of adequate ventilation with avoidance of hypoxemia or hyperoxia is recommended to maintain target oxygen saturation of 90–94%.
6. Maintenance of adequate perfusion of vital organs including brain by replacement of volume loss and use of inotropic agents as required to maintain blood pressure and adequate cerebral perfusion. However, systemic hypertension and volume overload, which can worsen cerebral edema, should be avoided.
7. Avoidance of polycythemia and hyperviscosity by maintenance of a target hematocrit below 65%.
8. When inborn error of metabolism is suspected, early treatment is crucial for intact survival. Feeds should be stopped, acidosis and hypoglycemia are corrected, and specific treatment such as vitamin supplementation or hemodialysis is considered after consultation with a specialist. Enteral nutriton

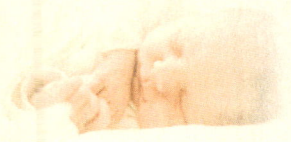

is started with expressed breast milk as soon as the neonate is hemodynamically stable and seizure free for 48 hours. Enzyme replacement therapy can be considered in specific enzyme deficiencies.

9. The commonly used anticonvulsants to control seizures include phenobarbital, phenytoin, and lorazepam. However, newer anticonvulsant levetiracetam can also be used as a first line agent, though high quality evidence is not available till date. Metabolic causes such as hypoglycemia and hypocalcemia should always be ruled out and managed before starting anticonvulsants.

10. In infants with persistent pulmonary hypertension, high frequency ventilation, inhaled nitric oxide (iNO), or extracorporeal membrane oxygenation (ECMO) are recommended to maintain oxygenation. When iNO is not available, sildenafil, milrinone or magnesium sulphate can be tried.

11. Laboratory investigations like complete blood count, sepsis screen including blood culture should be done to rule out sepsis. Coagulation profile, liver enzymes, blood urea and serum creatinine, chest and abdominal X-rays, abdominal ultrasonography and 2-D Echocardiography with color Doppler are useful to identify hypoxic damage to various end organs.

12. A lumbar puncture should be performed when there is concern for intracranial infection, as meningitis can mimic the signs and symptoms of neonatal encephalopathy.

13. Antibiotics should be started when infection is suspected. Acyclovir therapy should be initiated if Herpes simplex encephalitis is suspected.

14. Electroencephalography (EEG) or point-of-care aEEG is useful to identify electrical seizure activity to guide the initiation and duration of anticonvulsant therapy. Continuous or serial EEGs are helpful to define prognosis.

15. CUS and cranial MRI should be obtained, depending upon the feasibility.

16. Long-term treatment and follow-up should be provided by a multidisciplinary team consisting of neonatologist/pediatrician, pediatric neurologist, geneticist, occupational therapist, ophthalmologist, ENT specialist, cardiologist, counsellor and social worker.

Other Potential Neuroprotective Strategies

A variety of potential neuroprotective strategies to prevent the cascade of injurious events in neonates with hypoxic-ischemic encephalopathy are currently under trial and are listed in Box 19.1.

BOX 19.1 Emerging neuroprotective strategies for HIE

- Therapeutic hypothermia
- Erythropoietin
- Oxygen free radical scavengers
- Glutamate receptor antagonists
- Calcium channel blocking agents
- Monosialo-gangliosides growth factor and brain derived growth factor
- Nitric oxide synthase inhibitors
- Agents to block the pathway to apoptosis
- Anti-inflammatory agents
- Stem cell therapy

Prognosis

The possibility and extent of brain damage is directly related to the severity of neonatal encephalopathy. Most infants with mild encephalopathy have normal neuro-development, whereas infants with moderate to severe encephalopathy have a 20–35% risk of development of long-term neurologic sequelae. Severe MRI and EEG abnormalities are usually associated with poor outcome.

The neurologic sequelae may vary from mild, (learning difficulties or attention deficit disorder), to severe and disabling handicaps such as cerebral palsy, epilepsy, visual and hearing impairment, or severe cognitive and developmental disorders. Although there is an increased risk of cerebral palsy associated with neonatal encephalopathy, it is not an inevitable consequence. *In most cases of cerebral palsy or later developmental deficits, the cause is unknown or is related to conditions other than neonatal encephalopathy.*

Predictors of Poor Outcome

Clinical

- Neonates with mild encephalopathy and normal neurologic examination during first week of life are likely to have normal outcome.
- Neonates receiving therapeutic hypothermia may show a modest improvement in the combined incidence of death or neuromotor disability.
- Different scoring systems have been used to predict adverse outcome. Commonly used parameters indicative of poor prognosis include need for prolonged resuscitation, severe acidemia in umbilical cord blood and refractory seizures.

Neuroimaging

- Cranial MRI showing bilateral lesions in basal ganglia and thalami or an abnormal signal intensity in the posterior limb of the internal capsule obtained in the first two weeks of life are associated with adverse neurologic outcome or death.

- According to some studies, a watershed pattern of brain injury involving the boundary regions of the major cerebral vascular territories on cranial MRI is associated with long-term cognitive and motor deficits, with or without cerebral palsy.
- Diffusion-waited imaging (DWI) can detect the presence of acute brain injury occurring within past 7 to 10 days.
- MRS is useful to detect increased lactate and decreased N-acetyl aspartate (NAA) concentrations, indicating derangements of the metabolic state of specific regions of the brain indicating a poor prognosis. Elevated lactate/NAA ratios in the thalamus or basal ganglia are markers of poor prognosis with high sensitivity and specificity.
- In perinatal arterial stroke, presence of internal capsule and basal ganglia injury is associated with an increased risk of hemiparesis and long-term neurodevelopmental sequelae.

EEG

- An EEG or aEEG showing severe background abnormalities such as burst suppression, isoelectricity or extremely low voltage, predicts a high possibility of death or long-term neurological sequelae.
- Serial EEG examination is a useful predictor of progressive deterioration or recovery.

Biomarkers

Elevated serum interleukin (IL)-1β, IL-6, cerebrospinal fluid (CSF) neuron-specific enolase, and CSF IL-1β, measured before postnatal age of 96 hours are useful to predict adverse neurological outcome in survivors.

Key Messages

- Neonatal encephalopathy is a clinically defined syndrome characterized by disturbed CNS function during early days of life in an infant born at or beyond 35 weeks.
- No single etiology can explain neonatal encephalopathy. Common antecedents include peripartum hypoxia-ischemia, infection/inflammation, genetic, metabolic and toxic causes, either alone or in combination.

- Common clinical presentation includes low Apgar scores at 5 and 10 minutes, followed by an abnormal state of consciousness, diminished spontaneous movements, respiratory or feeding difficulties, poor tone, abnormal posturing, absent primitive reflexes and seizures.
- Diagnosis is based on the the clinical assessment as well as investigations. A cranial MRI is more reliable to establish the presence and pattern of CNS injury, and to predict neurologic outcome.
- Management is mostly supportive. In perinatal asphyxia with moderate to severe hypoxic ischemic encephalopathy, therapeutic hypothermia is the treatment of choice.

BIBLIOGRAPHY

American Collge of Obstetricians and Gynecologists (ACOG). Neonatal encephalopathy and cerebral palsy: executive summary. *Obstet Gynecol* 2004; 103(4):780–1.

Dammann O, Ferriero D, Gressens P. Neonatal encephalopathy or hypoxic-ischemic encephalopathy? Appropriate terminology matters. *Pediatr Res* 2011; 70(1):1–2.

Executive Summary: Neonatal Encephalopathy and Neurologic Outcome, second edition. Report of the American College of Obstetricians and Gynecologists' Task Force on Neonatal Encephalopathy. *Obstet Gynecol* 2014; 123(4):896–901.

Ferriero DM. Neonatal brain injury. *N Engl J Med* 2004; 351(19):1985–95.

Hayes BC, McGarvey C, Mulvany S, et al. A case-control study of hypoxic-ischemic encephalopathy in newborn infants at >36 weeks gestation. *Am J Obstet Gynecol* 2013; 209(1):29.e1–e19.

Kurinczuk JJ, White-Koning M, Badawi N. Epidemiology of neonatal encephalopathy and hypoxic-ischaemic encephalopathy. *Early Hum Dev* 2010; 86(6):329–38.

Locatelli A, Incerti M, Paterlini G, et al. Antepartum and intrapartum risk factors for neonatal encephalopathy at term. *Am J Perinatol* 2010; 27(8):649–54.

Martinez-Biarge M, Diez-Sebastian J, Wusthoff CJ, et al. Antepartum and intrapartum factors preceding neonatal hypoxic-ischemic encephalopathy. *Pediatrics* 2013; 132(4):e952–e9.

Nelson KB, Bingham P, Edwards EM, et al. Antecedents of neonatal encephalopathy in the Vermont Oxford Network Encephalopathy Registry. *Pediatrics* 2012; 130(5):878–86.

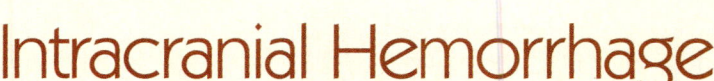

Intracranial Hemorrhage

Amit Upadhyay and Mohammed Sadique

Introduction

Intracranial hemorrhage (ICH) accounts for a significant proportion of neonatal morbidity and mortality. The recent advances in neonatology have enhanced the survival rate of very low birth weight and premature newborns, leading to an increase in the incidence of intracranial hemorrhage. The increased incidence of ICH is partly attributed to the higher detection rate with better investigation modalities. The actual incidence of perinatal ICH is not known because majority of cases are asymptomatic, and occur in otherwise healthy newborns. The clinical features, pathogenesis and severity of intracranial hemorrhage may vary according to the gestational age and site of hemorrhage. The intracranial bleed may occur at the subdural (SDH), subarachnoid (SAH), cerebellar (CH), intraventricular (IVH), other deep intracerebral and cortical areas of the brain (Figure 20.1). The salient epidemiological features and imaging modality of choice for various intracranial bleeds are summarized in Table 20.1.

SUBDURAL HEMORRHAGE

Subdural hemorrhage (SDH) denotes collection of blood between the dura and the arachnoid membrane.

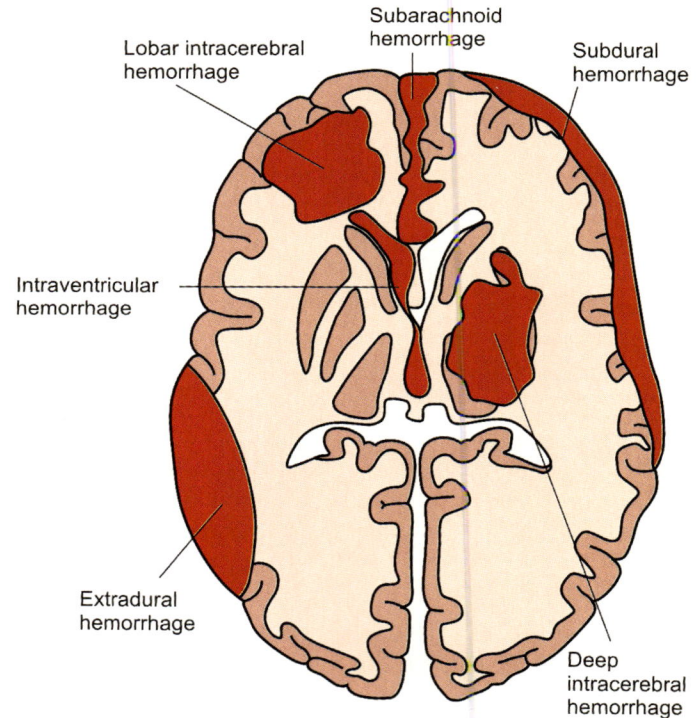

Figure 20.1 Location of different types of intracranial bleeds.

Table 20.1 The common types of intracranial hemorrhage				
Type of bleed	Gestation	Incidence	Investigation of choice	Prognosis
Subdural	Full term > Premature	Rare	MRI better than CT	Bad
Subarachnoid	Premature > Full term	Common	MRI better than CT	Good
Cerebellar	Premature > Full term	Rare	MRI better than cUSG (mastoid view)	Bad
Deep intra-parenchymal	Full term > Premature	Rare	MRI better than cUSG	Variable
Intraventricular	Premature > Full term	Common	The order of preference is cUSG, MRI, and CT	Grade I and II: Good Grade III and IV: Bad

cUSG; cranial ultrasonography, CT; computed tomography, MRI; magnetic resonance imaging

Subdural hemorrhage is relatively rare among various types of ICH. Term babies are more commonly affected than preterm. Based on location, it can be convexity subdural, supratentorial, infratentorial, occipital diastasis or falx laceration. The area where tentorium cerebri and falx cerebri join are the most common site for rupture of blood vessels.

Pathophysiology

The three types of injuries which can lead to SDH are rupture of unsupported subdural veins, tear of dural fold extending into venous sinuses and laceration of a sinus by margin of a fracture or separated skull bone. Most SDH occur due to difficult and assisted vaginal deliveries with some degree of cephalopelvic disproportion. These can cause extravasation of blood either in the supratentorial or infratentorial site, the latter being more common. The presence of coagulopathy like vitamin K deficiency, or intake of maternal drugs like phenobarbitone, phenytoin, warfarin can also contribute to development of SDH.

Clinical Features

The clinical features are variable depending upon the site, severity and progression of bleed. The infratentorial SDH has the worst prognosis because of involvement of brainstem (Figure 20.2).

Diagnosis

MRI is the best imaging modality for the diagnosis of SDH, as it provides better visualization of the posterior cranial fossa bleeds and also helps in detecting minor hemorrhage and coexisting parenchymal lesions. In case of non availability of MRI, or when patient is too sick and having metallic monitoring devices attached, CT scan can be done to identify the site and extent of bleed. Cranial ultrasonography (cUSG) is not useful in detecting SDH due to its peripheral location and because of acoustic interference by the overlying bone and near field transducer artifacts (Figure 20.3).

SUBARACHNOID HEMORRHAGE (SAH)

Subarachnoid hemorrhage is common during neonatal age group, second only to intraventricular hemorrhage.

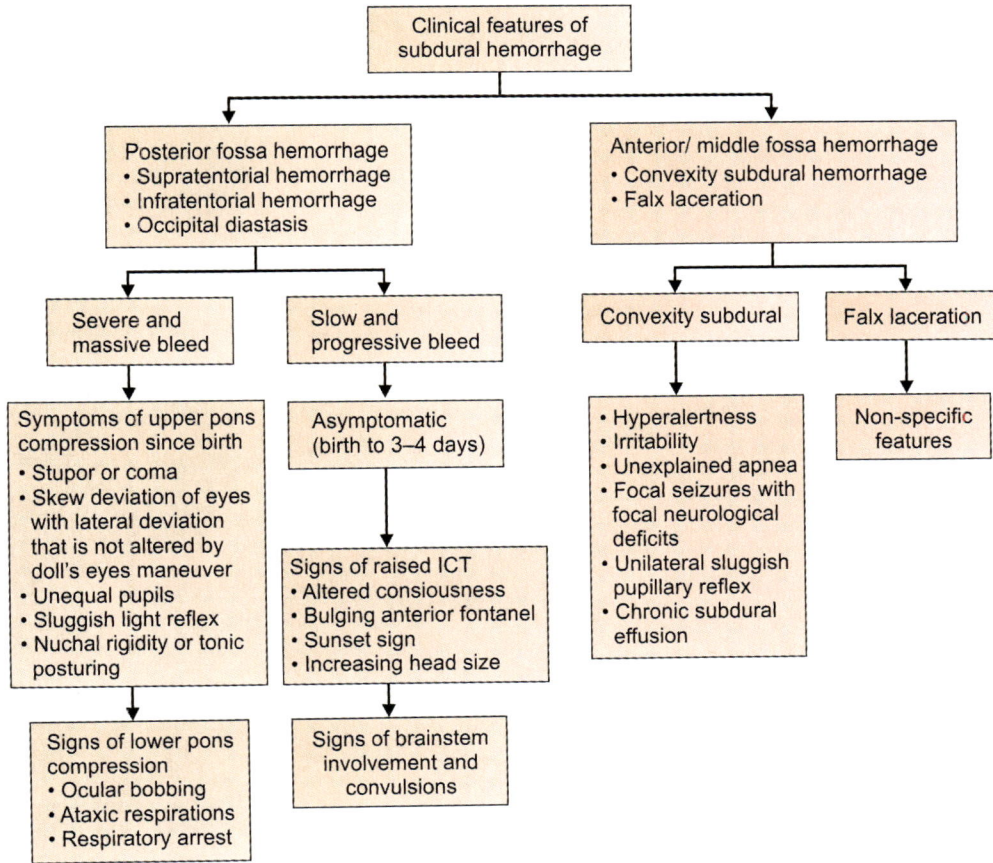

Figure 20.2 Clinical features of subdural hemorrhage.

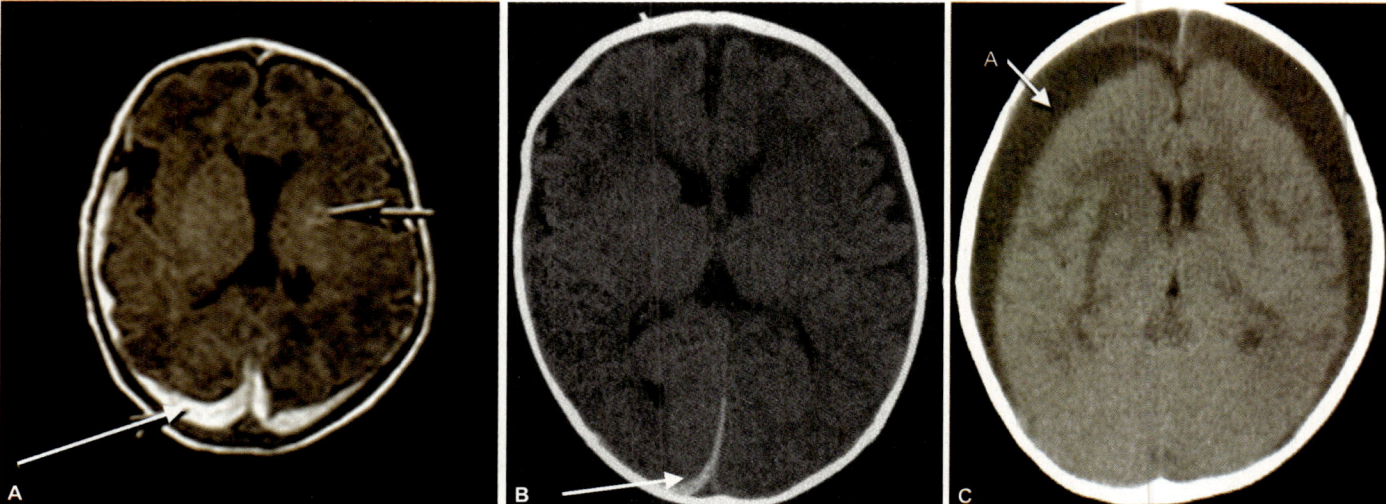

Figure 2.3 (A) MRI brain of a 4-day old newborn showing subacute subdural hemorrhage. See the hyperintense cresent shaped extra axial hematoma which is over riding the cranial sutures. (B) CT head of an infant showing acute subdural hematoma seen as hyperintense lesion involving the right occipital lobe and extending into the posterior interhemispheric sulcus. (C) CT head of an infant showing chronic bilateral subdural hematoma.

In subarachnoid hemorrhage there is collection of blood between arachnoid and pia mater. This space is normally occupied by CSF. Subarachnoid hemorrhage may seep into various cisterns. It may be primary SAH or secondary extension of other bleeds like SDH, IVH or cerebellar hemorrhage into the subarachnoid space. Most of SAH are asymptomatic and an incidental finding on autopsy.

Pathogenesis

The exact pathogenesis of neonatal SAH is not fully understood and it is believed to be related to trauma or hemodynamic events related to maturity. In term neonates, the pathogenesis is more commonly traumatic in origin as in case of SDH. The source of bleeding in subarachnoid hemorrhage may be due to leakage of blood from fine vessels of the leptomeningeal plexus or rupture of bridging veins within the subarachnoid space.

Clinical Features

In most cases SAH is asymptomatic. The classical presentation is occurence of seizure on 2nd to 4th day in an otherwise healthy looking neonate. In a rare case of severe subarachnoid hemorrhage, there is catastrophic clinical presentation with shock and death.

Diagnosis

The sensitivity of MRI or CT scan in detecting SAH is strongly influenced by the amount of subarachnoid blood and timing of hemorrhage. MRI can detect SAH as early as 12 hours, while hemorrhage is best visible on CT scan after 2 days. Normally the subarachnoid space is visible on CT as hypodense (black) due to presence of CSF. Acute hemorrhages are seen as hyperintensities (white) in CT scan which can vary according to timing of bleed. SAH is usually seen in CSF containing spaces like suprasellar cisterns overlying the circle of Willis (basal region), sulci over the cerebral convexities especially the Sylvian fissures and perimesenchephalic cistern around the brainstem (Figure 20.4). Cranial USG is relatively insensitive to diagnose SAH because of the normal increase in echogenicity around the periphery of brain.

CEREBELLAR HEMORRHAGE (CH)

Cerebellar hemorrhage is more common in preterm than term infants and usually involves unilateral

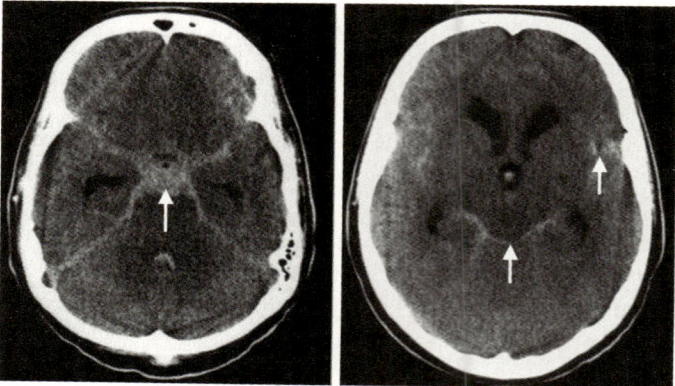

Figure 20.4 CT head showing hyperintensity in basilar cistern and Sylvian fissure due to SAH.

hemisphere. It can be primary cerebellar hemorrhage, or as a consequence of venous infarction (when bleeding extends from interventricular or subarachnoid hemorrhage) or traumatic laceration (with or without occipital diastasis). The clinical features depend upon the size of hematoma, progression of bleed and the gestational age. It can manifest as brainstem dysfunction or obstruction to CSF flow. The clinical features of posterior fossa hemorrhage are similar to SDH. In suspected cases, MRI or CT is done to look for the position, extent of the hematoma and other parenchymal abnormalities. Similar to other hemorrhages, cerebellar hemorrhage appears as areas of hyperintensities on CT scan within the cerebellar parenchyma, which may extend into the subarachnoid space or fourth ventricle. MRI gives better visualization because beam hardening and scattering are normal artifacts in posterior cranial fossa on CT scan. Conventional anterior fontanel view cranial USG can miss cerebellar hemorrhage and other posterior cranial fossa hemorrhages, so mastoid and posterior fontanel views should be taken.

Other Intraparenchymal Hemorrhages

These are more common in term babies and are mostly secondary to severe hypoxic ischemic encephalopathy. It can also occur due to rupture of arteriovenous malformation (AVM) or aneurysms, coagulopathies and extension from other compartments. Venous infarction due to obstruction of the superior sagittal sinus or its tributary veins results in a characteristic hemorrhagic lesion of cortex and subcortical white matter.

INTRAVENTRICULAR HEMORRHAGE

Hemorrhage into the germinal matrix/intraventricular hemorrhage (GM-IVH) is the most common cause of intracranial bleeding and neurological damage in very low birth weight babies and preterm babies. The germinal matrix lines the lateral ventricles and consists of fragile, unsupported immature capillaries. The germinal matrix hemorrhage result in intraventricular or parenchymal hemorrhage or both. The incidence is inversely related to the gestational age. In preterms, the origin of hemorrhage is mainly from the subependymal germinal matrix lying ventrolateral to lateral ventricles. More than three-fourths of GM-IVH occur near the head of caudate nucleus. In remaining cases, the site of hemorrhage is germinal matrix tissue adjacent to body and tail of caudate nucleus, lateral aspect of the lateral ventricle in the region of the trigone,

the lateral aspect of the occipital or temporal horns and the roof of the fourth ventricle. GM-IVH is less likely in term newborns because germinal matrix usually regresses by 36 weeks of gestation.

Pathogenesis

The exact pathogenesis of GM-IVH is not completely understood. It is probably multifactorial in origin. There is interplay between anatomical and physiological immaturity of developing cerebral vasculature of preterm babies exposed to hazards of perinatal hypoxia and its consequences. Risk factors for GM-IVH include immaturity, maternal infection/inflammation and hemorrhage, lack of administration of antenatal steroids, extraneous factors such as mode of delivery or neonatal transport to another hospital. The pathogenesis of GM-IVH can be best understood in terms of intravascular, vascular and extra vascular factors. In term babies, along with the above mentioned factors, trauma and hypocoaguable states are additional risk factors for intraventricular hemorrhage (Table 20.2 and Figure 20.5).

Clinical Features

Clinical features vary depending upon the severity and extent of hemorrhage. It can be asymptomatic, subtle or life-threatening. In preterms, GM-IVH is usually asymptomatic and detected by routine cUSG usually done at 3rd day of life. The risk period for the occurrence of IVH is highest in the first 3 or 4 days of life. Antenatal hemorrhages can occur, especially in the setting of neonatal alloimmune thrombocytopenia. Twenty-five percent of hemorrhages occur by the 6th hour and 50% during the first 24 hours of life. Intraventricular hemorrhage is rare in term infants and is usually asymptomatic. The clinical features of GM-IVH are summarized in Figure 20.6.

Table 20.2 Pathogenesis of germinal matrix intraventricular hemorrhage

Source of bleeding	Cause of bleeding
Intravascular	■ Rapid volume expansion
	■ Fluctuating cerebral blood flow
	■ Increase in cerebral blood flow
	■ Increase in cerebral venous pressure
	■ Platelet dysfunction and coagulation disturbances
Vascular	■ Tenuous, involuting capillaries with large luminal diameter
Extravascular	■ Deficient vascular support
	■ Excessive fibrinolytic activity

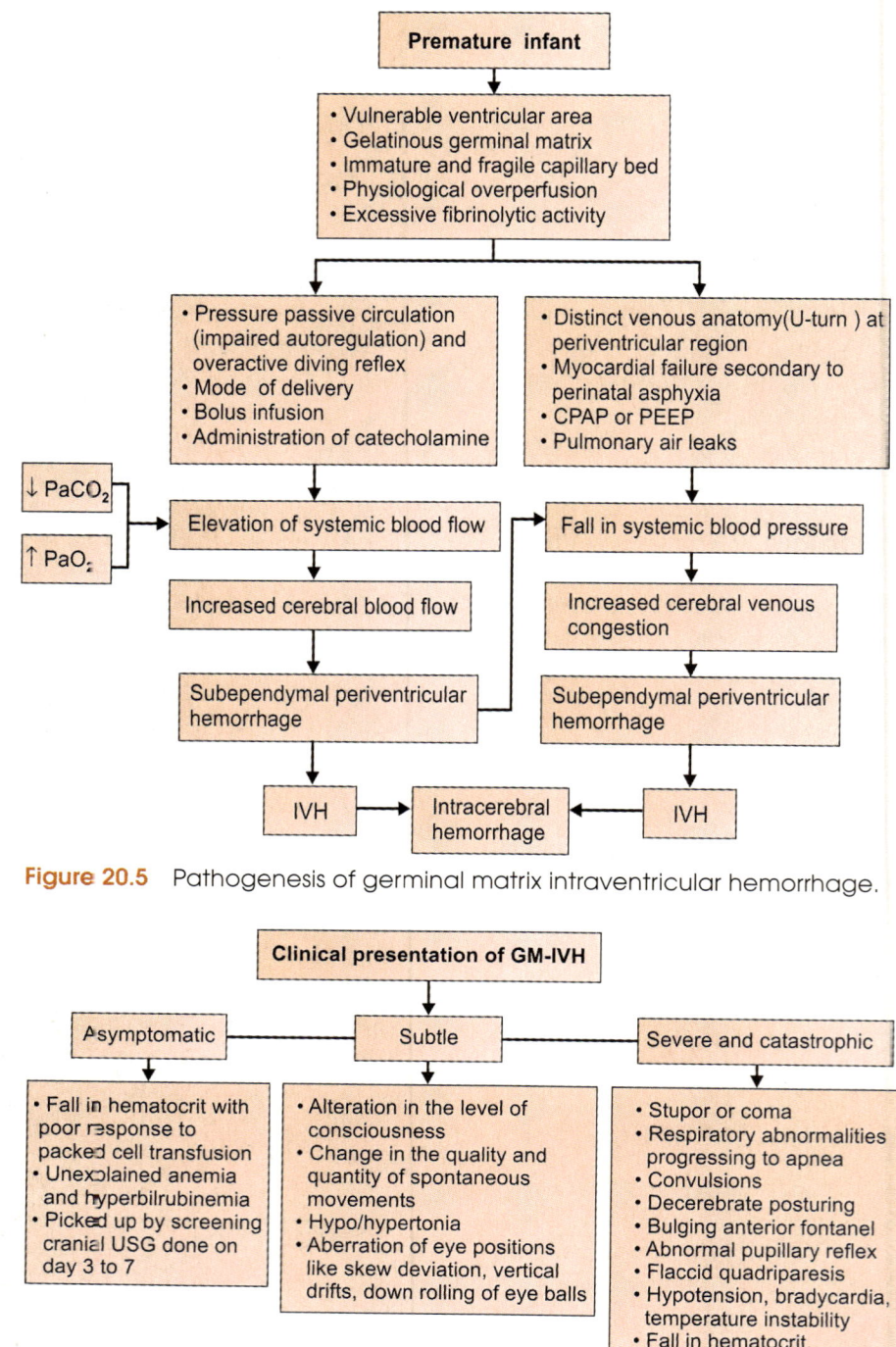

Figure 20.5   Pathogenesis of germinal matrix intraventricular hemorrhage.

Figure 20.6   Clinical features of germinal matrix hemorrhage.
SIADH; syndrome of inappropriate antidiuretic hormone.

Diagnosis

Unlike other intracranial bleeds, cranial USG (cUSG) is the investigation of choice for screening and assessment of the extent of IVH. Almost 50% cases of IVH are asymptomatic. The common signs and symptoms of

GM-IVH are summarized in Figure 20.6. Diagnosis can be confirmed by ultrasound scanning with portable high resolution sector scan using anterior fontanel as the acoustic window. Infants with a birth weight of <1500 g or gestational age of <32 weeks should be

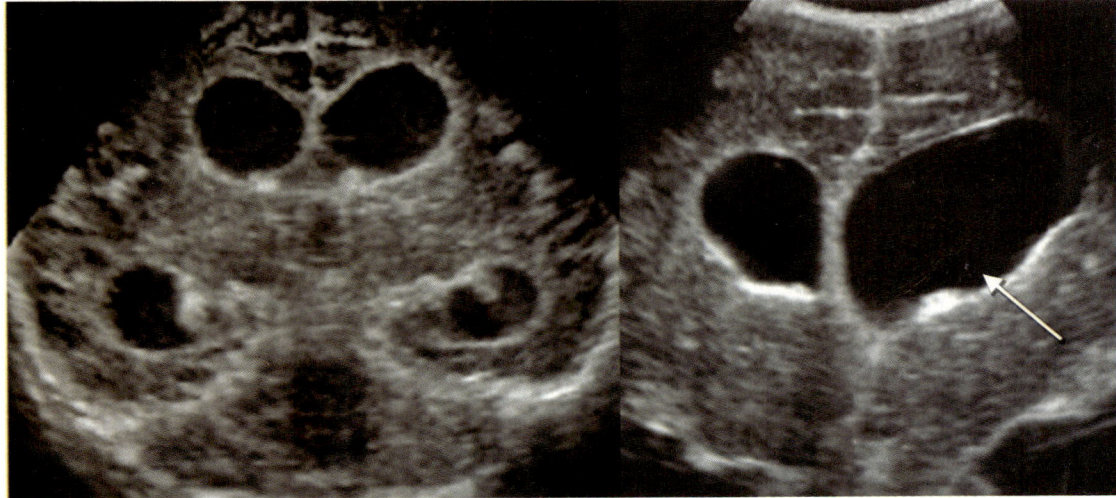

Figure 20.7 cUSG coronal view through anterior fontanel in 3 day old premature newborn showing grade III GM-IVH.

routinely screened by cUSG at the age of 3 days, 7 days, 21 days and before discharge from NICU. When repeated USG screening is not feasible, single screening on 7th day of life should be done. If head circumference is increasing by more than 1cm per week or anterior fontanel is full or cranial sutures are widely separated or there is unexplained clinical worsening, cUSG should be repeated to rule out GM-IVH or post hemorrhagic ventricular dilatation (PVD). When IVH is diagnosed, weekly cUSG is recommended till ventricular size is stabilized. Severity of GM-IVH can be graded as per findings of cUSG or CT head (Table 20.3). The

hemorrhage in the germinal matrix is identified as an echogenic focus over the head of the caudate nucleus and/or caudothalamic notch (Figure 20.7). The subependymal hemorrhage is generally bilateral. The hemorrhage may increase in size and rupture through the ependyma into the lateral ventricle to produce echogenic hematoma. Progressive post hemorrhagic hydrocephalus may occur because of obstruction in the posterior fossa by the particulate blood clot. The relative deficiency of fibrinolytic mechanism in the CSF of preterm infants is a contributory factor. In term babies with IVH, MRI should be done to rule out other coexisting parenchymal injuries in the brain.

Prevention of GM-IVH

Prevention of premature birth by identifying women at high-risk and early treatment of premature labor, primarily with tocolytic agents can decrease the incidence of GM-IVH. If premature delivery is inevitable, transportation *in utero* to a perinatal center specialized in the care of high-risk deliveries should be considered. Infants transported *in utero* have a lower incidence of IVH compared to infants transported after delivery. *Prenatal glucocorticoids to the mother is the single most effective pharmacological intervention for prevention of IVH.* It reduces both incidence as well as severity of GM-IVH.

Delivery of high-risk infant should take place in a specialized center where facilities for peripartum fetal monitoring are available to ensure early identification of fetal hypoxia and effective management of perinatal asphyxia. Postnatal measures include avoiding fluctuations in blood pressure due to excessive handling, rapid or bolus intravenous infusions, vigorous suctioning,

Table 20.3 Grading of IVH	
Papile grading of IVH on the basis of CT head	Volpe grading of IVH by cranial USG
I. Subependymal hemorrhage with minimal or no IVH	I. Germinal matrix hemorrhage with no or minimal intraventricular hemorrhage (<10% of ventricular area on parasagittal view)
II. Definite IVH without distension of the ventricles	II. IVH involving 10% to 50% of ventricular area on parasagittal view
III. Enlargement of the ventricles secondary to distension with blood	III. IVH involving >50% of ventricular area on parasagittal view, usually with distention of lateral ventricles
IV. Extension of the hemorrhage into the parenchyma	IV. Intraparenchymal echodensity due to periventricular venous or hemorrhagic infarct due to compression of deep terminal veins by an enlarged ventricle

administration of hypertonic fluids or drugs like sodium bicarbonate, and use of sedation and/or muscle relaxants to prevent asynchrony on ventilator support.

Management of Intracranial Hemorrhage

All babies with ICH should be evaluated closely for signs of deterioration of neurological status, especially for evidences of brainstem involvement. Most of the cases with ICH are self-limiting and can be managed conservatively. Close monitoring should be done for any neurological deterioration and repeat imaging may be required accordingly. There is no specific treatment for intracranial hemorrhage. Management largely consists of supportive care. Vitamin K should be given if it has been missed. Affected infant should be closely monitored to maintain optimal BP, oxygenation, circulatory volume and acid base status. Suctioning and handling should be gentle and kept to bare minimum. Severe anemia and bleeding manifestations should be managed by transfusion of packed RBCs. Thrombocytopenia and coagulation abnormalities should be corrected appropriately. Apnea should be managed with appropriate respiratory support. Seizures should be managed as per standard guidelines.

In some cases with massive infratentorial and posterior cranial fossa hematoma, clinical deterioration may be very rapid and decompression surgery may be required. In cerebral convexity SDH, the subdural taps are done only if the head circumference is growing fast or neuroimaging is showing significant progression.

Management of Posthemorrhagic Ventricular Dilatation (PVD)

Posthemorrahagic ventricular dilatation is more commonly seen in preterm infants as increasing head growth, bulging anterior fontanel, widening of sutures, decreased level of consciousness, impaired gaze or sun setting sign, apnea, worsening of respiratory status or feeding difficulties and vomiting. Progressive PVD may occur days to weeks following onset of GMH/IVH. Impaired CSF resorption and/or obstruction of the aqueduct, the foramina of Lushka and Megendie by particulate clot are the likely etiopathologic mechanisms.

Slowly progressive PVD which does not progress for more than 2 weeks and is associated with moderate ventricular dilatation and a stable resistive index (RI) requires only close monitoring of ventricular size by cranial USG, rate of head growth, clinical condition, baseline and serial RIs. Resistive index is calculated as systolic flow – diastolic flow/systolic flow. In most cases there is spontaneous arrest of hydrocephalus which is followed by total or partial resolution of

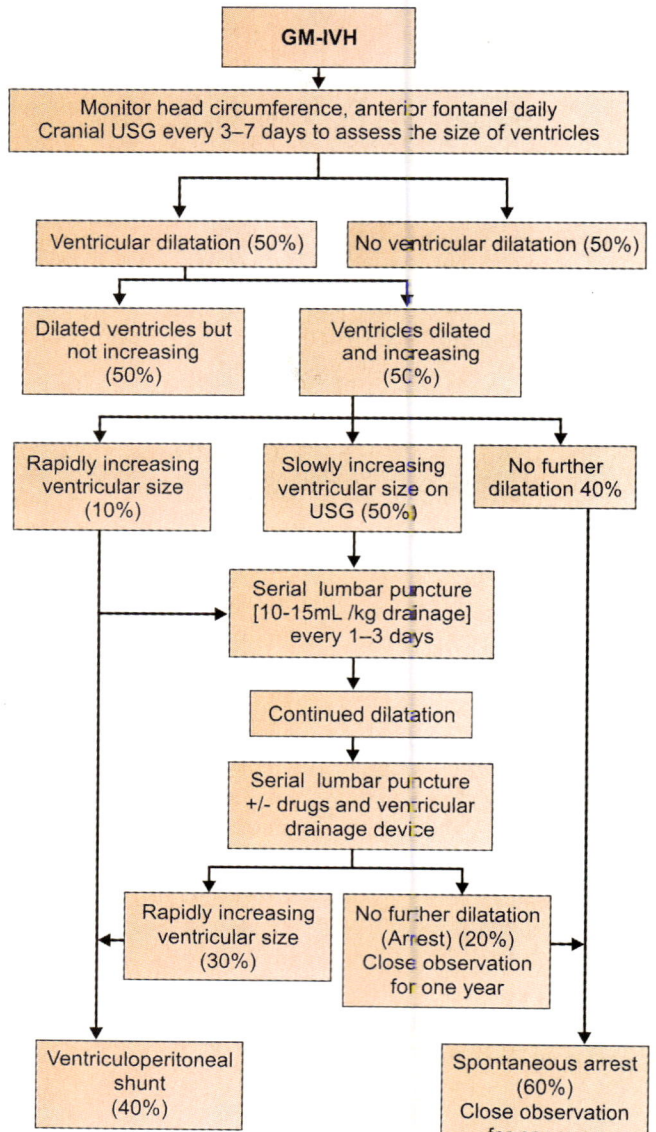

Figure 20.8 Algorithm for management of germinal matrix intraventricular hemorrhage.

ventriculomegaly. Rapidly progressive PVD is characterized by moderate to severe ventricular dilatation with excessive rate of head growth (>1 cm per week) and increase in RI. Serial lumbar punctures should be done and 10–15 mL/kg CSF should be removed (Figure 20.8). Ideally cranial USG should be done before and after the therapeutic lumbar puncture, although this may not be feasible at most centers. Communication between ventricles and lumbar subarachnoid space should be present to ensure better clinical outcome. The frequency of doing lumbar puncture is individualized depending upon the progression of PVD as suggested by cranial USG. Repeated lumbar punctures are cumbersome and associated with risk of infection.

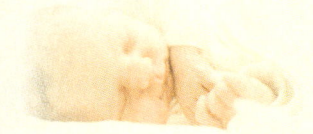

Table 20.4 Prognosis of GM-IVH according to the grading of hemorrhage

Grade of IVH	Birth weight	Short-term outcome (mortality rate and development of PVD)	Long-term outcome (neurological sequelae)
I	Any	Excellent	Excellent (15 %)
II	750–1500 g	PVD (5–15%)	Good (25%)
III	<750 g	Mortality (30%), PVD (75%)	Poor (50%)
	750–1500 g	Mortality (10%)	
IV	<750 g	Mortality (50%)	Dismal (75%)
	750–1500 g	Mortality (20%)	

In general, outcomes of Grade I and II IVH are similar to infants without IVH. PVD; progressive ventricular dilatation

Acetazolamide, a carbonic anhydrase inhibitor, in a dose of 50–100 mg/kg/day q 6 hr combined with furosemide (1 mg/kg/dose every 12 hr) are useful to arrest progress of hydrocephalus. The prolonged administration of diuretics is associated with risk of development of hypercalcemia, nephrocalcinosis and deafness. If serial lumbar punctures fail to decrease the RI, other ventricular drainage methods like direct external ventricular drain, tunneled external ventricular drain, subcutaneous ventricular catheter to reservoir or to subgaleal or supraclavicular space or a ventriculo-peritoneal shunt should be considered. Arrested progression is diagnosed when there is spontaneous arrest of ventricular dilatation or arrest following lumbar puncture. In such cases close surveillance for one year is recommended. There is a risk of development of hydrocephalus late in infancy in 5% babies in this group.

Prognosis

Irrespective of site of bleeding, prognosis of ICH depends on the location, size, and severity of hemorrhage and gestational age. Asymptomatic small SDH have good short-term survival rates and long-term neurodevelopmental outcomes, but SDH with massive posterior cranial fossa hemorrhage has a poor prognosis. Babies should be monitored for obstructive hydrocephalus and chronic subdural effusion. Subarachnoid hemorrhage is mostly asymptomatic with good prognosis. In mild cases presenting as neonatal seizures, up to 90% have no neurodevelopmental sequelae. Rarely SAH can lead to obstructive hydrocephalus. Mortality of intracerebellar hemorrhage is high in premature neonates. Preterm babies with intracerebellar hemorrhage are likely to have severe cognitive and neuromotor dysfunction and often succumb to systemic illness. Surviving babies are likely to develop cognitive deficits in 40% and autism spectrum disorder in 37% cases. In GM-IVH, the outcome depends upon the grade of IVH and gestational age of the infant (Table 20.4).

BIBLIOGRAPHY

Alan L, Karl CK, Linda VM, Marcello P, Elizabeth NA. Antenatal corticosteroids appear to reduce the risk of postnatal germinal matrix hemorrhage in intubated low birth weight newborns. *Pediatrics* 1993 Jun, 91:1083–88.

deVries L. Intracranial hemorrhage and vascular lesions in the neonate. In: Neonatal-Perinatal Medicine. Martin RJ, Fanaroff AA, Walsh MC, eds. 10th ed. *Philadelphia, PA: Elsevier Saunders*; 2015.

Janet SS. Neurological disorders: Intracranial hemorrhage. In: Manuel of Neonatal Care. Cloherty J P 7th edition pp 686–706.

Levene M. Intracranial haemorrhage at term. In: Roberton's Textbook of Neonatology. Martin RJ, Fanaroff AA, Walsh MC. Rennie JM (Ed.) *Philadelphia: Elsevier*; 4th Ed. 2005. pp. 1120–1128.

Papile LA, Burstein J, Burstein R, Koffler H. Incidence and evolution of subependymal and intraventricular hemorrhage: A study of infants with birth weights less than 1,500 gm. *J Pediatr* 1978; 92(4):529–34.

Volpe JJ, Intracranial hemorrhage: Subdural, primary subarachnoid, cerebellar, intraventricular (term infant), and miscellaneous. In: Neurology of the Newborn. 5th ed. *Philadelphia (PA); Saunders Elsevier*; 2008.

Wigglesworth JS, Pape KE. An integrated model for haemorrhagic and ischaemic lesions in the newborn brain. *Early Hum Dev* 1978; 2:179–99.

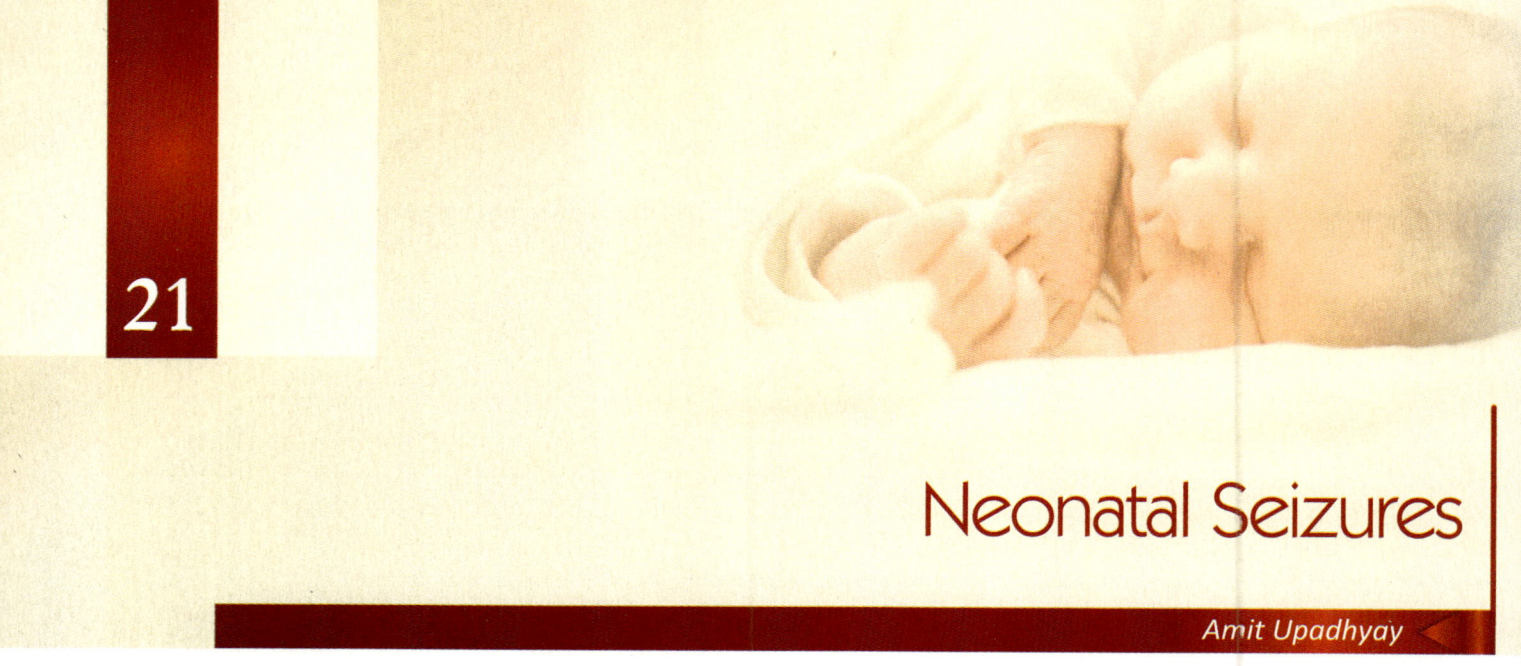

21

Neonatal Seizures

Amit Upadhyay

Seizures are one of the most common neurologic conditions managed by neonatal intensive care team. Neonates are at a higher risk for seizures compared to other age groups. The increased risk of seizures in neonates is multifactorial. It can be due to relative excitability of the developing brain, as well as high frequency of brain injury due to common neonatal problems like global hypoxia-ischemia, metabolic abnormalities, stroke and intracranial hemorrhage.

Epidemiology

The incidence of seizures depends upon birth weight and gestation. The incidence of neonatal seizures (NS) as per National Neonatal Perinatal Database (NNPD 2002–03), from 18 tertiary care units across the country, was 10.3 per 1000 live-births. Preterm infants had more than twice the incidence when compared to term neonates (20.8 vs. 8.4 per 1000 live births).

Definition

A seizure is a paroxysmal alteration caused by hypersynchronous discharge of a group of neurons. This alteration in neurologic function can be in motor, behavior and/or autonomic function.

Pathophysiology

Neonatal seizure activity results from an excessive synchronous electrical discharge (depolarization) of neurons within the central nervous system. The process of depolarization occurs by the inward migration of sodium (Na^+), and repolarization by the efflux of potassium (K^+). A potential is maintained across the membrane due to this ionic movement. It requires energy (adenosine triphosphate, or ATP-dependent pump), which extrudes Na^+ from cells and sucks in K^+.

Although the basic or fundamental mechanism of neonatal seizures is not entirely understood, but the excessive depolarization of neurons due to various neonatal causes is thought to be the most common mechanism (Figure 21.1).

The seizure activity of newborn differs from older children and adults. Unlike a child, newborns rarely have well-organised, generalised tonic-clonic seizures. The differences occur due to various neuroanatomical and physiological changes in the developing brain. Anatomical events like proper orientation, alignment, layering, i.e. lamination of cortical neurons, elaboration of axonal and dendritic ramifications, and establishment of synaptic connections mature with increasing gestation. The lamination is well-developed in the human newborn while neurite outgrowth and synaptogenesis are less developed. The cortical connectivity to propagate and sustain a generalised seizure does not occur in developing neonatal human brain. The enhanced excitability of neonatal brain is due to various factors. The neonatal period is a time of physiologic, use-dependent synaptogenesis, and both synapses and dendritic spine density are at their peak. In limbic and neocortical regions, there is greater development of excitatory mechanisms compared to inhibitory mechanisms. The N-methyl-D-aspartate (NMDA) receptors and and non-NDMA type ionotropic transmembrane a-amino-3 hydroxy-5 methyl isoxazolepropionic acid (AMPA) receptors are over expressed and exhibit multiple properties that enhance excitation. Also, gamma-amino-butyric acid (GABA), the primary inhibitory mechanism of the adult brain, can exert a paradoxical excitatory action in the developing brain. Moreover, the substantia nigra system which mediates inhibition of seizures is relatively underdeveloped in neonates.

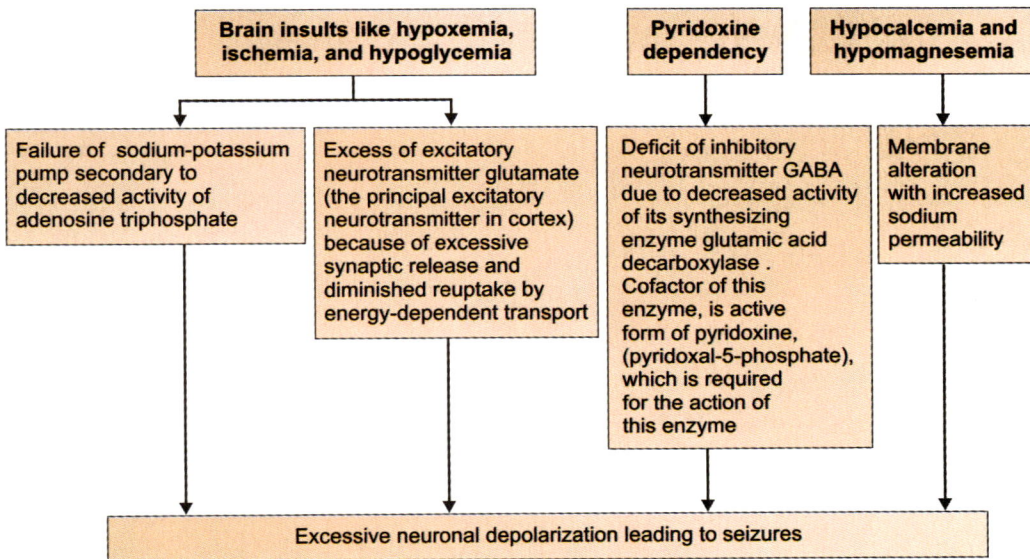

Figure 21.1 Pathophysiology of neonatal seizures.

Mechanism of Brain Injury Due to Seizures

Brain injury can also occur due to prolonged single or recurrent seizures or even following brief recurrent seizures. The most prominent feature of the former is neuronal loss, and of the latter is altered development. Although the threshold for seizure generation is lower in the developing brain than in the mature brain, developing neurons are less vulnerable to injury from single prolonged seizures compared to mature neurons. Repeated seizure activity can lead to increased metabolic demand of brain and hypoventilation and apnea leading to hypercapnia and hypoxemia. With repeated seizures, the brain glucose falls markedly along with rise in lactate levels. Systemic blood pressure rises to increase the cerebral blood flow, so as to meet the elevated metabolic demands of brain. Prolonged seizures also cause excessive release of glutamate and aspartate at excitatory amino acid synapses.

Recurrent seizures are associated with long-term functional, morphological, and physiological deficits. The most severe disturbances occur in the hippocampus and include dendritic spine loss in CA3 pyramidal cells and a distinctive pattern of synaptic reorganization of axons and terminals of the dentate granule cells (i.e. mossy fibers).

Etiology

The common causes of seizures include hypoxic-ischemic encephalopathy, metabolic disturbances (hypoglycemia, hypocalcemia and hypomagnesemia), intracranial hemorrhage and meningitis. Acute symptomatic causes like hypoxic-ischemic encephalopathy (HIE), transient metabolic disturbances, infection, stroke, or intracranial hemorrhage, are much more common than early-onset epilepsies due to malformation, fetal or neonatal brain injury, genetic or idiopathic causes. Inborn errors of metabolism, pyridoxine-responsive seizures and neonatal epilepsy syndromes must be considered in the setting of refractory seizures.

Etiology of seizures varies in preterm and term neonates. In term babies, HIE is the most common cause of neonatal seizures with onset within 24 hours while in preterm infants cerebrovascular events and intracranial hemorrhage are most common. In IUGR babies, hypoglycemia and polycythemia are predominant causes. Genetic and malformation related causes are also more common in IUGR babies. The timing of seizures and prognosis depends on the underlying cause. It is important to determine the cause of seizures as the specific treatment of the baby and future neurological outcome depends on it. The usual time of onset, and relative frequency seizures in premature or full-term infants are summarized in Table 21.1. The clinical features of neonatal seizures due to common causes are described below.

Hypoxic-ischemic encephalopathy consequent to perinatal asphyxia It is the most common cause of neonatal seizures in both full-term and premature infants. Seizures occurring within 4–6 hours of birth suggest intrauterine insult. Seizures commonly occur within 24 hours of birth in HIE. Though any type of seizure can occur but common variants include subtle

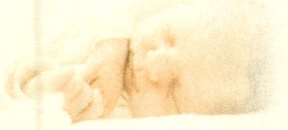

Table 21.1 Common causes of neonatal seizures and their relative frequency and age of onset

Cause	Frequency	Age of onset	Common clinical correlates
Hypoxic-ischemic encephalopathy	30–53%	1st 6–12 hr	History of delayed cry, poor Apgar score, dull baby, gaze and tone abnormalities are common
Metabolic disorders Hypoglycemia, hypocalcemia, hypomagnesemia, hypo-/hypernatremia	4–22%	1st 48 hours	IUGR, preterm, infants of diabetic mothers, exclusively breastfed baby with excessive weight loss and decrease in urine output
Intracranial hemorrhage	7–17%	2–3 days	Well baby with seizures, CT is diagnostic. cUSG is useful for intraventricular or parenchymal hemorrhage
Cerebral infarction	6–17%	Variable	Hemiplegia or monoplegia
Cerebral malformations	3–17%	Variable	Well baby with seizures, head size may be abnormal
Meningitis/septicemia	2–14%	Usually after 3 days	Associated with fever, bulging anterior fontanel, lethargy or excessive crying
Inborn errors of metabolism Pyridoxine dependency, folin c acid responsive seizures, glucose transporter defect, non-ketotic hyperglycinemia, propionic aciduria	3–4%	Variable	Refractory seizures with history of neonatal deaths and consanguinity. May be associated with hypoglycemia, metabolic acidosis or high ammonia levels
Kernicterus	1%	After 3–4 days	Severe jaundice due to Rh or ABO incompatibility and internal bleeding
Maternal drug withdrawal	4%	Usually first 3 days	History of maternal drug intake
Benign idiopathic neonatal seizures	1%	5th day	None
Neonatal epileptic syndromes	<1%	Variable	Benign sleep myoclonus
Congenital infections	2–5%	Variable	Associated IUGR, hepatomegaly, cataracts, calcifications in brain, osteochondritis, low platelet count
Idiopathic	2%	Variable	Family history of epilepsy

and clonic types. HIE is associated with low Apgar scores, delayed cry (for >3 min), low pH and high base deficit in arterial blood gas analysis.

Metabolic disturbances Hypoglycemia is most frequent in high-risk babies like preterm, small or large-for-gestational age. The onset is usually in first two days of life. The most critical determinants for the occurrence of neurological symptoms in neonatal hypoglycemia are the severity and duration of the hypoglycemia. It is diagnosed by screening with glucostix and confirmed by finding blood sugar of less than 40 mg/dL on standard glucose oxidase laboratory test.

Early-onset hypocalcemia occurs in first 3 days of life, most often in preterms, infants of diabetic mothers and babies with perinatal asphyxia. Late-onset hypocalcemia occurs in full-term infants who are fed on cow's milk with a suboptimal ratio of phosphorus to calcium and phosphorus to magnesium. The common clinical features include alert and well infant with jitteriness, tremulousness, brisk tendon jerks and jaw clonus. Hypomagnesemia is a frequent accompaniment

of hypocalcemia and should be considered in babies with refractory hypocalcemia.

Intracranial hemorrhage Seizures due to subarachnoid, intraparenchymal or subdural hemorrhage occur mainly in term neonates, while seizures secondary to intraventricular hemorrhage (IVH) occur in preterm infants. Most seizures due to intracranial hemorrhage occur between 2 and 7 days of age and are associated with severe brain lesion. In severe intraventricular hemorrhage, the most common seizure type is the generalized tonic variety. Subarachnoid hemorrhage often presents as seizures in a 'well baby' on 2nd or 3rd days of life. Subdural hemorrhage is often associated with birth trauma, which leads to cerebral contusion and the convulsive phenomena. The most common variety of subdural hemorrhage is the convex type, and the seizures are usually focal in nature.

Intracranial infection Seizures due to bacterial meningitis usually occur during later half of the first week. Most common bacterial pathogens include *Group B streptococci* and *Escherichia coli*. Seizures associated with Herpes simplex encephalitis also tend to occur after first week of life. Nonbacterial infections like neonatal encephalitides due to toxoplasmosis, rubella and cytomegalovirus infection may cause seizures within the first 3 days of life.

Developmental defects Aberrations of brain development can result in seizures, which begin at any time during the neonatal period. The common malformations of CNS include cerebral cortical dysgenesis and neuronal migration disorders (lissencephaly, pachygyria, and polymicrogyria). They are usually refractory to treatment and best diagnosed by MRI of brain.

Other metabolic disturbances They include hyponatremia, hypernatremia, hyperammonemia, amino acid and organic acid abnormalities, mitochondrial disturbances, peroxisomal disorders, pyridoxine dependency, folinic acid responsive seizures, and disorders of glucose transport.

Local anesthetic intoxication It occurs when local anesthetic is inadvertently injected into the infant's scalp during paracervical or pudendal block for episiotomy. Two distinguishing characteristics of local anesthetic intoxication include dilated and fixed pupils and absence of doll's eyes reflex. These infants improve during the first 24 to 48 hours and treatment with anticonvulsant drugs is of questionable value.

Drug withdrawal It is a rare cause of neonatal seizures in developing countries. The commonly involved drugs include narcotic-analgesics (methadone), sedative-hypnotics (short acting barbiturates), tricyclic anti-depressants, cocaine, alcohol, etc.

Epilepsy syndromes Epileptic syndromes include benign familial neonatal seizures, benign idiopathic neonatal seizures (fifth-day fits), early myoclonic encephalopathy, early infantile epileptic encephalopathy (Ohtahara syndrome)and malignant migrating partial seizures. Nonepileptic syndromes are benign neonatal sleep myoclonus and hyperekplexia, or exaggerated startle response.

Classification

Several classifications have been proposed, of which the classifications by Volpe and by Mizrahi and Kellaway are most widely used. Volpe has given a classification mainly based on the clinical characteristics of seizures which are likely to be associated with EEG seizure activity. Mizrahi and Kellaway classified seizures depending on the electroclinical characteristics of seizures into epileptic, nonepileptic and epileptic without clinical association. The Mizrahi classification

has the advantage that it takes the origin of events into account and includes clinically silent electroencephalographic seizures. Seizures can be classified into three broad categories.

- *Epileptic seizures* Clinical phenomena associated with corresponding EEG seizure activity, e.g. generalized clonic seizures
- *Non-epileptic seizures* Clinical seizures without corresponding EEG abnormalities, seizures due to metabolic causes, subtle seizures, most generalized tonic seizures, and the focal and multifocal seizures like myoclonic seizures (inconsistent electroclinical correlation/brainstem release phenomenon). These seizures probably originate from deep cortical structures (limbic region) or diencephalon (thalamus and hypothalamus), or brainstem region.
- *EEG seizures* There is abnormal EEG activity without any clinical correlation (electroclinical dissociation). They are common in immature neonates with subtle or no seizures and infants controlled on antiepileptic drugs.

The neonatal seizures are classified broadly into four clinical subtypes, i.e. subtle, tonic, clonic and myoclonic. They are further classified into focal; multifocal and generalized. Multifocal refers to clinical activity that involves more than one site, asynchronous, and usually, migratory in nature, whereas generalized refers to seizure activity that is diffusely bilateral, synchronous and non-migratory. Salient features of the Volpe classification of neonatal seizures are summarized in Table 21.2.

Conditions Mimicking Seizures

There are many conditions that mimic seizures and need to be identified. Some of the these conditions are described below.

Jitteriness or tremors Jitteriness is the most common condition mimicking seizures in neonates. They are known as rhythmic segmental myoclonus. They are commonly seen in hypoglycemia, hypocalcemia and in some normal neonates. These are characterised by rhythmic fast movements (4–6/sec) which are provoked or stopped by stimulus like gently pulling the leg or hand or by elicitation of startle or Moro's reflex. They are not associated with gaze abnormalities or any autonomic and EEG changes.

Benign neonatal sleep myoclonus The mechanism of the nonepileptiform myoclonus is unknown but may be related to a transient dysmaturity of the brainstem reticular activating system. It usually presents in the first week of life. It occurs only during sleep, and is

Table 21.2	Classification of neonatal seizures by Volpe		
Type of seizure	Clinical features	EEG abnormalities	Common causes
Subtle	More in preterm than in term infants Eye deviation, blinking, fixed stare, repetitive mouth and tongue movements, apnea, pedalling and cycling movements	+	Asphyxia and metabolic
Clonic	Rhythmic and usually slow (approximately one to three jerks per second at the onset, with the rate progressively declining). **Focal** Baby s usually conscious. It is common with metabolic encephalopathies and seizures do not cross the midline **Multifocal** Nonjacksonian march and do not cross the midline	+++	Asphyxia and metabolic
Tonic	Primarily in preterm, generalized being more common. **Focal** Sustained posturing of a limb, asymmetrical posturing of trunk or neck **Generalized** Mimics decerebrate/ decorticate posturing, autonomic phenomenon are prominent. Suggestive of severe ICH in preterm infants	+	Asphyxia, intracranial bleed and inborn error of metabolism
Myoclonic	They are distinguished from clonic movements because of the faster speed of the myoclonic jerk and predilection for flexor muscle groups. They occur commonly in severe neonatal epileptic and nonepileptic syndromes **Focal** Typically involve flexor muscles of upper extremity **Multifocal** Asynchronous twitching of several parts of the body **Generalized** Bilateral myoclonic jerks of upper and occasionally of lower limbs	+	Syndromic in nature

rapidly abolished by arousal. They are also induced by gentle rhythmic rocking or tactile stimuli. EEG is normal in this condition. The condition resolves spontaneously over weeks to months. Long-term outcome is good and epilepsy does not develop later in life. Early diagnosis is important because use of barbiturates or benzodiazepines worsen this condition, by triggering more sleep.

EVALUATION OF AN INFANT WITH NEONATAL SEIZURES

History

A detailed history should be taken regarding antenatal, perinatal, genetic and metabolic factors for the possible cause(s) of seizures.

Seizure morphology The details of seizure episode, like type, duration, autonomic phenomenon, relation to sleep and whether movements stop on restraining the infant should be looked for. Also check whether the abnormal movements can be induced by touch or any stimulus. Look for associated changes in respiration, heart rate, deviation of eyes or mottling of skin.

The day of life on which the seizures occurred may provide a useful clue to its etiology. The seizures occurring during 6–12 hours are mainly due to perinatal asphyxia, while those during first 72 hours may be related to intracranial hemorrhage and metabolic causes. Seizures occurring between 4–7 days or beyond may be due to sepsis, meningitis, metabolic causes and developmental defects.

Antenatal history Ask about any maternal symptoms suggestive of intrauterine infection, diabetes mellitus, hypertension, and any narcotic addiction. History of pre-eclampsia/eclampsia, antepartum hemorrhage, meconium stained liquor are recognized risk factors for intrauterine asphyxia. A history of sudden episodes of increase in fetal movements are suggestive of intrauterine convulsions. Ask whether mother received any supplementations of calcium and vitamin D during pregnancy.

Perinatal history Ask for history of perinatal asphyxia, fetal distress, decreased fetal movements, instrumental delivery, and need for resuscitation in the labor room. Apgar scores, abnormal cord pH (<7.0) and base deficit (>10 mEq/L) should be looked for as useful markers of birth asphyxia. Use of pudendal block for mid-cavity forceps may be associated with accidental injection of the local anesthetic into the fetal scalp. Check whether infant received vitamin K which is credited to reduce the risk of intracranial hemorrhage.

Post natal history Feeding history should be asked for any prelacteal feeds as it may lead to septicemia. Look for features like lethargy, poor activity, drowsiness, and refusal to accept feeds. The onset of seizures after initiation of enteral feeding is suggestive of inborn errors of metabolism (IEM). Late-onset hypocalcemia may occur as a consequence of hyperphosphatemia because of predominant cow's milk feeding.

Family history History of consanguinity, seizures or mental retardation in the family and early fetal/neonatal deaths are suggestive of inborn errors of metabolism. History of seizures in either parent or sibling(s) in the neonatal period may suggest benign familial neonatal convulsions (BFNC).

Physical Examination

Vital signs Heart rate, respiration, blood pressure, capillary refill time and temperature should be recorded in all infants.

General physical examination Gestation, birth weight, and weight-for-gestational age should be recorded. Anthropometry should be checked to identify preterm and growth retarded babies, who are at risk of developing hypoglycemia and polycythemia. Seizures on 2nd or 3rd day in full term 'well baby' may be due to subarachnoid hemorrhage while seizures in a large-for-dates baby may be secondary to hypoglycemia or intracranial hemorrhage (ICH). Malformations or dysmorphic features should be looked for. Presence of cleft lip/palate and genital abnormalities may associated with midline defects in the brain.

Systemic examination Presence of hepatospleno-megaly or an abnormal urine odor may suggest IEM. The skin should be examined for the presence of any neuro-cutaneous markers. Presence of sepsis, cataracts, hypoglycemia, jaundice, and hepatomegaly are charac-teristic features fo galactosemia. A detailed neurological examination including assessment of consciousness (alert, drowsy, comatose), tone (hypotonia or hypertonia), ocular examination for chorioretinitis and cataract should be done. Neurological states like lethargy, shrill cry and presence of a bulging anterior fontanel are suggestive of meningitis or intracranial hemorrhage. The separated sutures may point towards hydro-cephalus. The sequential neurological examination at 8–12 hourly interval is more important and revealing than a single one time examination. Rapid increase in head size is suggestive of ICH and hydrocephalus.

Diagnosis

The aim is to quickly identify the nature of seizure activity and its etiology. Ideally all electroencephalographic seizures should be abolished with treatment but availability of continous EEG monitoring is still a distant dream. Seizures should be treated as a medical emergency as they occur due a neurological dysfunction and may further cause secondary brain injury.

The choice of investigations should be individualised with an emphasis on early identification of a correctable metabolic cause. Blood sugar and serum electrolytes (Na, Ca, Mg) should be checked. Arterial blood gas (ABG) is mandatory to look for evidences of metabolic acidosis due to hypoxia and IEM. Examination of CSF is considered as an essential investigation but it may be withheld if there is severe cardio-respiratory compromise or even omitted in infants with severe birth asphyxia and HIE or a recognized metabolic disorder. In addition, bedside cranial ultrasonography (cUSG) and amplitude integrated electroencephalography (aEEG) are essential investigations. Additional investigations may be considered in neonates who do not respond to anticonvulsant drugs or when there are specific features or unusual clinical scenario. These include neuroimaging (CT, MRI), detailed screening for congenital infections (TORCH) and workup for IEM (glucose, ammonia, lactate, metabolic screening).

Identification of Seizures

Common methods for identifying neonatal seizures include clinical observation, continuous video clinical (cEEG) and amplitude-integrated electroencephalo-graphy (aEEG). Almost 50% of neonatal seizures can be identified at the bedside. It requires constant observation by the NICU staff. The subclinical or subtle seizures, which are the most common seizures in preterm neonates, can only be identified by EEG monitoring.

Treatment

As per WHO recommendations, all clinically apparent seizures of any phenotype lasting for more than 3 minutes or recurrent seizuress of brief duration should be treated. If continuous EEG monitoring is available, all electrical seizures should be treated even in the absence of clinically apparent seizures.

One should not initiate anticonvulsant therapy as soon as the seizures start. The initial management should focus on identification of type of seizures and determining its etiology by quick history and clinical examination. The infant should be stabilized by maintenance of body temperature, airway, breathing and circulation. Oxygen should be started, IV access should be secured, and blood sample collected for glucose, electrolytes and ABG. If glucostix shows hypoglycemia a 'mini bolus' of 2 mL/kg of 10%

dextrose should be given followed by a continuous infusion of dextrose @ 6–8 mg/kg/min. When hypoglycemia has been treated or excluded as a cause of convulsions, the neonate should be screened for hypocalcemia. If ionized calcium levels are suggestive of hypocalcemia (<4.8 mg/dL), or it cannot be tested immediately (ECG shows QoTc >0.2 sec), 2 mL/kg of 10% calcium gluconate diluted in distilled water is administered slowly over 10 minutes under strict cardiac monitoring. When hypocalcemia is confirmed, the neonate should receive calcium gluconate 8 mL/kg/d for 3 days. If hypocalcemic seizures are resistant to administration of calcium, serum magnesium should be tested. If hypomagnesemia is documented (serum magnesium <1.2 mg/dL), 0.25 mL/kg of 50% magnesium sulphate should be given intramuscularly every 12 hourly for 3 doses.

If seizures persist even after correction of glucose and electrolyte imbalance, antiepileptic drugs should be started. Based on current evidence, WHO recommends the use of phenobarbitone as the first line medication for management of neonatal seizures. The initial loading dose of phenobarbitone is 20 mg/kg and is given slowly over 20 minutes @ 1 mg/kg/min. If seizures persist, additional bolus dose of 10 mg/kg is administered till cumulative dose of 30 mg/kg. Repeated dosing may be avoided in infants with asphyxia because its metabolism is hampered due to hypoxic damage to the liver. In these cases, it is better to add phenytoin instead of giving additional loading dose of phenobarbital. Phenytoin, midazolam and lidocaine may be used as second line antiepileptic drugs (AED). Lidocaine is used with caution due its cardio-toxicity. Though limited data is available, levetiracetam has emerged as a useful second line drug due to its wide therapeutic index. In contrast to drugs like pheno-barbitone and phenytoin, levetiracetam does not appear to enhance neuronal apoptosis in animal models and may in fact have neuroprotective and antiepileptogenic effects.

In cases of refractory seizures, midazolam infusion, valproate and lidocaine can be used (Figure 21.2). If the underlying etiology is unknown, after initial labora-tory screening and imaging studies, a trial of pyridoxine, pyridoxal 5'-phosphate and folinic acid should be considered. Depending upon the etiology of seizures, response to anticonvulsant therapy and neurological status of the neonate, the AEDs are tapered (Figure 21.3). The dosages of commonly used anti-convulsants and their adverse effects are listed in Table 21.3.

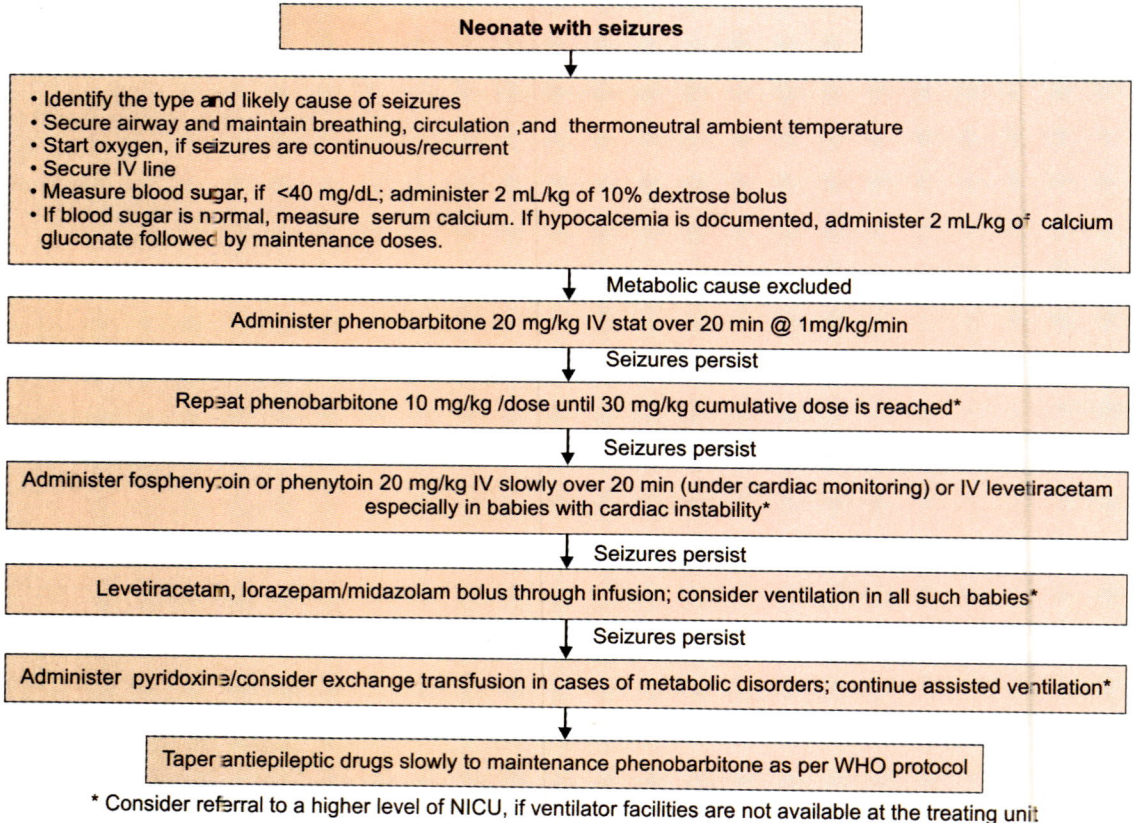

Figure 21.2 Algorithm for management of neonatal seizures.

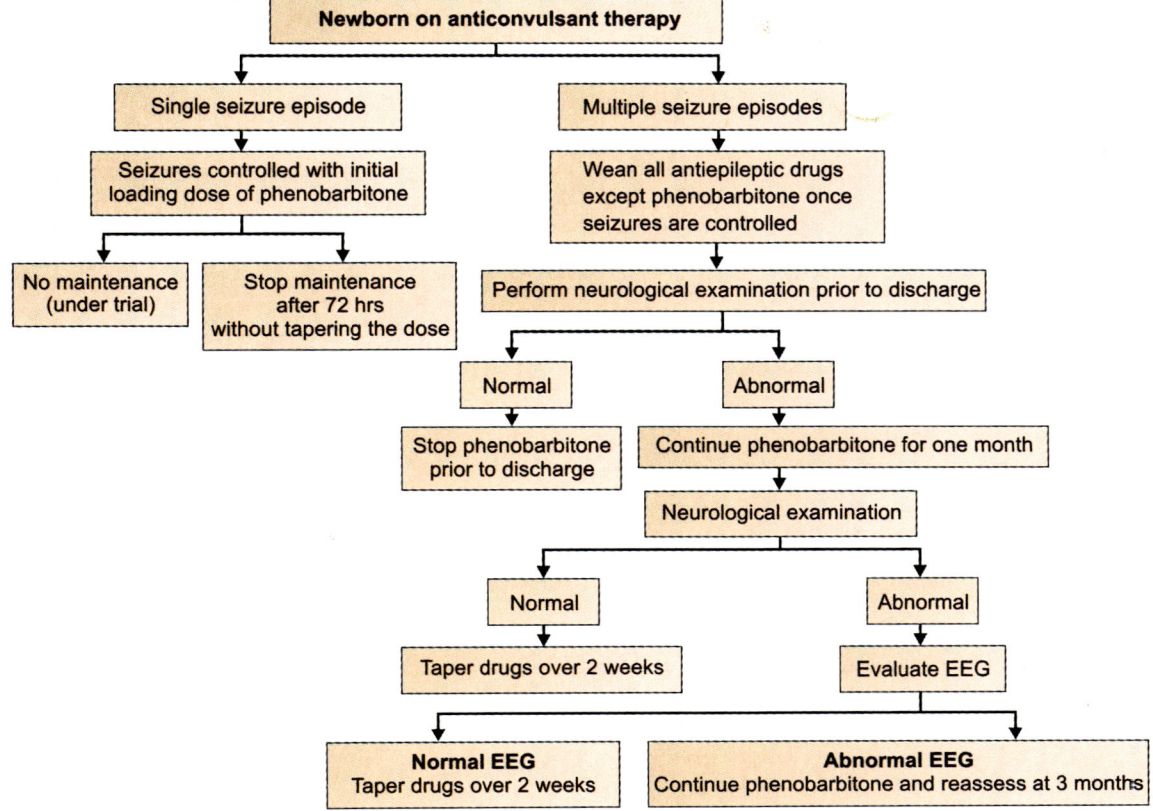

Figure 21.3 WHO protocol for tapering anticonvulsant drugs in neonates.

Table 21.3 Dosages and side effects of commonly used antiepileptic drugs		
Drugs	**Dosage**	**Adverse effects**
Phenobarbitone	Loading dose 20 mg/kg/ diluted to a concentration of 1:10 followed by 10 mg/kg/dose IV till maximum 30 mg/kg Maintenance dose 3–5 mg/kg/day q 12 to 24 hr PO Therapeutic blood level is 10–25 mg/dL	Hypotension, respiratory depression, dilated pupils and dolls' eye phenomenon. Long-term effect on attention, memory and cognition.
Phenytoin or fosphenytoin*	20 mg/kg IV (0.5–1.0 mg/kg/min) IV. Maintenance dose 3–4 mg/kg/day q 12 hr IV	Respiratory depression, hypotension or bradycardia or other cardiac abnormalities. Avoid oral route due to poor bioavailability. Rapid administration may cause cardiac arrhythmias including asystole
Levetiracetam	Loading dose 30–60 mg/kg IV @ 5 mg/kg/min. Maintenance dose 10 mg/kg/dose q 8–12 hr IV/ PO	Safe drug, wide therapeutic index. Monitoring of drug level not required
Lorazepam	0.05–0.10 mg/kg IV over 5 min	Respiratory depression, apnea, and bradycardia.
Midazolam	0.2 mg/kg, IV bolus; then, 0.1–0.4 mg/kg/hr	Advantage of less respiratory depression and sedation than lorazepam
Sodium valproate	20–25 mg/kg/d IV followed by 5–10 mg/kg q 12 hr IV/oral	Hepatotoxicity and elevated blood ammonia levels Avoid in IEM because it causes hyperammonemia
Lidocaine	4 mg/kg IV followed by infusion of 2 mg/kg/hr	Arrhythmia, hypotension and seizures
Paraldehyde	0.1–0.2 mL/kg/dose IM or 0.3 mL/kg/dose with coconut oil in 3:1 dilution per rectal	Respiratory disturbances (pulmonary hemorrhage, pulmonary edema, hypotension), secondary to pulmonary excretion of paraldehyde

(Contd...)

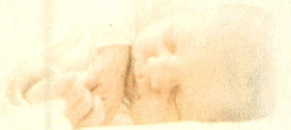

Table 21.3 Dosages and side effects of commonly used antiepileptic drugs (*Contd...*)

Drugs	Dosage	Adverse effects
Pyridoxine	1.0 ml neurobion® IM in both sides of gluteal region or in anterolateral aspect of thigh. Maintenance dose 50 mg single daily dose PO	Hypotension and apnea
Folic acid	Initial dose 15 µg/kg/dose IV (max 50 µg/kg/day) followed by maintanence dose 30–45 µg/24 hourly	High dose of folic acid may decrease absorption of phenytoin and may mask hematologic effects of vitamin B_{12} deficiency
Topiramate	Initial and maintenece dose of 3 mg/kg per day	Anorexia, weight loss, vomiting, diarrhea, and acidosis
Bumetanide	Add-on-drug with phenobaritone as it overcomes depolarizing action of immature neurons to GABA agonists	Ototoxicity

*1.5 mg fosphenytoin yields 1.0 mg phenytoin
IEM: inborn error of metabolism

Prognosis

The goal of management of neonatal seizures is not only to control the seizures but also to ensure satisfactory long-term neurodevelopment outcome. Data on animal studies showed that seizures in neonates impair the development of neuronal structure, its connectivity, synapses, and functions and thus adversely affect the whole process of neurogenesis. Recurrent seizures can cause further brain injury. It predisposes to cognitive, behavioral, learning or epileptic sequelae in later life.

The prognosis of seizures is basically determined by its etiology, the neurological status of newborn and the inter-ictal EEG pattern. The prognosis of hypocalcemic seizures, subarachnoid hemorrhage and familial neonatal seizures is excellent. Symptomatic hypoglycemia and meningitis have a 50% chance of sequelae in the survivors. In hypoxic ischemic encephalopathy, the prognosis depends on the grade of HIE, while CNS malformations generally have a poor outcome. Gestation also affects the neurological outcome as very low birth weight infants have poor outcome compared to term infants.

The inter-ictal EEG background pattern disturbances such as burst suppression is highly predictive of poor outcome, particularly when it persists beyond second week of life. The outcome of baby also depends on how judiciously the antiepileptic drugs are used. AEDs are known to have adverse effects on the developing brain. In animal models, phenobarbitone use is associated with increased neuronal apoptosis while levetiracetam is believed to be a neuroprotective drug. The duration of antiepileptic therapy also determines the neuro-developmental outcome, therefore there is a trend towards early weaning of AEDs.

BIBLIOGRAPHY

Agarwal R, Deorari AK, Paul VK. AIIMS Protocols in Neonatology, *New Delhi: CBS Publishers and Distributors Pvt Ltd.;* 1st edition 2015; p 48–61.

Bittigau P. Antiepileptic drugs and apoptotic neurodegeneration in the developing brain. *Proc Natl Acad Sci* 2002; 99(23): 15089–94.

Boylan GB, Stevenson NJ, Vanhatalo S. Monitoring neonatal seizures. *Semin Fetal Neonatal Med* 2013, 18:202–8.

Clancy RR. The contribution of EEG to the understanding of neonatal seizures. *Epilepsia* 1996; 37(Suppl 1):S52–S59.

Dulac O, Milh M, Holmes GL. Brain maturation and epilepsy. *Handbook Clin Neurol* 2013; 111:441–6.

Dzhala VI, Staley KJ. Excitatory actions of endogenously released GABA contribute to initiation of ictalepileptiform activity in the developing hippocampus. *J Neurosci* 2003; 23(5):1840–6.

Falsaperia R, Vitaliti G, Mauceri L, et al. Levetiracetam in seizures as first-line treatment: A prospective study. *J Pediatr Neurosci* 2017 May, 12:24–8.

Glass HC. Neonatal seizures: Advances in mechanisms and management. *Clin Perinatol* 2014; 41(1):177–90.

Guillet R, Kwon J. Seizure recurrence and developmental disabilities after neonatal seizures: outcomes are unrelated to use of phenobarbital prophylaxis. *J Child Neurol* 2007; 22(4): 389–95.

Hellstrom-Westas L, Blennow G, Lindroth M, et al. Low risk of seizure recurrence after early withdrawal of antiepileptic treatment in the neonatal period. *Arch Dis Child Fetal Neonatal Ed* 1995; 72(2):F97–F101.

Hill A. Neonatal seizures. *Pediatr Rev* 2000, Apr. 21(4):117–21.

Jensen FE. Neonatal seizures: an update on mechanisms and management. *Clin Perinatol* 2009; 36(4):881–900.

Lanska MJ. A population-based study of neonatal seizures in Fayette County, Kentucky. *Neurology* 1995; 45(4):724–32.

Mizrahi EM, Kellaway P. Characterization and classification of neonatal seizures. *Neurology* 1988 Jan, 37(12):1837–44.

Mizrahi EM, Kellaway P. Diagnosis and management of neonatal seizures. *Lippincott-Raven, Philadelphia* 1998, p181.

National Neonatal Perinatal Database. Report for the year 2002–03. http://www.newbornwhocc.org/pdf/nnpd_report_2002–03.PDF

Mruk AL, Garlitz KL, Leung NR. Levetiracetam in neonatal seizures: A review. *J Pediatr Pharmcol Ther* 2015, 20(2):76–89.

Painter MJ, Scher MS, Stein AD, Armatti S, Wang Z, et al. Phenobarbital compared with phenytoin for the treatment of neonatal seizures. *N Engl J Med* 1999; 341(7):485–9.

Pathak G, Upadhyay A, Pathak U, Chawla D, Goel SP. Phenobarbitone and phenytoin for treatment of neonatal seizures: An open label randomized controlled trial. *Indian Pediatr* 2013; 50:753–7.

Perveen S, Singh A, Upadhyay A, Singh N, Chauhan R. A randomized controlled trial on comparison of phenobarbitone and levetiracetam for the treatment of neonatal seizures: pilot study. *Int J Res Med Sci* 2016; 2073–8.

Rao LM, Marcuccilli CJ. Seizures in the preterm neonate. *Neo Reviews* 2017, 18(1):352–59, DOI: 10.1542/neo. 18-1-e52.

Sands TT, McDonough TL. Recent advances in neonatal seizures. *Neurol Neurosci Rep* 2016, 16:92.

Scher M. Seizures in neonates. In: Neonatal-Perinatal Medicine: Diseases of the Fetus and Infant. Richard J, Avroy A. Fanaroff MB, Michele C. Fanaroff and Martin's 9th Ed. *United States: Elsevier*; 2010.

Shellhaas RA, Chang T, Tsuchida T, Scher MS, Riviello JJ, Abend NS et al. The American Clinical Neurophysiology Society's Guidelines on Continuous Electroencephalography Monitoring in Neonates. *J Clin Neurophysiol* 2011; 28(6):611–7.

Volpe JJ. Neonatal seizures: current concepts and revised classification. *Pediatrics* 1989, 84(3):422–28.

Volpe JJ. Neurology of the newborn, Neonatal seizures. *Philadelphia; WB Saunders Elsevier*, 5th ed. 2008; pp 203–237.

Wasim S, Upadhyay A, Roy M, Saxena P, Chillar N. Serum phenobarbitone levels in neonatal seizures in term and near-term babies. *Indian Pediatr* 2016; 5:388–90.

Weeke LC, Boylan GB, Pressler RM, et al. Role of EEG background activity, seizure burden and MRI in predicting neurodevelopmental outcome in full-term infants with hypoxic-ischaemic encephalopathy in the era of therapeutic hypothermia. *Eur J Paediatr Neurol* 2016, doi:10.1016/j.ejpn.2016.06.003.

WHO Guidelines on neonatal seizures. Geneva: *World Health Organization,* 2012 *www.newbornwhocc.org.*

22

Metabolic Emergencies

N. Karthik Nagesh and Mrinal Pillai

ELECTROLYTE IMBALANCE

Excessive elevation or decrease in levels of electrolytes may be life-threatening which needs to be corrected rapidly. This should be followed by gradual correction till normal values are achieved. The underlying cause should be identified and treated.

Hyponatremia (Plasma sodium <135 mEq/L)

Hyponatremia may be classified into hypovolemic, euvolemic and hypervolemic depending on the volume status of the patient and the underlying cause of hyponatremia. Conditions associated with pseudohyponatremia (normal serum osmolarity, e.g. hyperlipidemia, hyperproteinemia) and factitious hyponatremia (high serum osmolarity, e.g. hyperglycemia, mannitol) must be excluded. Irrespective of whether hyponatremia is due to fluid overload or sodium deficit, rapid correction with 3% saline is indicated if serum sodium is <120 mEq/L with or without seizures/coma. The emergency administration of 3% saline (0.5 mEq/mL) intravenously over 4–6 hours in a dose of 2 to 4 mL/kg to increase serum sodium up to 120 mEq/L is life-saving.

In chronic hyponatremia (>48 hr) or in cases with unknown time frame, further increase in serum sodium up to 135 mEq/L is done slowly at a rate of 0.5 mEq/L over the next 48 hours. This is done to avoid osmotic demyelination syndrome. When chronic hyponatremia is established, brain cells extrude organic solutes from their cytoplasm, allowing intracellular osmolality to equilibrate with plasma osmolality without increase in cell water volume. This adaptation permits survival in chronic hyponatremia but makes the brain vulnerable to injury from overzealous therapy. When hyponatremia is corrected too rapidly, outpacing the brain's ability to recapture lost organic osmolytes, osmotic demyelination can result. Osmotic demyelination can lead to quadriparesis, dysphagia and movement disorder. It affects myelinated brain; therefore it is very rare in neonates. Nevertheless, it has been reported in infants as young as 40 days.

The cause of hyonatremia should be identified to determine the mode of treatment (Figure 22.1).

1. *Hypovolemic hyponatremia* It is treated with fluid and sodium supplementation to correct deficit, and provide maintenance and on-going losses. Calculate sodium deficit using the formula:

   sodium deficit = (135-plasma sodium) × 0.7 × body weight. (Assuming 70% of total body water as the distribution space of sodium). Replace two-thirds of deficit in 24 hours, and remaining one-third over subsequent 24 hours. Intravenous fluids with 5% dextrose and 0.45% to 0.9% saline is adequate as replacement fluid. In stable infants enteral sodium chloride can be used for correction and maintenance.

2. *Euvolemic hyponatremia* It is treated with water restriction to two-thirds of maintenance requirements.

3. *Hypervolemic hyponatremia* It is treated with both sodium and water restriction. Fluids administered to edematous hyponatremic infants should be less than the insensible water loss plus urine output. The most common cause of hyponatremia in sick neonates is excessive administration of fluids or retention of free water. The fluid excess can be calculated as follows:

   Excess fluid = TBW × [1-measured plasma sodium/expected sodium].

Hypernatremia (Plasma sodium >145 mEq/L)

Hypernatremia often occurs due to increased relative water loss compared to sodium retention and as a

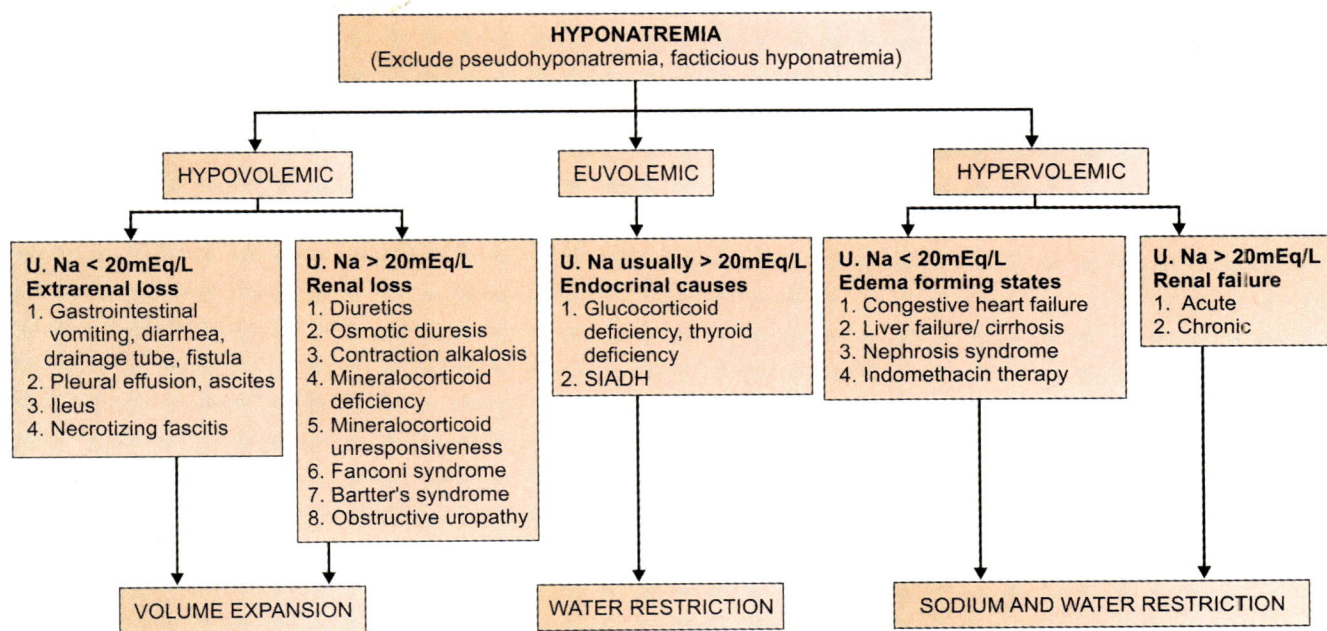

U.Na: urinary sodium, SIADH: secretion of inappropriate diuretic hormone

Figure 22.1 Algorithm for evaluation and treatment of hyponatremia.

consequence of trans-epidermal free water loss. Hypernatremic induced hypertonicity leads to shift of water from the intracellular compartment to extracellular compartment resulting in masking of clinical signs of dehydration. There is delayed onset of symptoms like lethargy, irritability, abnormal muscle tone, seizures, cardiovascular collapse and renal failure. It may be associated with venous sinus thrombosis, subdural hemorrhage or brain edema due to overzealous correction. In addition to hypovolemia, hypernatremia may be associated with normovolemia or hypervolemia (Table 21.1).

In chronic hypernatremia due to extracellular hypertonicity, central nervous system adapts by synthesis of osmoprotective aminoacids and organic solutes. These idiogenic osmoles help in maintaining normal brain cell volume. Rapid correction of hypernatremia may lead to rapid and abrupt fall in extracellular tonicity and shift of water into brain cells. Brain cells swell up, resulting in cerebral edema and

its deleterious consequences. The appropriate treatment of hypernatremia depends on the underlying cause.

Hypernatremic dehydration is the most common cause of neonatal hypernatremia. Treatment is divided in to two phases.

i. *Emergent phase* If the neonate is in shock or having reduced urine output, intravascular volume is restored by administration of 10 to 20 mL/kg of normal saline.

ii. *Rehydration phase* Remaining free water deficit and maintenance needs are provided evenly over at least 48 hours. The free water deficit is calculated by the formula:

Free water deficit (L) = 0.7 × body weight (kg) × [current plasma sodium level (mEq/L)/140-1], where 0.7 × body weight is estimation of total body water.

The correction of sodium level should be slow at a rate of 0.5 mEq/L/hr, it should decrease sodium level by 12 mEq/L over 24 hours period. Serial monitoring

Table 22.1 Causes of hypernatremia		
Hypovolemic hypernatremia	*Euvolemic hypernatremia*	*Hypervolemic hypernatremia*
■ Inadequate breast milk intake ■ Diarrhea ■ Radiant warmers ■ Excessive sweating ■ Renal dysplasia ■ Osmotic diuresis	■ Central diabetes insipidus ■ Nephrogenic diabetes insipidus ■ Reduced renal responsiveness due to extreme prematurity, renal insult, drugs such as aminoglycosides, amphotericin B	■ Improperly mixed formula or ORS ■ Bicarbonate administration ■ Saline boluses ■ Primary hyperaldosteronism

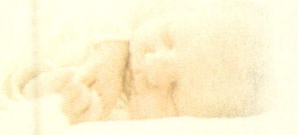

should be done every 4 hours until serum sodium level is less than 150 mEq/L. The free water needed to reduce the serum sodium by 1 mEq/L is 4 mL/kg for moderate hypernatremia (48 mL/kg to reduce by 12 mEq/L over 24 hours) and 3 mL/kg for severe hypernatremia with serum sodium level of 190 mEq/L (36 mL/kg to reduce by 12 mEq/L over 24 hours). The free water content of various IV fluids is given in Table 22.2.

The appropriate IV fluid concentrations used to correct hypernatremia of different severity is based on the relative free water content of the IV solution for a specific serum sodium value which is calculated by the formula:

Percentage of free water content = 1 – (Sodium level in IV fluid/serum sodium).

The sodium concentration of various fluids for treatment of hypernatremia of various severity is summarized in Table 22.3. If hyperglycemia accompanies the hypernatremia, it is should not be corrected with insulin because it can increase idiogenic osmoles in the brain. The associated hypocalcemia is corrected with calcium supplements.

Neonates who are volume overloaded and hypernatremic due to excess sodium intake are treated by withholding sodium administration and enhancement of sodium excretion by the use of hypotonic fluids along with diuretics in milder cases and by dialysis in severe cases especially when it is associated with oliguria.

Hypokalemia (Plasma potassium <3.5 mEq/L)

Hypokalemia is rarely symptomatic (except in neonates receiving digoxin) until serum potassium levels drop to less than 2.5 mEq/L. Electrocardiogram shows flat T waves, prolonged QT interval, or appearance of U wave. Severe hypokalemia can lead to arrhythmia, ileus and lethargy. The common causes of hypokalemia are listed in Table 22.4.

Rapid administration of potassium chloride intravenously is associated with life-threatening cardiac dysfunction and it is therefore not routinely recommended. Hypokalemia is treated by gradual potassium supplementation in IV fluids or orally. If hypokalemia is secondary to alkalosis, potassium intake is increased after correcting alkalosis. In extreme hypokalemia,

Table 22.2 Relative free water content in percentage at normal and high serum sodium concentration

Serum sodium concentration		5% dextrose	0.2% saline	0.45% saline	Ringer's lactate solution	0.9% saline
145 mEq/L	Isotonic (%)	0	22	50	86	100
	Water (%)	100	78	50	14	0
195 mEq/L	Isotonic (%)	0	17	39	68	79
	Water (%)	100	83	61	32	21

Table 22.3 The appropriate IV fluids to treat hypernatremia

Serum sodium level	IV fluid for replacement during rehydration phase	Relative free water content in percentage
≤165 mEq/L	0.45% DNS (77 mEq/L)	52% at serum sodium of 160 mEq/L
166–174 mEq/L	0.9% DNS (154 mEq/L)	9.4% at serum sodium of 170 mEq/L
≥175 mEq/L	3% saline (513 mEq/L) added to IV fluid so that sodium level in IV fluid should be 10–15 mEq/L less than serum sodium level	8.3% at serum sodium of 180 mEq/L when the sodium level of reconstituted IV fluid is 165 mEq/L

DNS: dextrose normal saline

Table 22.4 Causes of hypokalemia

Intracellular shift with normal K stores	Decreased potassium stores		Extra renal (urine K decreased)
	Renal (urine K increased)		
	Normal blood pressure	Hypertension	
1. Metabolic alkalosis	1. Renal tubular acidosis	1. Renovascular disease	1. Skin loss
2. Hyperinsulinemia	2. Fanconi syndrome	2. Excess renin	2. GI loss
3. Beta-2 catecholamines	3. Bartter syndrome	3. Excess mineralocorticoids	3. Malnutrition
4. Familial hypokalemic periodic paralysis	4. Antibiotics	4. Cushing syndrome	
	5. Diuretics		
	6. Amphotericin B		

potassium can be given over 30–60 min at a maximum rate of 0.3 mEq/kg potassium intravenously diluted in normal saline (1.0 mL KCl in 9 mL normal saline) and given preferably through central line.

Hyperkalemia (Plasma potassium >6 mEq/L)

Serum potassium greater than 6.5 mEq/L can cause life-threatening arrhythmias. ECG signs of hyperkalemia include peaked T waves (the earliest sign), prolonged PR interval, absent P waves, QRS widening/slurring, bradycardia, tachycardia, supraventricular tachycardia, ventricular tachycardia and ventricular fibrillation. The commonest cause of high potassium values in blood samples is hemolysis, and high potassium levels must be confirmed by ECG abnormalities and laboratory analysis of nonhemolysed blood sample. The causes of hyperkalemia in neonates include renal dysfunction, intraventricular hemorrhage, congenital adrenal hyperplasia, and metabolic acidosis (Table 22.5).

When hyperkalemia is diagnosed, potassium intake should be stopped and the ECG monitored. Therapy should preferably be started under ECG monitoring.

1. Calcium gluconate 1 mL/kg of 10% solution (100 mg/kg) is given intravenously over 5 minutes to stabilize the cardiac membrane. Intravenous calcium should be given under cardiac monitoring and it should be stopped if heart rate drops below 100/min.
2. Rapid cellular uptake of potassium is enhanced by following interventions:
   i. Alkali therapy with sodium bicarbonate 1–2 mL/kg (1–2 mEq/kg) by slow intravenous route over 0.5 to 1 hour. Hypernatremia, volume overload and hypertension may occur with excess bicarbonate use. Bicarbonate when given as a rapid bolus may cause intraventricular hemorrhage in preterm neonates.
   ii. Insulin 0.1 U/kg IV with 0.5 g/kg of 10% dextrose is given over 30 min. Blood glucose levels should be monitored to prevent hypoglycemia.

iii. Nebulized salbutamol 0.15 mg/kg is given in 3 doses every 20 min. It may cause tremors and tachycardia.
3. Remove all sources of exogenous intake of potassium.
4. Lower total body potassium stores.
   i. Furosemide 1–2 mg/kg/dose IV or oral every 12–24 hours.
   ii. Sodium polystyrene sulfonate (Kayexalate) 1 g/kg per rectum every 6 hourly may be used with caution in a neonate who has no gut pathology and is not very premature. It may lead to sodium overload. Calcium-potassium exchange resin may be used instead of kayexalate, which will not lead to sodium overload.
   iii. Peritoneal dialysis is life-saving in infants with unresponsive hyperkalemia.

Hypocalcemia (serum calcium <8 mg/dL in term and <7 mg/dL in preterm infants)

Hypocalcemia is defined as total serum calcium level of less than 8 mg/dL (ionic calcium <4.8 mg/dL) in term neonates and less than 7 mg/dL (ionic calcium <4 mg/dL) in preterm babies. Low ionized calcium levels decrease the threshold of action potentials in neurons leading to hyperexcitability in both sensory and motor nerves. Patients with hypocalcemia may be totally asymptomatic or may present with lethargy, poor feeding, vomiting, abdominal distension, seizures, tetany, cramps, laryngospasm or apnea. The ECG may show a prolonged QTc interval.

Infants with symptomatic hypocalcemia should receive a bolus dose of 10% calcium gluconate 2 mL/kg/dose diluted 1:1 with 5% dextrose over 10 minutes under cardiac monitoring. In severe hypocalcemia with poor cardiac function, calcium chloride 20 mg/kg may be given through a central line over 30 minutes (chloride unlike gluconate does not require hepatic metabolism for the release of free calcium). This should be followed by a continuous IV infusion of 80 mg/kg/day

Table 22.5 Causes of hyperkalemia		
Normal K+ stores	Increased potassium stores	
	Increased urine K+	Decreased urine K+
1. Leucocytosis	1. Transfusion with aged blood	1. Renal failure
2. Tumor lysis syndrome	2. Exogenous intake of K+ (e.g. salt substitutes)	2. Hypoaldosteronism
3. Metabolic acidosis	3. Pseudohypoaldosteronism	3. Aldosterone insensitivity
4. Type IV renal tubular acidosis		4. Decreased insulin
5. Rhabdomyolysis/crush injury		5. K+ sparing diuretics
6. Malignant hyperthermia		6. Congenital adrenal hyperplasia
7. Theophylline intoxication		

elemental calcium for 48 hours. The continuous infusion is preferred to IV bolus doses (1 mL/kg/dose q 6 hourly). Calcium infusion @ 50% of the original dose is given for the next 24 hours and then discontinued. The infusion may be replaced with oral calcium therapy on the last day. Normal serum calcium values should be documented for 48 hours before weaning the infusion. Calcium gluconate 10% contains 9.8 mg/mL or 0.45 mEq/mL of elemental calcium while calcium chloride 10% contains 27 mg/mL or 1.4 mEq/mL of elemental calcium and is thus more irritating to the tissues on extravasation.

Neonates who are at risk for early onset (within 72 hours of life) hypocalcemia (Preterm <34 weeks, sick infant of diabetic mother, and severe birth asphyxia with Apgar score at 1 min <4) should be screened at 24 and 48 hours. Those detected to have hypocalcemia on screening but who are otherwise asymptomatic should receive 80 mg/kg/day elemental calcium (8 mL/kg/day of 10% calcium gluconate) slowly through intravenous route for 48 hours (without bolus calcium). This may be reduced to 50% dose for another 24 hours and then discontinued. Neonates tolerating oral feeds may be treated with oral calcium (IV preparation can be given orally).

Bolus doses of calcium should be diluted 1:1 with 5% dextrose and given slowly (over 10 to 30 minutes) under cardiac monitoring because of danger of bradycardia and asystole. Hepatic necrosis may occur if the tip of the umbilical venous catheter (UVC) lies in a branch of the portal vein, hence it is mandatory to ensure that the tip of the catheter is positioned in the inferior vena cava. Accidental injection into the umbilical arterial catheter may result in arterial spasm and intestinal necrosis. Skin and subcutaneous tissue necrosis may occur due to extravasation. The IV site of administration of calcium should be closely watched for any extravasation.

Prolonged or Resistant Hypocalcemia

It should be considered in the following situations and evaluated for late-onset hypocalcemia (onset after 72 hours of birth)

1. Symptomatic hypocalcemia unresponsive to calcium therapy.
2. Infants needing calcium supplements for more than 72 hours of age.
3. Hypocalcemia presenting at the end of the first week of life.

The common causes of late-onset hypocalcemia are listed in Table 22.6. Treatment of late-onset hypocalcemia depends on the cause of hypocalcemia. The steps of management are listed below.

1. *High phosphate load* These neonates have hyperphosphatemia with near normal calcium levels. It occurs due to consumption of cow's milk which has high phosphate content. Exclusive breastfeeding is encouraged and cow's milk intake is discontinued. Avoid use of phosphate binding gels.

Table 22.6 Causes of late-onset hypocalcemia	
Causes	Investigations
Increased phosphate load Intake of cow milk, renal insufficiency	Serum calcium, phosphate, renal function tests
Hypomagnesemia	Serum magnesium level
Vitamin D deficiency Maternal vitamin D deficiency Malabsorption Hepatobiliary disease	Vitamin D level of the baby, maternal vitamin D status, maternal calcium, phosphate, alkaline phosphatase, liver function tests, X-ray wrist

Hypoparathyroidism
 	
1. Primary hypoparathyroidism: Hypoplasia/aplasia (Di George's syndrome), activating mutations of the calcium sensing receptors
2. Secondary hypoparathyroidism: Maternal hyperparathyroidism, metabolic syndromes (Kenny–Caffey syndrome)
   a. Parathyroid resistance
   b. Transient neonatal pseudohypoparathyroidism
	Parathyroid hormone level of the baby, maternal PTH level, X-ray/USG chest for thymus
	
	Serum calcium and parathormone level

Iatrogenic Administration of citrated blood products, lipid infusion, bicarbonate therapy, loop diuretics, glucocorticosteroids, phosphate therapy, aminoglycosides (mainly gentamicin), and phototherapy	Serum calcium, ECG and renal function tests

2. *Hypomagnesemia* Symptomatic hypocalcemia unresponsive to adequate calcium therapy is usually associated with hypomagnesemia. It may also present early within 3–4 days of life. It is treated with 50% magnesium sulfate 0.2 mL/kg 2 doses, 12 hours apart deep IM, followed by 0.2 mL/kg/day PO for 3 days.

3. *Vitamin D deficiency* These babies have hypocalcemia associated with hypophosphatemia due to intact parathyroid hormone effect on kidneys. Vitamin D_3 supplementation 1000–2000 IU/day for 4 weeks along with elemental calcium 40 mg/kg/day is recommended to prevent hungry bone syndrome.

4. *Hypoparathyroidism* These infants tend to be hyperphosphatemic with normal renal functions. Attempts should be made to reduce phosphate level (so as to keep the calcium and the phosphate product less than 55). These neonates are given supplements of calcium (50 mg/kg/day in 3 divided doses) and 1, 25(OH)$_2$ vitamin D_3 (0.5–1.0 µg/day) (alphadol, alfabol, alpha D_3 is available as 0.25 µg and 1.0 µg capsules). Therapy is stopped after 6 weeks in infants with hypoparathyroidism as a consequence of maternal hyperparathyroidism.

Hypercalcemia (Serum calcium >12 mg/dL)

Hypercalcemia is defined as total serum calcium of more than 12 mg/dL (>3 mmol/L) or ionized calcium >6 mg/dL (>1.5 mmol/L). Hypercalcemia suppresses parathyroid hormone secretion to regulate serum calcium. This regulatory effect is not so effective when serum calcium levels are below 7.5 mg/dL or above 11.5 mg/dL. At these levels, homeostasis is dependent on direct exchange of calcium between bone and extracellular fluid (ECF). A high ECF calcium concentration impairs the ability of the renal tubules to respond to ADH. This leads to polyuria, dehydration and azotemia.

The common causes of hypercalcemia and magnesium disorders in neonates are listed in Table 22.7. The predominant clinical features of hypercalcemia include nausea, vomiting, constipation, polyuria, polydipsia, dehydration, weight loss, renal failure, marked irritability and rarely seizures. There may be bradycardia, proximal muscle weakness, hypertension, pancreatitis, peptic ulcer disease, band keratopathy, metastatic calcification and renal stones. When calcium level exceeds 17 mg/dL, calcium phosphate may precipitate in the blood or tissues leading to cardiac arrest or coma. Besides calcium estimation, it is important to estimate phosphorus, alkaline phosphatase, paratharmone, 25 OH D_3 and 1–25 (OH)$_2$ D_3. Urinary calcium estimation and USG of abdomen for the presence of nephrocalcinosis is recommended.

The primary line of treatment is to augment urinary losses of calcium by saline diuresis with normal saline 20 mL/kg IV plus furosemide 2 mg/kg IV every 12 hourly. The fluids are administered at 1.5 to 2 times the maintenance requirement which reduces serum calcium by 1–3 mg/dL within a day. Serum electrolytes and urine output should be closely monitored. If serum calcium is more than 14 mg/dL, calcitonin 2–4 units/kg every 6 to 12 hours may be used. Biphosphonates such as pamidronate 0.5 to 1 mg/kg/dose IV over 4–5 hours or etidronate (5–10 mg/kg/day) PO can be used for 2 days. Biphosphonates have the potential toxicity of lowering serum phosphorus and can cause low grade fever, lymphopenia, myalgia and reversible hepatotoxicity.

Table 22.7 Causes of hypercalcemia and magnesium disorders

Hypercalcemia	Hypomagnesemia	Hypermagnesemia
Hyperparathyroidism	**Increased urinary losses**	**Renal failure**
Vitamin D intoxication	Diuretic use, renal tubular acidosis, hyper-	Hyoxic-ischemic encephalopathy,
Excessive exogenous calcium administration	calcemia, chronic adrenergic stimulants,	hypovolemia, shock, sepsis, obstructive
Malignancy	chemotherapy	uropathy
Prolonged immobilization	**Increased gastrointestinal losses**	**Excessive administration**
Thiazide diuretics	Malabsorption syndromes, severe mal-	Maternal magnesium administration for
Subcutaneous fat necrosis	nutrition, diarrhea, vomiting, short bowel	status asthmaticus, eclampsia/pre-eclampsia,
Williams syndrome	syndrome, enteric fistulas	cathartics, enemas, phosphate binders
Hyperthyroidism	**Endocrine disorders**	
Milk-alkali syndrome	Parathyroid hormone disorders, hyper-aldosterone states	
	Decreased intake	
	Prolonged parenteral fluid therapy with magnesium free solutions	

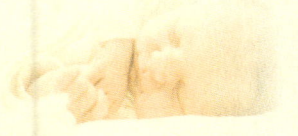

Biphosphonates have rarely been used in neonates. Oral glucocorticoids may play a role in vitamin D induced hypercalcemia by blocking GI absorption of calcium. In severe hypercalcemia, especially if associated with renal failure, dialysis may be life-saving. Surgical subtotal parathyroidectomy may be required in cases of primary hyperparathyroidism.

Hypomagnesemia (Serum magnesium <1.8 mEq/L)

The manifestations of hypomagnesemia include nausea, vomiting, lethargy, muscle cramps, neurologic and neuromuscular irritability. At levels less than 1 mEq/L there may be irritability, tremors, seizures, exaggerated deep tendon reflexes, carpopedal spasms, and tetany. Refractory ventricular tachycardia (Torsades de pointes) can occur in magnesium deficiency. Magnesium deficiency may lead to hypokalemia and hypocalcemia. Therefore decrease in any one of these electrolytes should prompt an evaluation of the other two electrolytes. ECG changes may be seen as prolonged PR, wide QRS, prolonged QT, ST depression, altered T waves, and low voltage.

Severe symptomatic hypomagnesemia with or without tetany, is treated by administration of magnesium 1 mEq/kg (0.2 mL/kg of 50% $MgSO_4$) 2 doses 12 hours apart, deep IM or slow IV (over 30 min, maximum @ 150 mg/minute) followed by a maintenance dose of 1.0 mEq/kg/day of magnesium, PO for 3 days. The mild asymptomatic cases can be managed by oral replacement with 1 mEq/kg/day of 50% $MgSO_4$. The total replacement dose is about 4 mEq/kg. In renal failure with documented hypomagnesemia, half the calculated amount should be given. The usual concentration of $MgSO_4$ that can be given intravenously ranges from 5 to 20%. Intravenous magnesium therapy is associated with potential risk of hypermagnesemia, hypocalcemia and hypotension. Careful monitoring of electrolytes and hemodynamics is required during IV magnesium infusion (50% $MgSO_4$ contains 4 mEq or 48 mg Mg^{++} per mL).

Hypermagnesemia (Serum magnesium >2.5 mEq/L)

Hypermagnesemia in neonates may occur due to renal failure and rapid mobilization from soft tissues following trauma, burns, shock and cardiac arrest. Maternal intake of magnesium sulfate for pregnancy induced hypertension is an important risk factor for development of hypermagnesemia in the neonate. Symptoms include nausea, vomiting, lethargy, weakness, dizziness, neuromuscular depression, hypotonia, absent deep tendon reflexes, respiratory depression, hypotension and altered sensorium. Hypermagnesemia can cause depression of the sino-atrial node, atrial fibrillation, widening of QRS, conduction delays, complete heartblock or asystole.

In severe or symptomatic cases, bolus dose of 10% calcium gluconate 2 mL/kg/dose diluted 1:1 with 5% dextrose over 10 minutes under cardiac monitoring is recommended because effects of magnesium on neuromotor and cardiac function are antagonized by calcium. Definitive treatment of hypermagnesemia requires increasing renal excretion of magnesium by administration of oral or intravenous diuretics when renal function is normal. When hypermagnesemia occurs due to acute kidney damage, it is managed by dialysis. In mild cases, withdrawing magnesium supplementation is often sufficient, to stabilize serum magnesium level.

ACID-BASE DISORDERS

Acid-base disorders are common in neonates and may occur due to metabolic, respiratory or mixed causes. The following protocol should be followed for rapid interpretation of arterial blood gases (ABGs):

1. **Check pH** pH of less than 7.35 is suggestive of acidosis while pH >7.45 indicates alkalosis.
2. **Acidosis** (pH < 7.35). Look for $PaCO_2$ and HCO_3^-.
   i. *Primary respiratory acidosis* There is elevation of $PaCO_2$ beyond 40 mmHg. In order to determine whether respiratory acidosis is acute or chronic, calculate $\Delta H^+/\Delta PaCO_2$ ratio. The ratio of >0.8 suggest acute respiratory acidosis while the ratio of <0.3 occurs in chronic respiratory insufficiency. In mixed or acute on chronic cases, the ratio varies between 0.3–0.8. The compensation of acidosis is assessed by estimation of HCO_3^-. In acute (<4 hr) cases, HCO_3^- increase by 1.0 mEq/L for every 10 mmHg elevation of $PaCO_2$ beyond 40 mmHg, while in chronic cases (>24 hr), HCO_3^- rises by 4 mEq/L for every 10 mmHg rise in PaO_2 beyond 40 mmHg.
   ii. *Primary metabolic acidosis* It is characterized by reduction in both $PaCO_2$ (due to compensatory rapid breathing) and HCO_3^-. The expected $PaCO_2$ can be calculated by the equation: $PaCO_2 = (1.5 \times HCO_3^- + 8) \pm 2$. When $PaCO_2$ is less than the expected level, it suggests concomitant respiratory alkalosis. In concomitant respiratory acidosis, actual PaO_2 is more than the expected or calculated $PaCO_2$. In metabolic acidosis, anion gap (AG) should be checked and infant classified into high AG acidosis or normal AG acidosis (hyperchloremic metabolic acidosis).

3. **Alkalosis (pH >7.45).** Look for HCO_3^- and $PaCO_2$.

   i. Primary respiratory alkalosis is characterized by low $PaCO_2$ due to wash out. It is classified as acute (<24 hr) when HCO_3^- falls by 2 mEq/L for every 10 mmHg fall in $PaCO_2$ below 40 mmHg and chronic (>24 hr) when HCO_3^- falls more than 5 mEq/L for every 10 mm Hg fall in $PaCO_2$ below 40 mmHg.

   ii. Primary metabolic alkalosis is associated with rise in both $PaCO_2$ and HCO_3^-. The expected $PaCO_2$ can be calculated by the equation $(0.7 \times HCO_3^- + 21) \pm 2$. When actual $PaCO_2$ is less than expected $PaCO_2$, it suggests concomitant respiratory alkalosis, while in concomitant respiratory acidosis, actual $PaCO_2$ is more than expected or calculated $PaCO_2$.

4. **Mixed disorders** In mixed disorders, $PaCO_2$ and HCO_3^- change opposite to each other. In combined respiratory and metabolic acidosis, $PaCO_2$ increases while HCO_3^- falls, while in combined respiratory and metabolic alkalosis, $PaCO_2$ falls while HCO_3^- rises.

Metabolic Acidosis

The outcome of metabolic acidosis depends on the underlying pathologic process, severity of acidosis and the response to treatment. The common causes of metabolic acidosis in neonates are given in Table 22.8. Most important aspect of treatment is to identify the cause and institute corrective measures. The cause of metabolic acidosis is divided into those with normal and increased anion gap.

Anion gap $= (Na^+ + K^+) - (HCO_3^- + Cl^-)$

Normal anion gap in neonates is 8–16 mEq/L. The efficacy of supportive therapy, by administration of sodium bicarbonate is unproven. If therapy with base is warranted, bicarbonate should not be used if ventilation and circulation are inadequate, because its administration will lead to increase in $PaCO_2$ and intracellular acidosis with clinical deterioration.

The dose of bicarbonate (mEq) $= 0.3 \times$ Body weight (kg) $\times$ Base deficit (mEq/L)

Table 22.8 Common causes of metabolic acidosis

Increased anion gap	Normal anion gap

▪ Lactic acidosis due to tissue hypoxia: Asphyxia, hypothermia, shock, sepsis, RDS
▪ Inborn errors of metabolism
▪ Renal failure
▪ Late metabolic acidosis
▪ Toxins like benzyl alcohol
	▪ Renal bicarbonate loss
	  a. Tubular bicarbonate loss due to prematurity
	  b. Renal tubular acidosis
	  c. Carbonic anhydrase inhibitors
	▪ Gastrointestinal bicarbonate loss
	  a. Small bowel drainage: ileostomy, fistula
	  b. Diarrhea
	▪ Extracellular volume expansion with bicarbonate dilution
	▪ Aldosterone deficiency
	▪ Excessive chloride in IV fluids

Bicarbonate is given slowly intravenously in 1:1 dilution with 5% dextrose solution. Half the dose is given over one hour and remaining half is given slowly based on subsequent blood gas measurements.

Sodium acetate may be used in prematurity related proximal renal tubular acidosis with bicarbonate wasting. Dose of sodium acetate is 2.5 to 4 mmol/kg/day. Tromethamine, another base, is associated with adverse effects such as respiratory depression, hyponatremia, hypoglycemia, hyperkalemia, diuresis followed by oliguria. Potassium levels should be monitored, because hypokalemia may become evident when acidosis is corrected and intracellular acidosis cannot be corrected until potassium stores are restored.

Metabolic Alkalosis

Metabolic alkalosis occurs when there is renal or extra renal loss of H^+, gain of HCO_3^- or depletion of extracellular volume with loss of Cl^-. The common causes of metabolic alkalosis in the neonatal period are listed in Table 22.9. If metabolic alkalosis is due to

Table 22.9 Causes of metabolic alkalosis

Loss of H^+	Gain of HCO_3^-	Loss of extracellular fluid (greater loss of chloride than bicarbonate)

1. Gastrointestinal loss
  ▪ Nasogastric aspiration
  ▪ persistent vomiting
  ▪ Congenital chloride wasting diarrhea
2. Renal loss
  ▪ Diuretics
  ▪ Congenital adrenal hyperplasia (certain forms)
  ▪ Hyperaldosteronism
  ▪ Bartter syndrome
	▪ Post hypercapnia
	▪ Drugs: Bicarbonate, tromethamine
	▪ Lactate, citrate, acetate in IV fluids and blood products
	▪ Hypokalemia
		▪ Contraction alkalosis
		▪ Diuretic phase of postnatal adaptation of preterm and term neonates

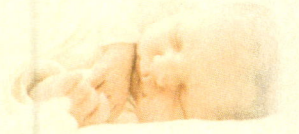

bicarbonate gain, it will rapidly clear because excretion of bicarbonate is not adversely affected in neonates. However, if alkalosis is severe and urine output is limited, carbonic anhydrase inhibitor (acetazolamide) may enhance excretion of HCO_3^-.

One of the most common causes of chronic metabolic alkalosis due to chronic lung disease in neonates include administration of long-term diuretics. Metabolic alkalosis is due to partial compensation of primary respiratory acidosis along with extracellular volume contraction and total body potassium depletion due to prolonged or aggressive use of diuretics. Hyponatremia occurs due to intracellular shift of sodium to compensate for low intracellular potassium. If alkalosis is severe, it can lead to hypoventilation. Potassium chloride supplementation in this situation, will correct hypokalemia and accompanying hyponatremia, hypochloremia, metabolic alkalosis and increase the effectiveness of diuretics. Close monitoring of serum sodium, potassium and chloride levels is indicated in neonates on long-term diuretic therapy.

Mild contraction alkalosis during the postnatal diuretic phase does not need any treatment. Contraction alkalosis due to other causes respond to replacement of intravascular volume with rehydration in conjunction with additional potassium supplementation to correct any potassium wasting. Primary problem of reduced glomerular filtration or elevated aldosterone must be treated to ensure resolution of alkalosis.

ENDOCRINE EMERGENCIES

Congenital Adrenal Hyperplasia

Congenital adrenal hyperplasia (CAH) in the neonatal period manifests as a salt-losing crisis, requiring prompt emergency medical care. The clinical features include dehydration, hyponatremia, hyperkalemia, hypoglycemia, hypotension and metabolic acidosis. If untreated, shock and cardiac arrest will result because of deficiency of adrenal hormones. The salt-wasting forms of CAH are listed below.

a. Classical form of 21-hydroxylase deficiency which is the most common disorder of CAH
b. Lipoid congenital adrenal hyperplasia
c. 3-β hydroxysteroid dehydrogenase deficiency.

The clinical diagnosis can be suspected in the presence of the following features:

1. Ambiguity of genitalia due to virilisation of a female infant in 21-hydroxylase deficiency. The absence of gonads in the scrotal sac, hyperpigmentation and the presence of uterus on pelvic ultrasonography are useful clues to make a correct diagnosis. A high index of suspicion is necessary to make a diagnosis of 21-hydroxylase deficiency in boys because of lack of any genital abnormalities.
2. Ambiguity of genitalia due to undervirilisation of a male infant (in case of b and c variants) may be seen.
3. Salt loss occurs in nearly 75% of cases with 21-hydroxylase deficiency, of which nearly half the cases present with the salt-losing adrenal crisis around 6–14 days of age. In others, the onset may be delayed to 6 to 12 weeks of age, often precipitated by infection or metabolic stress.
4. Hyperpigmentation of the nipples, umbilicus, genitalia or whole body may be seen. This finding may require distinction from the normal pigmentation of the neonate in case of parents with dark skin.
5. Unexplained vomiting and dehydration rapidly leading to shock.
6. Convulsions may occur because of hypoglycemia, and hyponatremia.
7. Previous history of sibling(s) with ambiguity of genitalia or unexplained deaths should be asked.

Management

Infant should be hospitalized and monitored for vital signs including blood pressure. Before starting intravenous fluids, blood samples should be obtained for serum electrolytes, cortisol, 17-hydroxyprogesterone (17-OHP), and dehydro-epiandrosterone sulphate (DHEAS) and plasma renin activity (PRA). Intravascular volume is restored with IV normal saline infusion, given rapidly at a rate of 20 mL/kg over 20 minutes to correct shock or hypotension. Following the initial therapy, dehydration should be corrected by assuming minimum deficit of 10% if the infant is in shock. Rapid correction of hyponatremia should be avoided. Hyperkalemia normalises, when serum sodium level rises and fluid volume is replaced. Severe hyperkalemia may be life-threatening. If hyperkalemia is persistent or associated with ECG changes, IV sodium bicarbonate, and calcium gluconate and rectal cation exchange resins are useful for rapid correction of serum potassium. Hypoglycemia should be treated with a bolus of 0.5 g of glucose/kg body weight.

Specific Therapy

Hydrocortisone in a dose of 25 mg/m^2/day is given orally in 3 divided doses. Fludrocortisone 100 µg tablet is crushed and given by nasogastric tube. Sodium chloride supplementation (1–2 gm/kg/day) is given in salt losing CAH. Frequent monitoring of serum electrolytes, hydration, body weight and blood pressure are required for optimizing treatment. Excessive

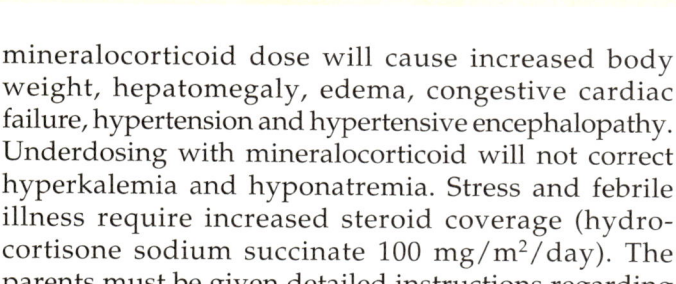

mineralocorticoid dose will cause increased body weight, hepatomegaly, edema, congestive cardiac failure, hypertension and hypertensive encephalopathy. Underdosing with mineralocorticoid will not correct hyperkalemia and hyponatremia. Stress and febrile illness require increased steroid coverage (hydrocortisone sodium succinate 100 mg/m²/day). The parents must be given detailed instructions regarding the nature of the disease and the need for regular follow-up and lifelong therapy.

Adrenal Insufficiency

Adrenal insufficiency may be primary, caused by destruction of adrenal cortex (Addison's disease), secondary to deficient ACTH secretion or tertiary because of deficiency of corticotropin releasing hormone (CRH) by the hypothalamus. When the infant is stable, short synthetic ACTH stimulation test may be carried out to confirm the diagnosis. Adrenal crisis may occur suddenly following adrenal hemorrhage. A high index of suspicion is necessary. Prompt treatment is life-saving. Mortality is high if untreated. Weakness, fatigue, weight loss, abdominal pain, anorexia, nausea, vomiting, confusion or coma may be the presenting clinical features. These nonspecific symptoms often go unnoticed unless a crisis occurs during an intercurrent illness or stress situation. Shock may be the initial presentation. The other features include hypoglycemia, hyperkalemia, hyperpigmentation and hypotension.

Management

Infant is immediately hospitalized and vital signs monitored including blood pressure. Shock is treated urgently with IV normal saline 20 mL/kg as a bolus followed by an infusion for correction of dehydration and for maintenance. Hyponatremia and hyperkalemia, if severe, will need special attention. Hydrocortisone 2–4 mg/kg/dose IV is given every 3–6 hourly. The hyponatremia is corrected slowly at a rate less than 0.5 mEq/L/hr. In the case of severe hyperkalemia, treatment with intravenous calcium and/or bicarbonate, potassium-binding resin, intravenous glucose and insulin infusion will be needed.

The precipitating cause of adrenal crisis needs to be identified and treated appropriately. Physiologic hormone replacement is given with hydrocortisone hemisuccinate 10–15 mg/m²/day in two or three divided doses and fludrocortisone 50–100 µg twice daily. In case of intercurrent illness, trauma or surgery, the infant who is already on physiologic replacement doses, is treated by giving 2–4 times the daily replacement dose. The dose is gradually decreased to maintenance dose over the next 3–4 days depending on the general condition of the patient and his ability

to tolerate orally. Infants who cannot retain oral hydrocortisone, may be given IV hydrocortisone sodium succinate 50 mg/m²/dose followed by 25 mg/m²/dose intramuscularly every 6–8 hourly.

Diabetes Insipidus

Diabetes insipidus (DI) manifests clinically with polyuria, polydipsia and hypotonic urine. It may be classified as central or hypothalamic, when there is inability to secrete vasopressin. In nephrogenic DI there is inappropriate renal response to vasopressin.

Hyperosmolarity, hypovolemia and hypotension are detected by osmoreceptors, volume receptors (in the cardiac atria and pulmonary veins) and baroreceptors in the carotid sinus. These stimulate the secretion of vasopressin and also induce thirst. Vasopressin acts on the collecting ducts of kidneys for increased reabsorption of water. In DI, because of the inadequate secretion or unresponsiveness to vasopressin, water does not get reabsorbed in the kidneys thereby failing to concentrate the urine. Diabetes insipidus may present with persistent polyuria, nocturia, increased thirst, polydipsia, irritability, weight loss, hyperthermia, weakness, lethargy, dullness, hypotension and coma. Early morning sample of urine specific gravity of <1.005; urine osmolality < 200 mOsm/kg; and elevated serum sodium suggest the diagnosis.

Fluid Management

Infant is provided liberal unrestricted water intake. A fine balance should be struck between the relatively benign course of DI and adverse consequences of overtreatment, the most dreaded being hyponatremia. In a conscious patient with free access to water, DI does not usually produce complications of hypernatremia. In a patient who presents with hypernatremic dehydration, it should be corrected with 0.45% saline with an aim not to reduce the serum sodium at a maximum 10 mEq/L/24 hr in order to avoid the risk of cerebral edema. 8-deamino D-arginine vasopressin (DDAVP) nasal spray 10 µg once or twice a day can be used for treatment of central DI. The urine specific gravity should be monitored at home before each dose of the nasal spray. Periodic monitoring of serum electrolytes may be done. Water retaining agents like chlorpropamide, indomethacin and natriuretic agents like thiazide diuretics, amiloride and indapamide may be tried. The treatment of congenital nephrogenic DI is difficult while the secondary nephrogenic DI (hypokalemia, hypocalcemia, aminoglycosides, tubular interstitial nephritis, bladder neck obstruction, renal dysplasia) is managed by treatment of the underlying cause. These infants should be provided with high calorie diet with minimal osmotic load. Thiazides or high dose of DDAVP may provide some relief.

Syndrome of Inappropriate Secretion of ADH Hormone

SIADH may be associated with euvolemic or hypervolemic hyponatremia. In this condition, the plasma level of vasopressin is elevated at a time during which its physiologic secretion should normally be suppressed. The net result is that the infant is unable to excrete water leading to water retention and hyponatremia. Along with increase in intravascular volume, more sodium is excreted in the urine in an attempt to normalize the blood volume. The diagnosis is confirmed by plasma hypoosmolality (<275 mOsm/kg), serum sodium <135 mEq/L, urine osmolality >100 mOsm/kg (but less than serum osmolality) with normal renal and adrenal functions and increase in urine spot sodium (>20 mEq/L) with normal salt and water intake. Hyperglycemia and pseudohyponatremia must be excluded.

Neurological symptoms like seizures appear when there is a rapid fall (within 48 hrs) in serum sodium to <120 mEq/L. These patients require immediate treatment with infusion of hypertonic (3%) saline or administration of normal saline along with furosemide. The latter combination has the advantage of not rapidly expanding ECF volume in an already volume expanded patient. The goal is to raise the serum sodium level above 125 mEq/L, at a rate of 10 mEq/L in 24 hours. When any of these end points are reached, slower acting therapy like fluid restriction and unrestricted salt intake should be advised. Close monitoring of serum sodium is essential for rational management of SIADH.

Congenital Hypothyroidism

Congenital hypothyroidism should be considered as a medical emergency, because the best outcome occurs when therapy is initiated within 2 weeks of life. Abnormal thyroid parameters on cord blood screening should always be confirmed with a venous sample. Thyroid functions should be tested in any infant with features of hypothyroidism such as postmaturity, macrosomia or widely open posterior fontanel at birth or prolonged jaundice, constipation, poor feeding, hypotonia, hoarse cry, umbilical hernia, macroglossia, or dry edematous skin in infancy. The common causes of congenital hypothyroidism are listed in Table 22.10.

Term as well as preterm infants with low T4 (<6.5 µg/dL) and elevated TSH (>20 µIU/mL) should be started on L-thyroxine as soon as the diagnosis is made. The initial dose of L-thyroxine should be 10–15 µg/kg/day with the aim to normalize T4 level at the earliest. Those infants with severe hypothyroidism (very low T4, very high TSH and absence of distal femoral and proximal

Table 22.10 Causes of congenital hypothyroidism	
Permanent hypothyroidism	*Transient hypothyroidism*
1. Thyroid dysgenesis (aplasia, hypoplasia or ectopia)	1. TSH binding inhibitory immunoglobulins
2. Thyroid hormone biosynthetic defects	2. Exposure to goitrogens (iodides or antithyroid drugs)
3. Iodine deficiency (endemic cretinism)	3. Transient hypothyroxinemia of prematurity
4. Hypothalamic-pituitary hypothyroidism	4. Sick euthyroid syndrome

tibial epiphyses on radiograph of knee) should be started with the highest dose (15 µg/kg/day). During follow-up, T4 should be kept in the upper half of normal range (10 to 16 µg/dL) or free T4 in the range of 1.4 to 2.3 µg/dL with the TSH suppressed and kept within normal range. Check T4 and TSH levels every 6 to 8 weeks during first 6 months. Avoid over treatment as it can lead to premature fusion of cranial sutures, acceleration of skeletal maturation and problems with temperament and behavior.

The best outcome occurs when L-thyroxine therapy is started within 2 weeks of age with a dose of 10 µg/kg or more per day, compared with lower doses or later start of therapy. Residual defects or sequelae include impaired visuospatial processing, selective memory loss and sensorimotor defects. More than 80% of infants given replacement therapy before three months of age have an IQ greater than 85 but may show signs of minimal brain damage, including impairment of arithmetic ability, speech, or fine motor coordination. When treatment is started between 3–6 months, the mean IQ is 71 and when therapy is delayed beyond 6 months, the mean IQ drops to 54.

Neonatal Hyperthyroidism

The diagnosis of neonatal thyrotoxicosis requires a high index of suspicion. The babies at high-risk for neonatal thyrotoxicosis are likely to have the following features in their mother:

1. More than 3 times normal thyroid stimulating immunoglobulins (TSIs) at 24–28 weeks of pregnancy.

2. Clinical thyrotoxicosis in third trimester of pregnancy (Grave's disease) or history of treatment with thionamides in third trimester.

3. Family history of TSH receptor mutation.

4. Features of fetal hyperthyroidism as evidenced by fetal tachycardia, fetal goiter, ascites, craniosynostosis, fetal growth retardation, maceration and hydrops fetalis.

Thyroid receptor antibodies (TRAb) are likely to be more than three times upper limit of normal on day 1–7 in infants who develop neonatal hyperthyroidism. In infants of mothers with thyrotoxicosis, cord blood, should be taken for Free T4, TSH and TRAb levels. Symptoms and signs of hyperthyroidism can be apparent at birth or may be delayed, but they are usually present by 10 days of life, rarely they can be delayed up to 45 days. Goiter is present in most cases. The central nervous system signs include irritability, jitteriness and restlessness. Eye signs like periorbital edema, lid retraction and exophthalmos may be seen. Cardiovascular system manifestations include tachycardia, arrhythmias, cardiac failure, systemic and pulmonary hypertension. Signs of hypermetabolism include voracious appetite, weight loss, diarrhea, sweating, and flushing. Other signs are acrocyanosis, hepatosplenomegaly, lymphadenopathy, and thymic enlargement. Bruising and petechial hemorrhages are secondary to thrombocytopenia. Advanced bone age, craniosynostosis and microcephaly may be evident both in fetus and newborn. Duration of neonatal throtoxicosis secondary to maternal Grave's disease is determined by transplacentally acquired thyroid-stimulating immunoglobulins (TSIs).

Neonates with thyrotoxicosis are generally very sick and require emergency treatment. The synthesis of thyroid hormone is blocked by carbimazole and propylthiouracil (PTU). In addition PTU blocks the peripheral de-iodination of T4-T3. The dose of carbimazole is 0.5–1.5 mg/kg/day and that of PTU is 5–10 mg/kg/day. Lugol's iodine acts by blocking the synthesis of thyroid hormones as well as blocking the release of the stored hormone. Lugol's iodine, which contains 5% potassium iodide is used in a dose of one drop every 8 hourly (each drop of Lugol's iodine contains 8 mg of iodine). Beta-blockers, like propranolol, which control the adrenergic symptoms and inhibit the peripheral iodination of T4-T3 are used in a dose of 0.27–0.75 mg/kg every 8 hourly. Steroids (prednisolone) act by inhibiting the peripheral de-iodination of T4-T3 and is given in a dose of 2 mg/kg/day. Sedatives help by alleviating restlessness. Supportive treatment is very important to manage respiratory distress, fluid and electrolyte imbalance, body temperature and high output heart failure. Specific treatment of congestive heart failure by diuretics and digoxin may be necessary. Oxygen therapy, noninvasive and invasive ventilation may be required. Diarrhea and hyperthermia may occur and patient may need intravenous fluids and thermoneutral environment. Sepsis may complicate neonatal thyrotoxicosis and may require administration of appropriate antibiotics.

Hypopituitarism

Neonates with hypopituitarism may present with features of midline facial defects (septo-optic dysplasia, cleft lip, cleft palate), deficiency of anterior pituitary hormones (ACTH, Growth hormone, FSH, LH, TSH), hypoglycemia, shock, micropenis, cryptorchidism, jaundice or features of central diabetes insipidus (polyuria, hypernatremia, dehydration). The common causes of congenital hypopituitarism are listed in Box 22.1.

Hypoglycemia and cortisol deficiency should be looked for and treated without delay. Patient should be evaluated for serum electrolytes, ACTH, cortisol, Growth hormone, FSH, LH, TSH, Free T4, and ADH. MRI brain is done to assess status of pituitary gland. Specific hormone replacement is started. Hypoglycemia may not resolve without Growth hormone therapy. Electrolyte disturbances may occur in neonates with hypopituitarism. Hyponatremia unassociated with hypovolemia and unresponsive to fluid restriction can develop. In contrast to the hyponatremia that occurs with the salt-losing crisis of 21-hydroxylase deficiency, serum potassium levels are typically low or within normal limits in hypopituitarism. The hyponatremia resolves with physiologic corticosteroid replacement. Hypernatremia secondary to excess free-water loss associated with uncontrolled diabetes insipidus may also occur.

Hypoglycemia

The operational threshold for hypoglycemia is defined as that concentration of plasma or whole blood glucose at which the clinician should consider intervention, based on the currently available evidence in literature. Operational threshold for hypoglycemia in a neonate has been defined as blood glucose level of less than 40 mg/dL (plasma glucose level less than 45 mg/dL). WHO defines hypoglycemia as blood glucose level of less than 45 mg/dL. Neonates at risk of hypoglycemia are screened at 1, 2, 3, 6, 12, 24, 48, 72 hours of age.

BOX 22.1 Causes of congenital hypopituitarism

1. Gene mutations: HESX1, LHX3, LHX4, PTX2, PROP1, PIT1
2. Pituitary agenesis/hypoplasia
3. Holoprosencephaly
4. Septo-optic dysplasia and other midline defects
5. CNS Infection
6. Hypovolemic shock
7. Birth injury and/asphyxia
8. Tumors/vascular abnormalities in the hypothalamic-pituitary region
9. Radiation to the head and neck region
10. Hydrocephalus

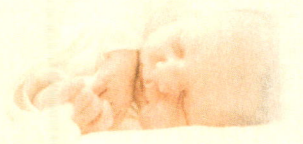

These high-risk neonates include low birth weight, preterm, small-for-gestational age, large-for-gestational age, infants of diabetic mothers, sick neonates (with perinatal asphyxia, sepsis, shock, polycythemia), and neonates on IV fluids/parenteral nutrition.

Clinical manifestations occur due to activation of the autonomic nervous system and include diaphoresis, tachycardia, hypothermia, pallor, episodes of cyanosis, apneic spells, tachypnea, nausea, vomiting, difficulty in feeding and rarely cardiac arrest. Neuroglycopenic signs of hypoglycemia include limpness and lethargy, weak and high pitched cry, jitteriness, tremors, apathy, stupor, convulsions, and or uprolling of eyes.

Treatment

Asymptomatic hypoglycemia with blood sugar 20–45 mg/dL

Trial of oral feeds (expressed breast milk or formula) and repeat blood test after 1 hour.

1. If repeat blood glucose level is >45 mg/dL, two hourly feeds are ensured with 6 hourly monitoring of blood glucose level for 48 hr. The target blood glucose value is 50 to 120 mg/dL.
2. If repeat blood sugar is <45 mg/dL, IV dextrose is started and further management is identical to infants with symptomatic hypoglycemia.

Blood sugar levels <20 mg/dL or symptomatic hypoglycemia or feeding is contraindicated/not tolerated or ineffective

10% dextrose is given as a bolus of 2 mL/kg followed by glucose infusion @ 6 mg/kg/min. Subsequently if glucose level stays below 45 mg/dL despite bolus and constant glucose infusion, glucose infusion rate (GIR) is increased in steps of 2 mg/kg/min every 15 to 30 min until a maximum rate of 12 mg/kg/min is reached. If there is persistent hypoglycemia, check the functioning of intravenous line, the intravenous fluid preparation and infusion rate. Central line is mandatory to infuse dextrose concentration of 12.5% or more. After 24 hours of IV glucose therapy, when two consecutive glucose levels are >50 mg/dL, the infusion rate can be tapered off at the rate of 2 mg/kg/min every 6 hours by keeping a close watch on blood glucose levels. Tapering should be accompanied by concomitant increase in oral feeds. Once a glucose infusion rate of 4 mg/kg/min is achieved, oral intake is adequate and the glucose levels are consistently >50 mg/dL, the infusion can be stopped.

Recurrent/Resistant Hypoglycemia

This condition should be considered when infant fails to maintain normal glucose level despite a GIR of

Table 22.11 Investigations of choice in infants with resistant hypoglycemia

Cause of resistant hypoglycemia	Investigations of choice
- Hyperinsulinemic states - Adrenal insufficiency - Congenital hypopituitarism - Galactosemia	- Serum insulin levels - Serum cortisol levels - Growth hormone levels - Urine ketones and reducing substances, galactose-1-phosphate uridyl transferase in RBCs
- Glycogen storage disorders	- Galactose-1-phosphate uridyl transferase levels
- Maple syrup urine disease - Mitochondrial disorders - Fatty acid oxidation defect	- Blood ammonia - Blood lactate levels - Urine and sugar amino-acidogram and free fatty acid levels

12 mg/kg/min or when stabilization is not achieved by 7 days of therapy. The common causes of resistant hypoglycemia and relevant investigations for various conditions are listed in Table 22.11. The blood sample should be collected when there is critical hypoglycemia. Insulinoma can be diagnosed on CT scan of abdomen.

Drugs that are used for treatment of resistant hypoglycemia are listed below.

1. Hydrocortisone hemisuccinate 5 mg/kg/day IV or PO in two divided doses for 24 to 48 hours.
2. Diazoxide can be given orally 10–25 mg/kg/day in three divided doses. Diazoxide acts by keeping the K_{ATP} channels of the beta-cells of the pancreas open, thereby reducing the secretion of insulin. It is therefore useful in states of unregulated insulin secretion because of insulinoma.
3. Glucagon 100 µg/kg subcutaneous, IM or IV (max 300 µg) upto maximum of three doses every 15 min can be tried. Glucagon acts by mobilizing hepatic glycogen stores, enhancing gluconeogenesis and promoting ketogenesis. These effects are not seen in small-for-gestational age infants. Side effects of glucagon include vomiting, diarrhea and hypokalemia and at high doses it may stimulate insulin release.
4. Octreotide (synthetic somatostatin analogue) in a dose of 2–10 µg/kg/day subcutaneously, 2–3 times a day is useful in resistent cases.

BIBLIOGRAPHY

Aschner JL, Poland RL. Sodium bicarbonate: basically useless therapy. *Pediatrics* 2008; 122(4):831–5.

Batra CM. Fetal and neonatal thyrotoxicosis. *Indian J Endocrinol Metabol* 2013 Oct; 17(Suppl1): S50–S54.

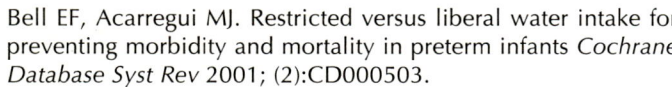

Bell EF, Acarregui MJ. Restricted versus liberal water intake for preventing morbidity and mortality in preterm infants *Cochrane Database Syst Rev* 2001; (2):CD000503.

Daly K, Farrington E. Hypokalemia and hyperkalemia in infants and children: Pathophysiology and treatment. *J Pediatr Health Care* 2013; 27(6):486–96.

Ellison, DH; Berl, T. The syndrome of inappropriate antidiuresis. *N Engl J Med* 2007, 356, 2064–72.

Forest MG. Recent advances in the diagnosis and management of congenital adrenal hyperplasia due to 21-hydroxylase deficiency. *Hum Reprod Update* 2004; 10(6):469–85.

Geffner ME. Hypopituitarism in childhood. *Cancer Control* 2002; 9(3):212–22.

Hsieh S, White PC. Presentation of primary adrenal insufficiency in childhood. *J Clin Endocrinol Metabol* 2011; 96(6):E925–E8.

Karaks HM, Erdem G, Yakinci C. Osmotic demyelination syndrome in a 40-day-old infant. *Diagn Interv Radiol* 2007; 13(3):121–4.

Kellum JA. Disorders of acid-base balance. *Crit Care Med* 2007; 35(11):2630–6.

Klien AH, Meltzer S, Kenny FM. Improved prognosis in congenital hypothyroidism treated before age three months. *J Fediatr* 1972; 81:912–5.

Lorenz J. Fluid and electrolyte therapy in very low birth weight neonate. *NeoReviews* 2008 9:e02.

Moe SM. Disorders involving calcium, phosphorus, and magnesium. *Prim Care* 2008 Jun; 35(2):215–6.

Ogilvy-Stuart AL. Neonatal thyroid disorders. *Arch Dis Child Fetal Neonatal Ed* 2002; 87:F165–F71.

Saborio P, Tipton GA, Chan JCM. Diabetes Insipidus. *Pediatr Rev* 2000; 21(4):122–9.

Sterns RH. Disorders of plasma sodium: causes, consequences, and correction. *N Engl J Med* 2015; 372:55–65.

Sweet CB, Grayson S, Polak M. Management strategies for neonatal hypoglycemia. *J Pediatr Pharmacol Ther* 2013; 18(3):199–208.

Vijayakumar M, Prahlad N, Nammalwar BR, Shanmughasundharam R. Subcutaneous fat necrosis with hypercalcemia. *Indian Pediatr* 2006; 43:360–3.

23

Neonatal Emergencies Due to Inborn Errors of Metabolism

Ratna Dua Puri and Shubha R. Phadke

Background

Inborn errors of metabolism (IEM) make a significant contribution towards neonatal and infant morbidity and mortality. Though individually rare, collectively the incidence of IEMs may be as high as 1 in 800 to 1 in 2500 births. Every neonatologist needs to have a working knowledge of diagnostic approaches, recent advances and availability of treatment options for this group of disorders. The clinical signs and symptoms of IEMs in neonates mimic those of common illnesses of the neonatal period and thereby a high degree of suspicion is essential to diagnose these disorders. The timely diagnosis can improve the outcome for treatable disorders. Some disorders are difficult to treat or are untreatable. However, accurate diagnosis is essential to provide genetic counseling to the family for risk of recurrence and prevention by prenatal diagnosis. Investigations on an urgent basis and storage of samples are needed, because the course in some cases is fulminant and fatal. The main aim of this chapter is to present a simplified approach through case studies to enable early recognition and investigations of inborn errors of metabolism in the neonatal period.

Inborn errors of metabolism (IEMs) are inherited disorders that occur due to deficiency of an enzyme, transporter or cofactor in the metabolic pathway. This leads to deficiency of the final product, or accumulation of metabolites proximal to the block (Figure 23.1). Some of the genetic metabolic disorders are limited to one system like hemophilia or congenital immuno-deficiency syndromes. The effects of the deficient enzyme or product are limited to the system of which the protein is a part. However, some enzymes are involved in basic metabolism (e.g. Kreb cycle) or metabolic derangements may affect multiple organs in

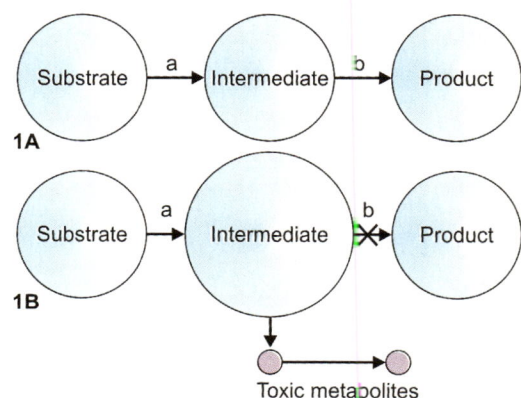

1A: Normal metabolic pathway
1B: Deficency of enzyme b in the metabolic pathway
a: enzyme in metabolic pathway, b: enzyme in metabolic pathway, x: deficiency of enzyme b

Figure 23.1 Pathophysiology of IEMs.

the body. This, latter group of disorders are traditionally grouped as IEMs and the discussion in this chapter is limted to these genetic disorders.

Small Molecule vs Organelle Disease

IEMs can be categorized into small molecule and large molecule disorders or organelle defects; the former have an acute presentation while large molecule disorders are more insidious in onset and progression. At the bedside, this classification is useful to decide the choice of investigations. The small molecule disorders include conditions where the defect occurs at a single step in the metabolic pathway of a water-soluble metabolite, such as an amino acid or monosaccharide. The diagnosis is made by evaluation of the metabolic intermediaries in physiological fluids, blood, urine and CSF. The organelle disorders are those where the defect is in an organelle specific enzyme or metabolic process

Table 23.1 The differences between small molecule disease and organelle defect

Feature	Small molecule disease	Organelle disease
Onset	Often sudden, and acute	Gradual
Course	Remissions and relapses	Progressive
Physical findings	Nonspecific	Characteristic
Histopathology	Nonspecific	Characteristic
Response to treatment	Often quick	Slow over a period of time
Common disorders	Aminoacidopathy, urea cycle disorders, organic acidemias, carbohydrate metabolism defects, disorders of nucleotides, porphyrins and trace metals	Lysosomal storage disorders, peroxisomal disorders, mitochondrial disorders, synthetic disorders like glycosylation defects, Smith-Lemli-Opitz syndrome

and they are usually associated with intracellular storage of metabolic substrates. Table 23.1 shows the differences between the two classes of IEMs. In general, the organelle diseases do not present in the neonatal period.

When to Suspect an IEM?

A high index of suspicion is important as the clinical features of many inherited metabolic diseases are non-specific and simulate those of a neonate with sepsis.

i. History of acute deterioration in the condition of a neonate after a brief period of normalcy after birth. The symptoms appear when enteral feeds are started.

ii. Exaggerated response to an intercurrent illness especially sepsis.

iii. Poor response to treatment of a co-morbid associated illness.

iv. Family history of consanguinity, similar illness in a sibling, or an unexplained neonatal death.

v. Progressive illness with signs of cerebral dysfunction such as poor sucking, limpness, vomiting, irritability, respiratory distress, lip smacking movements and hypothermia.

vi. Unusual odors from urine or sweat like maple syrup or burnt sugar, mousy, cabbage like smell, sweaty feet, etc. Abnormal urine odor is best identified on opening a container with urine that has been kept closed for a few minutes at room temperature.

vii. Intractable seizures.

viii. Persistent vomitings and hiccups.

ix. Persistent metabolic acidosis, ketosis, hypoglycemia. Hyperammonemia, and coagulopathy.

x. Cholestasis with or without hepatosplenomegaly.

xi. Involvement of multiple systems like, coarse facies, cataracts, alopecia, ambiguous genitalia, abnormalities of pigmentation, cardiovascular system and central nervous sytem.

Clinical Course of IEM in a Neonate

The neonate has a limited repertoire of responses to an illness and therefore a high index of suspicion is important to make a diagnosis of IEM. In the newborn period, most IEMs present as a life-threatening emergency closely mimicking a neonate with sepsis. The clinical manifestations can be categorized into following four groups.

1. Acute encephalopathy, e.g. urea cycle disorders, maple syrup urine disease (MSUD) and organic acidurias.

2. Liver disease, e.g. galactosemia, hereditary fructose intolerance, and tyrosinemia type I.

3. Cardiac failure, e.g. Pompe disease, fatty acid oxidation defects, and mitochondrial disorders.

4. Metabolic derangements like hypoglycemia and acidosis.

Acute encephalopathy with or without seizures is the commonest presentation of IEM in the neonatal period and infancy. Typically a term, good weight neonate, who is well for the first few days of life develops feeding difficulties, lethargy, vomiting, abnormalities of tone and consciousness. The progression of symptoms is extremely rapid and the neonate is transferred to the intensive care unit and started on assisted ventilation. A neonate with a metabolic disorder can also have associated sepsis, and therefore an high index of suspicion in a critically sick neonate is important to initiate investigations for an IEM. Typically five basic investigations are useful as a first step to differentiate the common categories of IEMs and facilitate an algorithmic diagnostic approach (Table 23.2).

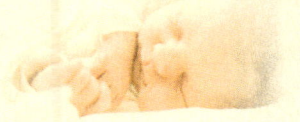

Table 23.2 Five basic investigations for screening of inborn errors of metabolism

Disorder	Acidosis	Ketosis	Lactate	Ammonia	Glucose
Maple syrup urine disease (MSUD)	N	++	N	N	N/↓
Organic acidemias	+	++	N/↑	N/↑	↓↓
Urea cycle disorders	N	N	N	↑↑	N
Lactic acidosis	+	+	++	N	N
NKH, sulfite oxidase deficiency, molybdenum cofactor deficiency, phenylketonuria, peroxisomal disorders	N	N	N	N	N
Galactosemia	N	N	N	N	↓/N
Glycogen storage disease 1	+	+ Post-prandial	+ Fasting	N	↓↓

NKH: nonketotic hyperglycinemia   N: normal

Typical case scenarios or clinical vignettes illustrating the diagnostic approaches to the above mentioned five metabolic derangements are presented below.

Case scenario 1. Acute encephalopathy with hyperammonemia

A female neonate, born at term, appropriate-for-dates, developed respiratory distress on day 2 of life. The blood glucose, electrolytes and sepsis screen were normal. The infant became lethargic and refused feeding. The arterial blood gases showed respiratory alkalosis and blood culture was sent before initiation of antibiotics. Despite treatment, she developed multifocal clonic seizures, became limp and had poor gag reflex and inability to suck. The resident on duty elicited a family history of parental consanguinity and death of a previous sibling on day 8 of life with suspected sepsis. He sent a blood sample for ammonia, lactate and urine for ketones, to rule out an IEM. There was no lactic acidosis or ketosis but ammonia was increased to 1450 µmol/L. A urea cycle disorder was suspected and the neonate investigated further. Quantitative amino acids by high performance liquid chromatography (HPLC), acylcarnitine profile analysis using Tandem Mass Spectrometry (TMS/MS), and urine organic acid estimation by gas chromatography-mass spectrometry (GC-MS) was performed. The plasma citrulline levels were high (1344 nmol/L); argininosuccinate and arginine were low and urine orotic acid was increased which were consistent with the possibility of Citrullinemia type I. The infant was managed with ammonia scavenging agents, peritoneal dialysis, IV dextrose, and intralipids. Despite aggressive life support management, she continued to be encephalopathic and died on day 7 of life. Molecular analysis for citrullinemia on the stored DNA sample confirmed the neonate to be homozygous for a nonsense mutation in ASS gene.

An elevated plasma ammonia level is an indicator of hepatocellular dysfunction due to any cause, most commonly due to inborn error of metabolism, infection or intoxication. Urea cycle disorders (UCDs) are the most common metabolic disorders with high ammonia levels. A hypotonic neonate with encephalopathy, respiratory alkalosis and hyperammonemia should alert to the possibility of a urea cycle disorder. The algorithmic approach for investigations and diagnosis of a urea cycle defect is illustrated in Figure 23.2. Central to this diagnostic algorithm is the quantitative analysis of amino acid levels in the blood and urinary orotic acid estimation by GC-MS. It is important and desirable to collect a free flowing blood sample for ammonia estimation and transport it to the laboratory in ice for immediate estimation. Transient hyperammonemia of the newborn (THAN) unlike UCDs occurs on the first day of life. Other disorders causing hyperammonemia due to secondary inhibition of the urea cycle pathway include pyruvate carboxylase deficiency, fatty acid oxidation defects, organic acidurias, lysinuric protein intolerance and hyperammonemia-hyperornithinemia-homocitrullinuria syndrome.

Case scenario 2a. Acute encephalopathy with metabolic acidosis

The family was from Jharkhand and the neonate (5th in birth order with a birth weight of 3.5 kg) was transferred when he developed lethargy and poor feeding on day 3 of life. At admission his sensorium was altered, he was dehydrated and had metabolic acidosis that persisted even after stabilization. The anion gap was 26, blood sugar 50 mg/dL, plasma ammonia 256 µmol/L, and plasma lactate was normal. Sepsis screen was negative. There was history of deaths of three siblings, two females and one male, all of them had presented in a similar manner. The family history of an autosomal recessive inheritance and presence of

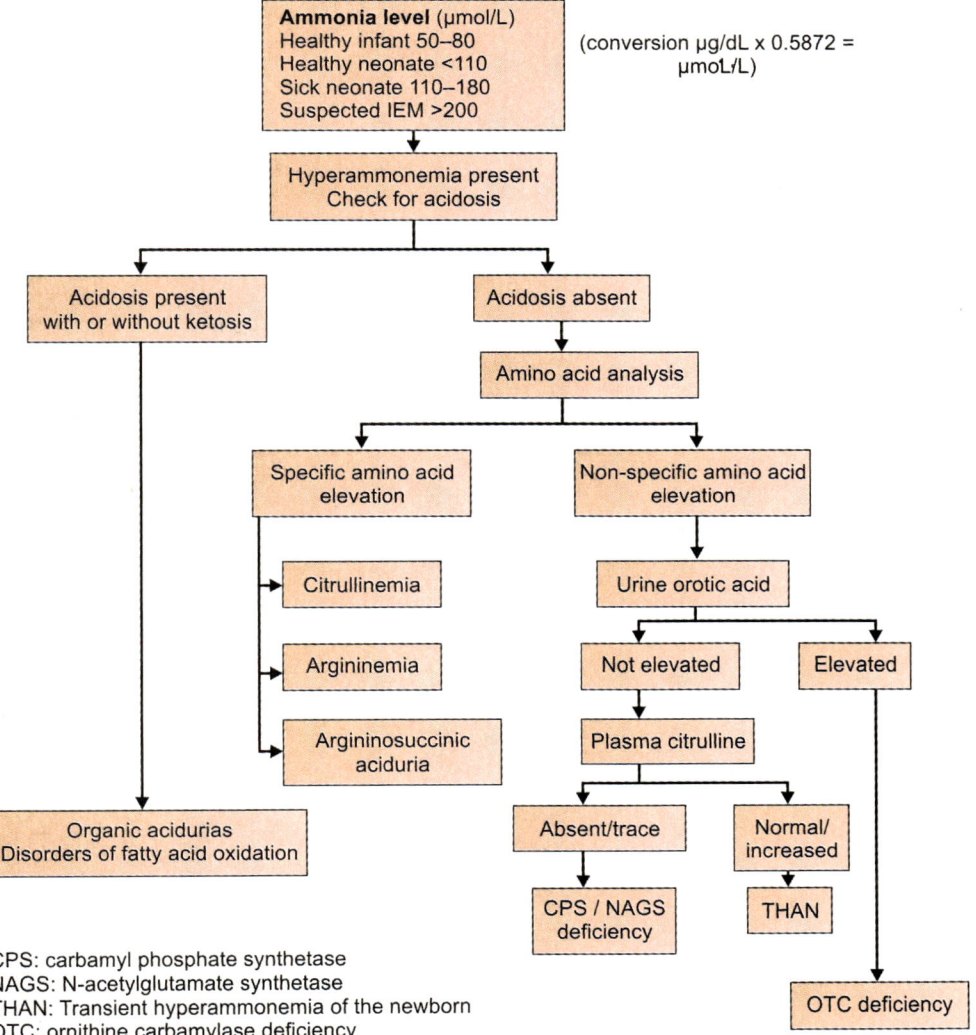

Figure 23.2 Evaluation and diagnosis of a child with high plasma ammonia.

high anion gap metabolic acidosis strongly suggested an IEM. Tandem mass spectrometry (MS-MS) showed elevated propionyl carnitine (C3) and urine GC-MS identified elevated 3-OH propionate, propionyl glycine and methycitrate. Propionic acidemia (PA) was diagnosed based on these reports. The neonate was started on an emergency protocol for management. However, in view of a worsening encephalopathy and guarded prognosis, the parents took the child home.

It is apparent from this family history that all the previous siblings had also died of propionic acidemia. Unfortunately, the possibility of a metabolic disorder had not been kept and appropriate investigations were not done to prevent recurrence or initiate timely management before the onset of encephalopathy. The information about the possiblity of prenatal diagnosis during next pregnancy of mother was provided and the need to store blood sample of the baby for detection

of mutation was stressed. Prenatal diagnosis can only be done if the mutation in the affected child is identified before the next pregnancy.

Most of the IEMs are autosomal recessive and there is 25% risk of recurrence in siblings. There can be two, or even more consecutive babies affected with the disorder as happened in this case. When prenatal diagnosis is made, the family can be offered the option of medical termination of pregnancy. Alternatively, when an affected baby is born, therapy can be instiued before appearance of encephalopathy.

Case scenario 2b. Acute encephalopathy with metabolic acidosis

In contrast to the case discussed above, Case 2b illustrates the utility of timely diagnosis and appropriate management of propionic acidemia. A second born male infant to nonconsanguineous parents was well till one month of age when he suddenly became sick following history of one day fever. He developed vomitings, lethargy and progressive encephalopathy. Investigations showed normal electrolytes, normoglycemia but persistent metabolic acidosis with an increased anion gap. His ammonia levels were 175 µmol/L. Urine was positive for ketones. A possibility of an organic acidemia was considered while awaiting the results of MS-MS and urine GC-MS analysis. He was started on the emergency protocol for management for organic acidemia with protein free high caloric feeds and carnitine supplementation. He improved on management and the diagnosis of propionic acidemia was confirmed by elevated levels of propionyl carnitine (8.0 nmol/mL) on MS-MS, acylcarnitine profile and increased methylcitrate and 3-hydroxy propionate in urine GC-MS testing. After stabilization, he was started on a diet restricted in isoleucine, valine, methionine and threonine with supplements of carnitine and administration of metronidazole. His clinical condition improved rapidly over next few days. He had one minor episode of decompensation after a viral illness during infancy which was managed successfully with an emergency regimen protocol. The important concern for this couple was to plan for their next pregnancy.

Propionic acidemia is an autosomal recessive disorder with a 25% risk of recurrence. Prenatal diagnosis is best performed at 11 weeks gestation by mutation analysis in a chorionic villus sample. The mutation in the proband was implicated in one of the two genes in PA. In our case the mutation was IVS1 + 5G > A and IVS3 + 2T > C in PCCB gene. Armed with this knowledge, prenatal testing was possible in the next pregnancy. The next fetus was not affected and family was happy to have a normal baby.

Organic acidurias may have vomiting as a prominent clinical manifestation and may be misdiagnosed as pyloric stenosis. The presence of metabolic acidosis should alert to the possibility of an organic aciduria because pyloric stenosis is usually associated with metabolic alkalosis. Metabolic acidosis is a common complication of almost any illness and is usually secondary to tissue hypoxia. However, if there is associated ketosis, high anion gap acidosis and normal plasma chloride; persistent acidosis even after correction of tissue perfusion, with or without previous history of similar complaints, metabolic disorder should be investigated as per the algorithmic approach presented in Figure 23.3. In acidosis due to IEM, urine pH is below 5 and differentiates it from renal acidosis.

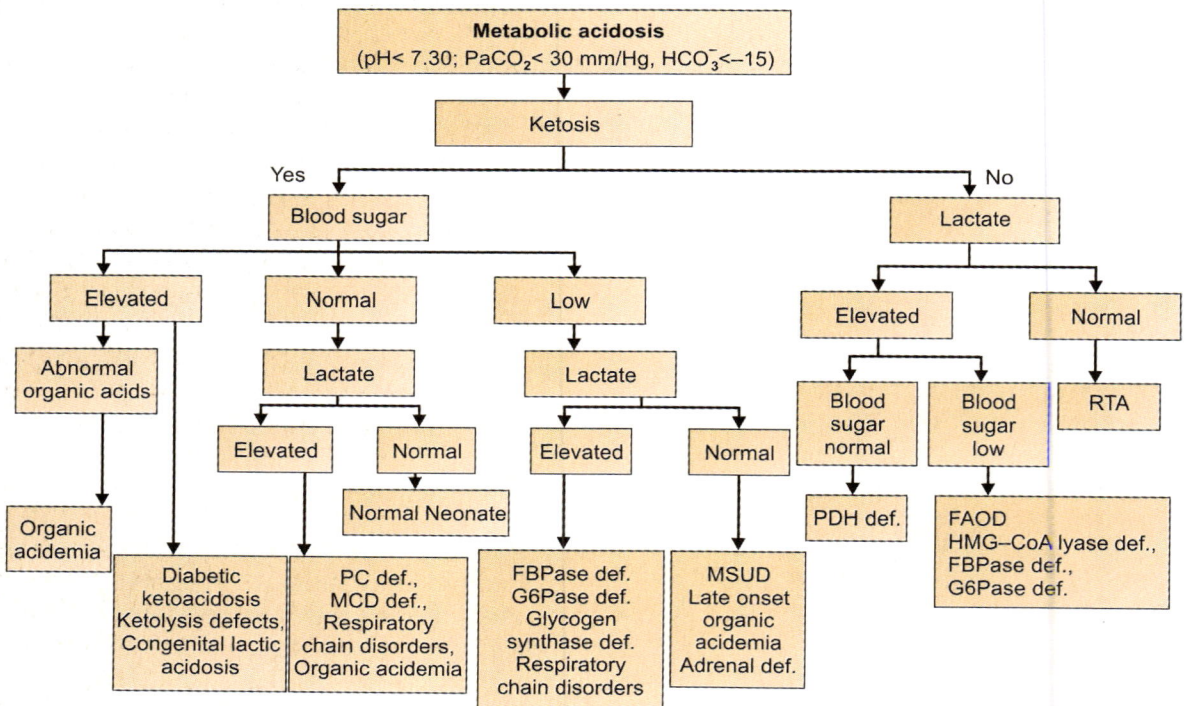

FAOD: fatty acid oxidation defects, FBPase: fructose-1,6-bisphosphatase deficiency; G6Pase: glucose-6-phosphatase deficiency, MCD: multiple carboxylase deficiency, MSUD: maple syrup urine disease, PC: pyruvate carboxylase, PDH: pyruvate dehydrogenase deficiency, HMG: 3-hydroxy 3-methylglutaryl, Def.: deficiency

Adapted from Saudubray, JM, van den, Berghe G, Walter, JH. Inborn Metabolic Diseases: Diagnosis and Treatment. 5th edition. *Springer-Verlag Berlin Heidelberg*; 2012

Figure 23.3 Approach to in a neonate with metabolic acidosis.

Collection of urine sample for estimation of organic acids by GC-MS and plasma acylcarnitine levels at the time of acidosis is useful to confirm or exclude the diagnosis of an organic acidopathy. The common organic acidurias prevalent in our country are maple syrup urine disease, methyl malonic aciduria, propionic aciduria, glutaric aciduria type I and multiple carboxylase deficiency.

DNA based testing for mutation detection is very important for providing prenatal diagnosis during next pregnancy. Two mL blood in EDTA vial should be stored for DNA testing and the sample can be transported at room temperature to a specialized laboratory.

Case scenario 3. Acute encephalopathy with ketosis

A 2500 gm male neonate was born at term and discharged home on day 2 of life. He was on breastfeeding. There were no adverse perinatal events. On day 5 he was readmitted with history of poor feeding and lethargy. He developed seizures, dystonic posturing of limbs and progressed to encephalopathy. There was significant respiratory distress for which he required ventilation. Investigations for sepsis were negative. Urine ketones were positive and there was no metabolic acidosis. It is important to note that presence of ketonuria in the neonate is always abnormal. The blood sugar was 78 mg/dL and electrolytes normal. The dinitro-phenyl-hydrazine (DNPH) test for ketones was positive. The quantitative amino acid analysis showed high levels of leucine 2900 µmol/L (normal 65–220 µmol/l), isoleucine 377 µmol/l (normal 26–100 µmol/L), valine 384 µmol/l (normal 90–300 µmol/L) and alloisoleucine 655 µmol/L (normal 0–5 µmol/L). This suggested the the possibility of maple syrup urine disease (MSUD).

The neonate was managed with a specific protein restricted feeds as recommended for MSUD and the emergency protocol was initiated whenever he showed decompensation. The mother was trained to do the DNPH test at home when she felt the child was unwell and was trained to initiate the emergency management at home. The baby did well with good metabolic control and normal developmental milestones. At 22 months of age, a liver transplant was performed. This was the first ever liver transplant in India for MSUD. The boy, now 9 years old, is without any dietary restrictions and doing well. This case illustrates that early diagnosis and educating the family about the disorder and appropriate management of the treatable IEMs can have a good outcome.

Coma in a neonate or infant is a common presentation for acquired as well as congenital metabolic disorders. A basic algorhithmic approach as presented in Figure 23.4 for a comatose neonate should be followed along with evaluation for the acquired causes of neonatal and infantile encephalopathy. Abnormalities of ammonia, arterial blood gas analysis, serum electrolytes and urine ketones are important screening tests to make a diagnosis and institute specific management.

Case scenario 4. A neonate with hypoglycemia and hepatocellular disease

A 40 days infant presented with failure to thrive, abdominal distension and mild jaundice. On examination he had bilateral cataracts, conjugated hyperbilirubinemia and elevation of transaminases. The blood sugar was 40 mg/dL and prothrombin and partial thromboplastin time were normal. The α-fetoprotein levels were normal. Benedict's test for reducing substances in urine was positive and the

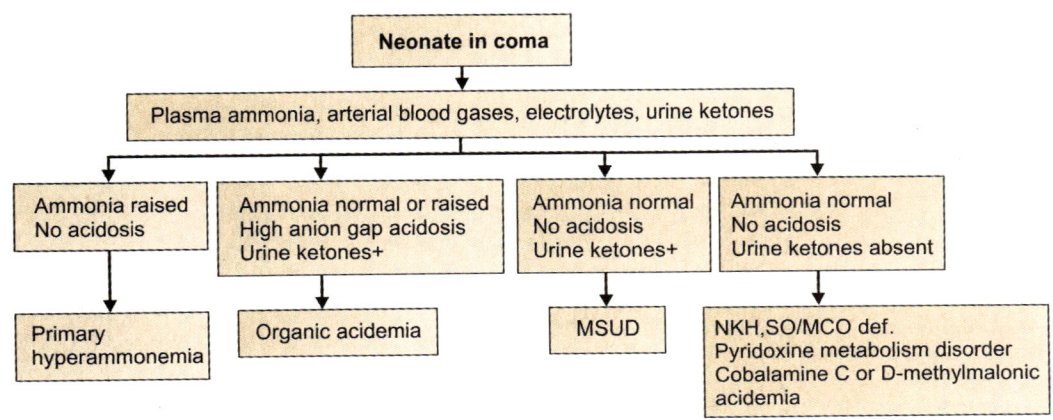

MSUD: maple syrup urine disease; NKH: non ketotic hyperglycinemia;
SO: sulfite oxidase deficiency; MCO: molybdenum cofactor deficiency

Figure 23.4 Approach to a neonate with coma.

glucose oxidase stix was negative suggesting the presence of non-glucose reducing substances in the urine. Plasma succinylacetone was normal. Plasma galactose and RBC galactose -1- phosphate levels were grossly increased to 6032.9 μmol/L (Normal <56 umol/L) and 4.5 mg/dL (Normal <1 mg/dL) respectively. Enzyme assay for galactose-1-phosphate uridyl-transferase enzyme (GALT) confirmed the diagnosis of galactosemia. Molecular analysis in GALT gene confirmed the presence of a homozygous mutation, CAT > CCT; c. A203C; p.H68P. The neonate was put on a galactose free diet. His cataract regressed spontaneously in 2–3 months. The metabolic parameters improved and on follow-up the levels of galactose and galactose-1-phosphate decreased. In infants with galactosemia, it is imperative to take blood samples for enzyme assays prior to blood transfusion. It is best to undertake analysis of the metabolites, galactose and galactose-1-phosphate along with GALT assay. This helps to interpret borderline values of enzyme and is useful to diagnose epimerase and galactokinase deficiency.

The protocol or algorithm for investigation of a neonate with hypoglycemia due to IEM is depicted in Figure 23.5. Investigations should be done at the time of hypoglycemia and it is prudent to store a blood and urine sample for future use if required. Additional features to be looked for at the time of assessment of

hypoglycemia include hepatomegaly, timing of hypoglycemia, lactic acidosis, and presence of ketones in urine and blood. Estimate the levels of insulin, cortisol and growth hormone to evaluate the endocrine causes of hypoglycemia. Hepatic functions should be checked for the possibility of acquired or inherited liver disease, as a cause for hypoglycemia. Hypoglycemia after a short period of fasting suggests a disorder of carbohydrate metabolism, while hypoglycemia after a prolonged fast signifies a disorder of fatty acid oxidation. Predominant hepatomegaly with hypoglycemia after a brief fast is suggestive of gluconeogenesis disorders and glycogen storage disorder type III. Hepatocellular disease seen in tyrosinemia type 1 may be accompanied with hypoglycemia. Respiratory chain defects and organic acidurias are associated with ketoacidosis. Early diagnosis is imperative as many disorders presenting with hypoglycemia such as glycogen storage disease I/III fatty acid oxidation defects, fructose 1, 6 bisphosphatase deficiency, 3-hydroxy-3-methylglutaryl (HMG) CoA lyase deficiency are easily treatable. Acute hepatocellular dysfunction can present with hepatomegaly, jaundice, hypoglycemia, elevated transaminases and abnormalities of coagulation. Metabolic disorders that should be considered in the differential diagnosis include galactosemia, tyrosinemia type 1, fatty acid oxidation defects, peroxisomal disorders, hereditary fructose intolerance, mitrochondrial respiratory chain defects, congenital disorders of glycosylation, Niemann-Pick disease, disorders of bile acid metabolism and neonatal hemochromatosis.

Case scenario 5. Acute encephalopathy with lactic acidosis
A second born male infant of consanguineously married couple developed poor feeding and lethargy with seizures on day 3 of life. The sepsis screen was negative. There was hypoglycemia and severe lactic acidosis. The serum ammonia was 78 μmol/L. Urine ketones were positive. Blood pyruvate analysis was not available. There was progressive deterioration of sensorium with requirement of ventilator support. The MS/MS analysis for acylcarnitines was normal. The urine organic acid estimation by gas chromatography-mass spectrometry (GC-MS) showed high lactate levels. A differential diagnosis of pyruvate carboxylase deficiency, pyruvate dehydrogenase (PDH) deficiency, disorders of gluconeogenesis like glucose-6-phosphatase dehydrogenase deficiency, fructose 1-6 biphosphatase deficiency and phosphoenolpyruvate carboxykinase (PEPCK) disorder was considered. There was a history of death of a male sibling in the neonatal period with undiagnosed encephalopathy and acidosis.

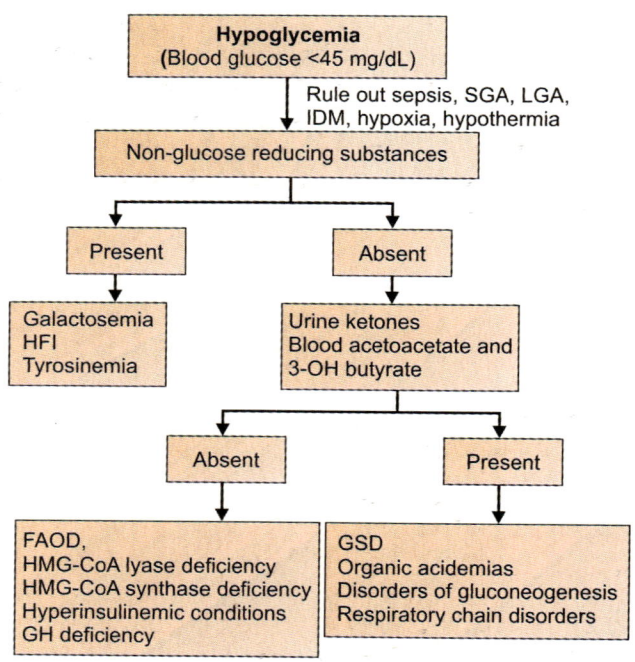

FAOD: fatty acid oxidation defects; GSD: glycogen storage disorders; HFI: hereditary fructose intolerance; IDM: infant of diabetic mother; SGA: small-for-gestational age, LGA: large-for-gestational age

Figure 23.5 Algorithm for identification of IEM on the basis of hypoglycemia.

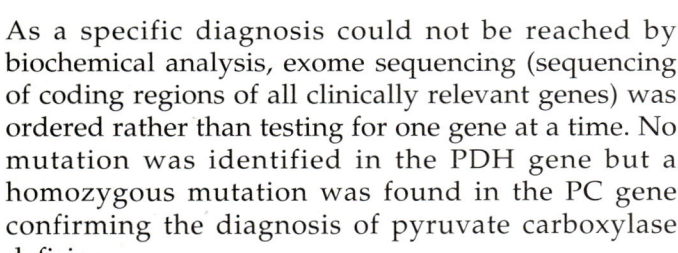

As a specific diagnosis could not be reached by biochemical analysis, exome sequencing (sequencing of coding regions of all clinically relevant genes) was ordered rather than testing for one gene at a time. No mutation was identified in the PDH gene but a homozygous mutation was found in the PC gene confirming the diagnosis of pyruvate carboxylase deficiency.

Once a high blood lactate is identified, the first step should be to exclude false elevation due to improper sampling technique. A high lactate level from a free flowing blood sample may occur because of acquired or genetically determined IEM. Acquired conditions associated with lactate accumulation include tissue hypoxia, circulatory collapse, diarrhea, sepsis, hepatic failure and hyperventilation. Presence of ketosis with high lactate suggests an IEM (exceptions include FAOD, PDH, GSD type1), as ketosis is less likely in acquired cases of hyperlactatemia. Among the IEMs, high lactate level may be seen secondarily in infants with organic acidurias, urea cycle disorders (esp. citrullinemia), and fatty acid oxidation defects. Primary lactic acidemia is a recognized feature of disorders of gluconeogenesis, glycolysis, pyruvate carboxylase deficiency, pyruvate dehydrogenase deficiency and disorders of mitochondrial respiratory function. Concomitant high levels of CSF lactate, and blood and CSF alanine levels support the diagnosis of a primary lactic acidemia. Fasting hypoglycemia and hyperlactatemia is seen in infants with glucose-6- phosphatase and fructose 1-6 biphosphatase deficiency. Postprandial hyperlactatemia suggests the possiblity of GSD type III/VI or glycogen synthase deficiency. In pyruvate dehydrogenase deficiency and disorders of respiratory chain function, the lactate levels are highest in the fed state and may be missed if blood sample is collected after an overnight fast. Lactate to pyruvate ratio (L/P ratio) measurements is useful to differentiate pyruvate carboxylase deficiency and respiratory chain disorders where the ratio is grossly increased (>30), as opposed to PDH deficiency, which is a characterized by normal or low L/P ratio.

Mutation detection confirms the diagnosis and is essential for making antenatal diagnosis in subsequent pregnancies. In situations where the metabolic profile does not provide a definite diagnosis or when a genetically heterogenous disorder like MSUD is suspected, an option of exome sequencing is found to be useful. Exome sequencing or whole exome sequencing (WES or WXS) is a test which sequences genes known for all monogenic disorders in one go by using the latest high-throughput sequencing technique known as next generation sequencing (NGS). This test has a 40 to 50% diagnostic yield in metabolic disorders and is of great importance when the clinical/biochemical diagnosis is not reached or gene for clinically suspected disorder is relatively large. In such situations, NGS test is useful and cost effective. It can be done even at a later date on a small volume (1.0 mL) of stored blood sample.

Case scenario 6. Neonate with unexplained seizures

At 36 hours of life a term neonate was noted to have increased irritability and abnormal seizure like activity of the face and limbs. There was no risk factor like hypoxia or sepsis and the investigation results were non-contributory. Serum electrolytes, and blood glucose were normal. Video EEG showed a burst suppression pattern. The seizures were refractory to anticonvulsant therapy. Injectable pyridoxine, 100 mg under cardiorespiratory and video EEG monitoring was promptly followed by cessation of the seizure activity. The clinical diagnosis of pyridoxine-dependent seizures was confirmed by molecular diagnosis by identification of mutation in the ALDH7A1 gene. Pyridoxine was continued orally and gradually the antiepileptics were tapered and stopped. This is another example that illustrates a good outcome of a treatable disorder if it is timely suspected and appropriately treated.

Seizures in the neonates commonly occur as a result of hypoxic-ischemic encephalopathy, metabolic disturbances, sepsis, cerebral dysgenesis, and cerebrovascular disorders. Neonatal seizures with or without associated biochemical derangements is an important manifestation of IEMs. A high index of suspicion is important to evaluate metabolic disorders presenting with isolated neonatal seizures. These include nonketotic hyperglycinemia, pyridoxine-dependent seizures, glucose transporter deficiency, sulphite oxidase deficiency, molybdenum cofactor defect, folinic acid responsive seizures, creatine deficiency syndromes, abnormalities of serine biogenesis and peroxisomal disorders. Peripartum onset of seizures, refractory to treatment or progressive worsening of seizure activity, electroencephalogram indicative of burst suppression pattern or hypsarrhythmia and magnetic resonance imaging of brain showing profound cerebral atrophy or hypoxic-ischemic injury without any obvious perinatal insult, mandates evaluation for an IEM. The diagnosis of the above mentioned disorders can be made by detection of the specific analyte in the urine, plasma and CSF. Specific molecular testing is important to confirm the diagnosis. Non-metabolic genetic disorders like pontocerebellar atrophy, and various forms of infantile epileptiform epilepsy, can also present with seizures. In these cases neuroimaging, family history and genetic studies are useful to confirm the diagnosis.

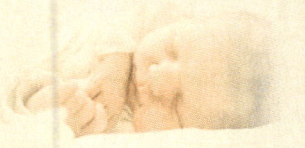

Miscellaneous Presentations of IEMs

Infants with IEM may present with stillbirth, ascites or non-immune hydrops fetalis, cardiomyopathy, dysmorphism, congenital malformations, and hypotonia during neonatal period.

Screening Tests

Table 22.3 lists the investigations to screen a neonate suspected to have an IEM. The need for specific investigations to confirm the diagnosis depends on the clinical picture and result of screening tests. Discussion with a geneticist/metabolic expert at the time of sampling is likely to improve the definitive diagnosis and appropriate treatment of neonates with IEMs. When there is a reasonable suspicion of IEM on the basis of screening tests, blood, body fluids and tissue samples can be sent to a reference laboratory for specialized tests and DNA studies. It is helpful to seek expert opinion and guidance of an experienced genetecist or metabolic expert for making a specific diagnosis and providing supportive and specific treatment.

Management

Many IEMs are treatable and specific dietary products and therapeutic options are now available in India. Early diagnosis and initiation of therapy is important for good outcome and intact survival. The therapy should be instituted without delay when there is suspicion of an IEM. The aims of management include removal of the toxic metabolite by reducing availability of substrate and enhancing excretion of toxic metabolite. Provision of adequate calories to prevent catabolism, administration of missing co-factor and supportive therapy are life-saving. Many sick neonates will also require circulatory and ventilatory support.

In all sick neonates, proteins are stopped for 24–48 hours and intaveneous 10% glucose and intralipid infusions is started to provide calories. If hyperglycemia occurs, do not decrease the glucose infusion but consider administration of insulin. Inadequate intake of calories promote catabolism and aggravation of the encephalopathy. Once the neonate improves, small amounts of protein are started orally after 24–48 hours (0.5 gm/kg/day) and gradually increased to 1 gm/kg/day.

The biochemical abnormalities like metabolic acidosis, hypoglycemia and hyperammonemia are treated promptly. Sodium benzoate, sodium phenylbutyrate/phenylacetate and arginine decrease ammonia levels and are best given through intravenous route. If the neonate continues to be comatose, dialysis should be initiated to decrease the blood levels of toxic products. Hemodialysis is more effective and life-saving but peritoneal dialysis is more widely available and feasible.

In neonates with a suspected organic acidemia, the acidosis is treated with sodium bicarbonate as per NICU protocol. In addition carnitine supplementation

Sample	Screening test
Blood	Complete blood count
	Glucose
	Electrolytes
	Arterial blood gas, anion gap $(Na^+ + K^+) - (HCO_3^- + Cl^-)$
	Ammonia
	Lactate and pyruvate
	Creatinine
	Calcium
	SGOT/SGPT, PT and APTT
	Uric acid
	Plasma amino acids by HPLC
	Carnitine and acylcarnitine profile by MS/MS
	Stored blood sample for DNA studies (3 mL blood in EDTA or a spot newborn screening filter paper)
Urine	Odor
	Ketones, sulfite, MPS screen
	Reducing substances by Benedict's reagent and glucose oxidase
	Organic acids by GC-MS
CSF	Glucose
	Lactate
	Amino acids

Table 23.3 Screening tests an infant suspected to have inborn error of metabolism

HPLC: High performance liquid chromatography; GC-MS: Gas chromatography–Mass spectrometry, MS/MS: Tandem mass spectrometry
MPS: Mucopolysaccharide

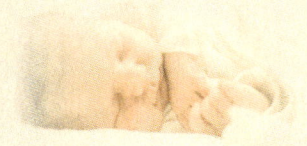

and co-factor therapy with biotin, vitamin B_{12} (vitamin B_{12} responsive methylmalonic acidemia), and thiamine (thiamine responsive MSUD) is initiated.

Intractable seizures in a setting of a suspected IEM are given a trial of pyridoxine. An initial dose of pyridoxine 100 mg is given intraveneously under EEG and ECG control. This can be repeated after 10 minutes if there is no response, up to a total dose of 200 mg. If the response is poor or partial, pyridoxine may be continued in a dose of 5–15 mg/kg/day orally up to 7 days to further evaluate the response. If seizures persist, folinic acid 5 mg/kg/day orally or IV in three divided doses, is given daily for 3 days. If still there is no response, pyridoxal phosphate 30 mg/kg/day for 3 days is tried. In a suspected glucose transporter defect, ketogenic diet is benificial.

The infants with life-threatening IEMs need high standard of nursing and supportive care to ensure provision of thermoneutral environment, hydration and electrolyte balance, treatment of associated sepsis and effective mechanical ventilation. *Sodium valproate should be avoided in infants with IEMs.* Specific long-term management after stabilization includes protein restriction and exclusion of specific amino acids depending upon the diagnosis. The special diets are now available in India. The indications and dosages of various co-factors and vitamins for treatment of specific IEMs are listed in Table 23.4.

Table 23.4 The life-saving medications for treatment of IEMs

Drug	Indication	Recommended dose	Route and frequency
Biotin	Biotinidase deficiency Multiple carboxylase deficiency Biotin responsive basal ganglia disease	5–20 mg /day	Oral/IV
Dextromethorphan	Nonketotic hyperglycinemia	5–7 mg/kg/day. Up to 35 mg/day have been used	Oral; 4 divided doses
Diazoxide	Persistent hyperinsulinemia	15 mg/kg/day in newborn 10 mg/kg/day in infants	Oral
Folinic acid	Remethylation defects DHPR deficiency Cerebral folate transporter defect	5–15 mg/day	Oral/IV
Hydroxycobalamin (vitamin B_{12})	Disorders of cobalamin metabolism	1 mg/day 10 mg/day	IM Oral
L-Arginine	Acute management of hyperammonemic crisis or urea cycle disorders except arginase deficiency	250–500 mg /kg /day	Oral/IV; 4–6 divided doses
L-Carnitine	Primary or secondary carnitine deficiency	Acute crisis: 100 mg/kg/dose Chronic: 100–200 mg/kg/day	IV/oral; 3–4 times daily Oral; 3 divided doses
N-carbamylglutamate	NAGS, CPS deficiency	100 mg/kg	Oral; 4 times a day
NTBC (Nitisinone)	Tyrosinemia type I, alkaptonuria	1 mg/kg	Oral; 1–2 divided doses
Pyridoxine (vitamin B_6)	Pyridoxine-responsive seizures, homocystinuria	100 mg IV with EEG monitoring or 30 mg/kg/day for 7 days Maintenance 5–10 mg per day	IV Oral/enteral Oral
Pyridoxal phosphate	Pyridoxamine 5-phosphate oxidase deficiency	40 mg/kg per day	Oral; 4 divided doses
Sodium benzoate	Hyperammonemia	250–500 mg/kg/day	Oral/IV; 4–6 divided doses or continuous IV infusion
Sodium phenylbutyrate	Hyperammonemia	250–500 mg/kg/day	Oral/IV; 4–6 divided doses
Thiamine (vitamin B_1)	Thiamine responsive variants of MSUD, PDH deficiency, Complex 1 deficiency	10–15 mg/day	Oral
Coenzyme Q10	Primary CoQ10 deficiency	2–15 mg/kg/day	Oral

CPG: carbamyl phosphate synthetase, NAGS: N-acetylglutamate synthase

DHPR: dihydropteridine reductase, MSUD: maple syrup urine disease; PDH: pyruvate dehydrogenase

NTBC: [2-(2-nitro-4-trifluoromethyl benzoyl)-1, 3,-cyclohexanedione]

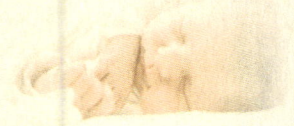

Biochemical Autopsy

Many a times, the neonate with suspected IEM is critically sick and it is not possible or feasible to undertake metabolic studies. In this situation, blood and urine samples should be preserved for diagnostic purposes. Pretransfusion 3–5 mL blood sample in an EDTA and plain vacutainer as well as on the newborn screening filter paper must be stored. Freeze 15 mL urine, CSF/tissue biopsy samples at –20°C or lyophilize them. Most of the IEMs have a 25–50% risk of recurrence and prenatal diagnosis in a subsequent pregnancy is not possible in the absence of a definitive DNA-based diagnosis. In the event of death, tissue samples should be collected as early as possible, preferably within 12 hours of death.

Genetic Diagnosis and Role of Newer Technology

Diagnosis of IEM is a challenging task for a neonatologist. High index of clinical suspicion is the first and most important step. Effective use of diagnostic algorithms and experience of the metabolic expert definitely improves the diagnosis and outcome. Many a times, definitive etiological diagnosis cannot be reached even if the possibility of IEM is strong. Lack of easy availability of GCMS and MS/MS technology, time lost in transport of sample, inappropriate timing of sample collection, metabolic profile modified by tissue hypoxia, and stoppage of enteral feeds adversely affect diagnostic yield of studies. DNA based diagnostic tests to identify the causative mutation, do not have some of these limitations and are more reliable.

DNA is not affected by timing of sample collection. The sequencing of the gene for the suspected IEM may be cumbersome because of several diagnostic possibilities. The newer technology of high-through put DNA sequencing known as Next Generation Sequencing (NGS) is of great help in these situations. This technology is used to sequence a panel of genes for the disorders with a similar clinical phenotype in one go or the whole genome can be sequenced and the data is analyzed to identify the genetic variation which may be the cause of the phenotype. NGS technology is commonly used to sequence all the coding regions of genes (Whole Exome Sequencing, i.e. WES) or sequencing all genes known to be associated with a variety of metabolic or genetic disorders. The diagnostic yield using WES in various clinical presentations may vary from 30 to 50%. The reporting time varies between 2 to 4 weeks but when a definitive diagnosis is made with the help of WES, it is of great help to institute rational therapy and improve the outcome. The detection of mutations is also of importance for facilitating prenatal diagnosis and should be pursued even if the child is unlikely to survive or has already died. In some situations where the proband has died and no sample for DNA studies has been taken, an attempt should be made to do WES of the parents to identify the carrier states for an autosomal recessive disorder or a heterozygous mutation for an X-linked disorder in the mother. WES has an advantage that in addition to IEMs, other genetic disorders presenting like an IEM can be detected; even when the clinician has not suspected it. Sometimes the results of WES are uncertain and due care must be exercised while providing genetic counseling. WES is also being evaluated as a first tier test for babies in the NICU for screening of asymptomatic babies with IEM. Availability of early diagnosis in an asymptomatic baby can revolutionize the management and intact survival of these babies.

BIBLIOGRAPHY

Bodian DL, Klein E, Iyer RK, Wong WSW, Kothiyal P, Daniel Stauffer, Huddleston KC, et al. Utility of whole-genome sequencing for detection of newborn screening disorders in a population cohort of 1,696 neonates. *Genet Med* 2015; 18:221–30.

Bruton BK. Inborn errors of metabolism in infancy: a guide to diagnosis. *Pediatrics* 1998, 102(6): E69.

Christodoulou JI, Wilcken B. Perimortem laboratory investigation of genetic metabolic disorders. *Semin Neonatol* 2004; 9: e275–e280.

Clarke JTR. Neurological syndromes. In: A Clinical Guide to Inherited Metabolic Diseases. 3rd Edn. Cambridge, Cambridge University Press, 2006; pp 28–87.

Fazeli W, Karakaya M, Herkenrath P, Vierzig A, Dotsch J, von Kleist-Retzow JC, Cirak S. Mendeliome sequencing enables differential diagnosis and treatment of neonatal lactic acidosis. *Mol Cell Pediatr* 2016 Dec; 3(1):22.

Filiano JJ. Neurometabolic diseases in the newborn. *Clin Perinatol* 2006; 33: of 411—79.

Gupta N, Kabra M. Acute management of sick infants with suspected inborn errors of metabolism. *Indian J Pediatr* 2011; 78:854–59.

Kabra M. Emergencies due to inborn errors of metabolism. In: Medical Emergencies in Children. Singh M. (Ed.) *New Delhi, CBS Publishers & Distributors Pvt. Ltd,* Revised 5th edition, 2016; pp 648–662.

Leonard JV, Morris AA. Diagnosis and early management of inborn errors of metabolism presenting around the time of birth. *Acta Paediatr* 2006; 95: 6e14.

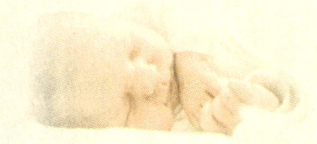
Nyhan WL. When to suspect metabolic disease? In: Inherited Metabolic Diseases. Hoffman GF, Zschocke J, Nyhan WL (Eds.). *Springer* 2010; pp 13–15.

Pitt JJ. Newborn screening. *Clin Biochem Rev* 2010; 31:57–68.

Pourfarzam M, Zadhoush F. Newborn screening for inherited metabolic disorders, news and views. *J Res Med Sci* 2013; 18(9):801–8.

Saudubray JM, Sedel F, Walter JH. Clinical approach to treatable inborn metabolic diseases: An introduction. *J Inherit Metab Dis* 2006; 29:261–74

Saudubray JM, van den Berghe G, Walter JH. Inborn Metabolic Diseases: diagnosis and Treatment. 5th Edn. *Heidelberg; Springer,* 2012.

Sharma S, Kumar P, Agarwal R, Kabra M, Deorari AK, Paul VK. Approach to inborn errors of metabolism presenting in the neonate. *Indian J Pediatr* 2008,75:271.

Singh M. Inborn errors of metabolism (IEM). In: Care of the Newborn. Singh M (Ed)., Revised 8th edition, *New Delhi, CBS Publishers & Distributors Pvt Ltd.* 2017; pp 481–492.

Tebani A, Abily-Donval L, Afonso C, Marret S, Bekri S. Clinical metabolomics: The new metabolic window for inborn errors of metabolism investigations in the post-genomic era. *Int J Mol Sci* 2016 Jul 20;17(7):1167 doi:10.3390/ijms 17071167.

Wilcken B. Expanded newborn screening: Reducing harm, assessing benefit. *J Inherit Metab Dis* 2010, 33 (Suppl 2): S205–S210.

24

Cardiac Emergencies

Kuntal Roy Chowdhuri , Nilanjan Dutta and Parvathi Unninayar Iyer

Background

Cardiac malformations are probably the most common of all birth defects and are responsible for majority of deaths due to congenital abnormalities. It is estimated that between 150,000 to 200,000 infants with congenital heart disease (CHD) are born each year in our country given the current prevalence of 4–8/1000 live births. Of these, about a third (~70,000 infants) would need some sort of cardiac intervention in the first year of life to reach their first birthday. *What is less well-recognized is that about 10–20% of newborns with cardiac defects (~30,000 neonates annually) have potentially lethal cardiac malformations which lead to cardiovascular collapse and death in the neonatal period if not appropriately managed.* Currently, unfortunately only a very small proportion of this number get any form of care in our country.

Thus, both the burden of congenital heart disease as well as the number of newborns with potentially life-threatening heart disease is huge in our country. Unfortunately, even today, the perception among both parents and many pediatricians is that *newborns with heart disease are doomed to die and that neonatal heart surgery or catheter intervention is a fancy and a futile exercise which is not feasible in India.* This myth exists despite the steadily improving outcomes of neonatal heart disease both in the high and low middle income countries like India. A recent report comparing neonatal surgical outcomes across the world reported a hospital mortality risk of less than 10%, i.e. a 90% survival of neonates with complex cardiac malformations. In our country, many centers today have similar results with surgical survival in dextro-transposition of great arteries (dTGA.IVS) and total anomalous pulmonary venous connexion (TAPVC). However, these outcomes are feasible with early diagnosis, appropriate stabilization and timely referral to advanced cardiac centers. Handling "cardiac emergencies" in the newborn infant can be a vexing and challenging experience particularly for the inexperienced resident in the emergency room.

The scope of this chapter is to discuss (i) common neonatal cardiac emergencies, (ii) to provide a systematic approach to a neonate with suspected critical heart disease, (iii) appropriate management of the critically ill cardiac neonate presenting to the emergency room, (iv) current prognosis and realistic expectations of various heart defects, (v) commonly missed neonatal heart defects, (vi) problems associated with delayed diagnosis, and (vii) need for early detection of neonatal heart disease to minimize circulatory collapse, and improve outcome.

Common Neonatal Cardiac Emergencies

Newborns are extremely delicate and vulnerable and tend to rapidly develop uncompensated low cardiac output state (LCOS) and dysfunction of multiple organs. This occurs because the neonatal myocardium is noncompliant and has a restrictive physiology. The newborns respond rapidly and profoundly to stress with drastic changes in pH, serum lactate, acid base status and glucose levels, becoming desperately unwell very quickly. They also tend to maintain blood pressures till the very end by intense vasoconstriction. The baby who has intense vasoconstriction is potentially a sick newborn, and requires urgent intervention.

Transitional Circulation and its Effects
(Figure 24.1a, b)

Most neonates with structural heart disease have *urgent or critical heart defects* and present in a dramatic fashion at the time of ductal closure and are thus called as *"duct*

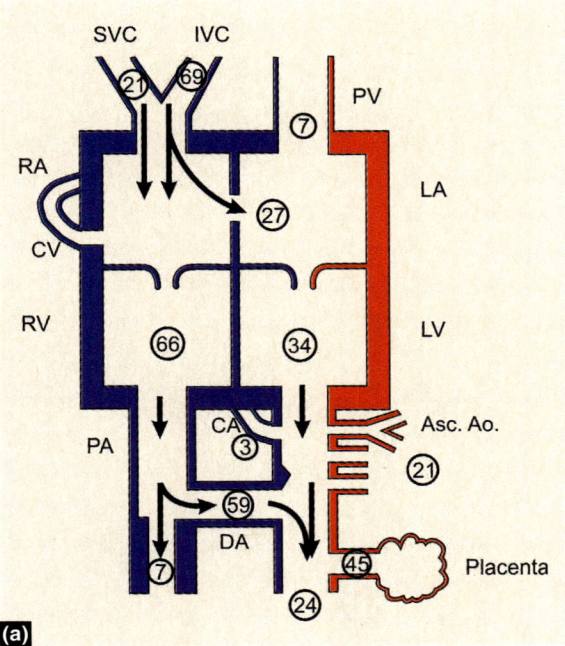

Figure 24.1a Fetal circulation showing relevance of ductus arteriosus and patent foramen ovale (PFO). A predominant ductal systemic circulation.

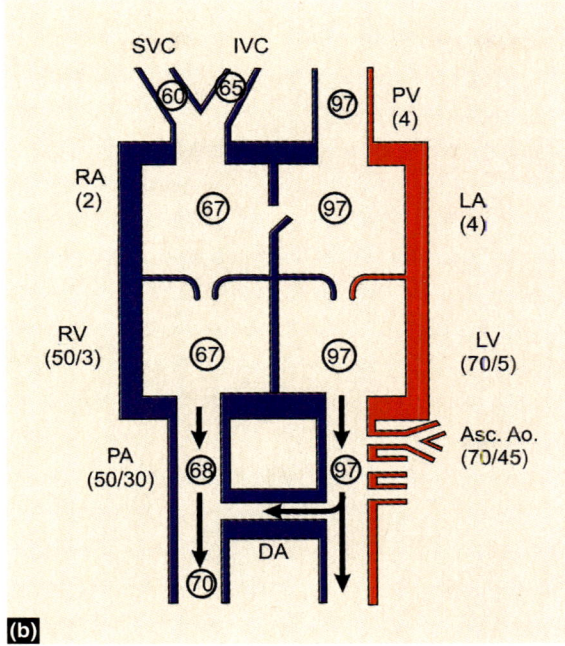

Figure 24.1b Transitional circulation at birth with closure of ductus arteriosus and foramen ovale.

dependent circulation". The first few days of postnatal life are associated with constriction of the ductus arteriosus followed by ductal closure. These changes in fetal circulation or transitional circulation causes profound hemodynamic instability in neonates who depend on adequate ductal flow for a stable circulation.

The sick cardiac neonate depends on a patent ductus arteriosus to ensure following hemodynamic changes to maintain stable circulation.

1. Adequate *intercirculatory mixing in parallel nonmixing circulations*, e.g. d-transposition of great arteries (dTGA) (Figure 24.2a,b,c).

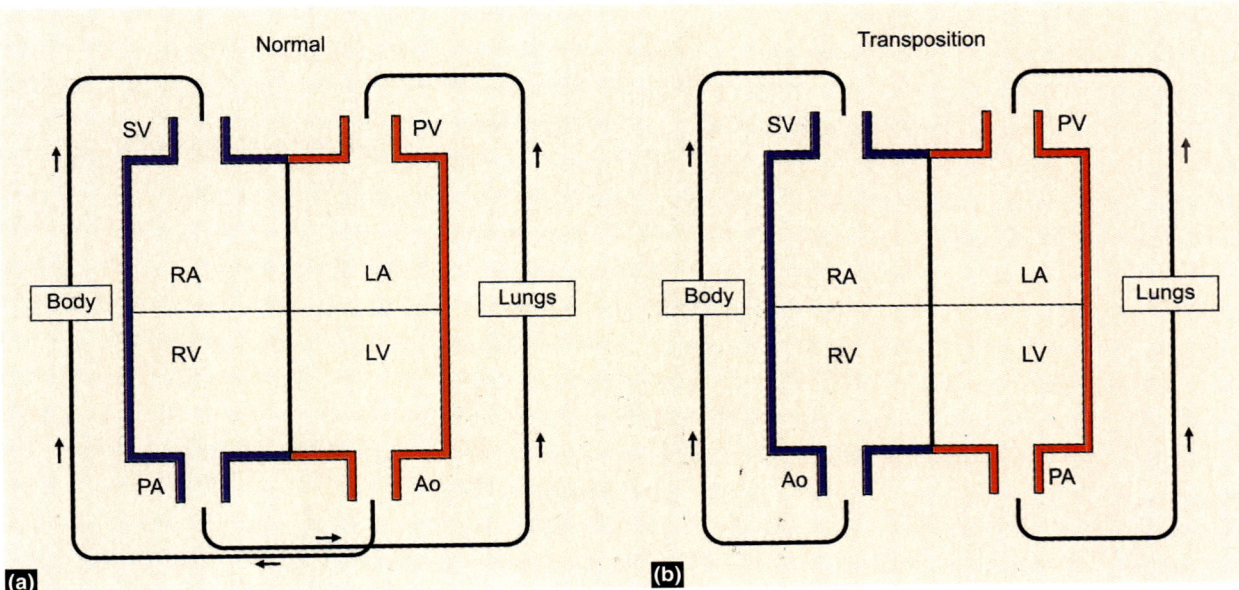

Figure 24.2a Normal circulation. 24.2b. Transposition of great arteries with two parallel nonmixing circulations leading to death.

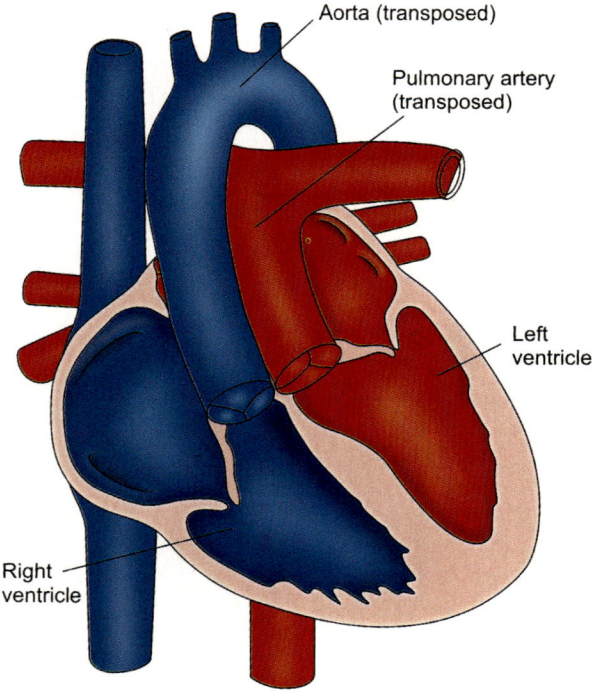

Figure 24.2c Transposition of great arteries.

2. Adequate *pulmonary blood flow* in right obstructive lesions (RVOTO), i.e. duct dependent pulmonary circulation (Figure 24.3 a, b).
3. Adequate *systemic perfusion* in left ventricular outflow tract obstruction (LVOTO) or aortic arch obstructive or hypoplastic lesions, i.e. duct dependent systemic circulation (Figure 24.4 a and b).

All these conditions worsen and deteriorate rapidly with ductal closure and present in a dramatic fashion to the emergency department if undetected before ductal closure. All pediatricians need to be familiar with these circulatory changes and consequent hemodynamic effects in order to provide immediate stabilization and speedy referral to a cardiac center.

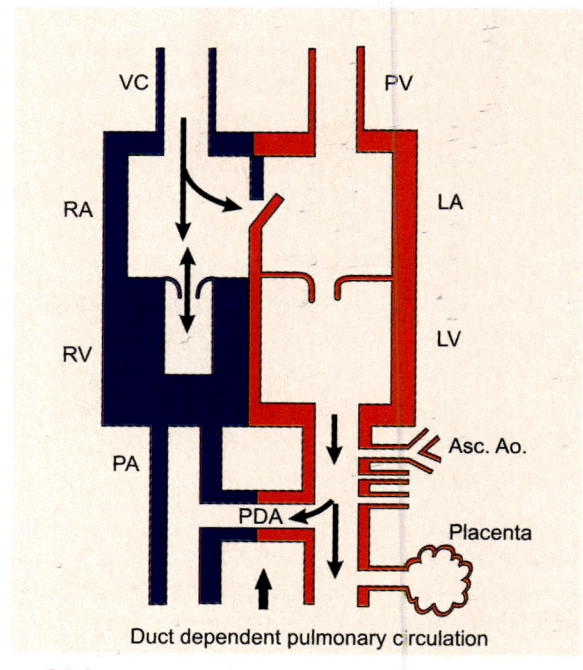

Figure 24.3a Pulmonary atresia with intact ventricular septum.

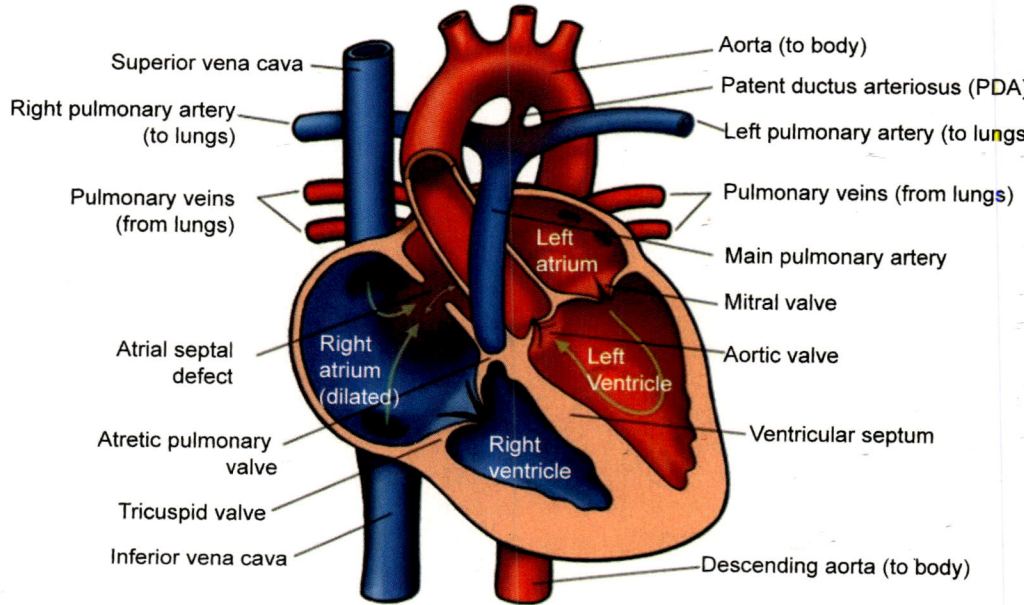

Figure 24.3b Pulmonary atresia with intact ventricular septum (IVS).

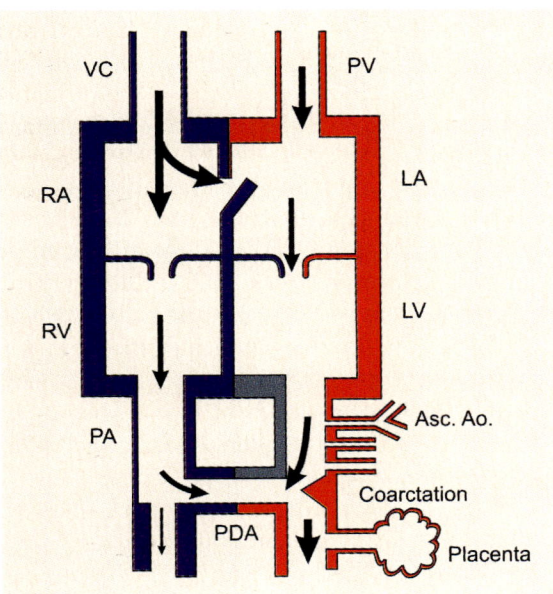

Figure 24.4a Neonatal aortic coarctation with duct-dependent systemic circulation.

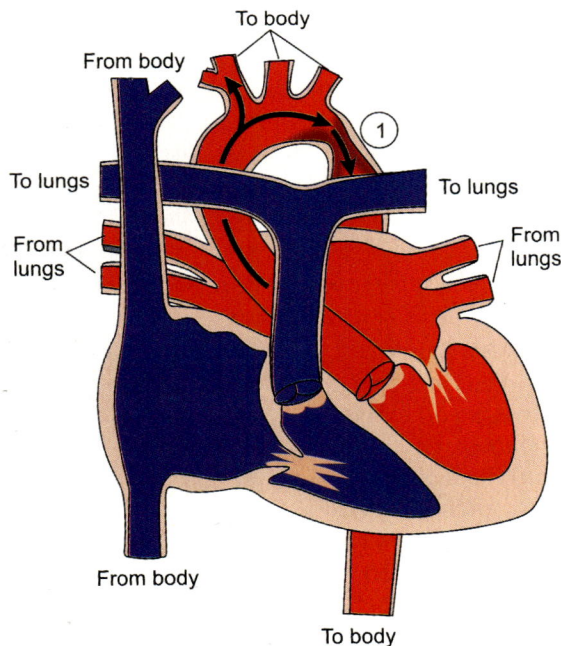

Figure 24.4b Neonatal aortic coarctation after origin of main arteries.

Other important neonatal cardiac emergencies which are *not duct dependent* but which may be both a diagnostic and management challenge include: (i) obstructed total anomalous pulmonary venous connexion (TAPVC), and (ii) destabilizing cardiac arrhythmias. Both of these situations are potentially lethal, but can be easily salvaged if diagnosed early and managed meticulously.

A SYSTEMATIC APPROACH TO A SICK CARDIAC NEONATE

The following is a simplistic and practical approach to a newborn with suspected critical heart disease.

Modes of Presentation of a Critically Ill Cardiac Newborn

The sick cardiac neonate typically presents to the emergency department with (i) marked cyanosis, (ii) respiratory distress and overt heart failure, (iii) cyanosis and respiratory distress, (iv) cardiovascular collapse or "shock" state and (v) arrhythmias. These symptoms often overlap and many newborns may have one or more of the above clinical manifestation. All of these constitute "critical or urgent heart disease" and need initial stabilization followed by some form of speedy intervention for survival.

Presentation with Cyanosis
(Figure 24.5 and Box 24.1)

Schematic diagrams and pictures of common cardiac lesions are given below. Visible and progressive cyanosis or blue baby is one of the most common symptoms reported by family members but most babies develop noticeable cyanosis only after discharge from the maternity ward. A pediatrician or neonatologist may

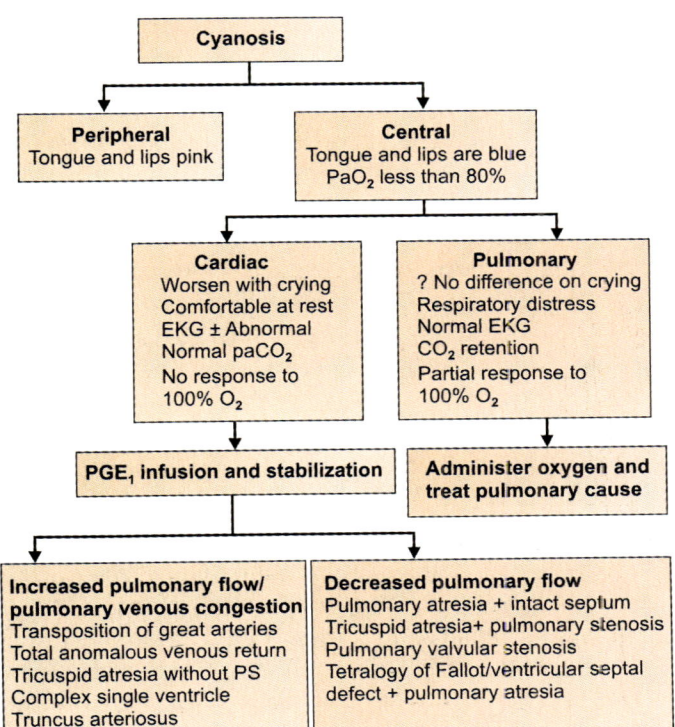

Figure 24.5 Approach to a cyanotic newborn.

> **BOX 24.1** Congenital heart diseases presenting with cyanosis
>
> - Transposition of great arteries (dTGA) is most common
> - Right ventricular outflow tract obstruction (RVOTO)
>   i. Pulmonary atresia with intact ventricular septum
>   ii. Tricuspid atresia with pulmonary atresia
>   iii. Tetralogy of Fallot
>   iv. Pulmonary atresia with ventricular septal defect
>   v. Ebstein's anomaly with functional pulmonary atresia
> - Total anomalous pulmonary venous connection (TAPVC)
> - Truncus arteriosus
> - Complex single ventricle

be the first to notice cyanosis if the baby is still admitted in the neonatal unit or during a routine postnatal outpatient visit. Not infrequently, the baby presents to the pediatric emergency room with deepening cyanosis and hypoxemia. Newborns who present with *worsening cyanosis* have either impaired intercirculatory mixing or reduced pulmonary blood flow. Impaired intercirculatory mixing occurs in transposition of great arteries (dTGA.IVS) where the pulmonary and systemic circulations are in parallel rather than in series as in the normal baby. dTGA is the most common cardiac malformation presenting with cyanosis in the neonatal period and comprises nearly 25–30% of all critical neonatal heart defects. Most infants with dTGA present in the first few hours of life with cyanosis, but the vast majority become symptomatic by the first few days of life. These babies tend to deteriorate rapidly and develop worsening hypoxemia with profound metabolic and lactic acidosis if the parallel circulations are allowed to continue without ensuring adequate mixing.

Clinically, the baby is relatively comfortable in the initial stages, i.e. has *"peaceful cyanosis"*, the second heart sound is split, a murmur may or not be audible, and the chest skiagram reveals cardiomegaly with increased pulmonary artery markings and a narrow mediastinum with a typical "egg on string" appearance. The X-ray chest may not always be typical or diagnostic, but the lung fields would show normal or increased vascularity. *Thus, in a cyanotic neonate , if the chest X-ray shows plethoric lung fields the probability is very high that the baby has a dTGA.*

Some babies with dTGA may have a tiny ductus at birth, or the ductus may have closed *in utero* either spontaneously or with maternal intake of medications like indomethacin. Thus, a newborn with dTGA and a tiny or closing ductus and a very small patent foramen ovale (PFO) at birth tends to deteriorate very rapidly immediately after birth due to inadequate mixing between the two parallel circulations. This subset of babies with dTGA become very sick quickly by

developing profound metabolic and lactic acidosis with severely impaired systemic perfusion and significant hypotension. It is of paramount importance that these critically sick babies with dTGA are diagnosed, stabilized and sent to a specialized cardiac unit without delay.

The instances of cyanosis with reduced pulmonary blood flow or right sided obstruction include (i) critical pulmonary valvular stenosis with right-to-left shunting, (ii) pulmonary valvular atresia with intact ventricular septum or functional pulmonary atresia, e.g. Ebstein's anomaly, (iii) tricuspid atresia with pulmonary atresia and a small ventricular septal defect and (iv) severe tetralogy of Fallot or pulmonary atresia with ventricular septal defect. The pulmonary stenosis in many instances may be so severe that the pulmonary artery is virtually atretic. These cardiac defects cause cyanosis and hypoxemia with progressive metabolic acidosis due to right-to-left intracardiac shunting. These lesions are dependent almost entirely on the ductus arteriosus (DA) *to* maintain blood flow to the lungs. When the DA finally closes, the baby suddenly becomes visibly and noticeably cyanotic since their pulmonary blood flow is duct dependent.

Most of these infants are not in cardiac failure, their second heart sound is single, and the chest skiagram reveals a normal sized or a small cardiac shadow with oligemic lung fields. If there is associated tricuspid atresia, the EKG shows left axis deviation. Thus, *if a cyanotic neonate has oligemic lung fields on chest skiagram with a normal or small heart size, the baby is likely to have duct dependent pulmonary circulation with significant pulmonary stenosis or atresia .*

When an infant has cyanosis, there is often a doubt whether it is due to an underlying respiratory disorder or due to a cardiac defect. The classical and traditional hyperoxia test may still be useful at times. If the PaO_2 is <150 mmHg on 100% oxygen, the infant is likely to have a cardiac defect with right-to-left shunting. Persistent pulmonary hypertension (PPHN) is an important differential and often mimics cyanotic heart disease. These babies often have a setting for PPHN, like meconium aspiration syndrome, or maternal diabetes mellitus. Babies with PPHN are often sicker and have greater respiratory distress. These are, however, only broad guidelines and it can be extremely difficult in an individual baby to differentiate between PPHN and structural heart disease. Some babies with severe PPHN may not show a good response to hyperoxia, and occasionally PPHN and dTGA may coexist. Thus, a definitive diagnosis may be extremely difficult in an individual baby.

In summary, the circulatory changes associated with transitional circulation are not well-tolerated by neonates who present predominantly with cyanosis. These babies become symptomatic during the first few days to weeks of life and become desperately unwell very rapidly. *Pulse oximetry is useful in confirming cyanosis, the oxygen saturation is usually less than 80–85%, and not infrequently in the 50s–60s in neonates who present late.* After deciding that the cyanosis is probably cardiac in origin, a swift clinical examination is done. If there is evidence of cardiac failure (puffiness and hepatomegaly), it is more likely to be a dTGA. IVS rather than due to reduced pulmonary blood flow. Chest X-rays and ECG are not diagnostic, but may be indicative. If the chest X-ray suggests oligemic lung fields, the baby is likely to have one of the conditions with reduced pulmonary blood flow, i.e. some form of RVOTO. On, the other hand, if the chest X-ray shows congested lung fields, the infant is more likely to have dTGA. The characteristic features of "egg on end" appearance on skiagram may not always be seen in dTGA. The diagnosis is readily confirmed by 2D echocardiography and color flow guided Doppler. Rarely a CT angiogram is needed if the pulmonary arteries are not clearly delineated on 2 D echo. It is useful to remember that the most common heart defect presenting with cyanosis in the newborn period is dTGA.IVS. Other causes of cyanotic heart disease are given in Box 24.1.

Respiratory Distress and Heart Failure

Many newborns with congenital heart disease present with tachypnea and respiratory distress. Skiagram of chest usually confirms or excludes major pulmonary pathology like pneumonia and aspiration. It is useful to determine if the baby has cyanosis by a baseline pulse oximetry and if needed a hyperoxia test may be done.

If there is no overt cyanosis or hypoxemia and pulmonary pathology has been reasonably excluded, the respiratory distress could be due to cardiac failure or left sided outflow obstruction. The causes of cardiac failure in the early neonatal period are given in the Box 24.2 and Table 24.1. Important causes include large patent ductus arteriosus (PDA), myocarditis, anomalous origin of coronary artery from pulmonary artery (ALCAPA) and various arrhythmias. An important and often missed cause of isolated tachypnea or respiratory distress include initial stages of coarctation of aorta or arch interruption before decompensation occurs. These babies typically present at 5–7 days of age and can be easily suspected by the discerning physician due to relatively impalpable femoral pulses. Unfortunately, many pediatricians do not routinely examine the femorals and often miss differential pulsations in upper and lower extremities.

BOX 24.2 Common causes of neonatal heart failure

- Large patent ductus arteriosus
- Congenital heart disease
- Birth asphyxia
- Hypoglycemia and hypocalcemia
- Severe anemia
- Sepsis
- Arrhythmias
- Myocarditis and cardiomyopathy
- Arteriovenous malformations
- Overtransfusion or overhydration

Table 24.1 Congenital heart diseases causing cardiac failure

- **Large L-R shunt (pulmonary over circulation) without cyanosis**
  - Large patent ductus arteriosus
  - Large ventricular septal defect
  - Left-to-right shunt at multiple levels
  - Complete atrio-ventricular canal
  - Aortopulmonary window
  - Arteriovenous malformations
- **Diminished left ventricular function**
  - Myocarditis
  - Dilated cardiomyopathy
  - Anomalous origin of left coronary artery from pulmonary artery (ALCAPA)
- **Pulmonary over circulation with cyanosis**
  - dTGA with ventricular septal defect and or coarctation
  - Truncus arteriosus
  - Complex single ventricle
  - Ebstein's anomaly

Babies with large left-to-right shunts develop heart failure once pulmonary over circulation occurs, i.e. when the pulmonary vascular resistance begins to fall. Thus, typically most large left-to-right shunts (ventricular septal defects, i.e. VSDs, VSDs with large PDA, large aortopulmonary windows) usually present after 6 weeks of age when the pulmonary vascular resistance falls to allow pulmonary overcirculation. Neonates with large VSDs who develop heart failure invariably have shunting at multiple levels or an associated severe coarctation or arch interruption causing severe heart failure and becoming dangerously unwell quickly. These infants need to be evaluated carefully and stabilized.

All these babies tire easily during feeds, nurse more frequently, are tachypneic at rest, have a diastolic apical flow rumble and frequently a gallop rhythm due to left ventricular failure. Babies with more florid cardiac failure have clinical signs of poor peripheral perfusion like decreased toe temperature and poor capillary refill.

In addition, babies with a VSD have a heaving precordium, a harsh holosystolic murmur while those with an atrioventricular septal defect (AVSD) or endocardial cushion defect have similar clinical findings but a fixed split of the second heart sound. Babies with an ASD have a soft systolic ejection murmur, a fixed split of the second sound with or without a diastolic rumble depending on the degree of shunting. Babies with a systemic AV malformation can present with very severe heart failure and shock like state, and may be symptomatic even in the first few hours of life if the systemic run off is very large. Careful examination in these babies usually reveals a cerebral bruit, or a bruit over the liver and sometimes bouncy pulses. The chest skiagram in all instances shows cardiomegaly, plethora and sometimes patchy atelectasis. *Differentiation on the basis of chest X-ray and EKG is seldom possible and once a left-to-right shunt is suspected it is best to confirm the exact nature of the defect by early echocardiography.* Likewise cardiomyopathy/myocarditis can also be diagnosed by a 2D echo study and confirmed by cardiac magentic resonance imaging.

Infants who have respiratory distress along with cyanosis are likely to have (i) dTGA.IVS with worsening acidosis, (ii) hypoplastic left heart syndrome (HLHS), (iii) obstructed TAPVC, and (iv) Ebstein's anomaly. Conditions which present after the first few weeks include dTGA.VSD, dTGA.VSD with coarctation or arch interruption, truncus arteriosus, and complex single ventricle. There is a small group of newborns who present with mild cyanosis and rapidly worsening heart failure. Some of these babies have total anomalous pulmonary venous connection (TAPVC), i.e. all the pulmonary veins are draining into the right side of the heart, the SVC, the right atrium or the IVC (Figure 24.6). *If the pulmonary venous drainage is obstructed, these babies can deteriorate very rapidly unless the pulmonary veins are surgically re-routed.* The common clinical features include a fixed split of the second heart sound, and a chest skiagram showing a normal heart size with pulmonary congestion with mottled look or diffuse haziness. Presence of these two features on chest X-ray should prompt an urgent echocardiographic study. The chest X-ray is often mistakenly diagnosed as hyaline membrane disease or meconium aspiration. Many term babies with obstructed TAPVC are often kept in the NICU and given multiple doses of surfactant due to the mistaken diagnosis of hyaline membrane disease in a term infant by an unwary pediatrician. The diagnosis is confirmed on 2D echocardiography based on a high degree of clinical suspicion.

A very unusual cause of structural heart defect in the newborn period include Ebstein's anomaly of the

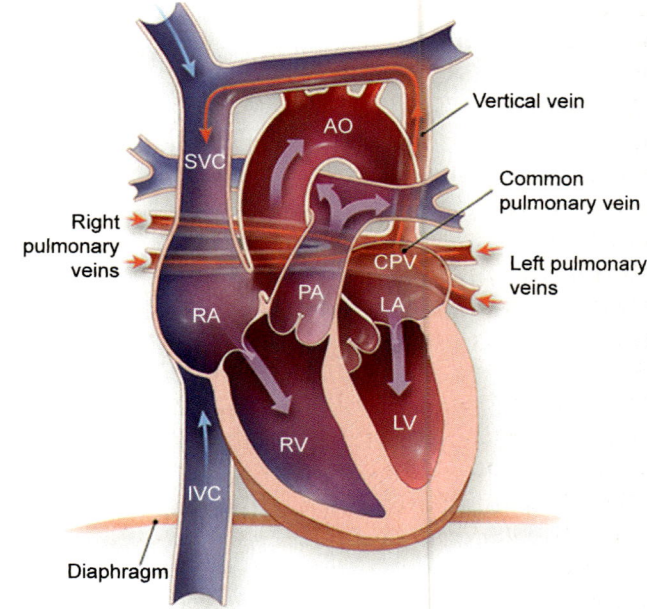

AO: Aorta   LA: Left atrium   RA: Right atrium
CPV: Common   LV: Left ventricle   RV: Right ventricle
    pulmonary   PA: Pulmonary artery   SVC: Superior vena cava
    vein

Figure 24.6 Supracardiac total anomalous pulmonary venous connexion.

tricuspid valve. These babies present with cyanosis, right heart failure, a systolic murmur of tricuspid valve regurgitation, loud third and fourth heart sounds, massive cardiomegaly on chest X-ray and right ventricular hypertrophy on EKG. In fact, this cluster of clinical findings in the presence of massive cardiomegaly is highly suggestive of Ebstein anomaly. Sometimes, they have functional pulmonary atresia due to elevated pulmonary vascular resistance.

The second group of babies with mild cyanosis and cardiac failure include babies with a truncus arteriosus who present with tachypnea with a prominent systolic murmur and a systolic ejection click. The pulses are usually bounding due to a run off into the pulmonary artery. These babies are usually symptomatic by three weeks or later, i.e. by the time the pulmonary vascular resistance drops with marked increase in pulmonary over-circulation. *Again, such a baby should be referred to a cardiac center well in time, because the early and long-term surgical outcome is best when surgery is performed in early infancy.*

Cardiovascular Collapse or Shock

Neonates who may present with cardiovascular collapse and lactic acidosis due to severely reduced peripheral circulation typically have or left ventricular outflow tract obstruction (LVOTO). The common cardiac malformations include severe coarctation of the aorta, aortic arch interruption, aortic valvular stenosis, and hypoplastic left heart syndrome (HLHS).

These babies have duct dependent systemic circulation and manifest features of greatly diminished peripheral circulation or shock as the ductus begins to close, i.e. during the first two weeks of postnatal life. This constitutes a serious medical emergency as these babies deteriorate rapidly by developing profound and irreversible multiorgan dysfunction. Early recognition, aggressive resuscitation and prompt intervention are essential for optimal outcome. Resuscitation is the priority and stabilization in these highly sick infants must be speedily accomplished even before definitive diagnostic evaluation is done to prevent ongoing further decompensation.

Initially, when the ductus is open and systemic perfusion adequate, the baby appears relatively well with normally felt central pulses, and is often discharged from the maternity ward. As the ductus begins to constrict, these infants become dull, lethargic and feed poorly. On examination, they are sick looking, tachypneic, tachycardiac and have a mottled grey color with cool, clammy peripheries and delayed capillary refill. The femoral pulses are feeble or impalpable and often all central pulses are poorly felt. *An important differential of severe LVOTO is fulminant sepsis.* These babies are often mistakenly diagnosed as septic shock and managed accordingly with disastrous consequences.

Duct dependent systemic circulation is mandatory for survival in nearly 50% of all neonatal critical cardiac defects. This important fact must be borne in mind when confronted with a shocky newborn. Coarctation of aorta and HLHS together account for 90% of all infants presenting as shock. Early clinical signs of coarctation or aortic arch interruption include brachio-femoral pulse discrepancy which is confirmed on recording the upper and lower limb blood pressures.

Skiagram of chest shows a normal heart or cardiomegaly with or without early pulmonary edema. If the coarctation is severe and has been undetected for a prolonged period, the left ventricle steadily becomes dysfunctional with ejection fractions as low as 10–15% at presentation.

Hypoplastic left heart syndrome (HLHS) is the most common cause of cardiac death in the first week of life. These babies have a dimunitive left ventricle, critical aortic stenosis or aortic atresia, and sometimes mitral stenosis or mitral atresia. In severe cases, there is extensive aortic atresia or hypoplasia. These babies present with cardiovascular collapse after ductal closure and are often critically ill. The chest skiagram reveals cardiomegaly and increased pulmonary artery markings, and the EKG shows diminished left ventricular forces. Prior to ductal closure, many of these babies have subtle problems which can be detected by the discerning pediatrician. These signs include tachycardia, tachypnea, cyanosis and sometimes steadily weakening peripheral pulses. Likewise, babies with critical aortic stenosis have severe compromise of the systemic circulation after ductal closure and present in a manner similar to babies with hypoplastic left ventricle. In addition clinically, the second heart sound is single, there is often a well audible ejection systolic murmur and a third heart sound. *The chest skiagram shows cardiomegaly, occasionally pulmonary edema and the EKG shows left ventricular hypertrophy.*

Arrhythmias (Figures 24.7 and 24.8)

A newborn infant may present predominantly with either a tachyarrhythmia (heart rate >200/min) or a bradyarrhythmia (heart rate <70/min). *Both may lead to profoundly low cardiac output state and shock if unrecognized.* Birth asphyxia, hypothermia, sepsis, hypothyroidism are often associated with rhythm disturbances. In many instances there is no underlying structural heart disease. Ventricular dysfunction and electrolyte imbalance may also lead to various ventricular arrhythmias. Thus, it is important to get an electrocardiogram (ECG) done in a sick newborn presenting to the emergency. Likewise, if an arrhythmia is suspected, an ECHO is useful to assess both ventricular function and to exclude structural heart disease.

Tachyarrhythmias are more common compared to bradyarrhythmias. Newborns who have tachyarrhythmia comprise a serious medical emergency since no newborn can sustain heart rates of over 200/min for long. The common cause of tachyarrhythmia is supraventricular tachycardia (SVT) or narrow ventricular complex tachycardia. This is suspected when heart rates are more than 200, typically over 250/min, with a narrow QRS complex and no beat to beat variability (Figure 24.7). If the baby is clinically stable, the standard vagal maneuvers may be attempted, by ensuring that the airway is uncompromised. The options of vagal stimulation like placing a cold pack on the forehead while protecting the eyes, insertion of anal thermometer or anal probe or a nasogastric tube should be tried. Eyeball pressure and carotid massage in newborns are no longer advocated. If there is no repsonse within 10–20 seconds, then adenosine (100 µg/kg rapid push) may be tried. Adenosine should be given through a large central vein or through the antecubital vein for maximum effect. If not effective, adenosine dose may

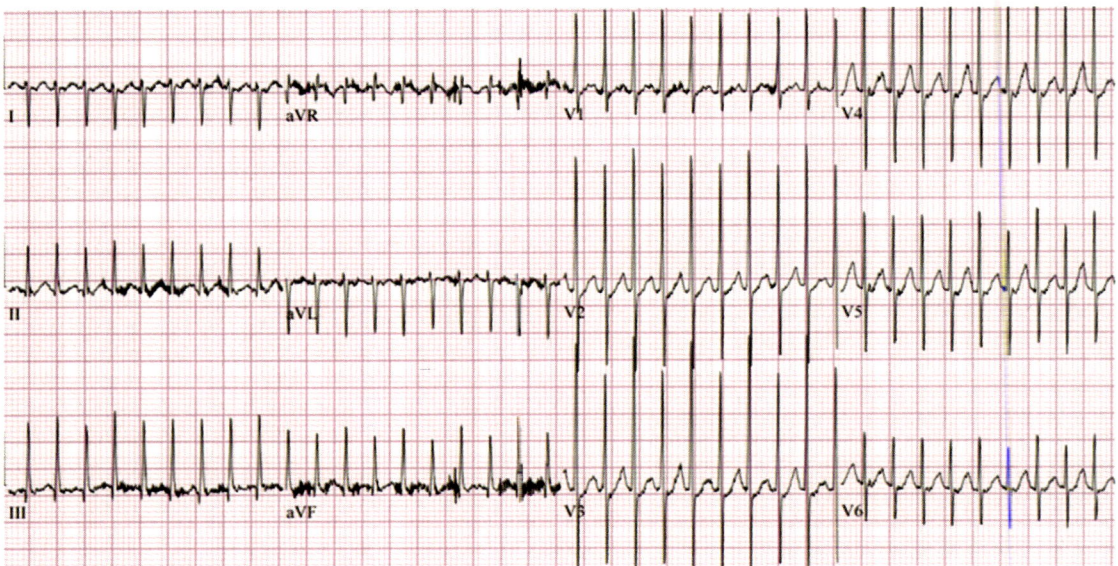

Figure 24.7 Supraventricular tachycardia in a neonate (HR >250/min).

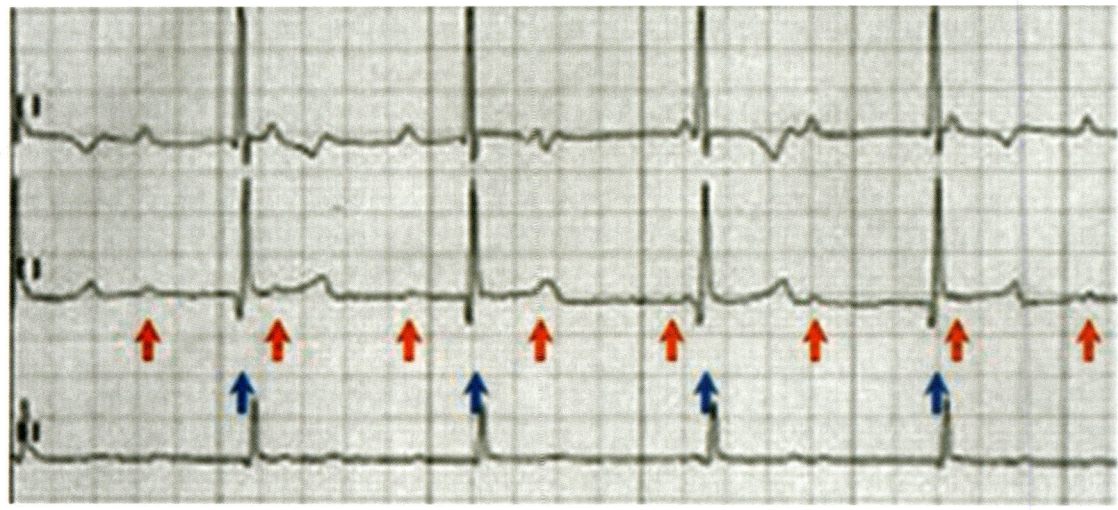

Figure 24.8 Congenital complete heart block (heart rate <60/min).

be increased in increments of 50 µg/kg up to a maximum of 500 µg/kg. Since adenosine acts by blocking the atrioventricular node, occasionally the baby may develop ventricular tachycardia needing resuscitation. If there is no response to adenosine, esmolol or amiodarone may be used. If the newborn with SVT is unstable at presentation, or if none of the above measures restore sinus rhythm, then synchronized cardioversion should be tried (Table 24.2).

All attempts should be made to restore sinus rhythm. Once sinus rhythm is restored it must be remembered that in many instances, the tachyarrhythmia recurs. The baby must be seen by a pediatric cardiologist and is likely to need long-term medications with a beta blocker like propranolol or metoprolol, and amiodarone or

Table 24.2 Therapeutic options for neonatal supraventricular tachycardia

1. Hemodynamically stable
   a. Vagal maneuvers (ice in plastic bag, anal thermometer)
   b. Adenosine 100 µg/kg rapid IV push; may be increased to 500 µg/kg in 50 µg increments until response occurs
   c. Esmolol bolus dose of 200 to 500 µg/kg over 10 minutes, followed by 50–100 µg/kg as maintenance
   d. Amiodarone bolus of 25 mg/kg/min infused over 60 to 90 minutes followed by continuous infusion of 5 to 15 µg/kg/min
   e. Synchronized DC cardioversion at 0.5 to 4 Joules/kg

2. Hemodynamically unstable
   a. Immediate synchronized DC cardioversion at 0.5 to 4 Joules/kg
   b. Transesophageal pacing if available

occasionally both. At present arrhythmia management is highly sophisticated and is done in close collaboration with an electrophysiologist and these aspects are beyond the purview of this chapter. Prognosis is often excellent and not infrequently there is spontaneous resolution by the second year of life. If there is sustained tachyarrhythmia, it is prudent to contact a pediatric cardiologist for a telephonic advice. Most pediatric cardiologists have experience with recurring or sustained tachyarrhythmias and will be able to effectively guide on the choice of immediate medications.

Bradyarrhythmias are typically due to congenital heart block occurring either *de novo* or due to maternal lupus erythematosus. These infants need to be speedily transferred to a cardiac unit where a permanent pacemaker can be placed if needed. Current indications for provision of a pacemaker in a newborn include (i) ventricular dysfunction, (ii) heart failure, (iii) heart rate <55–60/min. Pacemakers are placed surgically in the epicardial area and most surgical units today perform these procedures without any complications. These infants need ongoing review in a cardiac unit to ensure smooth pacemaker functioning and to detect early malfunction of the pacemaker.

MANAGEMENT OF THE CRITICALLY ILL CARDIAC NEONATE (Figures 24.9 and 24.10)

The initial management of a neonate with critical heart disease greatly impacts eventual surgical or interventional outcome. A baby who reaches a specialized unit in a stable condition has a much better chance of intact survival than a baby who arrives in a moribund, preterminal state. Delayed diagnosis of neonatal heart disease and presentation in a sick state with circulatory collapse, severe metabolic acidosis or organ dysfunction have been shown to be associated with both higher post operative morbidity and mortality.

It is useful to remember some unique aspects of neonatal physiology in order to manage these fragile neonates more effectively. Neonates are extremely intolerant to increased afterload as well as to diminished preload due to intravascular hypovolemia. They also respond badly to greatly increased preload which means that any volume augmentation has to be gentle, in small boluses (~5 mL/kg) and periodically reviewed for further volume requirements. Large boluses of 20–30 mL/kg are very poorly tolerated and many neonates may show catastrophic hemodynamic deterioration with such large fluid boluses. Newborns have increased pulmonary vascular resistance at birth, and they are prone to develop pulmonary hypertension.

The successful management of a neonate with a critical cardiac defect is based on a systematic meticulous approach. A high index of suspicion on the

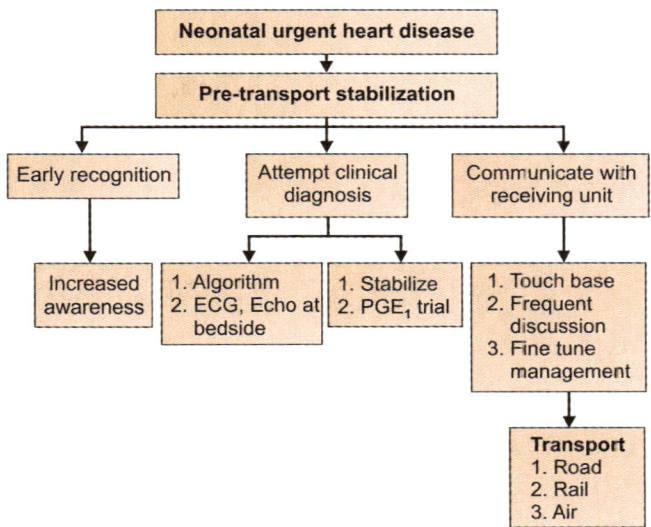

Figure 24.9 Approach to a critically ill cardiac newborn.

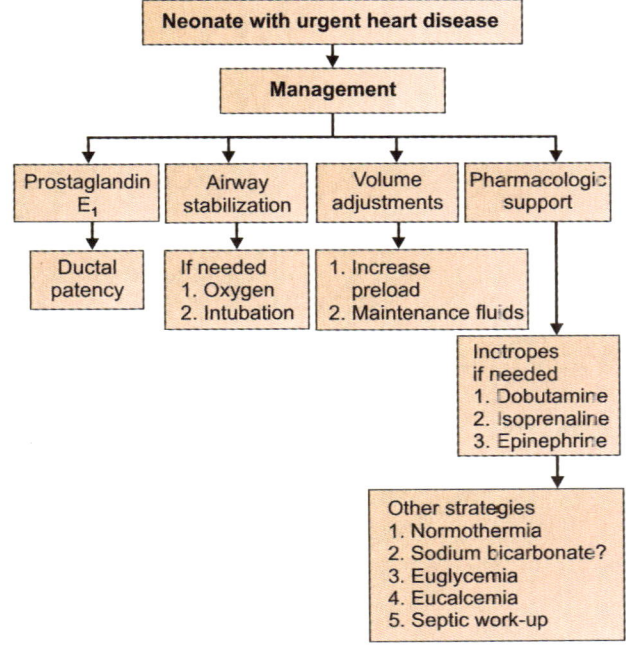

Figure 24.10 Stabilization of the critically ill cardiac newborn.

part of the pediatrician is essential for these chain of interventions to be initiated on an urgent basis.

1. *Prompt referral and safe transport to a tertiary center* is necessary. In many instances road transport may be feasible, but increasingly transfer by rail or air has been successfully accomplished in our country. The safety of transfer would depend on the nature of the cardiac defect, the clinical status of the neonate and the distance to be travelled. *Ideally transfer is best organized in close consultation with the receiving cardiac team, so that optimal stabilization, with the available resources of the referring doctor or team, is done prior to transfer.*

2. Accurate diagnosis is important and this is achieved by cross-sectional echocardiography with color Doppler which provides information both on the structural defect and the alterations of flow dynamics.

3. In many instances even today, immediate access to echo may not be feasible. In that situation, several measures need to be initiated even on clinical suspicion of critical heart disease for example a cyanotic or shocky neonate.

4. Essential principles of management include measures to improve cardiac output and tissue perfusion swiftly.

5. The following simple steps help to stabilize these babies in most instances.

a. *Restoration of ductal circulation* Stabilization involves in most instances timely restoration of ductal circulation to maintain systemic or pulmonary blood flow and enhance intercirculatory mixing. If the newborn is not too unwell, very often this is all that is needed to stabilize the baby. Ductal patency is maintained by initiation of prostaglandin E_1 (PGE_1) infusion in doses of 0.025–0.1 µg/min. PGE_1 is commenced on clinical suspicion, in a shocky neonate during the first week of life or in a neonate who is visibly cyanotic or who fails the hyperoxia test. A neonate should ideally be watched for 30–60 minutes prior to transport after commencing PGE_1. The common side effects include apnea (12%), vasodilatation (10%), fever (14%), bradycardia (7%), and seizures (4%). PGE_1 has been recently reviewed extensively and found effective to maintain oxygenation and ductal patency at doses of 0.003–0.02 µg/kg with lower rates of apnea at lower doses. PGE_1 has also been found to be effective even weeks after ductal closure. Therefore, it is worth a try even in the older shocky or cyanotic neonate.

Occasionally, clinical deterioration is noted following commencement of PGE_1. This may occur in the absence of a ductus, an unresponsive ductus or in the presence of obstruction at the foramen ovale or pulmonary veins. Structural heart defects associated with clinical deterioration with PGE_1 include obstructed total anomalous pulmonary veins, restrictive patent foramen ovale with dTGA and intact ventricular septum, hypoplastic left heart syndrome or mitral atresia with restrictive patent foramen ovale. *In the event of deterioration, PGE_1 should be immediately stopped and the baby re-evaluated by ECHO whenever possible.*

If the baby appears to stabilize, it is useful to use this window and swiftly organize a transfer to the receiving cardiac unit. The ongoing communication with the hi-tec unit cardiologist, or intensivist is the key to a stable and smooth transfer.

b. *Advanced life support including appropriate ventilation* The basic life support begins by ensuring good airway management. It is tempting to give supplemental oxygen to a cyanotic newborn. *However, oxygen has little benefit in a cyanotic neonate unless the baby has severe pulmonary hypertension due to total anomalous venous connection (TAPVC).* In fact, needless and inappropriate oxygen therapy may cause pulmonary overcirculation and pulmonary edema due to the pulmonary vasodilator effect of oxygen along with severely reduced peripheral circulation in HLHS and complex single ventricle situations where the goal of stabilization is to maintain a Qp: Qs ratio close to 1. Thus supplemental oxygen should be given only after consultation with a pediatric cardiologist, since it may not confer any benefit and may harm the neonate.

Intubation may be needed if the baby is apneic after PGE_1, deeply cyanosed or has respiratory distress. The potential complications of elective intubation prior to transport needs to be carefully balanced against the possible risks of accidental tube dislodgement, over ventilation, and air leaks.

c. *Maintain euvolemia* Normal or reduced maintenance fluids are needed in these neonates to maintain euvolemia. Additional volume augmentation may be required in many of these neonates due to the non-compliant neonatal myocardium or PGE_1 induced vasodilatory hypotension. Volume repletion may be achieved with normal saline, dextrose saline or albumin.

d. *Inotropic support to the myocardium* Myocardial support by inotropes is often needed to improve myocardial contractility and tissue perfusion once intravascular volume has been replenished. Delayed diagnosis is often associated with right ventricular or left ventricular dysfunction or biventricular dysfunction. Dobutamine is the preferred inotrope, occasionally epinephrine or isoprenaline is used in the presence of a slow heart rate.

e. *Correction of metabolic derangements* The negative inotropic effect of hypoglycemia, acidosis and hypocalcemia are often underestimated, and if uncorrected these metabolic derangements may lead to rapidly progressive irreversible deterioration. In fact profound and sustained hypocalcemia has been shown to cause severe, potentially lethal systolic and diastolic ventricular dysfunction which is easily reversed by restoration of normocalcemia. Likewise, hypoglycemia, hypothermia and hyperthermia need to be corrected due to their negative metabolic effects on the myocardium and the baby.

f. *Management of sepsis and other co-morbidities* Many critically sick neonates have coexisting Gram-negative, or positive bacterial or fungal sepsis. It is appropriate to initiate broad spectrum antimicrobial and/or antifungal therapy after drawing samples for blood cultures, so that window of timely management of sepsis is not missed. Later, if cultures are reported as negative, the receiving unit can stop antimicrobial therapy. Hypothyroidism is not uncommon in these infants, it should be identified and treated by replacement therapy. Additional malformations, like esophageal atresia, various syndromes or sequences and chromosomal abnormalities (Trisomy 21) should be looked for, and appropriately addressed.

The aforementioned measures usually help in improving perfusion and secondary tissue and metabolic acidosis. *Sodium bicarbonate correction is usually not required and may even be associated with poor outcome. In the event of refractory metabolic acidosis, half correction may be cautiously achieved.* Older neonates with heart failure should be managed with medications like diuretics, spironolactone and digoxin if needed. Acute deterioration may need admission and myocardial support with an inotrope and intravenous diuretics. If the baby tires while feeding, the infant may need assisted feeding through a feeding tube.

Prognosis

In this section, common and important cardiac conditions will be briefly reviewed, to acquaint a pediatrician with current advances in neonatal cardiovascular disorders, so that he or she is in a better position to guide, counsel and support families of babies with cardiac defects. The arterial switch operation (aorta is re-connected to the left ventricle (LV) and main pulmonary artery to the right ventricle) is the most physiologic solution for dTGA with intact ventricular septum. The morphologic left ventricle begins to regress rapidly after birth but it is uncertain when the regression becomes irreversible. Once the left ventricle regresses then it is not in a position to support the systemic circulation and such babies develop severe refractory unrelenting low output state postoperatively. *Thus in most instances, the arterial switch operation should be done in the first month of life and preferably in the first two weeks of life. It is important that babies with dTGA and intact septum are diagnosed, stabilized and referred to an appropriate center before this window period of one month, preferably within the first two weeks so that the optimal surgical option can be offered to these babies.* If an arterial switch is performed at the ideal age and under stable conditions, the current mortality of dTGA is as low as 0–5%. Long-term outcomes are also excellent with good quality of life and mainstream integration of the survivors.

Palliative balloon atrial septostomy to enhance intercirculatory mixing is rarely done in most units, instead corrective arterial switch operation is preferred by most cardiac surgeons. Occasionally, if the baby has florid sepsis or organ dysfunction, a balloon atrial septostomy is done to stabilize the baby and as a bail out, till corrective surgery can be offered. Infants with dTGA with ventricular septal defect may be successfully operated (arterial switch with ventricular septal defect closure) in the first 3 months. dTGA with ventricular septal defect and coarctation or arch interruption tend to be sicker, present earlier and need arterial switch with ventricular septal defect closure as well as repair of the coarctation. In the past, this subset of patients had high surgical mortality rates, but currently their surgical mortality is less than 5%.

Newborns with significant right sided obstruction (RVOTO with any underlying anatomy) urgently need an alternative source of pulmonary blood flow in the form of a surgically placed communication between the systemic and pulmonary circulation, most often a modification of the Blalock-Taussig shunt. In the event of isolated pulmonary valve stenosis, a balloon valvotomy (catheter intervention) is often enough and is usually life-saving. Early results depend on the underlying anatomy, those with tetralogy of Fallot do well both in the short-term and in the long-term. Infants with ventricular septal defect and pulmonary atresia need a shunt followed by a right ventricle to pulmonary artery conduit, i.e. creation of an artificial connection between the right ventricle and branch of pulmonary arteries. This means multiple lifelong surgeries, since the conduit needs replacement as the child grows and in the event of conduit calcification. Neonates with pulmonary atresia with intact ventricular septum, and tricuspid atresia with dimunitive right ventricle, need multiple staged palliative surgeries, the final surgery being the Fontan operation. These babies have effectively only a single ventricle and are called single ventricle physiology. These are not curative procedures, and they need lifelong palliative procedures, their current long-term 10 year and 20 year survival being about 75 % and 60% respectively. Thus, families need to be carefully counseled and told about the need for repeated surgical interventions with associated social and financial implications.

Newborns with critical coarctation and arch interruption are also relatively common critical cardiac defects presenting in the newborn period. Definitive surgery is possible in early life with excellent early outcomes.

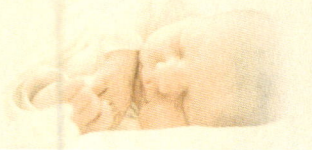

Many infants with a hypoplastic aortic arch tend to develop re-coarctation and may need repeat surgery or catheter ballooning. Likewise, infants with aortic valvular stenosis can be readily managed with ballooning of the aortic valve. In most infants repeated procedures are done, since the valve tends to re-stenose and about half need aortic valve replacement in later life.

The last two decades have witnessed improvements in the mangement of hypoplastic left heart syndrome (HLHS). This again falls into the group of single ventricle physiology, the functional ventricle being the right ventricle. Management involves multiple staged surgeries, hybrid procedures, with interstage attrition and finally culminating in the Fontan operation. Long-term studies have shown that HLHS is a significant risk for Fontan failure and long-term mortality and the current 5 year survival after multiple surgeries is 50–70%. Many centers in India do not offer these options to families and parents should embark on such procedures only if they are mentally prepared for the arduous path ahead. Many parents also opt for termination of pregnancy when HLHS is diagnosed *in utero*, therefore incidence of affected infants is gradually declining.

Babies with total anomalous pulmonary venous connection do not benefit from any form of stabilization. They need urgent surgical rerouting of the pulmonary veins to the left atrium. Initially, a high mortality procedure (nearly 20% surgical mortality) due to late diagnosis and severe postoperative pulmonary hypertension and low cardiac output, the current survival has improved to 90–95% because of improvements in surgical technique, cardiac intensive care and assisted ventilation support. Our early survival of these infants is currently 97%.

Commonly Missed Neonatal Heart Defects

Serious heart defects missed at the time of discharge from the maternity unit include dTGA. IVS, severe coarctation of the aorta including arch interruption and HLHS. Of these, about 40% of those discharged undiagnosed, tend to present later with circulatory collapse. Likewise, in the absence of pulse oximetry screening, nearly half of infants with dTGA. IVS, an entity with excellent outcome, are likely to leave the maternity ward undetected and present later with cerebral bleeds or other neuromotor sequelae. *The most common entity that gets commonly missed during newborn period is coarctation of the aorta, a condition with excellent early and long-term outcomes.* Another condition with a good surgical outcome that is often mistakenly treated as hyaline membrane disease is obstructed total anomalous pulmonary venous connection.

Complications Associated with Delayed Diagnosis

There are several issues associated with delayed diagnosis with subsequent adverse outcome. The delayed diagnosis of neonatal heart disease is associated with increased preoperative cardiovascular compromise and organ dysfunction which adversely affect the surgical outcome. The organs prone to be affected include kidneys, bowel, liver, heart and the brain with development of acute kidney injury, necrotizing entero-colitis, varying degrees of myocardial dysfunction and brain injury. Prolonged lactic acidosis has been shown to correlate well with neurological insults and brain injury. Delayed neonatal diagnosis has been shown to be associated with increased post operative mortality as well as increased duration of ventilation and post operative length of stay in the hospital.

Currently, there is renewed interest in neurological injury and neonatal heart disease. Preoperative brain injury in neonates with complex congenital heart disease (CHD) is widely prevalent, ranging from 26% to 41% in various studies and is associated with future neurodevelopmental disabilities. It is more commonly associated with HLHS and other cases of single ventricle physiology like transposition of great arteries (dTGA) and tetralogy of Fallot. The development of brain injury is multifactorial, contributed by intrauterine hemo-dynamic alterations, congenital brain abnormalities, and more importantly acquired brain injury related to prolonged hypoxia or significant hypoperfusion after birth. Balloon atrial septostomy (BAS) has also been shown to be a possible risk factor for preoperative focal brain injury (strokes) in neonates with TGA, but this has been challenged in subsequent studies.

Advances in medicine, including prenatal diagnosis, innovations in cardiothoracic surgical techniques and improvements in perioperative management have contributed to the greatly increased survival of infants with complex CHD but this is associated with an increase in neurodevelopmental morbidities. Our initial unit policy was to perform a brain ultrasound prior to neonatal cardiac surgery or catheter intervention. We have now moved to a screening CT scan or MRI brain to look for associated cerebral abnormalities and hypoxic ischemic injury before surgery or catheter intervention. When there are severe CNS abnormalities or diffuse ischemic brain injury preoperatively, infant is offered only palliative care.

The pediatricians and those caring for newborns need to be aware of these preoperative or pre catheter intervention "screening neuroimaging" practices being adopted worldwide as well as the well-founded reasons for these practices.

Early Detection of Neonatal Heart Disease

There is increasing evidence that prenatal diagnosis of complex CHD is associated with better post surgical morbidity and mortality as well as future neurocognitive outcomes. *Both coarctation of aorta as well as dTGA are difficult to diagnose antenatally unless the screening protocol is extremely detailed.* However, improved antenatal detection rates have been reported in recent times. When critical heart disease is suspected prenatally, ideally the delivery should be planned in a specialized unit or close to a cardiac center to obviate profound and needless hypoxemia with consequent injury to brain and other body organs.

In the absence of universal prenatal diagnosis, our goal should be early neonatal diagnosis of critical congenital heart disease. A prospective Swedish study published nearly eight years ago showed that a predischarge comprehensive neonatal screening (a thorough physical examination including femoral pulses + pulse oximetry screening) diagnosed more than 80% of duct dependent heart disease and 100% of duct dependent pulmonary circulation. The danger of leaving the hospital with undetected critical heart disease was nearly 30% without pulse oximetry screening. A pulse oximetry screening is considered positive if the preductal (right hand) or post ductal saturation (feet) is less than 95% or if the difference between preductal and post ductal saturations is >3%. In this Swedish study no baby with dTGA left the hospital undiagnosed as compared to *44% or nearly half of dTGA infants were not diagnosed at the time of discharge when oximetry was not used.* Unfortunately, over 25% of those undiagnosed either died or suffered serious cerebral bleeds or hypoxic-ischemic damage.

The most commonly missed duct dependent heart disease on pulse oximetry screening is critical coarctation and aortic arch interruption, both prone to cardiovascular collapse, reiterating *the need for a high index of suspicion of aortic arch obstruction in any critically sick newborn with shock.* Subsequent to several other studies, screening pulse oximetry has now become the standard of care in many countries in Europe, South East Asia as well as in USA after endorsement by the Department of Health and Human Services in 2011 for early diagnosis of neonatal critical heart disease.

Summary

Early and long-term survival both after surgery and catheter intervention has improved dramatically for most forms of critical neonatal heart disease over the last few years. Long-term prognosis for life-threatening defects like dTGA and various forms of aortic arch obstruction is good with reasonable quality of life. These facts underscore the importance of diagnosing potentially lethal cardiac defects before they present with circulatory collapse and their early and aggressive management. *The risk of missed cardiac diagnosis can be minimized by a comprehensive predischarge neonatal examination including pulse oximetry screening.* A systematic approach to a critically ill newborn enables a speedy diagnosis of cardiac defect and appropriate stabilization prior to transfer to a cardiac unit.

Key Points

- The burden of neonatal heart disease is huge in our country, about 150,000–200,000 neonates are born with cardiac malformations each year in India. Of these about 30,000 have potentially life-threatening heart disease leading to cardiovascular collapse and death if unrecognized.
- A sick cardiac newborn typically presents with cyanosis, respiratory distress, heart failure, cardiovascular collapse or arrhythmia.
- Those who present with cyanosis either have dTGA or cardiac defects with reduced pulmonary blood flow.
- The common neonatal critical heart diseases are dTGA and coarctation of the aorta. These two lesions have excellent early surgical survival and good long-term outcomes.
- Management of the cardiac neonate is no longer a futile exercise. Most surgical or catheter procedures in neonates are associated with 90–95% discharge survival.
- Critical neonatal heart disease usually has duct dependent systemic circulation or pulmonary blood flow or circulatory mixing and is called as duct dependent heart disease.
- Critical neonatal heart disease typically presents in a dramatic fashion at the time of ductal closure.
- Sick cardiac newborns may also have non-ductus dependent circulation, e.g. obstructed total anomalous pulmonary venous connection.
- Neonatal arrhythmias constitute an important neonatal cardiac emergency.
- A systematic approach to suspected neonatal heart disease is associated with reduced morbidity and improved survival.
- The conditions most commonly missed at discharge from a newborn unit are dTGA, coarctation of aorta and total anomalous pulmonary venous connection with catastrophic consequences. These conditions have good surgical outcomes.
- Comprehensive neonatal screening (examination of femorals and pulse oximetry screening) reduces the

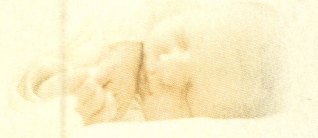

incidence of missed diagnosis. However, aortic arch obstruction or coarctation of aorta may still be missed.

- Delayed diagnosis is associated with adverse surgical outcome, organ dysfunction and brain injury.
- Single ventricle situations (HLHS and tricuspid atresia) are managed by multiple staged surgeries with 10 year survival being 50–75%.
- Early stabilization involves restoration of ductal circulation with infusion of PGE_1 along with other measures of advanced life support.
- Neonatal tachyarrhythmias have excellent prognosis and should be managed as per standard protocol.
- The outcome of neonatal heart disease is steadily improving, serious attempts should be made to detect them either prenatally or soon after birth to ensure prompt management.

BIBLIOGRAPHY

Abu-Harb M, Hey E, Wren C. Death in infancy from unrecognised congenital heart disease. *Arch Dis Child* 1994; 71:3–7.

Alwi M, Geetha K, Bilkis AA, Lim MK, Hasri S, Haifa AL, Sallehudin A, Zambahari R. Pulmonary atresia with intact ventricular septum percutaneous radiofrequency-assisted valvotomy and balloon dilation versus surgical valvotomy and Blalock Taussig shunt. *J Am Coll Cardiol* 2000 Feb; 35(2):468–76.

Bonnet D, Coltri A, Butera G, Fermont L, Le Bidois K, Kachaner J, Sidi D. Detection of transposition of the great arteries in fetuses reduces neonatal morbidity and mortality. *Circulation* 1999; 99(7): 916–18.

Brossard-Racine M, du Plessis A, Vezina G, Robertson R, Donofrio M, Tworetzky W, Limperopoulos C. Brain Injury in neonates with complex congenital heart disease: What is the predictive value of MRI in the fetal period? *Am J Neuroradiol* 2016; 7(37):1338–46.

Brown KL, Ridout DA, Hoskote A, Verhulst A, Ricci M, Bull C. Delayed diagnosis of congenital heart disease worsens preoperative condition and outcome of surgery in neonates. *Heart* 2006; 92:1298–1302.

Browning Carmo KA, Barr P, West M, Hopper NW, White JP, Badawi N. Transporting newborn infants with suspected duct dependent congenital heart disease on low dose prostaglandin E_1 without routine mechanical ventilation. *Arch Dis Child Fetal Neonat Ed* 2007; 92:F117–F119.

Calderon J, Angeard N, Moutier S, Plumet MH, Jambaque I, Bonnet D. Impact of prenatal diagnosis on neurocognitive outcomes in children with transposition of the great arteries. *J Pediatr* 2012; 161(1):94–98.

Fesseha AK, Eidem BW, Dibardino DJ, Cron SG, McKenzie ED, Fraser CD Jr, Price JF, Chang AC, Mott AR. Neonates with aortic coarctation and cardiogenic shock: presentation and outcomes. *Ann Thorac Surg* 2005; 79:1650–55.

Frank LH, Bradshaw E, Beekman R, Mahle WT, Martin GR. Critical congenital heart disease screening using pulse oximetry. *J Pediatr* 2013; 162(3):445–53.

Freed M, Heyman M, Rudolph A, Roehl SL, Kensey RC. Prostaglandin E_1 in ductus arteriosus dependent congenital heart disease. *Circulation* 1981; 64;889–905.

Granelli AD, Wennergren M, Sandberg K, Mellander M, Bejlum C, Inganas L, Eriksson M, Segerdahl N, Agren A, Ekman-Joelsson B, Sunnegardh J, Verdicchio M, Ostman-Smith I. Impact of pulse oximetry screening on the detection of duct-dependent congenital heart disease: a Swedish prospective screening study in 39,821 newborns. *BMJ* 2009; 8;338:a3037. http://dx.doi.org/10.1136/bmj.a3037

Hasegawa T, Masuda M, Okumura M, Arai H, Kobayashi J, Saiki Y, Tanemoto K, Nishida H, Motomura N. Trends and outcomes in neonatal cardiac surgery for congenital heart disease in Japan from 1996 to 2010. *Eur J Cardiothorac Surg* 2017; 51:301–07.

Huang FK, Lin CC, Huang TC, Weng KP, Liu PY, Chen YY, Wang HP, Ger LP, Hsieh KS. Reappraisal of the prostaglandin E_1 dose for early newborn care with patent ductus arteriosus–dependant pulmonary circulation. *Pediatr neonatal* 2013; 54:102–106.

Iyengar AJ, Winlaw DS, Galati JC, Wheaton GR, Gentles TL, Grigg LE, Justo RN, Radford DJ, Weintraub RG, Bullock A, Celermajar DS, d'Udekem Y. The extracardiac conduit Fontan procedure in Australia and New Zealand: hypoplastic left heart syndrome predicts worse early and late outcomes. *Euro J Cardio-Thorac Surg* 2014 Sep; 46(3):465–73.

Iyer PU, Kaur H, Awasthy N. Congestive heart failure: In PG Textbook of Pediatrics. Vol 2. (eds) Gupta P, Menon PSN, Ramji S, Lodha R. 1st edition, *New Delhi, Jaypee Brothers Medical Publishers Ltd*; 2015; pp 1909–18.

Jenkins KJ, Castaneda AR, Cherian KM, Couser CA, Dale EK, Gauvreau K, Hickey PA, Kupiec JK, Morrow DF, Novick WM, Rangel SJ, Zheleva B, Christenson JT. Reducing mortality and infections after congenital heart surgery in the developing world. *Pediatrics* 2014; 134(5):1422–30.

Kelle AM, Backer CL, Gossett JG, Kaushal S, Mavroudis C. Total anomalous pulmonary venous connection : Result for surgical repair of 100 patients at a single institution. *J Thorac Cardiovasc Surg* 2010; 139:1387–94.

Kuehl KS, Loffredo CA, Ferencz C. Failure to diagnose congenital heart disease in infancy. *Pediatrics* 1999; 103:743–47.

Kumar G, Iyer PU. Management of perioperative low cardiac output state without extracorporeal life support: What is feasible? *Annals Pediatr Cardiol* 2010; 3(2):147–58.

Kumar G, Iyer PU. Neonatal cardiac emergencies In : Principles of Pediatric and Neonatal Emergencies. Choudhury P, Bagga A, Chugh K, Ramji S, Gupta P. (Eds.) 3rd ed, *New Delhi : Jaypee Brothers Medical publishers (P) Ltd*; 2011. pp 579–590.

Mahle WT, Martin GR, Beekman RH 3rd, Morrow WR. Endorsement of health and human services recommendation for pulse oximetry screening for critical congenital heart disease. *Pediatrics* 2012; 129(1):190–92.

McQuillen PS, Hamrick S EG, Perez MJ, Barkovich AJ, Glidden DV, Karl TR, Teitel D, Miller SP. Balloon atrial septostomy is associated with preoperative stroke in neonates with transposition of the great arteries. *Circulation* 2006; 113:280–85.

Meckler GD, Lowe C. To intubate or not to intubate? Transporting infants on prostaglandin E_1. *Pediatrics* 2009; 123:e25–e30.

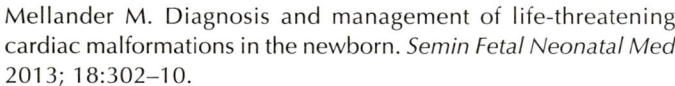
Mellander M. Diagnosis and management of life-threatening cardiac malformations in the newborn. *Semin Fetal Neonatal Med* 2013; 18:302–10.

Miller SP, C.M, McQuillen PS, Hamrick S, Xu D, Glidden DV, Charlton N, Karl T, Azakie A, Ferriero DM, Barkovich AJ, Vigneron DB. Abnormal brain development in newborns with congenital heart disease. *N Engl J Med* 2007; 357:1928–38.

Petit CJ, Rome JJ, Wernovsky G, Mason SE, Shera DM, Nicolson SC, Montenegro LM, Tabbutt S, Zimmerman RA, Licht DJ. Preoperative brain injury in transposition of great arteries in association with oxygenation and time to surgery, not balloon atrial septostomy. *Circulation* 2009; 119:709–16.

Prudhoe S, Abu-Harb M, Richmond S, Wren C. Neonatal screening for critical cardiovascular anomalies using pulse oximetry. *Arch Dis Child Fetal Neonatal Ed* 2013; 98(4):346–50.

Pundi KN, Johnson JN, Dearani JA, Pundi KN, Li Z, Hinck CA, Dalh SH, Cannon BC, O'Leary PW, Driscoll DJ, Cetta F. 40-year follow-up after the Fontan operation. *J Am Coll Cardiol* 2015; 66:1700–10.

Raju V, Burkhart HM, Durham LA, Eidem BW, Phillips SD, Li Z, Schaff H, Dearani JA. Reoperation after arterial switch : A 27 years Experience. *Ann Thorac Surg* 2013; 95:2105–13.

Saxena A. How to deliver the best: a call for action for congenital heart disease treatment in India. *Future Cardiol* 2014; 10:359–66.

St Louis JD, Harvey BA, Menk JS, Raghuveer G, O'Brien JE, Bryant R, Kochilas L. Repair of "Simple" total anomalous pulmonary venous connection: A review from the Pediatric Cardiac Care Consort um. *Ann Thorac Surg* 2012 July; 94(1):133–38.

Stevenson DK, Benitz WE. A practical approach to diagnosis and immediate care of the cyanotic neonate. Stabilization and preparation for transfer to level III nursery. *Clin Pediatr* 1987; 26:325–30.

Tobler D, Williams WG, Jegatheeswaran A, Van Arsdel GS, McCrindle BW, Greutmann M, Oechslin EN, Silversides CK. Cardiac outcomes in young adult survivors of the arterial switch operation for transposition of great arteries. *J Am Coll Cardiol* 2010; 56:58–64.

Wessel DL, Fraisse A. Preoperative care of the pediatric cardiac surgical patient. In: Rogers's Textbook of Pediatric Intensive Care. 4th ed. *Philadelphia: Lippincott Williams & Wilkins*; 2008: pp1149–1158.

Yates MC, Rao PS. Pediatric cardiac emergencies. *Emergency Med* 2013; 3(6):1–7.

Yoshimura N, Yamaguchi M. Surgical strategy for pulmonary atresia with intact ventricular septum: initial management and definitive surgery. *Gen Thorac Cardiovasc Surg* 2009; 57:338–46.

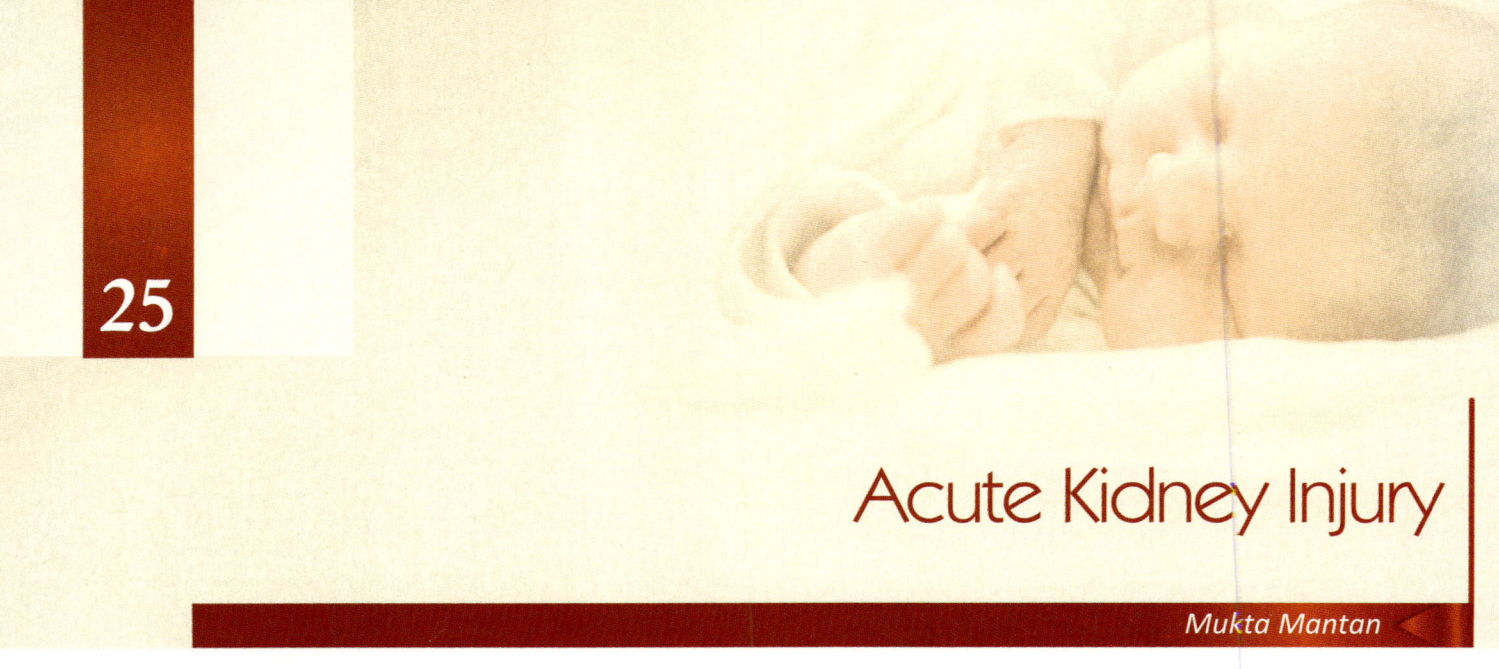

25

Acute Kidney Injury

Mukta Mantan

Acute kidney injury (AKI), previously known as acute renal failure (ARF), is an important emergency in neonates where prompt and appropriate management is life-saving. AKI usually occurs in neonates with previously normal renal function but may rarely be superimposed on pre-existing renal disease (acute-on-chronic renal failure).

Nomenclature and Classification

In the absence of a universally accepted definition and recognition that ARF comprises of a spectrum of clinical conditions, the term acute kidney injury (AKI) has recently been proposed for the entire spectrum of the syndrome. Acute kidney injury (AKI) is defined as an increase in serum creatinine by ≥0.3 mg/dL within 48 hours; or an increase in serum creatinine by ≥1.5 times of baseline, which is known or presumed to have occurred within the prior 7 days; or a urine volume of <0.5 mL/kg/hr for 6 hours. The AKI is further classified into 3 stages based on rise of serum creatinine or change in urine volume. It is recommended to use Kidney Disease: Improving Global Outcomes (KDIGO) classification for an early diagnosis of AKI so that necessary steps are taken to prevent the progression of the condition.

Staging of AKI based on glomerular filtration rate, serum creatinine and urine output has been proposed (Table 25.1), but it requires validation in neonates. In 2007 the AKIN (Acute Kidney Injury Network); a group comprising of experts from critical care and nephrology societies modified the staging (pediatric RIFLE) to suit the needs of the children and described the new classification as AKIN. A retrospective study from Brazil by Bezerra et al collected data from 312 neonates and found an association between urine output of <1.5 mL/kg/hr for 24 hours and mortality. Based on their findings they have proposed a neonatal RIFLE (nRIFLE) criteria where R stands for urine output <1.5 mL/kg/hr and injury as urine output <1.0 mL/kg/hr for 24 hours. However, till this classification is further validated it is suggested to use the KDIGO classification for neonates.

Table 25.1 KDIGO classification of acute kidney injury		
AKI severity	Serum creatinine	Urine output*
Stage I	1.5–1.9 times of baseline OR >0.3 mg/dL increase from baseline	<0.5 mL/kg/hr for 6–12 hr
Stage II	Increase by ≥2–2.9 times of baseline	<0.5 mL/kg/hr for ≥12hr
Stage III	Increase by 3.0 times of baseline OR Increase in serum creatinine to >4.0 mg/dL OR Initiation of renal replacement therapy OR In patients <18 years, decrease in eGFR to <35 mL/min per 1.73 m²	<0.3 mL/kg/hr for 24 hr or anuria for 12 hr

*Urine output criteria may not be very reliable in first 3 days after birth

Criteria for AKI in Infants

AKI is suspected in a neonate if any of the following criteria are met:

1. Plasma creatinine >1.5 mg/dL for at least 24–48 hours.
2. Rise in serum creatinine by 0.3 mg/dL over the baseline.
3. Serum creatinine fails to fall below the maternal levels by 5–7 days (in preterm babies it may take longer).
4. Oliguria defined as urinary output <1 mL/kg/hr after first day of life.

Criteria based on urine output may not be very reliable in first 3 days of life as newborns have a low GFR and the urine output is less during this period. Roughly about 17% neonates have their first void in the delivery room, 90% void urine by 24 hours and 99% by 48 hours. AKI can also present with normal urine output in one third of the cases especially in asphyxiated neonates. It is, therefore, essential to monitor plasma creatinine apart from urine output.

Neonatal Renal Physiology

Urine production by fetal kidneys begins by 12 weeks of gestation. The peak or maximum number of glomeruli are developed by 36 weeks of gestation and after that only the size of the glomeruli increases. There is a low mean arterial pressure (MAP) in the fetal period leading to low renal blood flow and a high renal vascular resistance. The primary mechanism for maintaining GFR in the presence of low MAP is a post-glomerular efferent vascular constriction mediated by angiotensin II. Due to this the newborns have a high plasma renin activity. Any inhibiton of angiotensin due to use of ACE inhibitors or angiotensin receptor blockers (ARBs) in the mother during the antenatal period can predispose to neonatal AKI. Endothelin is the second most potent vasoconstrictor and is expressed more in neonates and high levels are seen in the immediate postnatal period. The plasma atrial natriuretic peptide (ANP) levels are also elevated in first few days and it tries to reduce the expanded extracellular fluid volume. Also there are high circulating levels of vasodilatory prostaglandins. Any inhibition of these prostaglandins by use of drugs like indomethacin or ibuprofen in early neonatal period, for the closure of PDA especially in preterms, can predispose to neonatal AKI.

The GFR at birth is about 20 mL/min/m² in term neonates and there is a rapid increase in GFR in first 2 weeks after birth. The preterm infants have a slower rate of rise of GFR. Normal GFR values are attained by 1–2 years of age. Also the tubular development is slow in the first few months and this predisposes to decreased reabsorption of sodium and water resulting in higher fractional excretion of electrolytes and greater urinary volumes. The total body water in neonates is around 80% and the average urine output varies between 1–3 mL/kg/hr.

Epidemiology

Studies in critically sick children, using the RIFLE or its pediatric modification (pRIFLE) show that the incidence of AKI varies from 8–25%. Higher incidence has been reported from cardiac surgery neonatal units (upto 60% by AKIN or pRIFLE) especially in very low birth weight infants. A study from Thailand looked at the causes of neonatal AKI in developing world from 1984–2007 and reported sepsis as a cause in 30.9%, hypoxia in 18.7% and congenital anomalies of the kidneys and urinary tract (CAKUT) in 12.2%.

The etiology of AKI may be pre-renal, intrinsic renal or post-renal. Pre-renal failure occurs due to inadequate systemic and/or renal circulation. Pre-renal failure can be caused by either systemic hypovolemia or renal hypoperfusion. Hypovolemic pre-renal failure, if treated early, responds to a fluid challenge with resumption of normal urine output and resolution of azotemia. Post-renal failure occurs as a consequence of mechanical obstruction in the urinary collecting system. Both pre- and postrenal failure, when prolonged, may lead to parenchymal injury to the kidneys (intrinsic renal failure). Improved chances of survival of sick and low birth weight babies has resulted because of increased recognition of neonatal AKI in NICUs. Prerenal AKI because of perinatal asphyxia is an important cause of renal failure in preterm and term babies. Other causes include hypovolemia, septicemia, respiratory distress syndrome and intravascular volume depletion following surgery. Bilateral renal artery thrombosis may occur after umbilical artery catheterization. Commonly used medications like amino-glycosides, vancomycin, amphotericin-B, indomethacin, captopril and furosemide may contribute to the occurrence of neonatal AKI. Maternal use of NSAIDs or ACE inhibitors during the antenatal period may cause hypotension and AKI in the newborn. Urinary tract abnormalities, like posterior urethral valves, bilateral pelviureteral junction obstruction, multicystic dysplastic kidneys, and neurogenic bladder may also cause AKI. Post-renal AKI is primarily caused by the posterior urethral valves and is often relieved by catheterization.

History and Physical Examination

Specific history should be sought regarding the use of medications such as ACE inhibitors, angiotensin II receptor blockers (ARBs) and beta blockers by the mother in antenatal period. The use of these medications is associated with neonatal AKI. An antenatal ultrasound done during second or third trimester showing evidences of oligohydramnios along with hydronephrosis and/or distended bladder in the fetus is suggestive of an underlying obstructive structural defect. AKI is more common in neonates with birth asphyxia and sepsis. AKI may occur due to intrauterine anoxia requiring resuscitation after birth with an Apgar score of ≤6 at 5 minutes, with evidences of chorio-amnionitis in the mother leading to early onset sepsis in the baby or sepsis occurring later after 72 hours life. Family history of fetal or neonatal deaths or renal failure is suggestive of a familial etiology such as congenital cystic disease of the kidney, congenital nephrotic syndrome and tubulopathies.

The presence of single umbilical artery, lumbar meningomyelocele, bladder exstrophy, cloacal abnor-malities, and genitourinary abnormalities should be looked for. These conditions are commonly associated with renal dysfunction. Blood pressure should also be recorded to identify hypertension and shock.

Investigations

The blood investigations required to identify AKI and its complications include blood urea, serum creatinine, sodium, potassium, calcium, and phosphate levels. A venous blood sample should be collected for acid-base studies. In addition tests like C-reactive protein (CRP), calcitonin and micro-ESR are useful as screening tests for sepsis in neonates. Appropriate blood, urine and CSF samples should be sent for culture studies in infants suspected of sepsis. Investigations like urine osmolality and fractional excretion of sodium may be useful in differentiating pre-renal from renal AKI. The indices that help in differentiating pre-renal from renal AKI are given in Table 25.2.

A urinalysis is often normal in neonates with AKI but a culture may be positive if there is an underlying urinary tract infection. Radiological investigations like

X-ray chest is useful to detect cardiomegaly, effusions and pulmonary edema due to fluid overload. An ultrasound of the abdomen helps in identifying structural anomalies of the kidneys like hydronephrosis, posterior urethral valves, single kidney, etc. Investigations like micturating cystourethrogram may be done to identify lower tract anomalies. Antenatal ultrasounds of the mother, especially in the third trimester showing unilateral or bilateral hydronephrosis, are useful correlates of congenital structural renal anomalies.

Radionuclear scans like DTPA (diethylene triamine penatacetic acid), MAG-3 (mercapto acetyl triglycine) and DMSA (dimercaptosuccinic acid) should be delayed beyond 10–12 weeks of life as the low GFR during early infancy does not allow good dye uptake which results in poor films.

Recent research has focused on identifying early and more specific indicators of AKI, like plasma neutrophil gelatinase-associated lipocalin (NGAL) and cystatin C and urinary NGAL, interleukin 18 (IL-18), and kidney injury molecule-1 (KIM-1) which gets markedly upregulated in proximal tubules after ischemic injury. A rise of NGAL up to 10-fold has been seen within 6 hours of cardiac surgery in infants who later developed AKI. Elevated NGAL levels have been seen in neonates with birth asphyxia and they serve as a sensitive marker of asphyxia-related AKI. Elevated levels of NGAL are also seen in neonates with sepsis and interpretation of the levels may be difficult in complex situations when multiple etiologies are contributory to AKI. Kits are commercially available for detection of blood and urinary NGAL and serum cystatin. However, they are expensive and not routinely used in clinical practice.

Management

The management of neonatal AKI includes managing the associated complications and renal replacement therapy. Fluid and electrolyte imbalance is common because kidneys are the principal organ handling them to maintain homeostasis. Overhydration, pulmonary edema and congestive heart failure may result from excessive fluid retention due to a fall in GFR and inappropriate administration of fluids. Moreover, hypotension should also be avoided which is common in critically ill neonates with sepsis and shock.

Fluid Therapy

Intake of fluids must be restricted to insensible water loss plus urinary volume. The insensible water loss in a term neonate is around 25 mL/kg/day. In preterm neonates, this can vary between 40–100 mL/kg/day depending upon the gestation, postnatal age, use of

Table 25.2 Indices to differentiate pre-renal from established renal AKI

Indices	Pre-renal	Renal
Urinary sodium (mEq/L)	<20	>40
Urinary osmolality (mOsm/kg)	>500	<300
Blood urea-creatinine ratio	>20:1	<20:1
Urine-plasma osmolality ratio	>1.5	<1.0
Fractional excretion of sodium*	<1	>3

$$*FeNa\ (\%) = \frac{urine\ sodium \times serum\ creatinine}{serum\ sodium \times urine\ creatinine} \times 100$$

radiant warmers, phototherapy, etc. The insensible losses of water should be replaced with 5 or 10% dextrose solution. The urinary losses should be replaced with N/5 or 0.2 N saline. Potassium should be added to intravenous fluids only when hypokalemia is documented in the blood samples. The associated metabolic acidosis (serum bicarbonate levels <8 mEq/L), is corrected by administration of sodium bicarbonate added to 5 or 10% dextrose. Urine output should be carefully monitored by taking diaper weights. In boys urine can be collected in a test tube or condom. Catheterization should be avoided in neonates due to risk of infection.

Electrolyte Abnormalities

Hyponatremia

This is primarily dilutional and responds to fluid restriction. However, if there are seizures in association with severe hyponatremia, it should be corrected with 3% saline given over 2 hours. The rate of rise of serum sodium should not be more than 10–12 mEq/L every 24 hours. Rapid correction of hyponatremia predisposes to development of cellular dehydration especially of brain cells and may precipitate CNS symptoms and intracerebral hemorrhage.

Hypernatremia

Hypernatremia associated with AKI would require early initiation of peritoneal dialysis as extra free water administration may lead to fluid retention and cardiac failure.

Hyperkalemia

The life-threatening hyperkalemia with ECG changes is managed by administration of intravenous calcium gluconate (10%) 0.5–1.0 mL/kg over 5–10 minutes. This counteracts the effects of potassium on cardiac cells. Subsequently, nebulization should be started with salbutamol (β2 agonist) in a dose of 0.15–0.2 mg/kg. Salbutamol redistributes the K^+ in the body fluids by promoting its entry into the cells. The nebulization can be repeated at frequent intervals. Less urgent measures include administration of 7.5% sodium bicarbonate in doses of 1–2 mL/kg over 15 minutes or starting 10% dextrose 0.5–1.0 g/kg and insulin 0.1–0.2 U/kg neutralizing drip. Sodium bicarbonate should be administered very carefully in neonates as it has a high osmolality (1800 mOsm/L) and its rapid infusion is associated with risk of development of intracerebral hemorrhage especially in preterm infants. Calcium or sodium polystyrene (kayexalate) can be given orally in a dose of 1.0 g/kg every 12 hours, mixed with breast milk. They exchange potassium with sodium or calcium in the gut. However, the action of these resins is slow over a period of 4–6 hours. The management of complications of AKI is given in Table 25.3.

Nutrition

Infants require approximately 100 kcal/kg/d along with 1–2 gm/kg/d of proteins. In neonates with enteral feeds, expressed breast milk is the best. However, if enteral feeding is not feasible, total parenteral nutrition can be provided.

Role of Drugs

Diuretics

Diuretics mainly furosemide is commonly used in AKI. The rationale behind its use include increase in urine output and inhibition of Na-K ATPase, in order to limit oxygen consumption in already damaged tubules. However, recent studies have shown that the use of diuretics mostly helps in correction of fluid overload and ensure normal blood volume. There is no alteration either in mortality or need for renal replacement therapy with use of diuretics.

Mannitol

Mannitol in also ineffective in AKI and because of its hyperosmolarity may cause volume overload and precipitate congestive heart failure.

Vasopressors

AKI is frequently accompanied by septic shock in critically ill children. It should be managed by judicious use of fluids and vasopressors. Low doses of dopamine 1–5 µg/kg/min have been found to cause selective renal vasodilatation and found to increase urine output. However, recent studies have shown that it has no beneficiary role in clinical outcome and its use in AKI is no longer recommended. Fenoldopam mesylate, an oral dopamine agonist, is a newer drug in this category, which has lower side effects but there are no current guidelines for its use.

Theophylline

AKI occurs in 60% of neonates suffering from perinatal asphyxia. One of the mechanisms for development of AKI is adenosine mediated vasoconstriction. Theophylline being adenosine receptor antagonist, has been shown to have renoprotective action. When given during first hour of life, it is associated with improved GFR with greater clearance of creatinine. When given in low doses (5 and 8 mg/kg) theophylline has been found to be protective against post asphyxial AKI.

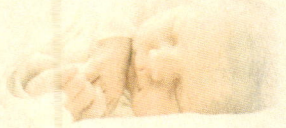

Table 25.3 Management of complications		
Complication	*Treatment*	*Remarks*
Fluid overload	**Fluid restriction** Insensible water losses (400 mL/m²/d); add urine output and other losses; 5–10% dextrose for insensible losses; N/5 saline for urine output	Monitor other losses and replace as appropriate, consider dialysis
Pulmonary edema	Oxygen; furosemide 2–4 mg/kg iv	Monitor CVP; consider dialysis
Hypertension	**Symptomatic** Sodium nitroprusside 0.5–8 mg/kg/min infusion; furosemide 2–4 mg/kg iv; nifedipine 0.3–0.5 mg/kg oral/sublingual **Asymptomatic** Nifedipine SR, amlodipine, prazosin or atenolol	In emergency, reduce blood pressure by one-third of the desired reduction during first 6–8 hr, 1/3 over next 12–24 hr and the final 1/3 slowly over 2–3 days
Metabolic acidosis	Sodium bicarbonate (IV or oral) if bicarbonate levels <15 mEq/L or pH <7.2	Watch for fluid overload, hypernatremia, hypo-calcemia; and consider dialysis
Hyperkalemia	**Emergency** Calcium gluconate (10%) 0.5–1 mL/kg over 5–10 minutes iv Salbutamol 5–10 mg nebulized **Less urgent** Sodium bicarbonate (7.5%) 1–2 mL/kg over 15 minutes Dextrose (10%) 0.5–1 g/kg and insulin 0.1–0.2 U/kg Calcium or sodium resonium (kayexalate) 1 g/kg per day	 Stabilizes cell membranes; prevents arrhythmias Shifts potassium into cells Shifts potassium into cells Requires monitoring of blood glucose Given orally or rectally, can be repeated every 4 hours
Hyponatremia	Fluid restriction; if there is sensorial alteration or seizures 3% saline 6–12 mL/kg over 30–90 minutes	Hyponatremia is usually dilutional; 12 mL/kg of 3% saline raises sodium by 10 mEq/L
Severe anemia	Packed red blood cells 3–5 mL/kg; consider exchange transfusion	Monitor blood pressure, fluid overload
Hyperphosphatemia	Phosphate binders (calcium carbonate, acetate; aluminium phosphate)	Avoid high phosphate products like milk products, and high protein diet

Based on the results of available studies, the KDIGO guidelines recommend the use of single dose of theophylline in neonates with severe birth asphyxia preferably within first hour after birth. The renal outcome improves with administration of theophylline but it does not have any protective effect on neuro-logical outcome.

Renal Replacement Therapy

AKI requiring dialysis can be managed with a variety of modalities, including peritoneal dialysis, intermittent hemodialysis, and continuous hemofiltration or hemodiafiltration. The choice of dialysis modality for management of a neonate with AKI is influenced by several factors, including age of the patient, the desired goals of dialysis, advantages and disadvantages of various modalities and institutional resources. In neonates and infants, peritoneal dialysis is the modality of choice. Due to small vessel size, access for hemo-dialysis and continuous renal replacement therapy (CRRT) is difficult in neonates.

The indications for initiating renal replacement therapy include severe or persistent hyperkalemia (K$^+$ >7 mEq/L), fluid overload (pulmonary edema, severe hypertension), uremic encephalopathy, and persistent severe metabolic acidosis (tCO$_2$ <10–12 mEq/L), hyponatremia (Na$^+$ <120 mEq/L or symptomatic) or hypernatremia (Na$^+$ >150 mEq/L). The decision to start dialysis should be based on an overall assessment of the patient keeping in mind the likely course of AKI. The access for peritoneal dialysis is achieved mostly using a stiff trocar catheter. The smallest size of a trocar for neonate should be used. The dialysis through the stiff catheter should not be continued beyond 48 hours because the risk of peritonitis rises exponentially after this period. Soft peel off catheters are available for neonates but are expensive. Tenckhoff soft catheters can also be surgically placed in neonates. The dialysate for neonates is available as dextrose (1.7%) and lactate based PD fluid. However, in presence of liver dysfunction and certain inborn errors of metabolism, lactate may not be converted to bicarbonate in the body. In such situations a bicarbonate based peritoneal dialysis fluid should be used. The fill volumes are generally kept between 20–30 mL/kg and the dwell time varies from 20–30 minutes. One mL of 10% KCl should be added to one liter of PD fluid once the serum potassium is normal or low. Electrolytes, blood sugar and calcium should be monitored after every 6–8 cycles. Serum creatinine can be monitored every 12–24 hours.

Prognosis

Nonoliguric AKI has a better prognosis in neonatal period. The mortality due to AKI varies betweem 25–75 % in oligoanuric AKI/sepsis. The risk factors for mortality include presence of intrinsic renal disease, prolonged anuria, use of ventilation, and need for RRT. The long-term abnormalities in GFR and tubular functions can persist in 25% of the neonates and may progress to chronic kidney disease (CKD). Therefore, all neonates with AKI should be followed up at least for one year for detection of chronic kidney disease. When there is established CKD, these infants need a long-term follow-up and at times kidney transplant.

BIBLIOGRAPHY

Agras PI, Tarcan A, Baskin E, Cengiz N, Gurakan B, Saatci U. Acute renal failure in the neonatal period. *Renal Failure* 2004; 26:305–9.

Akcan-Arikan A, Zappitelli M, Loftis LL, Washburn KK, Jefferson LS, Goldstein SL. Modified RIFLE criteria in critically ill children with acute kidney injury. *Kidney Int* 2007; 71:1028–35.

Bakr AF. Prophylactic theophylline to prevent renal dysfunction in newborns exposed to perinatal asphyxia–a study in a developing country. *Pediatr Nephrol* 2005; 20:1249–52.

Bellomo R, Ronco C, Kellum JA, Mehta RL, Palevsky P. Acute renal failure–definition, outcome measures, animal models, fluid therapy and information technology needs: The Second International Consensus Conference of the Acute Dialysis Quality Initiative (ADQI) Group. *Crit Care* 2004; 8:R204–12.

Bellomo R, Wan L, May C. Vasoactive drugs and acute kidney injury. *Crit Care Med* 2008; 36:S179–S86.

Bhat MA, Shah ZA, Makhdoomi MS, et al. Theophylline for renal function in term neonates with perinatal asphyxia: a randomized, placebo-controlled trial. *J Pediatr* 2006; 149:180–84.

Flynn JT, Kershaw DB, Smoyer WE, Brophy PD, Mc Bryde KD, Bunchman TE. Peritoneal dialysis for management of pediatric acute renal failure. *Perit Dial Int* 2001; 21:390–94.

Himmelfarb J, Joannidis M, Molitoris B, et al. Evaluation and initial management of acute kidney injury. *Clin J Am Soc Nephrol* 2008; 3:962–67.

Jenik AG, CerianiCernadas JM, Gorenstein A, et al. A randomized, double blind, placebo-controlled trial of the effects of prophylactic theophylline on renal function in term neonates with perinatal asphyxia. *Pediatrics* 2000; 105: E45.

Jetton JG, Askenazi DJ. Acute kidney injury in the neonate. *Clin Perinatol* 2014; 41:487–502.

Karlowicz MG, Adelman RD. Nonoliguric and oliguric acute renal failure in asphyxiated term neonates. *Pediatr Nephrol* 1995; 9:718–22.

Kidney Disease: Improving Global Outcomes (KDIGO). Acute Kidney Injury Work Group. KDIGO Clinical Practice Guidelines for Acute Kidney Injury. *Kidney international Suppl* 2012: 1–138.

Nguyen MT, Devarajan P. Biomarkers for the early detection of acute kidney injury. *Pediatr Nephrol* 2008; 23:2151–57.

Pannu N, Klarenbach S, Wiebe N, Manns B, Tonelli M; Alberta Kidney Disease Network. Renal replacement therapy in patients with acute renal failure: A systematic review. *JAMA* 2008; 299:793–805.

Van der Voort PH, Boerma EC, Koopmans M, et al. Furosemide does not improve renal recovery after hemofiltration for acute renal failure in critically ill patients: a double blind randomized controlled trial. *Crit Care Med* 2009; 37:533–38.

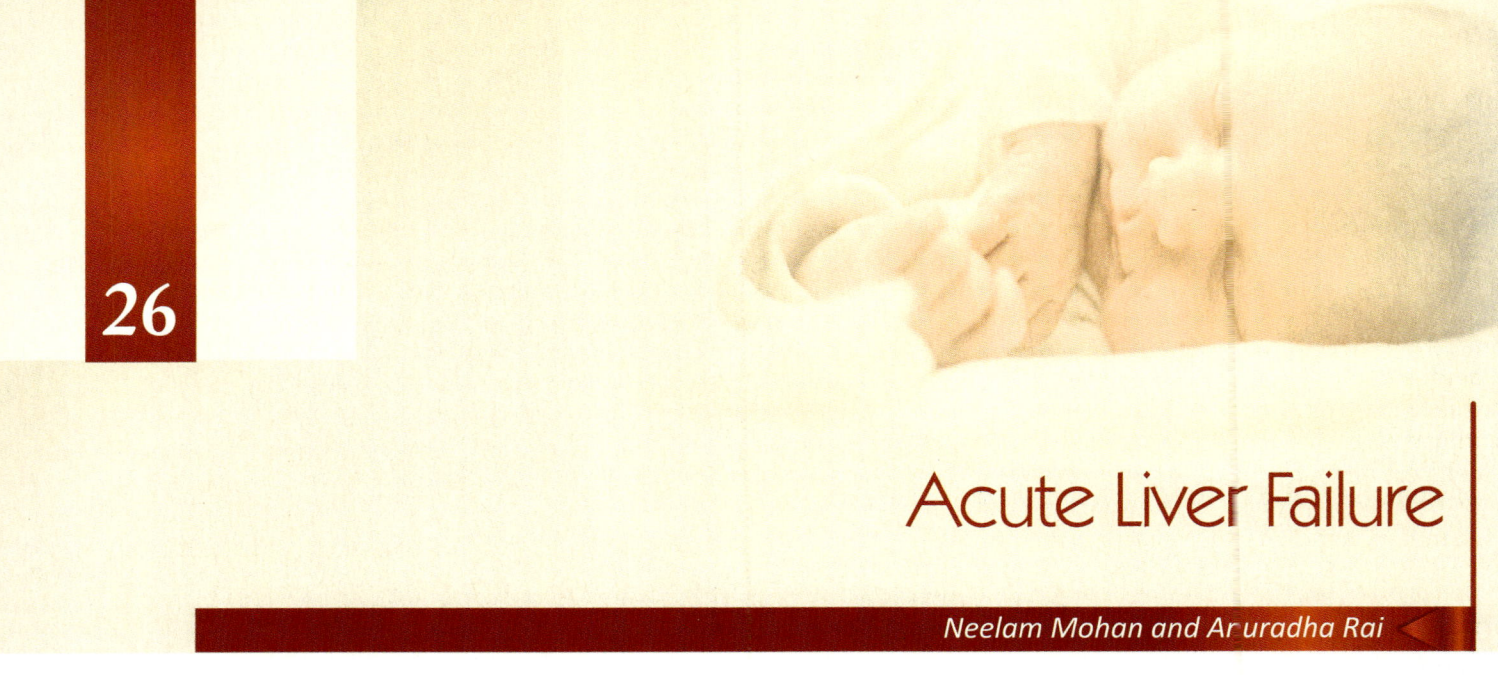

26

Acute Liver Failure

Neelam Mohan and Anuradha Rai

Introduction

Neonatal liver failure (NLF) is rare and carries high mortality if not treated promptly. The actual incidence of NLF is not well-known because of the difficulty in identifying liver failure in this group of population. There is relatively less published literature on NLF. Acute liver failure in general means absence of pre-existing liver disease and pathologically it is characterized by acute insult without significant fibrosis. The neonatal liver failure may be a continuum of fetal liver failure and presents with signs and symptoms of liver failure.

Definition

Acute liver failure (ALF) is defined in adults as bio-chemical evidences of severe hepatic dysfunction such as hyperbilirubinemia and prolonged prothrombin time complicated by hepatic encephalopathy that develops within 8 weeks of the onset of hepatic dysfunction. Hepatic encephalopathy is difficult to assess in infants and children and may never become clinically apparent in setting of ALF. The Pediatric Acute Liver Failure (PALF) study group redefined ALF as (i) hepatic based coagulopathy (PT ≥15 seconds or INR ≥1.5) not corrected by vitamin K with hepatic encephalopathy, or PT ≥20 seconds or INR ≥2 regardless of hepatic encephalopathy (ii) biochemical evidences of acute liver injury and (iii) no known evidence of chronic liver disease.

The above mentioned definition of PALF may not be appropriate for diagnosis of NLF because INR in normal newborns especially in preterm infants is normally up to 2 or more. It is suggested that in infants up to the age of 60 days, INR of ≥3 should be used as a cut-off for diagnosis of NLF.

Etiology

Common causes of NLF include gestational alloimmune liver disease (GALD)–neonatal hemochromatosis (NH), metabolic disorders, infections and hematological malignancies. GALD – NH, has been recognized recently as the most common cause of NLF. The various causes of NLF are enumerated in Table 26.1.

Table 26.1 Etiology of neonatal liver failure	
Immune mediated infection	GALD-NH Herpes simplex virus, Hepatitis B virus, Herpesvirus 6, Parvovirus B19, Enteroviruses like Echovirus 11, Coxsackievirus type A and B, Adeno-virus, Cytomegalovirus, and septicemia
Metabolic diseases	Galactosemia, tyrosinemia type 1, hereditary fructose Intolerance, inborn error of bile acid synthesis, mitochondrial cytopathy, fatty acid oxidation defect, Niemann–Pick disease type C
Hematological	HLH (Genetic and acquired due to infections), congenital leukemia neuroblastoma, Down syndrome associated with myeloproliferative disorders
Vascular disorders and congenital heart diseases	Hepatic vein thrombosis, shock, CHF, hypoplastic left heart, coarctation of aorta, right heart failure, acute myocarditis, severe asphyxia
Drugs	Valproate, acetaminophen (maternal overdose), isoniazid, nitrofurantoin
Idiopathic	'Le foie vide' (hepatic nonregeneration syndrome), giant cell hepatitis

GALD–NH: gestational alloimmune liver disease–neonatal hemachromatosis, HLH: hemophagocytic lymphohistiocytosis, CHF: congestive heart failure

The clinical variables that give clue about the etiology of NLF include age at presentation, evidence of any fetal insult, presence of patent ductus venosus, hepatomegaly, alanine aminotransferase (ALT) level, ferritin level, alpha-fetoprotein level, and persistent metabolic acidosis. Many patients with "indeterminate" NLF are due to giant cell hepatitis, a nonspecific response to liver injury with characteristic multinucleated syncytial giant cells on histology that can result from an intrauterine or postnatal event including infection or inborn error of metabolism.

Gald–NH

It is the most common cause of liver failure in the neonatal period which usually presents at birth and almost always within 3 days of birth. Recurrence risk during subsequent pregnancies is almost 80% and it is now well-understood that NH patients develop fetal liver disease as a result of gestational alloimmunity. GALD is now considered as the single most common disease causing NLF. GALD–NH is a frequently diagnosed entity when NH has been proved to be due to GALD. In GALD–NH, liver injury is of fetal onset and usually begins in mid gestation. It manifests with intra and extra hepatic iron storage while sparing the reticuloendothelial system. There may be antenatal history of maternal anemia, oligohydramnios (70–90%), intrauterine growth restriction (70–90%) or mega placenta. History of sibling death is common. Ascites seen on prenatal USG is suggestive of portal hypertension or fetal cirrhosis.

It clinically presents with jaundice, profound coagulopathy (INR 4–10), hypoglycemia, and hydrops fetalis (40–60%). However, splenomegaly is uncommon (10–20%) as most newborns maintain a patent ductus venosus (70–90%). Hepatomegaly is also uncommon (10–20%). ALT is typically low or normal and almost always <100 iu/L. Plasma iron and transferrin saturation are typically high, whereas transferrin levels are normal or low. Serum ferritin levels are elevated up to 800–7000 ng/mL in over 95% of patients. It is a sensitive marker of GALD-NH but this is not specific because it may be found in many neonatal liver diseases. Diagnosis is made by demonstration of extra hepatic iron deposits in the salivary glands of lips, sparing reticuloendothelial system . Intra-hepatic iron deposition is not diagnostic of GALD-NH because neonatal liver is physiologically iron overloaded. Liver histopathology reveals absence of normal hepatocytes; normal portal areas; numerous tubules in parenchyma; extensive parenchymal fibrosis; and replacement of hepatocytes with multinucleated giant cells. Retention of membrane attack complex (complement C5b-9 complex) in the remaining hepatocytes is considered as an evidence of alloimmune injury. However, it is not widely available for clinical use, and remains a research tool. Magnetic resonance imaging (MRI) of the abdomen may reveal iron deposition in the pancreas, but it is typically absent in the spleen.

When diagnosis of GALD is suspected, treatment with IVIG should be instituted immediately along with the use of an antioxidant cocktail (Box 26.1). After confirmation of the diagnosis, infant is treated with exchange blood transfusion followed by repeat high-dose IVIG. Liver transplant is indicated when there is no response to medical therapy. It is exceedingly important to make a proper diagnosis in these patients because of the high rate of recurrence of the condition in subsequent pregnancies. There is some evidence that recurrence can be prevented by administration of high dose IVIG during pregnancy.

Viral Infections

Viral hepatitis in the newborn usually presents after 1–2 weeks of age. Perinatal infection with Herpes virus, Parvovirus, Adenovirus and Hepatitis B may cause liver failure in neonates. Herpes simplex virus (HSV) type 1 induced liver failure is the most common among viral infections and carries a bad prognosis. It can present as localised skin disease or disseminated infection resulting in hepatitis, pneumonitis and intravascular coagulopathy. Characteristic vesicular skin rash is absent in 40% and early symptoms are nonspecific. The diagnosis should be considered in all sick neonates with raised transaminases and coagulopathy. Infants with hepatitis due to herpes virus should be started on intravenous acyclovir. Hepatitis due to perinatal viral infections typically present with acute hepatic necrosis. The amino-transferase levels are typically very high, often >1000 IU/L. Coagulopathy is usually moderate to profound, hepatomegaly, splenomegaly and hypoglycemia are common. Alfa-fetoprotein is almost always normal. The histopathology of liver shows global necrosis often with collapse. In HSV associated NLF, liver biopsy shows hemorrhagic necrosis and viral inclusion in

---

BOX 26.1 Anti-oxidant regime for treatment of GALD-NH

- Selenium 3 mg/kg/day intravenous
- Vitamin E 25 IU/kg/day per oral
- N-acetyl cysteine 100 mg/kg/day intravenous
- Prostaglandin E_1 0.4 mg/kg/h intravenous for 2 weeks duration
- Desferioxamine 30 mg/kg/day intravenous until ferritin level is <500 ng/mL

hepatocytes. Among other herpes viruses, Human Herpes Virus 6 (HHV6) has also been associated with NLF but is considered to be less ominous infection than HSV. CMV is very rarely associated with NLF, it usually produces chronic smoldering hepatitis with prominent cholestasis. Agents that typically produce mild illness in adults may also produce NLF such as enteroviruses. Recent diarrheal or respiratory illness in the mother should make one suspect enteroviral infection. Rarely liver failure has been reported in infants with dengue fever which may be fatal if treatment is not instituted early.

Sepsis Associated Liver Failure

Bacterial and fungal infections are common in neonates but they rarely lead to liver failure. Investigations should be directed towards work-up of sepsis including serum ferritin, and to look for secondary causes of liver dysfunction such as galactosemia, tyrosinemia, NH, hemophagocytic lymphohistiocytosis (HLH) and congenital leukemia. These infants are managed by administration of specific antibiotics, treatment of coagulopathy and management of all possible complications such as hemodynamic instability, shock and dialysis for renal failure.

Metabolic Disorders

They are an important cause of liver failure in the neonatal age group and must be promptly investigated because dietary modification or disease specific management may be life-saving. Common metabolic disorders known to cause hepatic dysfunction include galactosemia, tyrosinemia, hereditary fructose intolerance (HFI), fatty acid oxidation defects and mitochondrial respiratory chain defects.

Galactosemia is characterized by elevated galactose level in the blood. It may occur due to three types of enzyme defects such as galactose – 1-phosphate uridyl-transferase, galactokinase and uridine diphosphate galactose-4-epimerase, of which first one is the most common, and seen in 95% of affected newborns. It usually presents within the first month of life. The clinical picture is characterized by vomiting, jaundice, hypoglycemia, seizures, lethargy, irritability, feeding difficulty, poor weight gain, aminoaciduria, nuclear cataracts, hepatic failure, cirrhosis, and hepatosplenomegaly. They is an increased risk to develop *E. coli* sepsis. Screening is done by looking for reducing substances in urine when patient is receiving human milk, cow milk or any other lactose containing formula. Plasma galactose and RBC galactose-1-phosphate levels are grossly increased. Diagnosis is confirmed by assay of galactose-1-phosphate uridyl transferase enzyme

(GALT) in the erythrocytes. Treatment consists in elimination of galactose from diet by giving lactose-free formula.

Hereditary tyrosinemia Type 1 (HT-1) is caused by deficiency of fumaryl acetoacetase hydrolase (FAH), which results in accumulation of metabolites of tyrosine especially succinylacetone, which leads to hepatic damage. It may present as acute catabolic state in the form of fever, irritability, vomiting, hemorrhage, hepatomegaly, jaundice, elevated level of serum transaminases and hypoglycemia which may progress to liver failure. There is high lifetime risk of hepatocellular carcinoma. Diagnosis is made by elevated levels of succinylacetone in serum and urine of affected newborn. Serum tyrosine level may be increased, but is not specific and depends on diet. Alfa-fetoprotein is markedly increased with increased transaminase and decreased coagulation factors synthesized in the liver. When alpha-fetoprotein is increased in cord blood, it suggests intrauterine liver damage. Hereditary tyrosinemia Type 1 is treated by giving phenylalanine, and tyrosine restricted diet and administration of nitisinone (NTBC).

Hereditary fructose intolerance manifests after introduction of fructose or sucrose in the diet when solid foods are introduced. However, use of some non-cow's milk infant formulas with added sugars may trigger the onset of symptoms earlier. The clinical manifestations are similar to galactosemia which includes vomiting, lethargy, irritability, jaundice, hepatomegaly, and seizures. Laboratory parameters include prolonged clotting time, hypoalbuminemia, elevation of bilirubin and transaminases. Diagnosis is suggested by presence of reducing substances in urine and confirmed by fructose challenge test or assay of fructo aldolase B activity in the liver.

Mitochondrial hepatopathy includes respiratory chain defects, errors in fatty acid oxidation, and mitochondrial DNA depletion syndromes. The cells with high energy requirements such as neurons, skeletal and cardiac muscles are affected leading to encephalopathy and myopathy. It may present within first week to one month of life. History of sibling death is common. Polyhydramnios and intrauterine growth restriction may be seen in 20–30% cases. Multiorgan involvement specially of central nervous system, heart and skeletal muscles is common. They usually manifest as hypoglycemia, vomiting, coagulopathy, raised lactate, metabolic acidosis, hepatomegaly, cholestasis with or without neurological symptoms. Ascites, splenomegaly and patent ductus venosus are uncommon. Alanine transaminase (ALT) is typically high and often range between 100–500 IU/L. A suspicion for a mitochondrial disease is supported by metabolic distress, due to hypoketotic hypoglycemia with lactic acidosis. Screening is done by estimation serum and CSF lactate level, elevated ALT in plasma, abnormal lactate/pyruvate molar ratio with increased levels of Krebs cycle intermediates on urinary organic acid analysis. Brain MRI and spectroscopy are useful in suspected mitochondrial diseases with nonspecific neurological symptoms. Cardinal diagnostic procedure is muscle biopsy but it is relatively invasive. The liver pathology in these patients typically shows microvesicular or mixed macrovesicular and microvesicular steatosis, suggestive of the impairment of energy metabolism due to necrosis of liver.

Treatment is supportive by administration of ubiquinone 20 mg/kg/day, riboflavin 10 mg/kg/day and L-carnitine 100 mg/kg/day with high calorie diet. Rarely disorder of fatty acid oxidation and inborn errors of bile acid synthesis present with liver failure. Fatty acid oxidation defect presents as life-threatening coma and hypoglycemia induced by a period of fasting due to defective hepatic ketogenesis. The screening investigations include fasting blood sugar, and urinary ketones. The diagnosis is confirmed by tandem mass spectrometry (TMS) to detect characteristic acylcarnitines. Intravenous fluids containing 10% dextrose are given to prevent hypoglycemia. Long-term treatment includes avoidance of fasting, restriction of dietary fat and supplementation with carnitine.

Ischemic Injury

Acute liver dysfunction or shock liver syndrome in the neonate secondary to hemodynamic failure, is a known cause of ALF. In a case of circulatory failure and perinatal hypoxemia, the ductus venosus remains patent, which leads to significant reduction in blood flow to the right lobe of the liver compared with the left lobe. Shock liver can occur after a period of hypotension/hypovolemia, cardiac arrest or congestive cardiac failure. Ascites, hepatomegaly, coagulopathy and hypoalbuminemia may be present. Serum transaminase levels are markedly elevated but they normalize once the circulatory problem is stabilized. Treatment is supportive and symptomatic.

Hematological Causes

Hemophagocytic lymphohistiocytosis (HLH) and rarely congenital leukemia can present with NLF. HLH is a syndrome of excessive immune activation and is the most common malignant condition responsible for NLF. Age of presentation is variable, sometimes the condition may be present at birth. It can manifest in neonates in 10% of cases. It is of two types, genetic and acquired. Genetic type is further divided into familial and those associated with primary immunodeficiency syndrome. Acquired HLH may be associated with infections, malignancies, and autoimmune diseases. Various infectious causes include bacterial, parasitic, and viruses such as herpes simplex virus, adenovirus, dengue, parvovirus B19 and enterovirus. Clinical presentation in neonates is different from older children. In neonates, HLH can present as isolated liver failure. Fever is commonly absent, and hypertriglyceridemia has been reported in only 14% of neonates, which is due to age related differences in lipid metabolism. Hepatomegaly, splenomegaly, hypoglycemia, cholestasis are usually present.

Common laboratory findings are coagulopathy (moderate to profound), cytopenias, hypofibrinogenemia, hypertriglyceridemia, hyperbilirubinemia with elevated transaminases (often >1000 IU/L), raised ferritin (a cut-off of 10000 μg/L is 90% sensitive and 96% specific) and raised lactate dehydrogenase levels. Alfa-fetoprotein is almost always normal. 51-Cr release assay and measurement of sCD25 which measures NK cell activity and activated lymphocytes have 100% sensitivity. Hemophagocytosis of mature and immature hematopoietic cells in addition to myeloid and erythroid hypoplasia and variable megakaryocytic hyperplasia is a characteristic feature in the bone marrow. Liver histopathology usually reveals Kupffer cell hyperplasia with portal and sinusoidal cytotoxic T cell infiltrates expressing CD3, CD4 and granzyme B with variable hemophagocytic histiocytes.

The aim of treatment is to suppress exaggerated immune response which includes immune suppressive and immune modulatory agents, cytostatic drugs and biological response modifiers. Familial hemophagocytic lymphohistiocytosis, is managed by stem cell transplantation. In acquired type of HLH, immediate treatment of underlying disease is life-saving. Malignancy and massive blastic infiltration in leukemia causes liver failure by replacement of normal hepatocytes and therapy involves treatment of primary malignancy.

Drugs and Toxins

Various drugs such as valproic acid, acetaminophen, isoniazid, nitrofurantoin may cause liver damage and subsequently liver failure in newborns. Valproic acid when used to control seizures in infants with mitochondrial disorders such as Alpers disease may precipitate liver failure. Long-term total parenteral nutrition (TPN) can also lead to progressive and potentially life-threatening liver disease which manifests as jaundice and failure to thrive. TPN Initially leads to intrahepatic cholestasis but may progress to fibrosis and cirrhosis with prolonged intravenous alimentation. Cholestasis develops after 2 weeks of TPN and fibrosis of varying degree develops after receiving TPN for more than 6 weeks in majority of newborns. The harmful component of parenteral soyabean oil (w–6PUFAs) liberate pro-inflammatory mediators, leading to development of liver dysfunction because of increased plasma phytosterol and lipoproteins content in cell membranes. Treatment strategies include reduction in the dose of parenteral soyabean oil, replacement with fish oil, or mixed lipid emulsions.

Pathogenesis of NLF

In NLF, insult to the liver may occur in fetal life even before the liver is well-developed. Acute hepatic necrosis is the most common mechanism involved in neonates which usually occurs due to viral infections, toxins, ischemic injuries and some metabolic causes. In drug induced and hypoxic ischemic insults , sublobular necrosis with orientation of necrosis around central vein is seen. Aminotransferases are characteristically elevated in liver failure associated with necrosis.

HLH is also associated with hepatic necrosis. Replacement of hepatic parenchyma with non-functioning tissues such as massive hepatic hemangioma may sometimes lead to NLF. Absence of cell necrosis in association with liver failure implies organelle dysfunction, in which hepatomegaly is evident and jaundice is minimal. Failure of hepatocyte organelle function is not a common cause of liver failure in newborns. In inborn errors of metabolism (IEMs), hepatocyte necrosis is patchy and variable. Aminotransferases and serum bilirubin are moderately elevated. In diffuse hepatosteatosis and in some metabolic disorders like hereditary fructose intolerance (HFI), widespread functional impairment of hepatocytes without necrosis can cause liver failure. Failure of hepatic parenchymal development is a common underlying mechanism secondary to immune injury to developing hepatocytes in infants with GALD. Pathogenesis of NLF is summarized in Figure 26.1.

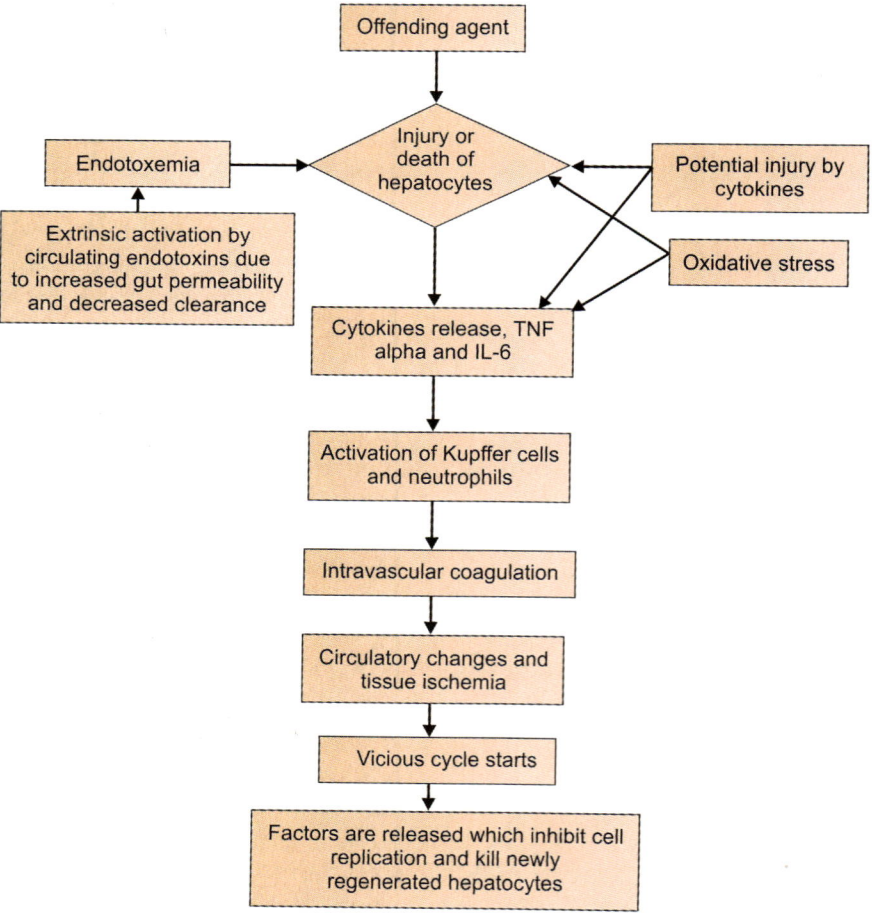

Figure 26.1 Pathogenesis of neonatal liver failure.

Clinical Features

The clinical features like age at onset, evidence of fetal insult, presence of patent ductus venosus, hepatomegaly, elevated alanine aminotransferase (ALT) level, ferritin level, alpha-fetoprotein level and persistent metabolic acidosis provide useful clues to the etiology of NLF. GALD-NH usually presents at birth and almost always within three days of birth. Viral infections present between 5–14 days after birth, HLH and mitochondrial hepatopathy may present between first week to few months after birth. Premature birth, oligohydramnios and intrauterine growth restriction are common (70–90%) correlates of GALD-NH. Liver failure in neonates usually manifests as multisystemic involvement and may be associated with hypotonia, hypoglycemia, hypotension, ascites, hepatosplenomegaly and cholestasis. Jaundice usually appears late which leads to delay in diagnosis. Presence of metabolic acidosis is suggestive of mitochondrial hepatopathy. Coagulopathy may be seen in association with liver dysfunction and moderate hyperammonemia. Encephalopathy is usually present but difficult to recognize in neonates. They may manifest as vomiting, hypotonia and convulsions. Physical examination and investigations of NLF are summarized in Table 26.2.

Management

General measures Patients with NLF should be nursed in a quiet environment with minimum handling to minimize sudden increase in intracranial pressure. General measures include intravenous dextrose to maintain blood glucose between 60–120 mg/dL, appropriate antibiotics and intravenous acyclovir, antifungal therapy, intravenous ranitidine to prevent gastric

Table 26.2 Salient clinical features and investigations in neonates with hepatic failure

History	Antenatal history of oligohydramnios, polyhydramnios, birth history, preterm, intrauterine growth restriction, age at presentation, and history of sibling death
Physical examination	Signs of multiorgan dysfunction, jaundice, hepatomegaly, splenomegaly, edema and ascites
Basic investigations	CBC, CRP, blood sugar, blood urea, serum creatinine, albumin and bilirubin, urine routine and reducing substance, culture and antibacterial sensitivity, SGOT/SGPT, GGTP, ALP, APTT, PT, INR, blood pH and lactate level
Specific investigations GALD-NH	Raised ferritin, extrahepatic iron deposition seen by MRI of pancreas or buccal biopsy, TIBC, transferrin saturation
Infections like Herpes virus, Echo virus, HHV6, Hepatitis B, Adenovirus, and Parvovirus	Viral serology and PCR
Hereditary tyrosinemia	Alfa-fetoprotein, urine succinylacetone, TMS, urine GCMS
Galactosemia	Red cell galactose-1-phosphate uridyl transferase, galactokinase, uridine diphosphate galactose-4-epimerase, serum galactose level
Hereditary fructose intolerance	Aldolase B
Mitochondrial hepatopathy	Lactate-pyruvate molar ratio >20, CSF and blood lactate, mitochondrial DNA, muscle and liver biopsy for quantitative respiratory chain enzyme determination
Fatty acid oxidation defects	Urinary ketones, fasting blood sugar, TMS
Hemophagocytic lymphohistiocytosis and congenital leukemia	Bone marrow examination
Septicemia and shock	Clinical evidences, vital signs and blood culture
Giant cell hepatitis with hemolytic anemia	Coomb's positive hemolytic anemia
Vascular malformations and congenital heart defect	Echocardiography
Maternal medications (paracetamol, isoniazid, valproic acid, nitrofurantoin)	History and drug levels

Abbreviations
GALD–NH: gestational alloimmune liver disease–neonatal hemochromatosis
CBS: Complete blood count, CRP: C-reactive protein, SGOT: aspartate aminotransferase, SGPT: alanine aminotransferase, GGTP: gamma-glutamyl transpeptidase ALP: alkaline phosphalase; APTT: activated partial thromboplastin time, PT: prothrombin time, INR: international normalized ratio, TIBC: total iron binding capacity; TMS: tandem mass spectrometry; GCMS: gas chromatography mass spectrometry; PCR: polymerase chain reaction

bleeding, and correction of coagulopathy with fresh frozen plasma if active bleeding is present. Hepatoprotective agent such as N-Acetylcystein may be started in a dose of 100 mg/kg/day. Once baseline and essential investigations have been conducted, galactose and protein should be excluded from the diet until the underlying diagnosis is confirmed or galactosemia is specifically excluded. Liver damage can be reversed in certain metabolic diseases by dietary alterations and in some infections by appropriate antimicrobial treatment, but when it is advanced, liver transplantation is the only hope.

Specific measures Prognosis and specific management depends on the cause of NLF. The etiology of NLF should be identified because it influences the management of the patient as well as the need for liver transplantation. Sepsis should be managed by early administration of appropriate antibiotics. Infants with hepatitis due to Herpes virus are treated with intravenous acyclovir. Patients diagnosed as GALD with coagulopathy but hemodynamically stable should be managed conservatively as liver injury from GALD can reverse over a period of time and liver transplantation can be avoided. Mitochondrial hepatopathy should be diagnosed early and considered for liver transplantation before multisystem involvement occurs. HLH is treated with chemotherapy.

Neonatal Liver Transplantation

Neonatal orthotopic liver transplantation (OLT) is performed in the first two months of life. The neonatal OLTs are performed for acute liver failure. Neonatal hemachromatosis (NH) is the most common specific indication for OLT. Giant cell hepatitis, hepatitis B, enteroviral, and echoviral hepatitis, total parenteral nutrition associated liver disease, and hepatic hemangioendotheliomatosis have also been considered for OLT. Liver transplantation in neonates pose unique challenges because of state-of-the-art need for medical and surgical techniques. High level of expertize is required by the transplant surgeons because the vascular structures in newborns are very tiny. Young age, functional immaturity and small size of transplant recipients is the main challenge encountered by medical and surgical team. Most of the cadaveric grafts from children may be relatively large for neonates. Similarly in the setting of live donor liver transplant (LDLT), the left lateral lobe is also rather large for newborn. The grafts are usually reduced by bench surgery to monosegment and then implanted which results in better outcome. Post-transplantation medical management is challenging as there is increased risk of bacterial and fungal infections. ABO incompatible liver transplantation can be successfully performed in neonates as they do not have prior sensitization to the major blood group antigens and they lack blood group specific antibody. Thus the patient or graft survival, complications such as biliary, vascular or rejection rates are not different from compatible transplants. However, the outcome of neonatal liver transplant is inferior compared to the older recipients.

Prognosis

Prognosis of NLF is poor with mortality rate of 70% without liver transplantation but survival improves to 54–70% with liver transplantation. Early recognition of hepatic failure with identification of underlying etiology and prompt initiation of supportive and specific treatment is the key to survival.

In our experience of more than 200 pediatric liver transplants, only one neonatal liver transplant was done for a 2.1 kg baby with NLF due to neonatal hemochromatosis with HLH. Infant underwent transplant at 8 weeks of age when medical therapy failed. Hyper reduced monosegment graft was used. Baby was discharged at 9 week post-transplant with normal liver and bone marrow functions and is doing well on a follow-up at 5 months of age.

BIBLIOGRAPHY

Alonso E, Squires R, Whitington P. Acute liver failure in children. In: Liver Disease in Children. Suchy JF, Sokol RJ, Balistreri WF, (eds). 3rd ed . Cambridge: *Cambridge university press*; p.71–96.

Asai A, Malladi S, Misch J, Pan X, Malladi P, Diehl AM, Whitington PF. Elaboration of tubules with active hedgehog drives parenchymal fibrogenesis in gestational alloimmune liver disease. *Hum Pathol* 2015 Jan, 46(1):84–93. DOI 10.1016/J Humpath 2014.09.010.

Bergounioux J, Abella SF, Monneret S, Essouri S, Jacquemin E. Neonatal ischemic liver failure: Potential role of the ductus venosus. *J Pediatr Gastroenterol Nutr* 2004 38:5.

Bhati V, Bavdekar A, Yachha SK. Management of acute liver failure in infants and children: Consensus Statement of the Pediatric Gastroenterology Chapter, Indian Academy of Pediatrics. *Indian Pediatr* 2013, 50:477–82.

Devictor D, Tissieres P, Durand P, Chevret L, Debray D. Acute liver failure in neonates, infants and children. *Expert Rev Gastroenterol Hepatol* 2011; 5(6):717–29.

Dhawan A, Vergani GM. Acute liver failure in neonates. *Early Human Development* 2005; 81:1005–10.

Fung STH, Tonf TF, Chow MPY. A case of early neonatal fulminant liver failure and haemophagocytic lymphohistiocytosis. *HK J Paediatric* (new series). 2009; 14:282–90.

Grijalva J, Vakili K. Neonatal liver physiology. *Semin Pediatr Surg* 2013; 22:185–89.

Gunson RN, Jackson A, Aitken C. A case of neonatal sepsis with acute liver failure. *Clin Virol* 2011; 50:266–69.

Jackson R, Roberts EA. Identification of neonatal liver failure and perinatal hemochromatosis in Canada. *Paediatr Child Health* 2001; May-Jun; 6(5): 248–50.

Lee WM. Acute Liver Failure. *N Engl J Med* 1993; 329:1862–73.

Ovchinsky N, Moreira RK, Lefkowitch JH, Lavine JE. The liver biopsy in modern clinical practice: A pediatric point of view. *Adv Anat Pathol* 2012 July; 19(4):250–62.

Rosado FGN, Kim AS. Hemophagocytic lymphohistiocytosis. *Am J Clin Pathol* 2013; 139:713–27.

Shanmugam NP, Bansal S, Greenough A, Verma A, Dhawan A. Neonatal liver failure : aetiologies and management – state of the art. *Eur J Pediatr* 2011; 170:573–81.

Squires RH, Shneider BL, Bucuvalas J, Alonso E, et al. Acute liver failure in children. *J Pediatr* 2006 May; 148(5):652–58.

Sundaram SS, Alonso EM, Whitington PF. Liver transplantat on in neonates. *Liver Transplant* 2003; 9(8):783–88.

Taylor S, Whitington P. Neonatal acute liver failure. *Liver Transplantation* 2016; 22:677–85.

27

Necrotizing Enterocolitis

Meharban Singh

Necrotizing enterocolitis (NEC) in the newborn has been recognized long since but of late there is an upsurge in its incidence in neonatal intensive care units throughout the world. It is one of the most common gastrointestinal medical/surgical emergency in preterm neonates. Its incidence is variable among different centers and even in a given center its occurrence varies from time to time depending upon the bacterial ecology of the neonatal intensive care unit (NICU), feeding practices, obstetric resuscitation procedures and other variables. At times, a number of cases appear in 'cluster' or as an outbreak. The overall incidence of NEC varies between 1 and 3/1000 live births or 5 to 10% of admissions to the NICU.

Epidemiology

The disease is mostly limited (90%) to low birth weight preterm babies because of the immaturity of the gastrointestinal tract. It affects about 10% of infants who weigh less than 1500 g. Preterm babies are vulnerable to develop NEC because of high incidence of perinatal distress factors, stasis of gut because of autonomic immaturity, poor barrier functions of gut or immune defences, lack of feeding with human milk and higher incidence of nosocomial infections. Among term infants with NEC, almost one-half are small-for-gestational age or dysmature. Various predisposing factors include prematurity (especially <34 weeks), perinatal hypoxia, active resuscitation, RDS/apnea or both, assisted ventilation, acidosis, hypoxia, shock, umbilical artery cathetrization, use of H_2 blockers or indomethacin and early or large-volume nasogastric formula feedings (Box 27.1). The protective role of human milk and probiotics for prevention of NEC is well accepted.

BOX 27.1 Risk factors for nectrotizing enterocolitis

- High-risk mother: Pregnancy-induced hypertension, absent or reversed end diastolic flow velocity and abruption, HIV-positive, substance abuse, and chorioamnionitis
- Preterm or very low birth weight (<1500 g) babies
- Genetic predisposition: upregulated TLR4 signalling and immune incompetence
- Infants with intrauterine growth retardation
- Low 5-minute Apgar score
- Use of umbilical catheters
- Exchange or packed cell transfusion
- Mechanical ventilation
- Enteral formula feeding
- Bacterial colonization of gut, sepsis and/or shock
- Administration of histamine H_2 receptor antagonists, prolonged antibiotics, indomethacin, xanthine derivatives, and vitamin E
- Excessive fluid administration with development of patent ductus arteriosus

---

Pathogenesis

The exact etiology of NEC is unknown and its pathogenesis is multifactorial and complex. The disease is by and large limited to preterm and very low birth weight babies (VLBW). In VLBW babies, the gastrointestinal host defences including intraepithelial lymphocytes and secretory IgA are markedly impaired. Many biochemical factors such as lactoferrin, epidermal growth factor (EGF), heparin binding (HB)-EGE, transforming growth factor, insulin like growth factor, oligosaccharides, and polyunsaturated fatty acids (PUFAs) are either deficient or absent. NEC most commonly affects the terminal ileum and proximal ascending colon. It would appear that intestinal mucosal injury due to or as a consequence of ischemia is the core pathogenetic mechanism. Perinatal hypoxia, hypovolemia

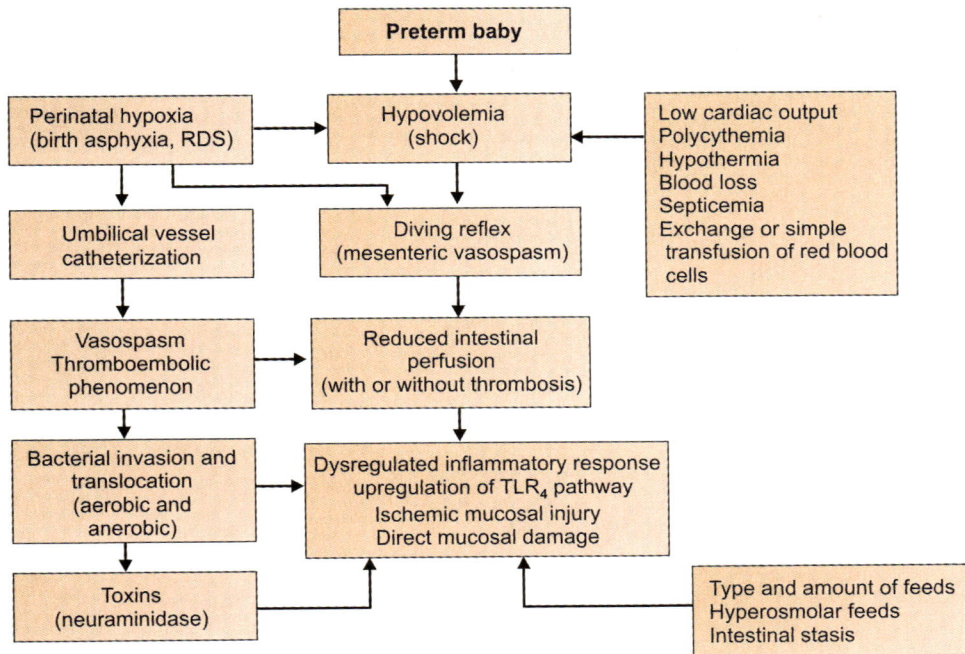

Figure 27.1 Pathogenesis of necrotizing entercolitis. Perinatal hypoxia and shock appear to initiate intestinal mucosal ischemia in a preterm neonate

or shock due to various predisposing factors leads to a situation akin to "diving reflex" resulting in mesenteric vasospasm in order to divert the blood to vital organs to enhance their perfusion. The net reduction in intestinal perfusion with or without mesenteric vasospasm or thrombosis, leads to ischemic mucosal and transmural necrosis of intestine (Figure 27.1).

Additional or direct mucosal damage due to large volume of intragastric feedings and bacterial toxins (neuraminidase) elaborated by invasion of anerobic microorganisms aggravate mucosal injury. Recent evidence suggests that NEC develops as a consequence of intestinal hyper responsiveness to microbial ligands upon bacterial colonization in preterm infants. A number of drugs like xanthine derivatives, indomethacin, antacids and vitamin E have been implicated to initiate and aggravate NEC. There is increasing evidence to support the critical role of platelet activating factor (PAF) and other inflammatory mediators, like leukotrienes, interleukins and tumor necrosis factor, thromboxanes, oxygen free radicals and nuclear factor kappa B (NF_KB). Accumulation of ileal bile acids cause significant injury to small intestine by acting in concert with Toll-like receptors (TLR 4 pathway) in the pathogenesis of NEC. Cellular protective mechanisms such as epidermal growth factor (EGF), transforming growth factor β_1 (TGF-β_1), and erythropoietin are downregulated, further compromising the infant's ability to mount a protective response. Subsequent release of

norepinephrine and vasoconstriction result in splanchnic ischemia, followed by reperfusion injury. The mucosal necrosis leads to intestinal dysfunction with functional intestinal obstruction characterized by delayed gastric and small gut emptying, bilious vomiting and abdominal distension.

Feeding with large volume of hyperosmolar feeds (formula feeds, 10% dextrose, human milk fortifier, vitamin E, calcium gluconate, etc.) at this stage would aggravate mucosal damage and may be associated with leakage of undigested protein antigens into portal circulation. The hepatic Kupffer cells may be unable to contain or eliminate these antigens, resulting in systemic endotoxemia and shock with further aggravation and perpetuation of ischemic damage to intestinal mucosa. Mucosal necrosis and bleeding manifests as fresh or occult blood in stools. Enteric bacteria cause fermentation of undigested feeds leading to production of hydrogen gas which enters through mucosal breaks to produce blebs of pneumatosis intestinalis and portal venous gas.

Clinical Features

Preterm or sick newborn babies should be closely watched for development of NEC. It typically develops in the second or third week of life in an infant who is premature and has been formula fed. The symptoms may appear after 96 hours of initiation of oral feeding. Disease may occur anytime during neonatal period but

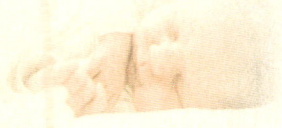

Table 27.1 Modified Bell's staging criteria for NEC				
Stage	*Systemic signs*	*Abdominal signs*	*Radiologic signs*	*Treatment*
IA-Suspected NEC	Temperature instability, apnea, bradycardia and lethargy	Elevated pre-gavage residuals, mild abdominal distension, emesis, guaiac-positive stool	Normal or intestinal dilatation, mild ileus	NPO, antibiotics for 3 days pending culture report
IB-Suspected NEC	Same as above	Bright-red blood per rectum	Same as above	Same as above
IIA-Definite NEC (Midly ill)	Same as above	Same as above, plus absent bowel sounds	Intestinal dilatation, ileus, pneumatosis intestinalis	NPO, antibiotics for 7–10 days
IIB-Definite NEC (Moderately ill)	Same as above, plus metabolic acidosis and thrombocytopenia	Same as above, plus absent bowel sounds, definite abdominal tenderness, abdominal cellulitis or right lower quadrant mass	Same as IIA, plus portal vein gas, doubtful ascites	NPO, antibiotics for 14 days, sodium bicarbonate for acidosis
IIIA-Advanced NEC (Severely ill, bowel intact)	Same as IIB, plus hypotension, bradycardia, severe apnea, combined respiratory and metabolic acidosis, disseminated intravascular coagulation, neutropenia	Same as above, plus signs of generalized peritonitis, marked tenderness and distension of abdomen	Same as IIB, plus definite ascites	Same as above, plus 200 mL/kg fluids in 24 h, inotropic agents, assisted ventilation, paracentesis
IIIB-Advanced NEC (Severely ill, bowel perforated)	Same as IIIA	Same as IIIA	Same as IIB, plus pneumoperitoneum	Same as above, plus surgical intervention

NPO; nil oral or nothing by mouth
Source: Walsh MC, Kliegman RM. *Pediatr Clin North Am* 1986; 33:179–201.

majority of cases occur within first 10 days of life. The onset may be insidious or explosive and at times delayed. Functional intestinal obstruction as evidenced by abdominal distension and retention of milk in the stomach in a sick-looking LBW baby is the earliest marker of the disease. Early signs are indistinguishable from neonatal sepsis. *The full blown clinical picture is characterized by triad of abdominal distension, gastrointestinal bleeding and pneumatosis intestinalis (air in the bowel wall) on abdominal radiography.*

Further progress of the disease can be arrested, if oral feedings are withheld at this stage. The clinical picture is characterized by progressive abdominal distension and blood-streaked loose stools or occult blood in stools in a sick preterm baby. Gastric emptying is delayed and peristalsis is reduced or absent. Bilious vomiting may afford decompression, if gastric aspiration is delayed. Infant looks sick, pale and lethargic with circumoral grayish discoloration. Thermal instability and hypotension are frequent. Apneic attacks, generalized bleeding (due to DIC) and sclerema herald poor outcome. About one-half of patients develop transmural necrosis and perforation resulting in peritonitis

and free air under the right dome of the diaphragm. The presence of ascites, erythema and edema of abdominal wall and localized mass or rigidity over right lower quadrant of abdomen should alert to the possibility of intestinal perforation. Candidemia produces an identical clinical picture and must be excluded. The modified Bell's staging criteria for NEC along with treatment options are shown in Table 27.1.

Investigations

Leukocytosis, thrombocytopenia, metabolic acidosis and hyponatremia are commonly associated. Neutropenia (absolute neutrophil count <1500/μL) is strongly suggestive of sepsis. Hyponatremia (Na$^+$ < 130 mEq/dL) and metabolic acidosis are commonly present. Elevated C-reactive protein, proinflammatory cytokines such as TNFα, IL-6, IL-8, and intestinal fatty acid binding protein biomarker in the urine are commonly seen. Serial skiagrams of abdomen, supine, cross-table lateral and oblique views, should be taken every 12-hour during the course of NEC. Depending upon the stage of the disease, gaseous distension, dilated fixed loops of bowel, pneumatosis intestinalis, portal vein gas, and pneumoperitoneum may be seen on X-rays (Figures 27.2 and 27.3). Pneumatosis intestinalis, the pathognomonic feature of NEC, is present in 85% of patients. Abdominal ultrasonography is useful to identify areas of loculation, free air and fluid in the peritoneal cavity. Overt or occult blood in the stools is invariably present. Elevated hydrogen gas in the breath is a useful marker of the disease. Reducing substance (positive stool clinitest) due to unabsorbed lactose in stools may be positive.

Following perforation, meconium pigments may be absorbed in the bloodstream and excreted in the urine. The meconium pigment is different than bilirubin and gives a specific absorbance at 405 nm. Spectrophotometric examination of urine may show meconium index of more than 1.0. At times, urine may appear dark-brown or green when large amounts of meconium pigment is excreted. Urine should be examined for budding yeasts and hyphae to rule out systemic candidiasis. Serological test for identification of T-antigen in blood would confirm the co-existence of anerobic bacterial infection in the gut. Elevated alpha-fetoproteins are indicative of associated hypoxic damage to the liver. Electrolytes, hematocrit, and coagulation status should be monitored during the course of therapy. Prolonged prothrombin time (PT) and activated partial thromboplastin time (aPTT), decreasing fibrinogen and rising fibrins split products are suggestive of consumptive coagulopathy due disseminated intravascular coagulation (DIC). Serial measurements of C-reactive protein (CRP) are helpful in the diagnosis and assessment of response to therapy. Blood and stool cultures for aerobic and anerobic organisms are mandatory.

Differential Diagnosis

The insidious onset, characteristic clinical picture and radiological findings of pneumatosis intestinalis are diagnostic. The triad of thrombocytopenia, persistent metabolic acidosis and intractable hyponatremia is usually present. Feeding intolerance in a sick preterm baby may be confused with early stage of NEC. Sepsis and pneumonia may cause ileus without NEC. Acute surgical abdomen due to malrotation with midgut volvulus, intussusception, gastric perforation and thrombosis of mesenteric vessels may present rather acutely as a catastrophe. The presence of diarrhea and blood in stool is suggestive of infectious enterocolitis due to *Campylobacter* species rather than NEC. Candidemia may mimic early features of NEC and must be excluded by appropriate culture studies.

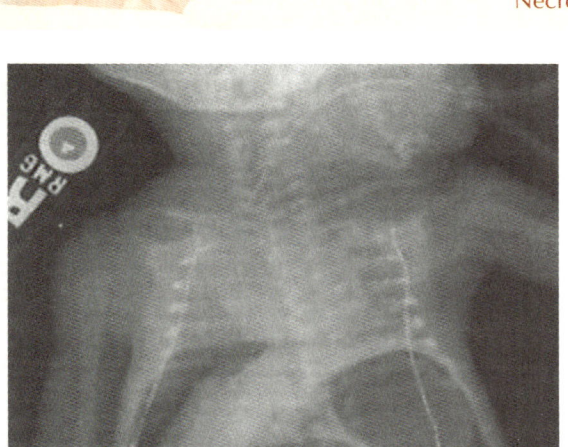

Figure 27.2 Plain X-ray abdomen erect showing gas under the diaphragm in a preterm infant with necrotizing enterocolitis

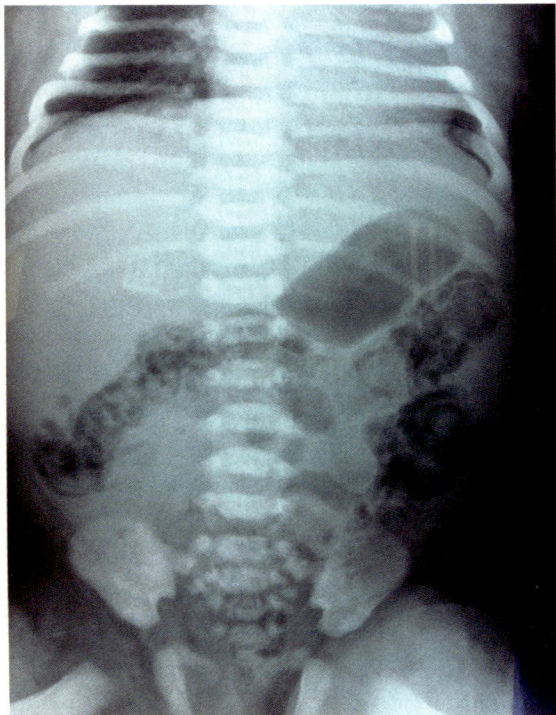

Figure 27.3 Typical appearances of pneumatosis intestinalis in an infant with necrotizing enterocolitis

Treatment

Early recognition of NEC and vigorous medical management has reduced the need for surgery. Nevertheless, the condition should be managed under close guidance and supervision of a pediatric surgeon so that when indicated surgery is not unnecessarily delayed. If there are any umbilical catheters, they should be promptly removed. Intravenous line should be established to administer fluids, electrolytes and drugs. Pharmacological support with low doses of dopamine (3–5 µg/kg/min) is useful to improve splanchnic and renal blood flow. The fluid requirements are markedly increased due to abdominal fluid sequestration (3rd space losses), peritonitis and septic shock. Oral feedings should be stopped for 7 to 14 days and gastric aspiration preferably by slow continuous suction with a wide-bored catheter (Fr 10 or 12) is advised. Total parenteral nutrition (TPN) is instituted and by and large outcome in cases of NEC is related to the feasibility and availability of TPN. Systemic antibiotics, depending upon the prevailing spectrum of bacterial pathogens in a particular NICU, are administered intravenously. Piperacillin-tozabactam is a useful broad-spectrum antibiotic and can be used as a single agent. The role of oral colistin (10–15 mg/kg/dL) or gentamicin is controversial. Metronidazol 15 mg/kg IV loading dose followed by 7.5 mg/kg/dose every 12 hours should be administered to treat associated anerobic infection. Fresh frozen plasma (10 mL/kg/day) is recommended on every alternate day to provide complement, humoral immune factors, coagulation factors and to improve blood volume to correct shock. The blood lost through glastrointestinal bleeding or through sampling should be replaced.

Diluted enteral feedings with EBM are started in small amounts when abdominal distension disappears, gastric aspirate is negligible, intestinal peristalsis is audible and there is no occult blood in the stools. The stomach should be aspirated before each feed and next feed should be omitted or its volume reduced, if aspirate contains bile/milk or exceeds 5 mL. The weaning from intravenous to oral alimentation in cases of NEC should be extremely slow, cautious and controlled. Most cases of NEC can be managed conservatively but surgery is indicated in following situations:

1. Doppler ultrasound is useful to assess perfusion of the intestinal wall to determine the need for surgical intervention.
2. Bowel perforation as evidenced by pneumoperitoneum or portal venous gas on plain abdominal radiograph.
3. Full thickness necrosis of bowel wall with impending perforation as evidenced by dilated loop of intestine that remains unchanged in position and shape for more than 24 hours on serial radiographs.
4. Peritonitis as suggested by ascites, abdominal mass, induration and erythema of abdominal wall and localized abdominal rigidity. Aspiration of brown-colored or meconium-stained ascitic fluid (or ascitic fluid showing bacteria on Gram's stain) is indicative of intestinal gangrene and perforation.

The necrotic portion of the gut is excised and end-to-end anastomosis is established or enterostomy is performed. The abdomen is closed after placing a drain in the peritoneal cavity. The conservative therapy is continued and oral feedings are initiated with extreme caution in operated cases. The convalescence is extremely slow and infants with NEC are likely to stay in the NICU for several weeks. In ELBW (<1000 g) or unstable babies, peritoneal drainage is established under local anesthesia and exploratory laparotomy is delayed.

Prognosis

Early NEC without perforation is likely to have outcome akin to neonatal sepsis. Depending upon the stage of the disease, quality of supportive care and availability of parenteral nutrition, the case fatality rates vary between 20% and 50%. Infants requiring surgical intervention are likely to have growth retardation, osteopenia, neuromotor delay and parenteral nutrition-related complications. Common gastrointestinal sequelae include strictures, enteric fistulas, short bowel syndrome, malabsorption and chronic diarrhea.

Prevention

Even following aggressive therapeutic efforts, the mortality in cases of established NEC varies between 15% and 30% in the West. Due to greater awareness of predisposing factors and current understanding of pathogenetic mechanisms underlying NEC, it has been possible to reduce the incidence of the condition. Antenatal administration of corticosteroids, when labor starts prematurely, is credited to reduce the risk of NEC. Perinatal hypoxia, RDS/apnea, hypovolemic shock and other predisposing situations should be prevented and managed promptly to circumvent "diving reflex". Oral feeding should be delayed in sick LBW babies and whenever poor perfusion of bowel is suspected. The enteral feedings should be small, iso-osmolar (preferably human milk) and their volume should be increased gradually and cautiously. Human milk is protective against NEC by virtue of macrophages, lymphocytes, secretory IgA, lysozymes, lactoferrins, L-arginine, epidermal growth factor, erythropoietin, oligosaccharides, PUFA and various enzymes that modulate host immunity, inflammation and mucosal protection. The stomach should be aspirated before each feed and next feed should be omitted or reduced, if aspirate contains bile/milk or if its volume exceeds 50% of the amount of the last feed.

The double-blind controlled trials have failed to demonstrate any prophylactic utility of administration of oral antibiotics to high-risk LBW babies for prevention of NEC. Recently, it has been shown that oral administration of immunoglobulins (75% IgA and 25% IgG) to high-risk preterm infants may reduce the incidence of NEC. Trials are being conducted to assess the role of platelet aggregating factor (PAF) antagonists to reduce the incidence of NEC. Administration of probiotics to preterm babies are credited to reduce the risk of NEC. Studies are ongoing to determine which friendly organisms are most effective and their safety and side effects. There is some evidence that supplementation with L-arginine and zinc may reduce the incidence of NEC. Other novel therapeutic modalities include administration of TLR4 modulators, short chain fatty acids (SCFs) and fecal transplantation from healthy neonates.

BIBLIOGRAPHY

Aceti A, Gori D, Barone G, et al. Probiotics for prevention of necrotizing enterocolitis in preterm infants: Systemic review and meta-analysis. *Italian J Pediatr* 2015, 41:89.

Bell MJ, Ternberg JL, Feigin RD, et al. Neonatal necrotizing enterocolitis. Therapeutic decisions based upon clinical staging. *Ann Surg* 1978, 187:1–7.

Bohnhorst B. usefulness of abdominal ultrasound in diagnosing necrotizing enterocolitis. *Arch Dis Child Fetal Neonatal Ed* 2013, 98(5): F 445–50.

Caplan MS, Jilling T. New concepts in necrotizing enterocolitis. *Curr Opin Pediatr* 2001, 13(2):111–15.

Choi YY. Necrotizing enterocolitis in newborn: update in pathophysiology and newly emerging therapeutic strategies. *Korean J Pediatr* 2014, 57(12):505–13.

Gephart SM, McGrath JM, Halpren MD. Necrotizing enterocolitis risk. *Advances Neonat Care* 2012, 12(2):77–89.

Hammerman C, Kaplan M. Germ warfare: Probiotics in defence of the premature gut. *Clin Perinatal* 2004, 31:489–500.

Howart JM, Wilkinson AW. Functional intestinal obstruction in the neonate. *Arch Dis child* 1970, 45:800.

Kasivajjula H, Maheshwari A. Pathophysiology and current management of necrotizing enterocolitis. *Indian J Pediatr* 2014, 81(5):489–97.

Kastenberg ZJ, Sylvester KG. The surgical management of necrotizing enterocolitis. *Clin Perinatal* 2013, 40:135–48.

Kliegman RM, Fanaroff AA. Necrotizing enterocolitis. *N Engl J Med 1984*, 310:1092.

Kosloske AM. Surgery of necrotizing enterocolitis *World J Surg* 1985, 9:277.

More K, Athalye – Jape G, Rao S, Patole S. Association of inhibitors of gastric acid secretion and higher incidence of necrotizing enterocolitis in preterm and very low birth weight infants. *Am J Perinatol* 2013, 30:849–56.

Muss R, Dimmitt RA, Barnhart DC, et al. Laparotomy versus peritoneal drainage for necrotizing enterocolitis and perforation *N Engl J Med* 2006, 354:2225–34.

Neu J, Walkar WA. Necrotizing enterocolitis. *N Engl J Med* 2011, 364:255–64.

Neu J. Necrotizing enterocolitis: The search for a unifying pathogenic theory leading to prevention. *Pediatr Clin North Amer* 1996, 43(2):409–32.

Nino DF, Sodhi CP, Hackam DJ. Necrotizing enterocolitis: new insights into pathogenesis and mechanisms. *Nat Rev Gastroenterol Hepatol* 2016, 13(10):590–600.

Thompson AM, Bizzarro MJ. Necrotizing enterocolitis in newborn: pathogenesis, prevention and management. *Drugs* 2008, 68(9):1227–38.

Toulikian RJ. Neonatal necrotizing enterocolitis. *Surg Clin N Am* 1976, 56:281.

Walsh MC, Kliegman RM. Necrotizing enterocolitis: treatment based on staging criteria. *Pediatr Clin North Am* 1986, 33: 179–201.

28

The Surgical Neonate

Meharban Singh

MEDICAL MANAGEMENT OF SURGICAL NEONATES

The improved survival rates for complex surgical conditions of the newborn babies have been achieved by improvements in the skills of pediatric surgeons, increased understanding regarding the problems of homeostasis and physiological needs of sick preterm babies and availability of noninvasive technology for continuous monitoring of vital parameters in neonates. The specific details regarding management of various surgical conditions are not discussed but broad principles governing the perioperative management of a surgical neonate are discussed in this chapter. A close cooperation and coordination between the pediatric surgeon, neonatologist, anesthetist, neonatal nurses, respiratory therapist and pharmacist is essential to improve the outcome of the surgical neonate. The medical management is directed to ensure stable body temperature (normothermia), adequate ventilation (and oxygenation), satisfactory tissue perfusion (effective circulation), thermoneutral environment, supply of adequate amounts of fluids, electrolytes and calories, maintenance of biochemical homeostasis and prevention of nosocomial infections (Table 28.1).

Preoperative Management

Early diagnosis of a surgical condition in the neonate is important because operative success and outcome is directly related to the time taken to diagnose and prepare the infant for surgery. *It needs to be emphasized that one-day-old infant is a good surgical risk and no preoperative management may be required in such cases.* Delay in the diagnosis is likely to lead to complications, disturbances of fluids and electrolytes and compromised status of tissue perfusion and oxygenation depending upon the nature of the developmental defect. The condition of the infant should be stabilized by parenteral administration of fluids and electrolytes to provide maintenance needs, correct any deficits and replenish on-going concurrent losses. The third-space fluid losses are known to occur in a variety of abdominal conditions, such as NEC, peritonitis, gastroschisis, omphalocele and intestinal obstruction. Inadequate replacement of these losses (which are difficult to quantify) can lead to hypovolemia and shock. Infusion of 5% albumin, plasma and whole blood may be required to maintain blood pressure.

Fluid losses due to vomiting and nasogastric aspiration should be replaced as 0.45% saline in dextrose (N/2 saline-dextrose solution). Persistent and protracted vomiting due to pyloric stensosis can lead to hypochloremic alkalosis with hypokalemia which is corrected by administration of sodium chloride and potassium chloride. Apart from adequate hydration and satisfactory perfusion, status of ventilation (as evidenced by normal arterial blood gases and pH) and biochemical parameters (electrolytes, calcium, glucose and BUN) should be within normal limits before undertaking major surgery. *Vitamin K 0.5–1.0 mg IV or IM must be given to all neonates before surgery.* A suitable antibiotic should be administered to an infected neonate and those requiring major abdominal surgery. Adequate amount of crossmatched blood should be arranged. The infant should be taken to the operation theater in a transport incubator to ensure that his body temperature and ventilation are normal before induction of anesthesia. Hypothermia should be avoided because of risk of several complications like respiratory embarrassment, metabolic acidosis, hypoglycemia, hypoxia, cardiac disturbances, coagulopathy, increased risk of wound infection and sepsis.

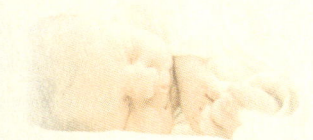
Table 28.1 Principles governing perioperative medical management of newborns

1. Ensure adequate ventilation
- Maintain pH 7.35–7.45, arterial PO_2 50–80 mmHg, PCO_2 35–45 mmHg.
- Ensure optimal position, posture, suction, open airways, relieve abdominal distension, provide oxygen with head box, CPAP and ventilation.
- Monitor breathing rate, color, apneic attacks and oxygen saturation.

2. Maintain satisfactory tissue perfusion
- Ensure adequacy of cardiac contractions and circulating blood volume.
- Check losses due to vomiting, nasogastric aspiration, intestinal obstruction (third space losses), gastroschisis, bleeding, and operative blood loss and ileostomy fluid losses, etc.
- Monitor pulse, capillary filling time (<2 sec over upper chest), blood pressure*, pH, central venous pressure.

3. Provide thermoneutral environment
- Nurse and operate under servo-control system.
- Avoid unnecessary exposure, give fluids, blood and blood products after warming to body temperature.

4. Supply fluids, electrolytes and calories
- Establish a reliable intravenous access.
- Check sources of fluid and electrolyte losses and assess status of hydration.
- Provide maintenance needs of fluids, electrolytes and calories, replenish deficits and concurrent on-going losses.
- Monitor weight, hydration status, urine output, plasma and urine osmolality and serum electrolytes.
- Start total parenteral nutrition if starvation is prolonged beyond 5 days.
- Give vitamin K before surgery.

5. Maintain biochemical homeostasis
- pH, acid-base parameters, electrolytes, calcium, glucose, BUN and bilirubin should be monitored.

6. Prevent nosocomial infections
- Strict asepsis and handwashing
- "Septic screening" for early diagnosis of sepsis
- Prophylactic or early administration of antibiotics following major surgery or during assisted ventilation

*It is useful to maintain mean arterial blood pressure just above the gestation of the baby in weeks, i.e. around 32 mmHg in a baby of 32 weeks gestation.

Intraoperative Management

The aim of surgical management is not merely to correct the abnormality but also to ensure that minimal metabolic stress is imposed during the procedure. The main concerns during surgery include the risk of cold stress and need for making an accurate assessment of blood loss and third-space losses of fluids to prevent hypovolemia and shock. During major surgery, infant should be attached to an electronic thermometer, ECG oscilloscope, noninvasive blood pressure monitor and pulse oximeter. The baby should be placed on a circulating warm water mattress or enclosed in a fiberoptic hot pipe system to create a warm microenvironment during surgery. The circulation of hot air under the drapes and microprocessor controlled circulating water mattress (Allon system), which heats or cools the recirculating water contained in a garment covering the patient is useful for maintaining perioperative normothermia. The overhead radiant warmer is ineffective because baby is covered with thick drapes and it interferes with OT lights and movements of the anesthetist and surgeon. Fluids, blood and blood products must be warmed to 37°C before infusion. Accurate estimate of blood loss during surgery should be maintained preferably by weighing dry and blood soaked guaze pads on an accurate electronic weighing scale. It must be remembered that loss of 20 mL of blood in a 1500 g infant amounts to a loss of 15% of his blood volume (equivalent to 750 mL of blood loss in an adult).

During surgery, the maintenance fluid requirement should be provided by infusion of one-fourth saline-dextrose solution at a rate of 4 mL/kg/hour. The infusion rate of glucose should not exceed 4–6 mg/kg/minute to prevent the risk of hyperglycemia. In addition to the maintenance fluid needs and blood loss, the third-space fluid losses due to translocation of tissue fluid by surgical dissection and damage must be replaced. During major abdominal surgery, third-space losses are replenished by administration of a dextrose-free solution like Ringer's lactate at a rate of 10–15 mL/kg/hour. Transfusion of large volumes of blood can lead to hyperkalemia and hypocalcemia which should be specifically looked for on the ECG monitor. During a prolonged surgical procedure, frequent monitoring of hematocrit, pH, glucose and electrolytes is mandatory.

Postoperative Management

Infant should be transferred to NICU and attached to a vital sign monitor, electronic thermometer, non-invasive blood pressure monitor and pulse oximeter. Urine bag must be attached and urine output maintained between 1 and 3 mL/kg/hr with an osmolality between 150 and 400 mOsm/L or specific gravity 1005–1015. The infant should be nursed in an intensive care incubator or open care system with a facility for servo-controlling the body temperature. Hematocrit, electrolytes, glucose, calcium, blood gases and osmolality should be checked as soon as possible after the surgery. *Acidosis in the presence of normal arterial oxygen and carbon dioxide tension, is a very sensitive index of unsatisfactory tissue perfusion in a neonate.* It should be promptly treated by rapid administration of 20 mL/kg of physiological saline or fresh frozen plasma (FFP) over a period of one hour. Sodium bicarbonate can be administered as a slow infusion over 4 to 6 hours. Postoperatively, many infants demonstrate hyponatremia and fluid retention because of inappropriate secretion of antidiuretic hormone which is released during surgery in response to hypoxia, hemorrhage, hypotension, anesthesia and pain. During first 48 hours postoperatively, maintenance fluids should be restricted to two-thirds of the recommended volume. The gastric aspirate should be replaced by one-half strength physiological saline while ileostomy losses are replenished with physiological saline. Tissue breakdown and catabolic state during surgery may be followed by hyperkalemia which needs to be monitored by keeping a close watch on the ECG tracing. The supplements of potassium should be withheld till adequate urine flow is established.

The infant should be closely watched clinically and by periodic septic screening to identify occurrence of nosocomial infection as early as possible. The role of administration of large doses of immune globulins for prevention of bacterial infections is controversial. Fresh frozen plasma should be administered on every alternate day to provide proteins, complement, lysozyme, and coagulation factors. There is no significant difference in the rates of amino acid oxidation, protein degradation or synthesis and caloric needs during pre- and postoperative period in newborn babies. When enteral feeding cannot be established by fifth postoperative day, it is desirable to start total parenteral nutrition to reverse the catabolic state in order to promote healing and growth. Adequate supplements of vitamins and calcium is essential during postoperative management.

The emotional and physical needs of the surgical neonate should not be overlooked in the maze of catheters and sensors. It is often forgotten that newborn babies also feel pain. Infact they feel more pain because they are more delicate but they are unable to complain and the tiny ones cannot even cry. A number of adverse physiological and biochemical consequences have been demonstrated in neonates after giving them painful stimuli. Pain is associated with rise in blood pressure, increase in heart rate, elevation of intracranial pressure and fall in arterial oxygen saturation. Depending upon the nature of the surgical procedure, pain can be safely controlled by administration of morphine in a loading dose of 50 µg/kg followed by continuous infusion of morphine at a rate of 10–15 µg/kg per hour. Fentanyl in a loading dose of 10 µg/kg followed by constant infusion at a rate of 1–5 µg/kg/hour also provides adequate analgesia and sedation. The toxic side effects of both morphine and fentanyl can be effectively reversed by administration of naloxone.

OPTIMAL TIMING FOR SURGERY

Life-threatening Surgical Conditions

Early diagnosis and rational medical management of congenital malformations is crucial to enhance survival. Immediate or early surgery is life-saving in following life-threatening surgical conditions. Most of these malformations are present in fetal life and surgical correction is required to save life or prevent complications. However, the condition of the baby should be stabilized before undertaking major surgery.

1. Diaphragmatic hernia
2. Esophageal atresia with/without tracheo-esophageal fistula
3. Tension pneumothorax
4. Lobar emphysema
5. Intestinal obstruction, fetal perforation, supralevator anorectal malformation
6. Gastroschisis
7. Ruptured omphalocele
8. Leaking meningomyelocele
9. Acute abscesses
10. Necrotizing enterocolitis with perforation

Various other surgical conditions can be subdivided into following two groups depending upon the need for urgent or elective surgery. In several situations, surgery may not be requried because the condition may get corrected spontaneously, viz. umbilical hernia, hydrocele, sternomastoid tumor, hemangioma and ventriculoseptal defect. At times, extensive surgery is postponed till baby can withstand the procedure or when organs are fully developed for best cosmetic results.

Emergency Surgical Conditions

Infants with inguinal hernia, cystic hygroma, meningomyelocele with thin sac should be operated as soon as diagnosed. Sacrococcygeal teratoma should be operated within two weeks after birth and infant with congenital hypertrophic pyloric stenosis is operated around 4–5 weeks of age. The surgical correction of congenital biliary atresia should not be delayed beyond 12 weeks due to risk of development of biliary cirrhosis. Infants with talipes equinovarus and congenital dislocation of hips should receive physiotherapy and special plaster

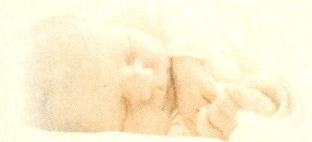

Table 28.2 Elective surgical conditions with optimal timing for their surgery			
Condition	Timing for surgery	Condition	Timing for surgery
▪ Biliary atresia, congenital	4–6 weeks (preferably within 12 weeks)	▪ Hemangioma	5–6 years
▪ Cleft lip	Usually at 2–3 months. Ideally it should be operated in the neonatal period for good cosmetic results.	▪ Hirschsprung's disease	Between 12 and 15 months (body weight 10 kg) or 6 months after colostomy
▪ Cleft palate	9–18 months	▪ Hydrocele	After 2 years
▪ Ectopic anus in the vestibular region	2–3 months	▪ Indirect inguinal hernia	In preterm babies at corrected age of 2 months. At the time of diagnosis in healthy term babies
▪ Hypospadias		▪ Perineal ectopic testis	At the time of diagnosis
• Meatotomy	Any time after birth	▪ Phimosis*	
• Chordee correction	Around 6 months	• Prepucial separation	Around one year of age
• Urethroplasty	18–24 months	• Circumcision	After 2–3 years
▪ Epispadias		▪ Sternomastoid tumor	Physiotherapy soon after birth and tenotomy around one year of age, if torticollis persists
• Chordee correction	Around one year of age		
• Urethroplasty	6 months to one year after chordee correction	▪ Syndactyly	1–2 years
▪ Exstrophy bladder		▪ Tongue-tie**	Around one year, if parents insist
• Bladder closure	Within 48 hours	▪ Umbilical hernia	After 4–5 years
• Bladder neck repair and anti-reflux surgery	After 2 years	▪ Undescended testes	12–15 months. Surgery may be done earlier, if it is associated with inguinal hernia
• Urethroplasty	After achieving continence		
• Augmentation cystoplasty	8–10 years		

*Application of steroid cream after gentle retraction of prepuce for 3–4 weeks corrects the abnormality by breaking the adhesions in most infants.
**Dentist can snip it with laser

casts within first week after birth. The casts would need removal and refixing every 1–2 weeks depending upon the severity of abnormality.

Elective Surgical Conditions

Surgery can be delayed for optimal cosmetic results till the deformed organs can be handled and resected with ease. A number of conditions are self-limiting and may resolve spontaneously while a delay in surgical correction in others may lead to irreversible organ damage and permanent sequelae. Table 28.2 gives the list of common developmental disorders with optimal timing for their surgical correction.

BIBLIOGRAPHY

Agarwala S, Mitra DK. Timing of surgery for common pediatric surgical conditions. *Indian J Pediatr* 1996, 63:769–74.

Anand KJS. Consensus statement for the prevention and management of pain in the newborn. *Arch Pediatr Adolesc Med* 2001, 155(2):173–80.

Bajwa SJS, Swati. Perioperative hypothermia in pediatric patients: diagnosis, prevention and management. *Anaesth Pain Int Care* 2014, 18(1):97–100.

Carbajal R, Rousset A, Danan C, *et al*. Epidemiology and treatment of painful procedures in neonates in intensive care units. *JAMA* 2008, 300(1):60–70.

Dillon PW, Cilley RE. Newborn surgical emergencies. *Pediatr Clin North Am* 1993, 40:1289.

Gupta DK, Sharma S, Azizkhan RG (Eds). Pediatric Surgery: Diagnosis and management, volume I and II. *New Delhi, Jaypee Bros Medical Publishers*, 2009.

Higgins RD, Patel RM, Josephson CD. Preoperative anemia and neonates. *JAMA Pediatr* 2016, 170(9):835–36.

Mathew PJ, Mathew JL. Assessment and management of pain in infants. *Postgrad Med J* 2003, 79:438–43.

Pani N, Panda CK. Anaesthetic considerations for neonatal surgical emergencies. *Indian J Anaesth* 2012, 56(5):463–69.

Richardson WR. Surgical emergencies on the day of birth. *Am J Dis Child* 1961, 102:164.

Taneja B, Srivastava V, Saxena KN. Physiological and anesthetic considerations for the preterm neonate undergoing surgery. *J Neonatal Surg* 2012, 1:14.

29

Parenteral Nutrition

Umesh Vaidya and Ketki Falak

Introduction

Parenteral nutrition (PN) or intravenous nutrition is an important component of critical care in the NICU. Nutritional support prevents a catabolic state that is associated with a life- threatening illness and hastens recovery. Most sick infants in the NICU are unable to feed adequately by the enteral route. Parenteral nutrition thus supports their nutritional needs till adequate enteral nutrition is established.

Incomplete and erratic availability of nutrients, lack of awareness regarding need for PN, lack of knowledge, constraints of financial and human resources and risk of complications are the main reasons for inadequate use of PN in NICUs. At our NICU in KEM Hospital, Pune we have been running the PN program successfully over the last 25 years. This has involved developing trained TPN nutritionists, establishing standard procedures, developing innovations and interacting with the industry regarding the need for suitable parenteral nutritional products. The KEM Hospital has also been involved in conducting training workshops on a regular basis to propagate this expertise across the country.

In the last decade, with the sprouting of tertiary NICUs and expanded neonatology training programs, more and more NICUs are using PN. The National Neonatology Forum (NNF) and Indian Academy of Paediatrics (IAP) have included PN as a mandatory criterion for accreditation of Level II and Level III neonatal units. Clinical practice guidelines for neonatal PN have been published.

This chapter will discuss the PN protocol which will facilitate calculation of parenteral nutrients and their administration. Information is based on the current availability of nutrient products in India and certain adaptations in the techniques for their administration.

Setting up PN Facility in NICU

All level II and Level III NICUs should have the facility for providing PN. This involves trained personnel to prepare PN, space for preparation, protocol for PN administration and monitoring. Box 29.1 shows the list of requirements for setting up PN facility.

Indications for PN

The primary aim of PN is to prevent a catabolic state. With higher nutrient doses, it is also able to achieve a positive nitrogen balance and promote physical and mental growth. Common indications of PN in the NICU are shown in Box 29.2. These indications would vary depending on the strength of the facility (personnel and workload) and availability of financial resources. At our NICU, all babies less than 1500 g are routinely started on PN (amino acids and lipids) on day 1 and if possible immediately after birth. In eligible neonates, PN should be started as early as possible. PN can be stopped once enteral nutrition provides 75% of the caloric needs.

BOX 29.1 Requirements for setting up parenteral nutrition in the NICU

1. Avalability of dedicated trained personnel like nutritionist, pharmacist, nurse, infusionist and medical staff
2. TPN room (150 to 200 sq feet)
3. Laminar flow system to prepare parenteral nutrients
4. Refrigerator
5. Computer with a printer
6. PN calculation software
7. Infusion pumps (two per patient)
8. Nutrient solutions (macro and micronutrients)
9. Provision for central venous access
10. Disposables (Infusion sets, connectors, filters)
11. Scrub linen, gowning, mask, gloves, antiseptics
12. Laboratory support with microchemistry facilities

BOX 29.2 Indications for parenteral nutrition

- Preterm neonates <28 weeks and/or <1000 g
- Preterm infants <32 weeks and/or <1500 g who are unable to achieve full enteral feeds by day 3
- Preterm neonates >32 weeks and/or >1500 g who are unable to achieve at least 50% enteral feeds by day 5
- Necrotising enterocolitis (stages II and III)
- Surgical neonates (exomphalos, gastroschisis, intestinal surgery)
- Short bowel syndrome
- All neonates with catabolic states (weight loss, poor muscle mass) where enteral feeding is limited, not feasible or not tolerated

Nutrients Needed for PN

PN comprises of macronutrients (dextrose, proteins and lipids) and micronutrients (vitamins and minerals). For several years, the availability of suitable products and volume of the commercial pack (mL) remained a concern in our country. Intravenous phosphates, trace elements, pediatric multivitamin solutions and newer lipid emulsions are not readily available in our country. In spite of the incomplete nutrient armamentarium, it is still possible to provide reasonable PN to majority of preterm and sick neonates. Table 29.1 summarises the list of parenteral nutrients currently available in India.

Steps in Starting PN

1. Identify the patient.
2. Discuss the nutritional requirements based on birth weight, postnatal age, medical condition, presence of comorbidities, and biochemical profile.
3. Calculate the PN requirements (manual/software).

4. Preparation of PN solution with available formulations (compounding)
5. Administration via central/peripheral route
6. Monitoring (clinical and biochemical).

Protocols and Doses of Parenteral Nutrients

Energy Minimum energy needs are met by providing 50–60 kcal/kg/day. The energy requirements for growth of preterm and term neonates on PN are 110–120 kcal/kg/day and 90–110 kcal/kg/day respectively. It should be ensured that minimum of 30 kcal/kg/day are provided for every g/kg of protein. This is calculated as calorie nitrogen ratio (CNR), which is discussed later.

Dextrose Dextrose as a part of PN is based on the standard guidelines of intravenous fluids. It is started on day 1 and calculated on the basis of glucose infusion rate (GIR). It is usually started @ 6 mg/kg/min and increased daily as per glucose tolerance. Maximum GIR for preterm and term neonates is 12 mg/kg/min and 13 mg/kg/min respectively. Glucose should provide 60% of the caloric intake on PN.

Amino acids Recently, the role of early (day 1) protein supplementation in adequate doses (up to 3.5 g/kg/day) has been shown to be beneficial and safe for preterm infants. Early and adequate protein intake leads to better nitrogen retention, satisfactory postnatal physical and head growth, and reduced incidence of broncho-pulmonary dysplasia. As per current guidelines, preterm babies should be started with a minimum of 2 g/kg/day of proteins on day 1 (desirable 2.5 to

Table 29.1	The formulations of parenteral nutrients available in India		
Constituent	Preparation	Manufacturer	Volume of the commercial pack (mL)
Dextrose	Dextrose 5%, 10%, 25%, 50%	Freely available*	25, 100, 500
Amino acids	Aminoven infant 6%, 10%	Fresenius Kabi India Pvt Ltd	100
Lipids	Intralipid 10% PLR	Fresenius Kabi India Pvt Ltd	100
	Intralipid 20% PLR	Fresenius Kabi India Pvt Ltd	100
	Clinoleic 20%	Baxter Healthcare	500
	SMOF 20%	Fresenius Kabi India Pvt Ltd	100
Sodium	Concentrated Ringer lactate	T. Walker's Pharmaceuticals Pvt Ltd	20
	0.9% Normal saline	Freely available*	10, 25, 100, 500
	Ringer lactate	Freely available*	500
Potassium	Potassium chloride 15%	Freely available*	10
Calcium	Calcium gluconate 10%	Freely available*	10
Magnesium	Magnesium sulphate 25%, 50%	Freely available*	2
Vitamins	Multivitamin infusion (MVI)	NBZ Pharma Ltd	10
Trace elements	Celecel 4, Celecel 5	Claris Lifesciences Ltd	1, 3, 10
	T- pres	Bharat Serums and Vaccines Ltd	3

*Several manufacturers produce these solutions of various concentrations, PLR: phospholipid reduced, SMOF: soyabean oil medium-chain triglycerides, olive oil and fish oil

3 g/kg/day). Amino acids are gradually increased on consecutive days to a maximum of 3.5 g/kg/day). For term infants, amino acids are started @ 2.5 g/kg/day and slowly increased up to 3.5 g/kg/day.

Restricted doses of amino acids may be needed in fluid restricted states, renal impairment, acidosis, hyperammonemia and PN associated liver disease. In general, doses up to 1.5 g/kg/day are safe and well-tolerated in most situations. The calorie-nitrogen ratio (CNR) ensures availability of adequate calories for the amount of proteins being given. It is calculated as follows:

Calorie nitrogen ratio (CNR)

$$= \frac{\text{Non-protein calories (dextrose + lipids)}}{0.16 \quad \text{proteins (g)/d}}$$

The CNR should be maintained between 150 and 250. At times CNR of more than 250 is acceptable and indicates that protein intake can be increased if necessary. The CNR of <150 indicates the need to increase non-protein sources of calories or decrease intake of proteins. The PN calculation software calculates the CNR and provides alerts on out of range CNR values.

Lipids Lipids are energy dense and iso-osmolar. They should provide 30% (range 25–40%) of the caloric intake on PN. Apart from calories, lipids provide essential fatty acids (linoleic and linolenic acids) which are necessary for cell metabolism particularly brain and retinal development. In preterms, lipids can be started on day 1 of life with a minimum dose of 1 g/kg/day (desirable up to 3 g/kg/day). Lipids are always infused over a 24-hour period by a syringe pump. The maximum dose of lipids for a preterm and term newborn is 3 g/kg/day and 4 g/kg/day respectively.

Tolerance of lipids is assessed on the basis of serum triglyceride level which should be maintained below 200 mg/dL. In the past, there were concerns regarding the use of lipids in neonates with jaundice, sepsis and thrombocytopenia. Recent studies have shown that lipids are safe in these conditions if proper dosage and administration guidelines are followed. Lipids in a dose of 1 g/kg/day are sufficient to prevent deficiency of essential fatty acids (EFAs). 20% lipid emulsions are better tolerated by neonates by virtue of the lower phospholipid content. Lipid infusions are protected from light by covering the infusion line with aluminium foil to prevent peroxidation. Amber colored special infusion sets are also available for the same purpose.

Soybean oil-based lipid emulsions have been used for many years. Newer lipid emulsions with olive oil and fish oil or combo formulations are now available and claimed to be anti-inflammatory because of less peroxide formation. A special lipid preparation containing soybean-medium chain triglycerides-olive oil- fish oil (SMOF, Fresenius Kabi) is available in India and is being used in our unit regularly. Omegaven (Fresenius Kabi) is a pure fish oil-based lipid which is given along with standard soybean-based lipid emulsion. Though benefits have been shown in older children and adults, especially in PN-related cholestasis, this product is not currently approved for neonatal use.

Vitamins Multivitamin preparation (MVI) is added to the PN infusion from day 1. As per ESPGHAN recommendations, vitamins are added to the lipid emulsion during formulation of TPN solution. In India, pediatric MVI is not available and adult MVI is used as a substitute. This preparation has a higher vitamin A content, lacks vitamin K and is alcohol based. It also contains benzoic acid as a stabiliser, which is not suitable for neonatal use. Presently, till appropriate solutions are available, we use adult MVI in a dose of 0.5 mL/kg. It is added to the amino-acid dextrose infusion because we are not sure about its stability with the lipid infusate.

Electrolytes and minerals Sodium, potassium, chlorides, calcium, phosphorus and magnesium are part of the PN infusions. Doses of these electrolytes are based on recommendations similar to standard intravenous fluids. Table 29.2 shows the recommended doses of electrolytes. The doses are decided on a daily basis, considering the postnatal day of life, clinical condition of the baby and the biochemical values.

The various PN solutions available in India are shown in Table 29.1. Intravenous phosphate (Potphos, Neon laboratories) was available till recently. Because of risk of precipitation of phosphates we infuse calcium gluconate separately in 3 daily doses through a separate intravenous line when phosphates are added to the PN.

Trace elements Trace elements are started after 10 days when of TPN is required for more than 15 days.

Table 29.2 Doses of minerals used in PN infusates	
Sodium	0–3 mEq/kg/day
Potassium	0–2 mEq/kg/day
Chloride	0–5 mEq/kg/day
Calcium	42–120 mg/kg/day (preterm), 32 mg/kg/day (term)
Phosphorus	28–64 mg/kg/day (preterm), 14 mg/kg/day (term)
Magnesium	5 mg/kg/day

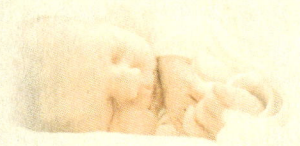

Table 29.3 Manual calculation of TPN

Name of patient

Date of birth

Day of TPN

Weight of the patient

1. TPN fluid volume (TFV)

   _____ mL/kg/day * _____ kg = ——————— mL/day

2. TPN volume (TPNV)

   TFV _____ — feed volume (FV) _____ mL

   + losses _____ mL = ——————— mL/day

3. Fat volume (FAT-V)

   _____ g/kg/day * _____ kg ÷ 0.1 or 0.2 (lipid concentration) = ——— mL/day

4. Hyperalimentation solution volume (HAV)

   TPNV _____ mL — FAT-V _____ mL = ——————— mL/day

5. Prepared volume:

   HAV * Overfill Factor = ——————— mL

6. Additive volume (AV)

   Aminoacid _____ g/kg *_____ kg* _____ (B/A) ÷ (aminoacid conc.) = ——— mL

   Sodium _____ mEq/kg *_____ kg* _____ (B/A) ÷ (sodium conc.) = ——— mL

   Potassium _____ mEq/kg *_____ kg* _____ (B/A) ÷ (potassium conc.) = ——— mL

   Phosphorus _____ mg/kg* _____ kg* _____(B/A) ÷ (phosphate conc.) = ——— mL

   Calcium _____ mEq/kg *_____ kg* _____ (B/A) ÷ (calcium conc.) = ——— mL

   Magnesium _____ mEq/kg *_____ kg* _____ (B/A) ÷ (magnesium conc.) = ——— mL

   MVI _____ g/kg *_____ kg* _____ (B/A) = ——— mL

   Heparin 0.1 mL/ 100 mL (1000 I.U/ 1 mL) = ——— mL

   Sum of additive volume _____ mL

7. Dextrose volume (DV)

   PV _____ mL minus AV_____ mL = ——————— mL

8. Dextrose concentration (DC)

   Need to add _____ g dextrose in remaining vol _____ mL (DV) (PV—AV)

   _____ g ◁ D10 _____ mL _____ g

   D25 _____ mL _____ g   DC = [   ]

   D50 _____ mL _____ g

   $$CNR = \frac{(Fat\ Cal + glucose\ Cal)}{AA\ in\ gm \div 6.25} = ——————— = ——————— (150–250)$$

   TPN final constitution

   D10 _____ mL + D50 _____ mL + AA _____ mL + Na _____ mL + K _____ mL

   + Ca _____ mL + MVI _____ mL + Mg _____ mL + Heparin _____ mL

   Lipid infusion = ——————— mL of lipid ÷ 24 hrs = ——————— mL/hr

Presently T-Pres (Trace element injection 5) is being used in TPN solution which includes zinc, copper, chromium, manganese and selenium.

Calculation of PN Needs

Nutritional requirements of premature babies should be calculated accurately to facilitate growth and to avoid complications. Manual calculation is difficult, time consuming, needs training and validation before execution of the order. Prescription errors up to 27.9 %

have been reported. Automating the process of undertaking the repetitive task of tedious calculations is likely to prevent errors thus improving the safety of PN administration. None the less, it is important to learn the manual calculations in order to acquire basic knowledge of the nutrient dosing (Table 29.3).

Software Calculations

Software for PN calculations is now available. The software is accurate, validated and reduces errors of

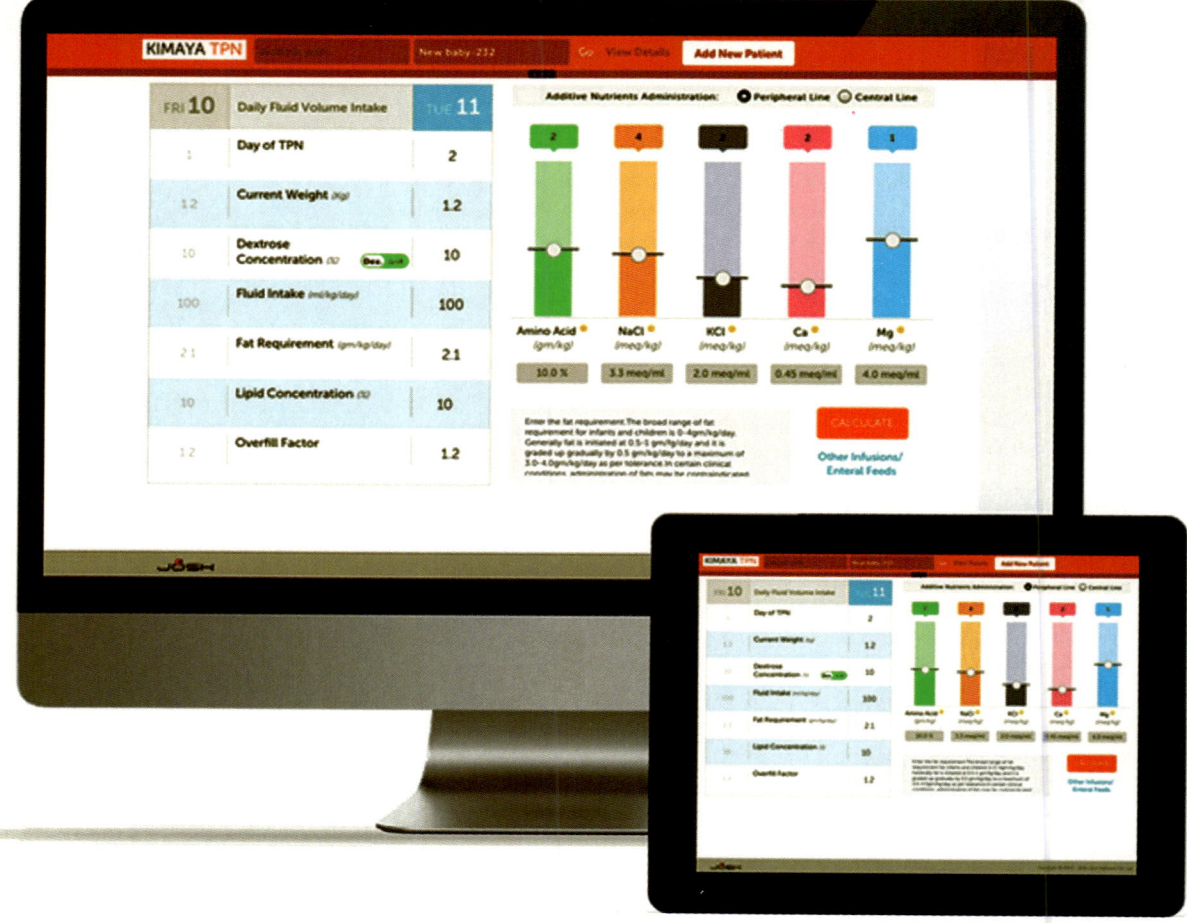

Figure 29.1 Nutrition calculation software.

calculation and compounding. It is used to keep track of patient's nutritional status on a serial basis. In our NICU, we have developed a user friendly software named 'Kimaya NICU software', which is in regular use (Josh Software Pvt. Ltd, Pune; E-mail: info@joshsoftware.com, website: *kimayanicu.com*).

Kimaya-TPN application, developed over a 15-year period and updated five times till now, is doctor-friendly and has resulted in a huge increase in calculation speed and accuracy compared to the manual calculations. This cloud-based application allows calculating right mix of nutrients, infusion rate and CNR to avoid complications. It provides information on various nutrients and gives safety alerts when doses are out of range. Printouts of calculations are generated for patient records as well as labels for infusates. The application archives can assess the progress of each infant on a day-to-day basis, thus allowing the health staff to plan administration of nutrients over a period of time. Kimaya NICU software is a domain specific neonatal health care technology provider (Figure 29.1).

Compounding of TPN

Compounding means mixing and preparing the PN solutions for administration once the calculations have been done. A strict sterile aseptic technique is essential for preparation and administration of the TPN. There are two methods of compounding the TPN, automated compounding machines and manual compounding.

Automated compounding machines Automated compounding is done by a system on a wider scale. It is expensive and currently not used in India. It involves the precise combination of nutritional compounds such as dextrose, amino acids and electrolytes under sterile conditions, to create patient-tailored parenteral nutrition solutions. These machines provide a complete TPN management system comprising of both a compounding machine and an advanced management software. It accurately measures and combines up to nine nutritional compounds in one go, reducing overall set-up time to less than 15 minutes, and prepares one liter of TPN solution in less than one minute.

Manual compounding Manual compounding implies preparation of PN solution by the nutritionist/nurse/doctor under laminar flow system (Figure 29.2). Manual compounding mainly involves preparing the solutions in a chamber using a HEPA (high efficiency particulate air) filter. These filters ensure that the circulating air is free of contaminants and particulate matter thereby reducing the risk of sepsis in patients receiving the TPN. During manual compounding, the HEPA filter and the room in which this is kept should be sterilized for 45 minutes under UV light. Maintenance of the machine in aseptic condition is very important because it is likely to be contaminated by yeasts, fungi and bacteria due to spillage of solutions.

Once the PN solutions are prepared under the laminar flow system, it is ready for administration. Dextrose, aminoacids, electrolytes, vitamins and trace elements are mixed in one bottle, whereas the lipids are administered separately through a syringe based infusion pump over a period of 24 hours.

Compatibility and Stability of PN Solutions

The PN formulation is a complex mixture containing different chemical components that may cause problems with stability and compatibility of various ingredients. The stability refers to the risk of loss or degradation of the various nutrients over a period of time. The compatibility refers to the physical and chemical interaction between the nutrients. A small degradation of nutrients is expected with any compounded solution. However, incompatibilities between nutrients or other components may be harmful to the patient. There are examples of 'All in One' PN mixes where all nutrients including lipids are infused together through one bottle. Stability and compatibility issues are especially important for such 3-in-1 or total nutrient admixtures. Destabilization of the lipid component of a formulation

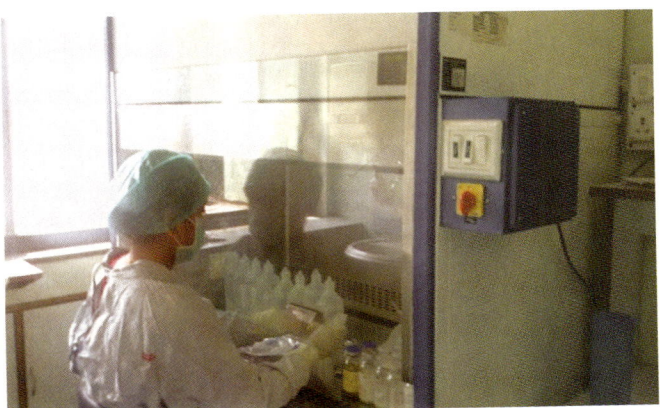

Figure 29.2 Manual compounding of TPN under laminar flow.

BOX 29.3 Factors affecting stability of various nutrients

1. Amino acid constituents
2. pH of the formulation (maintain final pH of 5.0 or above)
3. Dextrose concentration (keep the final dextrose concentration at 3.3% or greater)
4. Concentration of the electrolytes
5. Sequence of mixing
6. Calcium-phosphate ratio. Calcium and phosphorus are essential electrolytes in PN solutions. If mixed in too high a concentration, calcium and phosphorus may form an insoluble precipitate of calcium phosphate. Pulmonary emboli secondary to calcium phosphate precipitates have been reported as a fatal complication.
7. The osmolarity of the final PN formulation dictates the route of administration. Osmolarity is primarily dependent on the dextrose, amino acid, and electrolyte content.

can occur under certain conditions. We do not practice 'All in One' PN modality due to stability issues and lack of robust research in this area. A large number of factors are known to adversely affect the stability of various nutrients (Box 29.3).

Photo protection of PN Peroxide oxidation of PN is now considered an important issue that needs attention. The sources of peroxide in PN include amino acids (tryptophan, tyrosine, methionine, cysteine and phenylalanine), multivitamins (riboflavin), trace elements, lipid emulsion (PUFA) and additives used for stabilization of PN. Peroxides infused with PN may interfere with lipid metabolism causing hyper-triglyceridemia and impair glucose uptake in the muscles and fat. Photo exposure of TPN contributes to high blood glucose and plasma triglycerides. Peroxides in PN disrupt cell membrane integrity, mediate tissue injury, and change quality of PN and cause loss of potency of PN by reducing levels of some vitamins and amino acids. Photo protection of PN reduces peroxide load on the newborn and reduces risk of broncho-pulmonary dysplasia (BPD). Photo protection of PN solution can be achieved by wrapping the infusion lines with aluminium foil or by using special amber-colored infusion sets (Vygon).

Quality Control of TPN Preparations

The TPN should be checked visually for any precipitation or particulate matter. Biological integrity of the product should be checked on a periodic basis by collecting random samples of 5 mL to 10 mL of TPN solutions under strict precautions. They are sent to the microbiology lab for sterility testing. Aerobic, anerobic and fungal cultures are done to ensure that the TPN infusates are sterile.

HEPA filter hood swabs for culture should be taken from working surface of the hood. Generally, a swab is taken before preparing first TPN and after preparing the last TPN while the HEPA hood is running. The air circulating in the HEPA hood is taken by exposing a culture dish to the air flow inside the HEPA hood and then observing any growth after incubation. HEPA filter hood must be tested for its efficiency once every 6 months.

Setting up of TPN

TPN solutions must be administered using an IV-infusion set with a filter. Do not add any medication to a TPN solution. Never piggy back a TPN solution with any other biochemical agent due to physical, chemical and biological incompatibility. Use of Y connectors or triple lumen connectors can be used for administration of amino acid solution and intralipid from the same line (Figure 29.3). Alternatively, some units infuse aminoacid-dextrose-electrolyte solution and lipids through two separate infusion lines established at different sites. The infusion sets must be changed daily while bacterial filters are changed every 3 days.

Routes and Techniques of PN Administration

TPN can be administered through the peripheral or central lines (umbilical or central venous route). Use of peripheral line is safer when PN is needed for less than 10 days. Percutaneous inserted central catheter (PICC) is used to reduce the risk of phlebitis when concentration of glucose exceeds 12.5%, osmolarity of solution is >900 mOsm/L and when TPN is required for more than 10 days. The position of the tip of the catheter should be in a large vessel preferably the superior or inferior vena cava outside the heart and its position confirmed by X-ray prior to use. Single lumen central lines are preferred over multiple lumen catheters due to reduced risk of sepsis. PN lines should be handled minimally and with due aseptic techniques.

Monitoring during TPN

A flowchart should be maintained to record daily changes in weight, status of hydration, urine output and intake of fluids, calories and its sources. Serum electrolytes, BUN, glucose, hematocrit, blood pH, plasma and urinary osmolality should be checked daily. Plasma osmolality should be maintained between 285 and 300 mOsm/L. Plasma should be inspected daily to look for turbidity due to fat emulsion. Liver function tests, serum proteins and fatty acids should be checked once every week (Table 29.4). An accurate record of amount of blood removed for biochemical monitoring should be maintained.

Complications

They may be related to the catheter or to the infusate. Inflammation and sloughing of skin at infusion site is alarming. Hospital-acquired infection (HAI) is a common life-threatening complication and should be prevented by use of effective aseptic precautions like use of laminar flow for mixing of PN solutions, use of bacterial filter in amino acid-glucose line and daily change of infusion sets. The metabolic complications include competitive displacement of albumin-bound bilirubin by free fatty acids, and alterations in the concentration of a variety of blood constituents such as glucose, acid-base status, sodium, potassium, chloride, calcium, magnesium, phosphorus, BUN, essential amino acids, vitamins and trace elements. Hyperglycemia with osmotic diuresis and dehydration can occur among ELBW babies receiving hyperosmolar infusates. A constant clinical and chemical monitoring

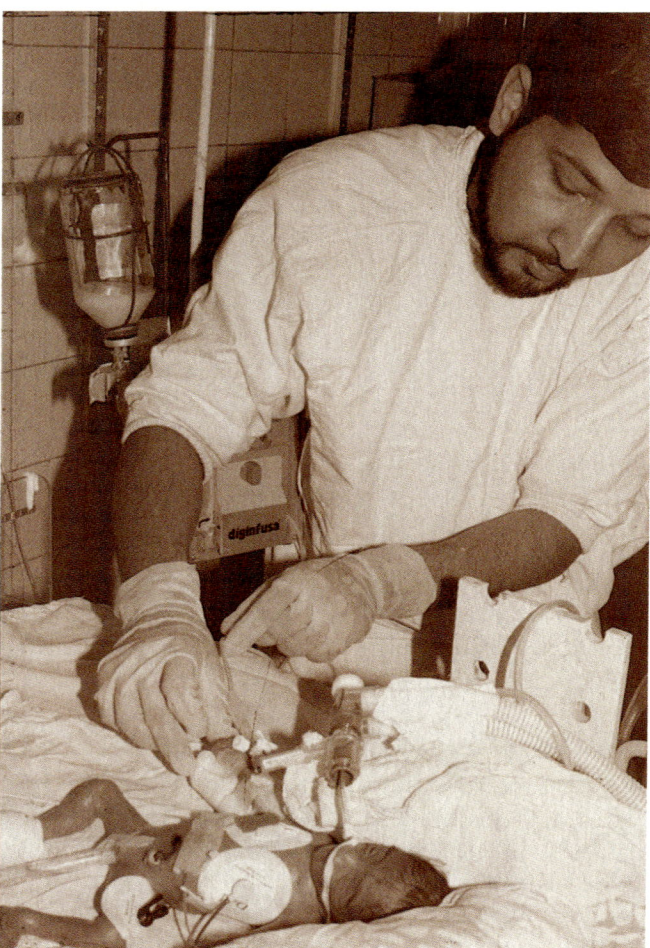

Figure 29.3 Setting up 3-way stopcock for administration of TPN with strict aseptic precautions.

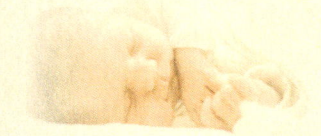

Table 29.4 Monitoring schedule for neonates receiving parenteral nutrition

Parameter	Frequency
*Anthropometry**	
Weight (g)	Daily (same time each day)
Length (cm)	weekly
Head circumference (cm)	Weekly
Biochemistry	
Urine glucose and specific gravity	8 hourly first week, then once daily
Inspection of plasma sample for lipemia	Once daily
Blood glucose	6 hourly initially, 12 hourly when glucose infusion rate is static
Serum sodium and potassium	Daily initial 3–4 days, then twice weekly
BUN, creatinine	Daily initial 3–4 days, then twice weekly once protein intake becomes static
Blood pH	Daily initial 3–4 days, then twice a week once protein intake becomes static
Hemogram	Weekly
Serum calcium, phosphorus, magnesium, proteins, triglycerides, liver function tests	Weekly

*The target anthropometric gains during TPN include weight gain 15–18 g/d (1.0% of body weight/d), length gain 0.75–1.0 cm/week, and head circumference gain 0.75 cm/week.
Note: Daily intake of fluids (mL/kg/d), urine output (mL/kg/hr), energy intake (kcal/kg/d), glucose infusion rate (mg/kg/min), protein intake (g/kg/d) and lipids (g/kg/d) should be recorded. Catheter-related complications including hospital acquired infection (HAI) should be looked for. Eosinophilia is a useful marker of allergy to intralipid. Blood transfusion is mandatory as soon as 10% of blood volume has been removed by sampling.

with the aid of a micro chemistry laboratory support is essential for early diagnosis and prompt management of metabolic alterations.

Hepatomegaly with cholestasis and jaundice is a frequent complication of TPN in very LBW babies. TPN-associated hepatic dysfunction is possibly related to disorder in bile secretion due to toxic effect of certain amino acids, deficiency of essential fatty acids or associated sepsis. The deficiency of essential fatty acids is managed by cutaneous application of sunflower oil, oral administration of sunflower oil 2.5–5.0 mL/day and intermittent plasma transfusion. Intralipid administration is contraindicated in infants with jaundice and bleeding manifestations. Rapid infusion of intralipid in tiny preterm babies may cause reduction in pulmonary diffusion capacity producing dyspnea and cyanosis. Thrombocytopenia and hypercoagulability of blood are rare complications.

BIBLIOGRAPHY

Brans YW, Dutton EB, Andrew DS, Menchaka EM, West DL. Fat emulsion tolerance in very low birth weight neonates: effect on diffusion of oxygen in the lungs and on blood pH. *Pediatrics* 1986; 78:79–84.

Brown CL, Garrison NA, HutchisonAA. Error reduction when prescribing neonatal parenteral nutrition. *Am J Perinatol* 2007; 24:417–27.

Chaudhari S, Vaidya U. Total parenteral nutrition in India. *Indian J Pediatr* 1988; 55:935–40.

Chessex P, Harrison A, Khashu M, Lavoie JC. Is the risk of developing bronchopulmonary dysplasia influenced by the failure to protect total parenteral nutrition from exposure to ambient light? *J Pediatr* 2007; 151:213–14.

Chessex P, Laborie S, Lavoie JC, Rouleau T. Photoprotection of solutions of parenteral nutrition decreases the infused load as well as the urinary excretion of peroxides in premature infants. *SeminPerinatol* 2001; 25:55–59.

Deshpande G, Maheshwari R. Intravenous lipids in neonates. In: Nutrition for the Preterm Neonates: A Clinical Perspective, Patole S, (Ed) *Springer Publication* 2014, 215–32.

Gilbertson N, Kovar IZ, Cox DJ, Crowe L, Palmer NT. Introduction of intravenous lipid administration on the first day of life in the low birth weight neonates. *J Pediatr* 1991; 119:615–23.

Havranek T, Ambrecht E, Scavo LM. Compassionate use of omegaven in preterm neonates with parenteral nutrition associated direct hyperbilirubinemia *J Pediatr Neonatal Care* 2014, May 16, 1(1):00004. DOI:10.15406jpnc.2014.01.00004.

Ibrahim HM, Jeraidi MA, Baier RJ, Dhanireddy R, Krouskop R. Aggressive early total parenteral nutrition in low birth weight infants. *J Perinatol* 2004; 24: 482–6.

Koletzko B, Gaulet O, Hunt J, Krohn K, Shamir R. Guidelines on Paediatric Parenteral Nutrition of the European Society of Paediatric Gastroenterology, Hepatology and Nutrition (ESPGHAN) and the European Society for Clinical Nutrition and Metabolism (ESPEN), Supported by the European Society of Paediatric Research (ESPR) *J Pediatr Gastroenterol Nutr* 2005, Nov (Suppl 2), 41:S1–S4.

Porcelli PJ, Sisk PM. Increased parenteral amino-acid administration to extremely low birthweight infants during early postnatal life. *J Pediatr Gastroenterol Nutr* 2002; 34:174–79.

Raimbault M, Thibault M, Bussieres J-F. Automated compounding of parenteral nutrition for pediatric patients: Characterisation of workload and cost. *J Pediatr Pharmacol Ther* 2012, 17(4):389–94.

Saini J, Macmohan P, Morgan JB, Kovar IZ. Early parenteral feeding of amino acids. *Arch Dis Child* 1989; 64:1362–66.

Simmer K, Rao SC. Early introduction of lipids to parenterally-fed preterm infants. *Cochrane Database of Systematic Reviews* 2005, Issue 2. Art. No.: CD005256. DOI: 10.1002/14651858.CD005256.

Tagare A, Vaidya U. Parenteral nutrition: Current guidelines. *J Neonatol* 2007; 21:186–88.

Thureen PJ, Melara D, Fennessey PV, Hay WW. Effect of low versus high intravenous amino acid intake on very low birth weight infants in the early neonatal period. *Pediatr Res* 2003; 53:24–32.

Vaidya U, Hegde VM, Bhave SA, Pandit AN. Reduction in parenteral nutrition related complications in the newborn. *Indian Pediatr* 1991; 28:477–84.

Ziegler E, Carlson S. Early nutrition of VLBW infants. *J Maternal Fetal Neonatal Med* 2009; 22:191–97.

30

Transport of Sick Neonates

Neelam Kler, Anup Thakur and Poonam Singh

Introduction

Regionalized neonatal intensive care facilities and availability of transport facilities for sick neonates is crucial to enhance their survival. *In utero* transport of a high-risk neonate is ideal but preterm delivery, perinatal complications and congenital malformations are not always predictable. A well-organized transport system can expeditiously and safely transport sick infants from home or a basic health set-up to a higher level of intensive care. Emergency transport has been working successfully in developed countries but development and implementation of such a program needs meticulous planning and involves expenditure. Availability of adequate transport facilities for sick children are in an evolving phase in developing countries.

In India, approximately 60% of the deliveries occur in rural areas (NFHS-3) with minimal facilities for care of sick newborns. With the development of Special Newborn Care Units (SNCU) at the district level, newborns delivered at home or primary care facilities may need to be transported to avail higher level of newborn care. The common indications for transport of sick neonates include prematurity, hyaline membrane disease, sepsis and birth asphyxia. In India, the onus of transport of a sick baby usually lies with the parents, who are ill informed about the condition of their baby, need and timing for transfer. The neonates are usually brought to the emergency department wrapped in cotton (24.5%), blanket (25.4%), quilt (11.8%) or just in towels without any external source of warmth and emergency life support measures during transport. This scenario highlights the need to develop facilities to safely transport the sick neonate to a regionalized tertiary care center. Transportation of the sick or preterm babies to a center with a higher level of expertise and facilities for the provision of multi-organ intensive care has been shown to improve the outcome of critically sick neonates.

Regionalization of Intensive Care of Newborn

According to American Medical Association, regionalization of neonatal care has two goals. It includes programs for timely identification of high-risk pregnancy, delivery at hospitals which are adequately staffed, and equipped for optimal perinatal care. The other goal is to promptly transport high-risk or critically sick neonates to a higher level of care with due safety and urgency. Implementing the concept of regionalization of perinatal care has a potential to strengthen neonatal care, by facilitating referrals and transport resulting in improved neonatal survival. There are several regionalized neonatal transport systems all over the world. Among them, the popular ones are the New South Wales Emergency Transport System (NETS), regionalized transport systems in United Kingdom and United States of America. In India, regionalization is at a nascent state. Ganapathy Venkata Krishna Reddy Emergency Management and Research Institute (GVK EMRI) established country's first emergency service facility under the public private partnership model. It provides emergency medical services and quality pre-hospital care to any sick person, pregnant mothers, and sick neonates. The GVK EMRI use general ambulances for transport of sick and premature infants, they are not specifically equipped for care of neonates and they do not have transport incubator or ventilator. Specially designed neonatal ambulances were first introduced in public sector by the state of Tamil Nadu. They started with three ambulances in 2011 to cover two districts in the state. This number has grown to 66 ambulances by

May 2015, covering all 32 districts of the state. The neonatal transport services are utilized more by the rural population (70%) than the urban population. There are also upcoming private companies and hospitals in India which are trying to develop organized transport services for critically sick patients. For example, Life Savers Ambulance Services in Northern part of India has official tie up with tertiary private care patient institutes and hospitals. Sporadic efforts have been made to develop road transport system in Hyderabad with specially designed ambulances. Authors have reported that biochemical and temperature disturbances are more common in self-transported neonates compared to those who utilized the specialized transport services. We have also published feasibility and comparable outcomes of infants transported from long distance compared to those shifted from within the city.

Indications for Neonatal Transport

Sick neonates are transported from the referring treating unit to a specialized NICU either for evaluation of a rare disease or for providing high level technology based neonatal care. The indications of neonatal transport depend upon the level of care provided by the treating and the referral unit. The common indications for transport of high-risk and sick neonates are listed in Box 30.1.

Neonatal transfers may occur from home to hospital, intra-hospital transport (including delivery rooms, operation theaters, neuro-imaging and special proce-dures) or to provide specialized intensive care to the neonate in a regional center for cardiac, neurological, renal or surgical management.

BOX 30.1 Indications for neonatal transport

- Very Low birth weight Infants (<1500 g)
- Prematurity with gestational age <32 wk
- Respiratory distress or apnea requiring supplemental oxygen or bag and mask ventilation
- Hypoxic ischemic encephalopathy requiring intubation and assisted ventilation or having seizures or acute kidney injury
- Sepsis with multiorgan dysfunction
- Active bleeding from any site
- Severe jaundice with potential for exchange blood transfusion
- Refractory or persistent hypoglycemia
- Life-threatening surgical conditions
- Congenital heart disease (antenatal diagnosis or suspected after birth)
- Heart failure or arrhythmia
- Suspected inborn error of metabolism
- Severe abnormalities in electrolytes

Source: NNF Practice Guidelines, 2014

Transport facilities are also needed for "reverse transport" from the referral unit back to the referring unit once the baby is stabilized and out of danger.

Types of Transport

Neonatal transport can be classified into two main categories depending on the level of sophistication.

Basic neonatal transport Mild to moderately ill infants can be transported without any provision for intensive care or life support measures during the journey. They can be successfully shifted to a facility along with their mothers while maintaining their body temperature by warm clothing and kangaroo mother care. In addition a low cost device "Embrace Infant Warmer" developed by a non-profit organization, can be used for the maintenance of temperature of premature and low birth weight babies during the transport. It is a portable and reusable insulated wrap fabricated with heat releasing phase change material that can keep the infant warm for 4–6 hours. In short distance transport, the pad is heated before the journey. The Embrace India Program serves under-resourced health care centers in states like Uttar Pradesh, Bihar, Karnataka, Gujarat and Uttrakhand by donating infant warmer pads for care of low birth weight babies. Their staff also provides health educa-tion to the mothers and health care workers for keeping the babies warm. Apart from temperature maintenance, euglycemia is maintained by feeding the baby during the transport. A vast majority of babies require only simple and affordable low cost transport facilities.

Advanced neonatal transport Babies with life-threatening complications and requiring life support measures are provided intensive care during trans-portation. This requires a well-equipped ambulance with a transport incubator, ventilator, oxygen supply, suction, syringe pumps, etc. simulating a mini mobile NICU (Figure 30.1). Doctors and specially trained

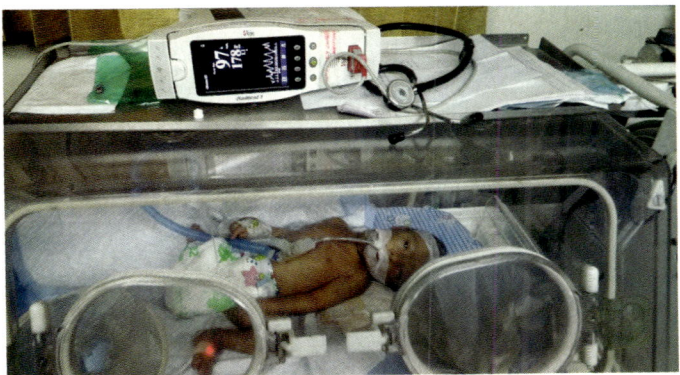

Figure 30.1 Baby in a transport incubator.

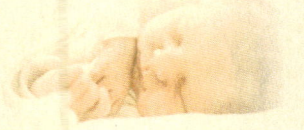

paramedic who can provide effective neonatal resuscitation, accompany the sick neonate. There is a need to develop cost-effective models of neonatal transport in a phased manner throughout the country.

Modes of Transport

The mode of transport (ground or air) should be determined by transferring institution in consultation with the referral hospital. The thumb rule is to use the safest and fastest means of transport that is available. The vehicle used would depend upon the local terrain, condition of the neonate, distance to be travelled, safety and cost. The transport vehicle should be compatible with weather and traffic conditions. Ground transport is satisfactory for distances upto 250 km, beyond which an aircraft is desirable to ensure speedy transfer.

Organization of Transport

Organization of transport includes preparation of components of transport system (human resource, ambulance and equipments), pre-transport stabilization, care during transport and communication and support to the family.

The referring hospital should communicate to the parents about nature and severity of illness, need for transport, facilities available at the referral hospital including infrastructure and names of the key personnel. The type and mode of transport, time needed to reach the referral hospital, possible need for emergency procedures during transport and cost involved should be explained. Parents of a sick child are under marked stress and they can be supported by compassionately responding to their queries regarding baby's condition, chances of survival, anticipated procedures, operations or clinical studies likely to be undertaken at the referral hospital. Parents should have an opportunity to touch and caress their baby prior to the transport and should preferably accompany the baby.

1. Components of a Neonatal Transport System

Transport note The referral unit should write a detailed note about the clinical condition of the baby, biochemical indices, medications and life support measures being provided (*see* sample documentation sheet).

Sample referral note and documentation sheet for neonatal transport

Date _____   Time _____

Address and telephone number of key person _____
(Referring hospital)

_____

Baby's name _____   Mother's name _____   Father's name _____

DOB _____   TOB _____   Sex _____

Duration of pregnancy_____   LMP _____   EDD _____

Antenatal risk factors - PIH/GDM/PROM/maternal disease _____

Antenatal steroids (in case of prematurity)   Yes/No

Birth Details

Mode of delivery _____   Place of delivery _____

Apgar score 1 min ___   5 min ___   10 min ___

Resuscitation details: Initial steps/bag and mask ventilation/chest compressions/medications

Birth weight _____ gm

Clinical summary ....

....

....

Reasons for transfer: LBW / Respiratory distress/ Convulsions/ Jaundice/ Malformation/ Any other

Examination Findings

Present weight _____

Vitals: HR _____, Respiratory rate _____, CRT _____, BP _____, Temp _____, SpO_2 _____

Blood sugar _____

Ventilatory settings

Ionotropes requirements

ET fixed at

IV cannula length   Site

Central line if any   Yes/No   Site

Any specific findings

Medications and IV fluids

....

....

....

Investigations with dates

....

....

....

Diagnosis ....

The possible needs for emergency medications and procedures during the transport _____

_____

Duly signed consent form by parents   Yes/No

Mode of transport _____ Accompanying persons _____

Name, address and phone number of key person at the referral hospital _____

_____

Signature

Name

Date and Time

Human resource A physician trained in neonatal resuscitation and competent to undertake emergency procedures in a sick neonate serves as a leader of the transport team. A person like a specially designated trained nurse or physician can serve as a manager of the team. He/she can control the day-to-day management, budget and maintenance of equipment. Other team members include neonatal-trained nurse, anesthetist, respiratory therapist and paramedic. In case of rural transport, the team may be constituted by ASHA worker, ANM, a trained/untrained paramedic and a family member. They should be guided to provide essential newborn care during transport, identification of danger signs and their immediate management. Trained paramedics are not available in India and most advanced transports are undertaken by pediatric residents or neonatal fellows. There is a need to develop a cadre of trained paramedics in our country who can assist to provide neonatal transport.

Transport vehicles Most ambulances in India are makeshift commercial vehicles like a van, SUV or mini truck, modified to the designed specifications of the purchaser. The van or mini-truck is suitable for transport up to distance of 300 km (6–10 hours). Long SUV or Minivan is good enough for moving the baby up to a distance of 100–150 km. The ambulance should be equipped to provide essential requirements for basic life support to the neonate. The vehicle must provide secure fixation of the transport incubator, and equipped with independent power source or batteries to operate other monitoring and supportive devices. The national guidelines state that the speed of the ambulance should not exceed more than 15–20 km/hr over the designated speed limit.

Equipment The transport team must check the list of equipments mentioned in Table 30.1. All the equipments must be fully charged, should have a battery

Table 30.1 Equipments required during transport

Thermal support equipment and supplies
- Transport incubator
- Thermometer and/ or temperature monitor and probes
- Plastic wrap, insulating blankets, heat shield

Respiratory support equipment
- Oxygen and air cylinders with appropriate indicators of in-line pressure and gas content
- Flow meters, oxygen tubing and adapters
- Oxygen hood, neonatal size masks and cannulae
- Oxygen analyzer, pulse oximeter
- Neonatal positive pressure bags
- Continuous positive airway apparatus with nasal prongs or endotracheal tube
- Mechanical ventilator with back up circuit
- Endotracheal tubes: 2.5 mm, 3.0 mm, 3.5 mm, 4.0 mm
- Laryngoscope with 00, 0 and 1 size blades
- Laryngoscope batteries and extra lamps
- Endotracheal tube holders and tape to secure ET tube

Suction equipment
- Mucus suction trap
- Suction catheters (5, 6, 8, 10, 12 Fr)
- Regulated suction with a gauge limiting <100 mmHg.
- Feeding tube (8 Fr) and 20 mL syringe for oro-gastric decompression
- Sterile gloves
- Sterile water or normal saline for rinsing

Monitoring equipment
- Stethoscope, cardiac monitor, pulse oximeter
- Glucometer for blood sugar evaluation

Parenteral infusion equipment
- Intravenous catheters (24, 26 gauge)
- Syringes (2, 5, 10, 20, 50 mL)
- Splint, transparent dressings or micropore
- Three way stopcocks, IV chamber sets/micro drip sets and infusion pumps
- Intravenous administration tubing compatible with infusion pump

Source: NNF Practice Guidelines, 2014

backup and provided with a power backup. Gas cylinders should be filled prior to start of journey and arrangements should be made for spare cylinders depending upon the duration of journey. As most babies are referred for respiratory support, CPAP, mini ventilators, T-piece device or self/flow inflating resuscitation devices should be available. Some of the commercially available transport systems have ventilators that are integral to the incubator system (Air-Shields Globetrotter TI500, Draeger Medical) or standalone systems (Pneupac® babyPAC™, Smiths Medical). It is important to secure the neonate inside the incubator with the help of a neonatal harness that is commercially available (Neo-restraint, Paraid Medical) and consists of a series of foam wedges and straps, that can be adjusted to the position and size of the infant within the transport incubator. Syringe infusion pumps with battery backup are best suited to deliver maintenance fluids and drugs. A multi-parameter monitor is preferable but portable pulse-oximeter is a good alternative in resource constraint situations. Pulse oximeters with Massimo technology help to minimize motion artifacts. End-tidal CO_2 ($EtCO_2$) monitoring is a useful device to assess the placement and patency of an endotracheal tube. It also helps to identify accidental tube dislodgement during transport.

2. Pre-transport Stabilization

Metabolic derangements like hypoglycemia, hypothermia, poor perfusion and oxygenation are reliable predictors of mortality in transported neonates. Pre-transport stabilization basically includes maintenance of vitals and correction of metabolic derangements before start of journey. There are acronyms like STABLE (Sugar, Temperature, Artificial breathing, Blood pressure, Laboratory work-up, Emotional support) and TOPS [Temperature, Oxygenation (airway and breathing), Perfusion, Sugar] which are useful to remember important steps of pre-transport stabilization. The STABLE program is a widely accepted pre-transport neonatal stabilization educational and clinical tool. TOPS, a simplified assessment of neonatal acute physiology also gives a good prediction of mortality in sick neonates.

Airway

This includes maintaining a neonate's head in a slightly extended position or intubating the baby depending upon the respiratory and neurological status of the neonate. An infant can be transported without intubation if the gestation is greater than 30 weeks, vital signs have been consistently stable in an FiO_2 of <0.5 and $PaCO_2$ is normal. If the infant is extremely preterm (<30 weeks), clinically unstable, has high oxygen requirement (FiO_2 of 0.5 or more), and rising $PaCO_2$, with recurrent apneic attacks, endotracheal intubation and respiratory support must be provided during the transport. If an infant is already intubated, it is better to transport the baby with a tube *in situ* and endotracheal tube position confirmed radiologically or by $EtCO_2$ monitoring. It is better to sedate an intubated baby during transport to prevent accidental tube dislodgement.

Breathing

Breathing is assessed by chest movements and good bilateral air entry. A ventilator in a good working condition is required to provide assisted breathing to an intubated infant. The blood gas parameters like PaO_2, $PaCO_2$, pH and SaO_2 should be satisfactory before commencement of journey. If an infant with pneumothorax is being transported, it is important to make sure that the chest drain is functioning.

Circulation

Sick infant should have secure and dependable venous access. A well positioned umbilical venous catheter is a safe and reliable route for the delivery of fluids and drugs, especially inotropes and prostaglandins. Baby's perfusion (color, capillary refil time, blood pressure) should be assessed prior to transport. Bolus of normal saline and inotropes should be initiated as per need. Severe anemia should be corrected by administration of packed RBCs. Arterial access is required for infants who are ventilated or who have an unstable circulation for invasive blood pressure and ABG monitoring. The umbilical artery, radial and posterior tibial arteries are the preferred sites. All lines and connections must be visible and marked with the site of insertion and details of the infusates and drugs being administered.

Temperature

Small and sick preterm infants rapidly lose heat. Hypothermia increases oxygen consumption and caloric requirements with increased risk of hypoxia, hypoglycemia, acidosis and intraventricular hemorrhage. It is important to warm the transport incubator to the correct temperature before the start of journey. After placing the infant in the incubator, affix the temperature sensing probe over right hypochondrium. On arrival at the referral hospital, connect the transport incubator to the mains supply, set the desired temperature and keep the access ports closed. Bubble sheet or polythene wraps can be used to cover smaller infants but without obscuring the sites of probes and cannulae.

Metabolic

Before transporting the baby, it is important to stabilize the sugar, electrolytes, blood gases and acid-base status. In the presence of metabolic acidosis, baby's perfusion should be assessed and shock should be managed. Antibiotics should be started when sepsis is suspected on clinical grounds or screening tests.

3. Care during Transport

The aim of ideal transport is to provide a similar standard of care during the transport which is provided in the NICU. Temperature, airway, breathing and circulation should be maintained as during pre-transport stabilization. Vital signs should be recorded every 15 min and infusion rates checked every 30 min. Oxygen saturation, end-tidal CO_2 and blood pressure (invasive or noninvasive) should be recorded when advanced transport facilities are utilized. If the infant needs interventions like reintubation or insertion of a chest drain, the ambulance needs to be stopped in a safe place until the procedure is successfully completed. Interventions and changes in the baby's condition and vital signs should be documented. Referral unit should be informed about baby's condition beforehand so that necessary preparations and facilities are organized.

4. Communication and Family Support

The transport team should maintain an effective communication between the referring (sending), receiving units and parents. The availability of bed must be confirmed before starting transport and referral hospital must be informed in advance. The referring unit must provide the referral unit and transporting team with patient's demographic details, antenatal, perinatal and birth history, laboratory reports and treatment received in the referring unit and reasons for transfer. The transport team should intimate the referral unit about any deterioration and interventions done during the journey and likely interventions required immediately on arrival so that necessary preparations can be made by the referral unit. The approximate time when the baby is likely to reach the referral hospital should be intimated. After intensive care at the referral unit, once the baby is improved and stable, the infant is transported back (reverse transport) to the parent hospital for ongoing care and follow-up.

Special Clinical Circumstances

The basics of organization of transport and monitoring remain the same with some specific components of care during special clinical situations as mentioned below.

Respiratory distress syndrome Infant should be provided with CPAP through nasal prongs or intubated and provided assisted ventilation during transport. FiO_2 should be adjusted to maintain SpO_2 between 85–90%. Resuscitation facilities and adequate supply of oxygen should be available for the duration of transport. The referral unit should be fully prepared to administer surfactant as soon as the neonate is received.

Congenital diaphragmatic hernia Baby should preferably be intubated and ventilated during transport with large bore nasogastric tube *in situ* for continuous decompression of stomach. These infants should never be ventilated with a bag and mask. If baby is having features of persistent pulmonary hypertension and shock, inotropes should be started.

Spina bifida with myelomeningocele Position the infant either prone (preferable) or on the side and dress the lesion with a sterile non-adhesive dressing and cover with a sterile gauze.

Necrotizing enterocolitis Fluid resuscitation, antibiotics, securing the airway and ventilation are important interventions when transferring babies with NEC. Bowel should be decompressed and continuous nasogastric drainage is mandatory. A tension pneumoperitoneum should be aspirated prior to transfer to allow adequate ventilation.

Esophageal atresia and tracheo-esophageal fistula During transfer, the proximal pouch is decompressed using a sump drain (10 Replogle tube) with continuous suction.

Gastroschisis or exomphalos Nasogastric decompression should be done. The exposed herniated bowel is a source of heat and fluid loss. The baby should be covered with a cling film and bowel wrapped with sterile gauze. To prevent stretching or twisting of the mesentery and possible vascular compromise, the infant should be nursed in lateral decubitus.

Congenital heart disease During first few weeks of life, the duct-dependent cardiac malformations present as worsening cyanosis, hypoxemia, metabolic acidosis and shock. In these infants, it is critical to maintain patency of duct by prostaglandin infusion. It is preferable to intubate and ventilate these infants because of risk of apnea during prostaglandin infusion.

Cooling during Transport

Therapeutic hypothermia is the standard treatment to decrease adverse consequences of hypoxic-ischemic encephalopathy and improve the survival of infants with moderate to severe birth asphyxia. Because hypothermia must be initiated within first six hours of life, cooling during transport is an important issue in developing countries when infant is born in a peripheral center and needs to be transported to a tertiary care center for further management. As per 2015 NRP recommendations, therapeutic hypothermia in resource limited settings may be considered and offered but only under clearly defined protocols and in facilities having capabilities for multidisciplinary care and long-term follow-up. Servo-controlled active cooling improves thermal control, avoids temperature fluctuations and reduces stabilization time compared to passive cooling. If active cooling facilities are not available, passive cooling with continuous rectal temperature monitoring is advocated during transport.

Air Transport

Air transport assures expedient and high quality care, and safe delivery of a critically sick infant to a tertiary care center. The first civilian hospital-based air medical helicopter service was established at St Anthony's Hospital in Denver, Colorado, in 1972. The two primary modes of air transport are helicopters (or rotor-wing aircraft, RWA) and airplanes (fixed-wing aircraft, FWA) with their own merits and demerits. Specialized air ambulances are not available in India and a modified nine seater FWA is used for air transport because of safety, availability of pressurization, less noise and vibrations and feasibility for its use during long distance transport of 800–1500 km.

Air medical physiology Air transport is associated with changes in body physiology by virtue of altitude, noise and vibrations. As altitude increases, barometric pressure decreases requiring adjustments in FiO_2. Air expands at higher altitude. It is mandatory that pneumothoraces are drained and a chest drain is *in situ* during air transport. Abdomen should be decompressed before transporting the infant in an aircraft. Because of changes in heart rate and peripheral vasoconstriction due to noise, it is desirable to insert ear muffs before the start of journey. Special precautions should be taken to harness the incubator firmly during take off and landing.

Equipment issues during air transport Hospital-based equipment may cause electromagnetic interference with aircraft navigation or communication system. Ventilators must have the operational tables, indicating changes in performance and corrective actions required at various altitudes. The oxygen analyser must have an altitude conversion table, indicating equivalent oxygen

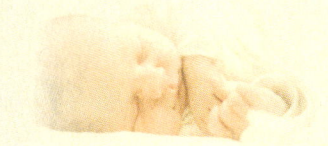

percentage concentrations at different altitudes. Non-invasive blood pressure readings may be inaccurate in a helicopter transport posing therapeutic issues. Pressure changes in intravenous solution containers can affect flow rates of fluids, intravenous lines should be operated on volume-regulated infusion pumps. All monitoring equipment and displays must be clearly visible from a variety of heights and angles by the transport personnel.

Complications during Transport

Complications during transportation of sick neonates on life support measures may arise either due to failure of equipment, excessive movement and worsening of the clinical condition of the baby. The common complications encountered during transport are listed below.

- Hyperventilation during manual ventilation may cause respiratory alkalosis, cardiac arrhythmias and hypotension.
- The loss of PEEP may result in hypoxemia.
- Inadvertent disconnection of intravenous drugs like inotropes or prostaglandins may lead to hypotension or hypoxemia.
- Movements due to rough ride may result in accidental extubation, disconnection from ventilator support, dislodgement of vascular access and bleeding.
- Equipment failure, and exhaustion of oxygen cylinder may occur.

Medico-legal Issues Associated with Transport

Excellent communication between transporting team and the parents is important to avoid any medico-legal issues. In case of cardiorespiratory arrest during transport, ambulance should be stopped and baby should be resuscitated according to the NRP guidelines. In case of the death of the baby, team should approach a nearby health facility and a death certificate should be issued by the transporting team after emergency admission. Parents should be constantly kept informed.

Quality Assurance

Quality management program should be an integral part of development of transport system. It assesses all the aspects of transport including patient care, communication, training of manpower, maintenance of required certifications, ambulance maintenance, safety issues and establishment of patient care guidelines. The institution providing transport services should have predefined quality indicators and should follow local standards of operation and regional standards of care.

Conclusion

In order to launch regionalization of neonatal care in our country, a well organized transport system is essential to provide continuum of care to high-risk neonates from home or primary set-up to tertiary care level. There is a need to train personnel at all levels for providing effective resuscitation of sick neonates and establishment of effective transport system. Specialized ambulances equipped with neonatal ventilators and incubators apart from other essential monitoring equipments are crucial to establish a robust transport system. Quality management program should be an integral part of development of transport system to maintain the high standards of transport for optimal outcomes.

BIBLIOGRAPHY

Agostino R, Fenton AC, Kollée LAA. Organization of neonatal transport in Europe. *Prenat Neonatal Med* 1999; 4 20–34.

Britto J, Nadel S, Maconochie I, Levin M. Morbidity and severity of illness during inter-hospital transfer: impact of a specialized pediatric retrieval team. *BMJ* 1995; 311:836–39.

Dalal E, Vishal G, Solanki D. Study on neonatal transport at tertiary care centre. *Int J Science and Res* 2013; 2(12):289–91.

Kempley ST, Sinha AK. Census of neonatal transfers in London and the South East of England. *Arch Dis Child Fetal Neonatal Ed* 2004; 89:F521–F526.

Kumar PP, Kumar CD, Shaik F, Yadav S, Dusa S, Venkatlakshmi A. Transported neonates by a specialist team - How STABLE are they? *Indian J Pediatr* 2011; 78(7):860–2.

Kumar PP, Kumar CD, Venkatlakshmi A. Long distance neonatal transport: The need of the hour. *Indian Pediatr* 2008; 45(11):920–22.

Kumutha J, Rao GV, Sridhar BN, Vidyasagar D. The GVK EMRI maternal and neonatal transport system in India a mega plan for a mammoth problem. *Semin Fetal Neonatal Med* 2015; Oct, 20(5):326–34.

Mathur NB, Krishnamurthy S, Mishra TK. Evaluation of WHO classification of hypothermia in sick extramural neonates as predictor of fatality. *J Trop Pediatr* 2005 Dec; 51(6):341–45.

Mir NA, Javied S. Transport of sick neonates: Practical considerations. *Indian Pediatr* 1989; 26:755–64.

NNF Practice Guidelines downloaded from http://www.cntop-in.org/ontop-pen/Week-12-13/Transport20.pdf.Last accessed May 12, 2016.

Rashid A, Bhuta T, Berry A. A regionalized transport service, the way ahead? *Arch Dis Child* 1999; 80:488–92.

Schierholz E. Flight physiology: science of air travel with neonatal transport considerations. *Adv Neonatal care* 2010; 10(4):196–9.

Singh H, Singh D, Jain BK. Transport of referred sick neonates: how far from ideal? *Indian Pediatr* 1996; 33(10):851–3.

Yu VYH, Dunn PM. Development of regionalized perinatal care. *Semin Neonatol* 2004; 9:89–92.

31

Assisted Ventilation

Panagiotis Kratimenos and Vineet Bhandari

Introduction

The primary objective of assisted ventilation is to provide support to breathing until the neonate's respiratory efforts are sufficient and sustainable. Ventilation may be required during immediate care of the infant who is depressed or apneic or during prolonged periods of respiratory failure. It is divided into invasive and noninvasive mechanical ventilation depending on the use of an artificial airway in the administration of breathing support. Although the use of invasive mechanical ventilation has been the standard of care for preterm infants with respiratory failure, non-invasive respiratory support is being increasingly employed in neonatal units, because of ease of availability and reduced risk of complications.

Noninvasive Ventilation (NIV)

Noninvasive ventilation (NIV) can be defined as a ventilation modality that supports breathing without the need for endotracheal intubation or surgical airway and may be provided through following interfaces.

- Nasal intermittent positive pressure ventilation (NIPPV) which can be synchronized NIPPV (SNIPPV) or neurally adjusted ventilatory assist (NIV-NAVA) or non-synchronized (NIPPV)
- Continuous positive airway pressure (CPAP) and bi-level CPAP (BiPAP)
- High flow nasal cannula (HFNC)

Nasal Intermittent Positive Pressure Ventilation (NIPPV)

NIPPV is a form of noninvasive ventilatory assistance using a nasal interface to deliver IPPV to provide respiratory support. It is a mode of noninvasive respiratory support that combines NCPAP and intermittent mandatory ventilation (IMV). Any ventilator capable of providing NCPAP and IMV modes of ventilation in neonates can be used for the NIPPV mode of respiratory support.

- *NIPPV may be synchronized (SNIPPV) or non-synchronized (NIPPV) with the infant's breathing efforts.*
  - The main benefits/mechanisms of action of SNIPPV are the decrease in thoraco-abdominal motion asynchrony and flow resistance through nasal prongs, with improved stability of the chest wall and pulmonary mechanics.
  - The use of SNIPPV achieves increased intermittent distending pressure above positive end expiratory pressure (PEEP) with increased flow delivery in the upper airway by providing peak inspiratory pressure (PIP) above the PEEP.
  - SNIPPV may be associated with increased tidal and minute volumes when compared with NCPAP in the same infant.
  - SNIPPV may recruit collapsed alveoli, increase functional residual capacity (FRC) and decrease work of breathing.
  - SNIPPV mode in the Infant Star ventilator uses a pressure transducer (Graseby capsule) to detect abdominal movements (secondary to diaphragmatic motions) to synchronize with the infant's breathing efforts.
  - SNIPPV mode in the Giulia neonatal ventilator uses synchronization via its flow sensor. The Giulia flow sensor detects every spontaneous breath of the neonate despite the amount of leak from the nasal prongs. The reliability of flow sensors in NIV is a common issue as it can be influenced by variable leaks from the infant's nostrils and mouth.

- The use of SNIPPV relative to NIPPV may not have a significantly different impact on the clinical outcome of bronchopulmonary dysplasia (BPD)/death, though prospective randomized clinical trials are needed to definitively confirm or refute this conclusion, which is based on a retrospective study.
- *NIPPV is used in the primary and secondary modes.*
  - Primary mode is the use of NIPPV soon after birth with or without a short period (≤2 hours) of intubation for administration of surfactant, followed by extubation.
  - Secondary mode is the use of NIPPV after a longer period (> 2 hours to days or weeks) of intubation.

Indications

NIPPV is **NOT** a replacement for endotracheal ventilation. It should be viewed as an enhancement over NCPAP. It can be considered for preterm infants soon after birth or after extubation with ongoing apneic attacks, and/or previous extubation failure. Non-synchronized NIPPV may not sufficiently increase the tidal volume, and intubation and ventilation should be considered for infants with inadequate oxygenation and/or high or increasing CO_2 despite maximal NIPPV settings.

Contraindications

- Diaphragmatic hernia
- Tracheoesophageal fistula
- Choanal atresia
- Cleft palate
- Cardiovascular instability and poor cardiac function
- Poor or no respiratory drive
- Infants with rapidly progressing respiratory failure with increasing CO_2, decreasing pH, and progressive hypoxemia.

Interface

Short bi-nasal prongs are recommended.

Initial Settings

(S)NIPPV (Primary Mode)

Frequency	30–40 per minute
PIP	4 cm H_2O > PIP than that required during manual ventilation; adjust PIP to ensure effective aeration on auscultation
PEEP	4–6 cm H_2O
Inspiratory time (IT)	0.45s
Fraction of inspired oxygen (FiO_2)	FiO_2 should be titrated to maintain SpO_2 between 88–92% (87–93% alarm limits)
Flow	10–12 L/min

(S)NIPPV (Secondary Mode)

Frequency	15–25 per minute
PIP	2–4 cm H_2O > IMV settings (pre-extubation PIP); adjust PIP to ensure effective aeration on auscultation
PEEP	5 cm H_2O
FiO_2	The FiO_2 should be titrated to maintain SpO_2 between 88–92% (87–93% alarm limits)
Flow	10–12 L/min

(S)NIPPV Weaning to NCPAP to Nasal Cannula (NC)

Minimal (S)NIPPV settings

- Frequency ≤20 per minute
- PIP ≤14 cm H_2O
- PEEP ≤4 cm H_2O
- FiO_2 ≤0.3
- Flow 8–10 L/min
- Blood gases within normal limits

Wean to

- NCPAP of 6 cm H_2O. Wean progressively to NCPAP of 4 cm H_2O, and then to 2 cm H_2O
- NC adjust flow (1–2 L/min)
- Adjust FiO_2 to maintain SpO_2 between 88–92% (87–93% alarm limits)

Maximal (S)NIPPV Settings *Primary and Secondary Modes*

≤1000 g birth weight infants: Mean airway pressure (MAP) 14 cm H_2O

>1000 g birth weight infants: MAP 16 cm H_2O.

Considerations for re-intubation

1. pH <7.25; $PaCO_2$ ≥ 60 mmHg
2. Single episode of apnea requiring bag and mask ventilation
3. Frequent (>2–3 episodes per hour) apnea/bradycardia (cessation of respiration for >20s associated with a heart rate <100 per minute) not responding to theophylline/caffeine therapy
4. Frequent desaturation (<85%) ≥3 episodes per hour not responding to increased ventilatory settings.

Practical Tips

- Compared with NCPAP, synchronized or non-synchronized NIPPV has been shown to be superior in keeping infants extubated.
- Pilot randomized controlled trials have suggested that use of SNIPPV or NIPPV, with or without early surfactant (<2 hours of life), may decrease the risk of BPD.

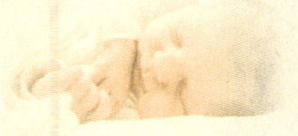

Noninvasive Ventilation—Neurally Adjusted Ventilatory Assist (NIV-NAVA)

NAVA is recently introduced innovation to mechanical ventilation which is based on neural respiratory output. With NAVA, the electrical activity of the diaphragm (Edi) is captured through the placement of the Edi catheter (in the esophagus) that represents the diaphragmatic electromyography (EMG). The Edi represents the neonate's neural respiratory effort, which is fed to the ventilator and used to assist the patient's breathing in synchrony with, and in proportion to the neonate's own efforts.

NAVA is available for both invasive and noninvasive (NIV) modes. In NIV, inspiratory assist is provided via nasal prongs or a mask. It is synchronized to the patient's effort independent of the size of the leak around the prongs and mask. The ventilator (SERVO-i) basically functions as an "accessory diaphragm", controlled by the patient, in order to generate adequate pressures.

If the baby is apneic or the Edi signal is undetectable, the ventilator will automatically provide backup breaths until the Edi signal is re-detected and it returns back to NAVA mode. The ventilator will also flow trigger in NAVA mode if the catheter does not detect the Edi signal.

Indications

It is used when there a need for synchrony during noninvasive assisted ventilation.

Contraindications

- Diaphragmatic hernia
- Tracheoesophageal fistula
- Choanal atresia
- Cleft palate
- Cardiovascular instability and poor cardiac function
- Poor or no respiratory drive
- Infants with rapidly progressive respiratory failure with increasing CO_2, decreasing pH, and progressive hypoxemia
- Paralysis and heavy sedation

Settings

Placement of the Edi catheter, which is a functioning gastric feeding tube, either in nasogastric (NG) or oro-gastric (OG) site	The retro cardiac EKG, seen on the catheter positioning screen, should have the largest P-waves and QRS complexes in the upper lead and minimal to absent P-waves and small QRS complexes in the lower leads. At times, the superimposed blue color of the Edi signal will drift from the middle 2 leads to the upper or lower leads, but this does not seem to have an impact on the effectiveness of NAVA.
NAVA number	The NAVA number is the factor that determines i. How much work the patient does compared to the ventilator and ii. How much support the patient will receive. Start at a low NAVA level (0.5–1 cm H_2O/mcV) and observe the Edi peak and the patient's work of breathing. If the Edi peak is consistently high (>15–20 cm H_2O) and/or the patient is having significant retractions, increase the NAVA level every few minutes in increments of 0.2–0.5 H_2O/mcV. The adequate NAVA level will be at the point where the Edi peak remains steady.
Edi trigger	The Edi trigger is the increase in Edi that should be achieved by the ventilator to support the spontaneous breaths. The default for the Edi trigger is 0.5 mcV which is a good starting point.
Peak pressure alarm	Upper pressure limit (UPL) is initially set at 10 cm H_2O above previous PIPs. The patient will alarm and breath will be terminated at 5 cm H_2O below UPL. If the "regulation pressure limited" warning appears frequently, consider increasing UPL in increments of 5 cm H_2O. If UPL continues to alarm and the limit appears to be excessive, re-evaluate patient's clinical status to allow for occasional recruitment breaths.
Apnea time	The apnea time is the maximum time the neonate will be without any ventilation. For example, setting the apnea time at 5 seconds guarantees a minimum rate of 12 breaths per minute. After 5 seconds of apnea the neonate goes into backup ventilation at the backup rate set in the NAVA set up screen.
NAVA apnea	This alert notifies the operator that the patient is in backup ventilation by flashing the words "No Patient Effort" or "No Consistent Patient Effort" on the screen with an audible beeping. The audio alarm delay can be set between 0 and 30 seconds on the alarm screen. This backup alert should be set for all neonates whether they are having apnea or not.
Tidal volume	4–6 mL/kg
Backup respiratory rate (apnea)	5–10 to 30–60 bpm

Practical Tips
- Asynchrony during ventilation has the potential for adverse effects including the need for increased MAP and FiO$_2$ as well as fluctuations in blood and intracranial pressures.
- NIV-NAVA provides inspiratory assist which is synchronized to the patient's effort independently of the size of the leak around the nasal prongs and masks.

Weaning

If the patient is clinically stable consider weaning by
  i. Increasing the apnea time
 ii. Decreasing the backup settings
iii. 'Loading' the respiratory muscles by decreasing the NAVA number in increments of 0.2 to 0.5 cm H$_2$O/mcV.

Continuous Positive Airway Pressure (CPAP)

CPAP is used to maintain continuous positive airway pressure during both inspiratory and expiratory phases when the infant is breathing spontaneously. Bubble CPAP (B-CPAP) and ventilator-derived CPAP (V-CPAP) are the two most popular CPAP modes.

- In V-CPAP, a variable resistance valve is adjusted to provide resistance to the flow of air.
- In B-CPAP, the positive pressure in the circuit is achieved by simply immersing the distal expiratory tubing in a water column to a desired depth rather than using a variable resistor (Figure 31.1).

The B-CPAP system consists of three major components:

  i. *Gas source* An oxygen blender is connected to a source of oxygen and compressed air is used to supply an appropriate concentration of inspired oxygen (FiO$_2$). The humidified blended oxygen is then circulated through corrugated tubing.

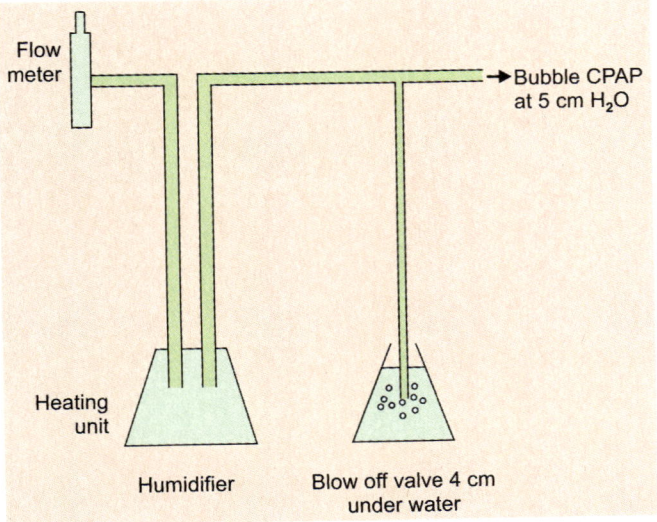

Flow meter

Bubble CPAP at 5 cm H$_2$O

Heating unit

Humidifier

Blow off valve 4 cm under water

Figure 31.1 Bubble CPAP set-up.

 ii. *Pressure generator* Pressure in the B-CPAP system is created by placing the distal expiratory tubing in water. Designated pressure is determined by the length of tubing immersed in water.
iii. *Patient interface* Short bi-nasal prongs are used as the nasal interface between the circuit and the infant's airway.

Therapeutic Benefits of CPAP

- Increase in FRC leading to an increase in PaO$_2$
- Increased pulmonary compliance
- Increase in spontaneous tidal volume with reduced respiratory effort
- Decrease in alveolar-arterial oxygen pressure gradient
- Prevents alveolar collapse
- Increase in airway diameter
- Conserves surfactant
- Splints the airway
- Splints the diaphragm
- Reduces mechanical obstruction (e.g. secondary to meconium aspiration)

Indications

- Evidences of significant respiratory distress.
  - Tachypnea
  - Flaring
  - Grunting
  - Retractions
  - Cyanosis
  - Increased oxygen requirement (FiO$_2$ should be titrated to target SpO$_2$ between 88–92%)
- PaO$_2$ less than 50–60 mmHg.
- Need for increased level of respiratory support but not severe enough to require NIPPV or intubation.
- Increased frequency or severity of apnea, yet episodes not severe enough to warrant NIPPV or intubation.
- PaCO$_2$ >60–70 mmHg and mild acidosis (pH 7.2–7.25).
- Diseases with low FRC.
  - Respiratory distress syndrome (RDS)
  - Transient tachypnea of the newborn
  - Pulmonary edema with left-to-right shunt
- Meconium aspiration syndrome.
- Airway closure disease.
  - Bronchopulmonary dysplasia (BPD)
  - Bronchiolitis
  - Apnea and bradycardia of prematurity
- Weaning from mechanical ventilation.
- Tracheomalacia.
- Atelectasis on X-ray chest.

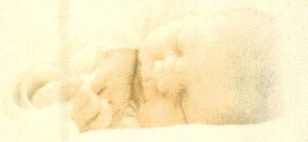

Contraindications

- Diaphragmatic hernia
- Tracheoesophageal fistula
- Choanal atresia
- Cleft palate
- Cardiovascular instability and poor cardiac function
- Poor or no respiratory drive
- Infants with rapidly progressive respiratory failure with increasing $PaCO_2$, decreasing pH, and progressive hypoxemia
- Patients with persistent pulmonary hypertension (PPHN)
- Increased intracranial pressure that can cause intraventricular hemorrhage (IVH)

CPAP Settings

Flow	6–10 L/min
Initial pressure	5 cm H_2O. Higher pressure (up to 9 cm H_2O) may be used with caution keeping in mind the risk for air leak syndromes
FiO_2	FiO_2 should be titrated to target SpO_2 between 88–92%

Interface

- Usually short bi-nasal prongs are used
- Nasal mask may be used

Weaning

The weaning is started when
- Respiratory rate <70 breaths/min
- FiO_2 is <0.3
- Reduced work of breathing

> **Practical Tips**
> - Make sure that CPAP circuit is complete (bubbling if B-CPAP is used) before applying it to the neonate
> - Apply a snug fitting hat

Bi-level positive airway pressure (BiPAP; when synchronized, it is called SiPAP)

BiPAP is a variant of NCPAP with the additional ability to utilize small pressure differences with the help of Infant Flow SiPAP Comprehensive (CareFusion, San Diego, CA) ventilator (available in Europe and Canada, but not in the United States). It is a bi-level device providing higher and lower pressures with much longer inspiratory times (up to 1s) compared with SNIPPV mode. The PIPs generated by the SiPAP device are typically 9 to 11 cm H_2O. It is not universally accepted modality of ventilation because of lack of robust efficacy data.

Settings

- Inspiratory or IPAP range is set between 6–25 cm H_2O, with typical settings of 8 to 16 cm H_2O.
- Expiratory or EPAP range is 2–20 cm H_2O, with usual settings of 5 to 10 cm H_2O.
- Use the desired respiratory rate or a backup rate. The cycle may be fixed as a function of time, or it may be triggered by the patient's inspiratory flow.
- BiPAP may be provided by a traditional ventilator set to an appropriate bi-level pressure support settings.

> **Practical Tips**
> - Attention should be paid to the selection of the interface.
> - Consider lower end expiratory pressures for patients with congenital cardiac conditions.

High Flow Nasal Cannula (HFNC)

HFNC is utilized in the NICU for infants with mild respiratory dysfunction. The system provides, warm and humidified flow of air and/or air-oxygen mixture (via a blender) to the neonate. HFNC provides some degree of end distending pressure; however, it is debatable as to how much end distending pressure exactly is being delivered. Although HFNC may provide some end distending pressure, but its main purpose is to flush the expired CO_2 from the anatomical dead space and supply a fresh flow of gas at the desired FiO_2.

HFNC may be better tolerated by infants who may be agitated with use of CPAP, and it leads to less gastric distension than CPAP. Nippling (bottle or breastfeeds) and kangaroo-mother-care are more feasible with HFNC than CPAP.

Indications

HFNC should only be used after due consideration in following situations.
- At least 30 weeks corrected gestational age
- Infant needs FiO_2 of <0.3
- Infant is not stable in room air.

Contraindications

- Diaphragmatic hernia
- Tracheoesophageal fistula
- Choanal atresia
- Cleft palate
- Cardiovascular instability and poor cardiac function

- Poor or no respiratory drive
- Infants with rapidly progressive respiratory failure with increasing $PaCO_2$, decreasing pH, and progressive hypoxemia.

Settings

Flow	>2–5 L/min
	(It has been used up to 8 L/min in some centers)
FiO_2	FiO_2 should be titrated to target SpO_2 88–92%

Weaning

- Once a neonate is stable on HFNC, the FiO_2 is gradually weaned to 0.3, and then the flow is weaned over a number of days.
- Once the flow has been weaned to <2 L/min, it is considered as Low-Flow. The warm and humidified air-oxygen mixture is continued till the flow is <300 mL/min.

NEONATAL CONVENTIONAL MECHANICAL VENTILATION (CMV OR INVASIVE VENTILATION)

There are three main characteristics of conventional mechanical ventilation (Figure 31.2).

1. The initiation of inflation

- Assisted ventilation mode
  - Synchronized intermittent mandatory ventilation (SIMV)
  - Assist/control (A/C)
  - Pressure support ventilation (PSV)
- Controlled ventilation mode

The inflation may be synchronized with the patient's respiratory efforts (assisted ventilation mode) or it may be independent of the infant's efforts (controlled ventilation mode).

The assisted ventilation mode is used in awake patients in whom inflations are triggered by the patient's respiratory effort. It is subdivided into the following three modes:

i. *Synchronized intermittent mandatory ventilation (SIMV)* SIMV is a time-cycled, pressure-limited mode that provides a set number of mechanical inflations which are synchronized with the neonate's spontaneous respiratory efforts, because it may be associated with uneven tidal volume and potentially high work of breathing during weaning because spontaneous breaths in excess of the set rate are not synchronized.

ii. *Assist/control (A/C)* A/C is a time-cycled, pressure-limited mode, in which every spontaneous breath and controlled breath is equally supported by the ventilator. This approach results in more uniform tidal volumes and decreased work of breathing. In A/C, the patients will receive a preset minimum number of breaths per minute whether they initiate them or not.

iii. *Pressure support ventilation (PSV)* PSV is a flow-cycled, rather than time-cycled, pressure-limited mode that supports every spontaneous breath. When flow declines to a preset threshold of 10% to 70% of peak flow, the inflation is terminated, although this is mainly ventilator specific. This mode provides optimal synchrony as it avoids a prolonged inflation time. PSV is often used to support spontaneously breathing infant with low-

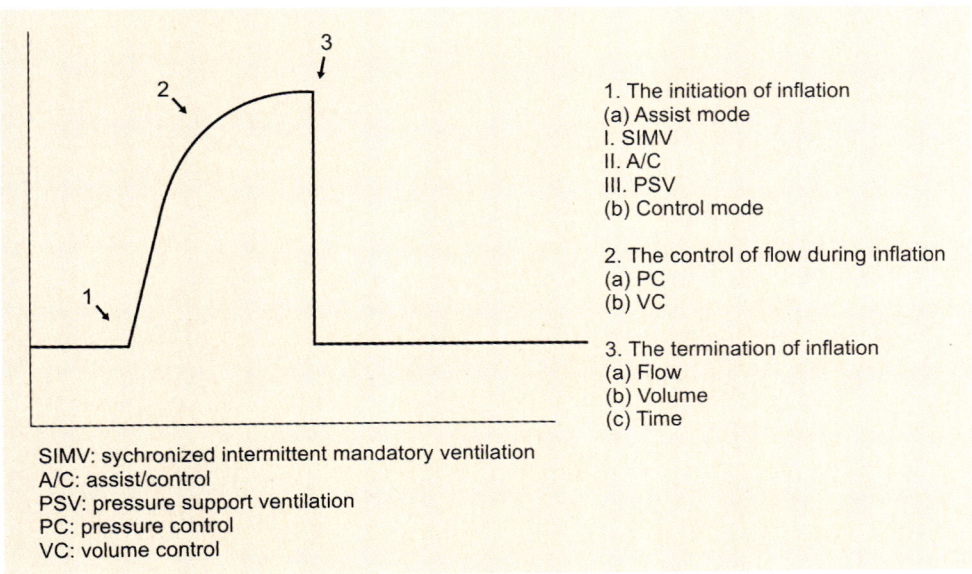

1. The initiation of inflation
(a) Assist mode
I. SIMV
II. A/C
III. PSV
(b) Control mode

2. The control of flow during inflation
(a) PC
(b) VC

3. The termination of inflation
(a) Flow
(b) Volume
(c) Time

SIMV: sychronized intermittent mandatory ventilation
A/C: assist/control
PSV: pressure support ventilation
PC: pressure control
VC: volume control

Figure 31.2 Modes of invasive mechanical ventilation.

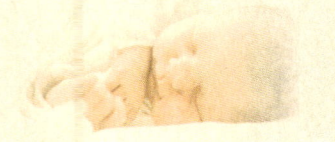

rate SIMV to overcome the problems associated with inadequate spontaneous respiratory efforts and high endotracheal tube (ETT) resistance.

The controlled ventilation mode is initiated at a fixed rate without regard to patient's inspiratory effort and is used in patients who are heavily sedated or paralyzed.

2. The control of flow during inflation

The primary control variable for gas flow during inflation is provided either by increasing pressure or tidal volume.

- Pressure control (PC)
- Volume control (VC)

3. The termination of inflation

Inflation termination occurs when inflation flow decelerates to a certain percent of peak flow, when a set tidal volume is delivered or when a set inflation time has elapsed.

- Flow
- Volume
- Time

Most ventilators designed for infants utilize pressure-controlled ventilation (PCV). The volume controlled ventilation (VCV) is a newer mode which is being increasingly used for ventilation of neonates.

Pressure-Controlled Ventilation (PCV)

Intermittent positive pressure ventilation using time-cycled, pressure-limited ventilators remains the most widely used mode of neonatal ventilation.

Pressure-limited

A pressure-limiting valve limits the maximum pressure exerted against the patient's airway during the inspiration. This is called the peak inspiratory pressure or PIP. Another valve maintains a set level of positive pressure during the expiratory phase. This is called the positive end-expiratory pressure or PEEP. The level of PIP is one of the determinants of the delivered tidal volume and is changed as needed to alter ventilation. Due to the influence of PIP on mean airway pressure (MAP), PIP can also affect oxygenation. MAP is the average pressure exerted on the airway and lungs from the beginning of inspiration until the beginning of the next inspiration. Unlike volume controlled ventilators, pressure-limited ventilators deliver a variable tidal volume depending on the patient's lung compliance. As lung and thoracic compliance worsens, the pressure limit must be increased to maintain the same tidal volume. Conversely, as compliance improves, the pressure limit must be decreased to avoid excessive ventilation as well as barotrauma and/or volutrauma. Tidal volume (VT), as it pertains to mechanical ventilation, is the amount of gas entering the patient's lungs during the inspiratory phase of ventilation.

Time-cycled

Inspiratory time (IT) is set to cycle off the inspiratory breath. This time determines how long the gas is in contact with the alveoli for gas exchange. IT and frequency or rate of ventilation determine the I:E ratio. There is a delicate balance between inspiratory to expiratory time to maintain good oxygenation and ventilation and prevent air trapping. Rate or frequency is the number of inspirations that will be delivered in one minute. During mechanical ventilation of the infant, generally a 1:2 ratio is maintained between inspiratory and expiratory time. Inspiratory time usually range from 0.3–0.5 seconds. There are no definitive studies to determine the appropriate inspiratory times for infants, but the trend is to use the shorter times. Longer inspiratory times increase the MAP, which in turn increases the chance of barotrauma.

Volume-Controlled Ventilation (VCV)

Volume controlled ventilation deliver a constant preset tidal voume (VT) with each inflation. In theory, the volume controlled ventilators allow the operator to select VT and rate, thereby directly controlling minute ventilation. The ventilator delivers the preset VT into the circuit, generating whatever pressure is needed, up to a safety pop-off, which is generally set at >40 cm H_2O. A maximum inflation time is also set as an additional safety measure. Inflation ends when the set VT has been delivered or when the maximum inflation time has elapsed. The latter ensures that with very stiff lungs, the ventilator does not maintain inflation for a prolonged period trying to deliver the set VT. The major limitation of volume-controlled ventilators is that what they really control is the volume injected into the ventilator circuit, not the VT that enters the patient's lungs, because the VT measurements do not account for compression of gas in the circuit/humidifier and distention of the compliant lungs Furthermore, the variable leak around uncuffed endotracheal tubes makes accurate control of delivered VT very difficult with traditional volume-controlled modes.

Indications

- Increased $PaCO_2$ (>60 mmHg) with a pH of less than 7.20–7.25, PaO_2<50 mmHg despite the use of CPAP/NIPPV and FIO_2 0.6 or greater along with grunting, flaring, chest retractions, and cyanosis.

- Neurologic conditions that compromise the drive for spontaneous breathing.
  - Apnea of prematurity (AOP)
  - Intracranial hemorrhage (IVH or ICH)
  - Drug depression
- Congenital neuromuscular disorders
- Respiratory distress syndrome (RDS)
- Meconium aspiration syndrome (MAS)
- Pneumonia
- Bronchopulmonary dysplasia (BPD)
- Bronchiolitis
- Diaphragmatic hernia
- Sepsis
- Decreased lung volume as seen on chest X-ray
- Persistent pulmonary hypertension (PPHN)
- Post-resuscitation stabilization
- Congenital heart disease
- Shock
- Postoperative neonate with impaired ventilatory function.

Settings

The parameters set during ventilation of the infant depend on the mode of ventilation being used by the clinician and the clinical situation. We suggest following initial settings during assisted ventilation:

PIP	15–20 cm H_2O
PEEP	3–5 cm H_2O
Respiratory rate	30–40 bpm
FiO_2	0.4 to 1.0
Flow rate	6–8 L/min
IT	0.3–0.5s
I:E ratio	1:2

Protocol for Weaning

- Nutritional support is mandatory for successful weaning of chronic ventilator-dependent babies.
- When using controlled mechanical ventilation (CMV), gradual stepwise reductions in ventilator rate should be instituted after FiO_2 and MAP have been decreased.
- Improved compliance as noted on the pressure/volume loops, on the ventilator screen.
- Increased urine output (diuretic phase seen in RDS).
- Low $PaCO_2$ allows you to decrease the PIP, ventilator rate, PEEP or IT.
- At least four hours prior to extubation, feedings should be stopped or a NG tube inserted to decompress the stomach in order to prevent aspiration.

- The infant should be started on caffeine therapy prior to extubation.
- Ensure that the hematocrit level is ≥35% prior to extubation.

Extubation CMV Settings [During secondary mode NIPPV (Recommended) or NCPAP]

Frequency	15–25 per minute
PIP	≤16 cm H_2O
PEEP	≤5 cm H_2O
FiO_2	≤0.35

Practical Tips

- Small infants have poorly compliant lungs with limited muscle strength and are not capable of generating strong inspiratory flow or pressure. Changes in compliance may occur rapidly in the immediate postnatal period with resorption of lung fluid, optimization of lung volume and administration of exogenous surfactant.
- The major drawback of pressure-limited ventilation is that tidal volume (VT) varies with changes in lung compliance. Hyperventilation and lung injury from excessively large VT may occur. It is important to recognize that high inflation pressures may cause lung injury due to excessive VT.
- It is important to measure both inspiratory and expiratory tidal volumes as leaks occur mainly during the inspiratory phase. Uncuffed ETTs are used in mechanical ventilation and some degree of leak around the ETT during inflation reduces the risk of pulmonary air leaks.

HIGH FREQUENCY VENTILATION (HFV)

The main advantage of HFV is to provide higher MAP at a lower peak pressure compared to conventional ventilation. This is achieved by delivering hundreds of breaths per minute and providing a baseline distending pressure. The lower pressures and volumes generated decrease the possibility of lung injury. HFV is not effective for high resistance respiratory failure. There are two principal types of HFVs.

1. High frequency oscillatory ventilation (HFOV, rate 300–3000/minute)
2. High frequency jet ventilation (HFJV, rate 100–600/minute).

Indications

- Inadequate ventilation due to poor lung compliance despite high ventilatory rates and tidal volume.
- When extremely high MAPs are required for adequate oxygenation with continuous mandatory ventilation (>12–14 cm H_2O).
- Infants complicated with air leak syndromes (pneumothorax or pulmonary interstitial emphysema).

Differences between HFOV and HFJV

- HFOV uses VT that are less than the dead space ($\approx$ 1.5–3.0 mL/kg) compared with HFJV. As a result, the use of low VT minimizes the risk of barotrauma and thus reduces the morbidity associated with ventilator management of common neonatal pulmonary conditions such as RDS.

- The expiratory phase in HFOV is active, compared with HFJV in which it is passive due to elastic recoil.

- High frequency jet ventilator (Bunnell Life Pulse), when used in conjunction with a conventional ventilator, is capable of delivering PEEP and sigh breaths for alveolar recruitment. The high frequency oscillatory ventilator (Sensor Medics 3100A), cannot deliver PEEP and sigh breaths.

Settings for HFOV Sensor Medics 3100A

Frequency	Term infants: 10 Hz (600 BPM) Premature infants: 15 Hz (900 BPM)
IT	Set initially at 33% (e.g. 22 milliseconds at 15 Hz, 41 milliseconds at 8 Hz, 55 milliseconds at 6 Hz)
I:E ratio	1:2 for 3–15 Hz at 33% IT
Amplitude (Delta-P)	Start with a numerical value 2–4 higher than the PIP on the conventional ventilator and adjust to achieve adequate "wiggling" of the chest
MAP	2–4 cm above the MAP on conventional mechanical ventilation
Manual ventilation	When hand bagging is necessary, PIP should not exceed 8–10 cm H_2O above the MAP and PEEP 6–8 cm H_2O

Practical Tips

- If necessary, total IT should only be increased by decreasing frequency and keeping the I:E ratio constant. The percent of IT should never be increased because it will lead to air trapping and barotrauma. IT can be decreased to 30% to promote resolution of airleaks.
- Hand bagging should be avoided due to the risk of barotrauma because of over distention. Suctioning should be performed using an in-line suctioning catheter to avoid disconnection of the ventilator circuit.

Weaning

Once oxygenation is adequate and the patient is ready to be weaned, the following steps should be followed:

1. The first step is to wean FiO_2 until it is $\leq$0.50–0.60, unless the lung fields are hyper-inflated.

2. Once FiO_2 is $\leq$0.50–0.60 or chest inflations >8–9 rib spaces, decrease MAP by 1 cm H_2O every 4–8 hours. When oxygenation falls during weaning, increase MAP by 3–4 cm H_2O to restore lung volumes and begin weaning again, but proceed more slowly with decreases in MAP.

3. When minimal MAP $\approx$ 8–16 cm H_2O with FiO_2 $\leq$0.40–0.50 is achieved, at this point one can revert back to CMV or remain on HFOV while the patient continues to recover and grow (8–12 cm H_2O for those <2.5 kg weight, 13–16 cm H_2O for those $\geq$2.5 kg weight). In the latter situation of HFOV modality, the infant can be extubated directly to NIPPV or NCPAP.

Settings for HFJV (Bunnell Life Pulse High Frequency Jet Ventilator – 2006)

Frequency	7 Hz (420 BPM 6 Hz (360 BPM) if either air leaks or air trapping is a concern
IT	20 milliseconds (range 20–34 milliseconds) The IT should never be increased above 20 milliseconds (0.02 sec) without the approval of neonatologist. Any increase in IT will greatly increase the risk of air trapping and pneumothorax
I:E ratio	1:6, at 20 milliseconds IT and at 7 Hz (420 BPM)
PIP	8–50 cm H_2O **Change over from conventional ventilation**: Set PIP to a value that is 2 cm H_2O lower than the conventional ventilation. If ventilation is not satisfactory, set PIP equal to the PIP on the conventional ventilator **Change over from HFOV:** Set PIP approximately 1–2 cm H_2O below the measured PIP that is generated by the HFOV amplitude. If ventilation or oxygenation is not satisfactory, set PIP on the jet equal to the measured PIP generated by the amplitude of the high frequency oscillatory ventilator
PEEP	2–4 cm H_2O below the MAP on either CMV or HFOV after the conversion
MAP	MAP on the jet should equal the MAP on either the CMV or the HFOV prior to conversion. After conversion, if Jet MAP is >2 cm H_2O above the CMV/HFOV MAP before conversion, then decrease PEEP 1 cm H_2O at a time until the MAP on the jet is equal to the MAP before conversion or stop at a MAP 1 cm H_2O higher if there is a need to improve oxygenation

Practical Tips

- HFV should primarily be used as a rescue therapy in neonates in whom CMV has failed, or when high ventilator pressures are required for effective ventilation, which are likely to cause lung injury.
- High frequency ventilation allows for effective ventilation with smaller tidal volumes than a conventional ventilator with reduced risk of air leaks and BPD.

Weaning

Once oxygenation is adequate and the patient is ready to be weaned, the following steps should be followed for weaning:

- Start weaning when FiO_2 is ≤0.50, unless the lung fields are over-inflated.
- Once FiO_2 is ≤0.50 and $PaCO_2$ levels are acceptable, decrease PEEP and PIP by 1 cm H_2O every 4–8 hours and when FiO_2 ≤0.30–0.35, decrease PEEP and PIP by 1–2 cm H_2O every 2–4 hours to avoid over-inflation.
- Simultaneously decrease PIP of conventional sigh breaths by the same amount that you decrease the PEEP (e.g. PIP 16 cm H_2O and PEEP 10 cm H_2O should be decreased to PIP 15 cm H_2O and PEEP 9 cm H_2O).
- Minimal PEEP or MAP ranges from 3–7 cm H_2O with FiO_2 ≤0.40. The minimal PIP on jet ventilation is <20 cm H_2O. At this point, one can revert back to IMV at low rates (15–20 bpm), or stay on HFJV while the patient recovers (anti-apnea settings) and grows, or infant is extubated to NIPPV or NCPAP mode.

INHALED NITRIC OXIDE (iNO)

iNO is a pulmonary vasodilator that is useful for the the regulation of vascular muscle tone. It is widely used in the treatment of PPHN which is usually recognized in term or near-term neonates. It is characterized by persistently high pulmonary vascular pressure with resultant right-to-left shunting of blood which can lead to hypoxemic respiratory failure. iNO improves oxygenation and may decrease the combined outcome of death or need for extracorporeal membrane oxygenation (ECMO) in infants ≥35 weeks' gestational age at birth.

Indications

iNO is indicated to improve oxygenation and reduce the need for ECMO in term and near-term (≥35 weeks gestation) neonates with hypoxic respiratory failure associated with clinical or echocardiographic evidences of pulmonary hypertension in conjunction with adequate ventilatory support and other appropriate cardiovascular support.

Dose

The usual dose of iNO for term infants is 20 ppm or less. Doses in excess of 20–40 ppm have the potential to increase toxicity without conferring any additional benefits.

Weaning from iNO

- Weaning should be started when infant is stable and adequately oxygenated for 4–6 hours. FiO_2 should be <0.6 or the oxygenation index [OI = (FiO_2 × MAP)/PaO_2)] is <10.
- When OI is <10, decrease the dose of iNO by 50% every 4–6 hours intervals.
- Once a dose of 5 ppm has been achieved, further decrease in dosing should be done cautiously @ 1 ppm every 4 hours. iNO is discontinued when infant is stable and well-oxygenated with a iNO dose of 1 ppm at FiO_2 of <0.6.

Practical Tips

- iNO use in the term infant with severe hypoxic respiratory failure improves oxygenation and decreases the need for ECMO.
- Its role in the management of preterm infants has not been established.

Extracorporeal Membrane Oxygenation (ECMO)

ECMO is an advanced modality of life support for critically sick neonates. Veno-venous (VV) and veno-arterial (VA) ECMO with percutaneous cannulation are increasingly used for cardiorespiratory support during severe respiratory and cardiac failure, respectively. Venous drainage is always passive from the patient to the ECMO circuit. Automatic shutdown of the circuit occurs by cessation of venous drainage, preventing air leakage into the circuit.

Veno-arterial (VA) ECMO

The blood is drained from a vein (internal jugular vein, femoral vein) and returned into the arterial system (internal carotid artery). This extracorporeal right-to-left-shunt unloads the failing heart by preload reduction. In order to ensure circulatory support, VA cannulation is performed. It is indicated for primary cardiac failure or respiratory failure combined with secondary cardiac failure. The patient's total cardiac output (CO) is the sum of the native CO and the pump flow generated by the circuit.

Veno-venous (VV) ECMO

During VV ECMO deoxygenated blood is drained from a large vein, it is oxygenated and decarboxylated in the extracorporeal device and returned to the right atrium. The blood is drained and returned to the jugular vein through a double-lumen cannula. The internal jugular vein has to be large enough for a 14-Fr double-lumen cannula. VV ECMO supports only the respiratory system and is indicated for isolated respiratory failure. It can be considered for respiratory failure combined with hypotension and cardiovascular instability, if hypoxemia is the sole cause of the hemodynamic instability. VV ECMO is changed to VA modality if infant develops hypotension, cardiac failure or metabolic acidosis or when there are technical difficulties because of large recirculation in the venous cannula.

Indications

- *Respiratory failure*
  - PaO_2 <40 mmHg for more than 2 hours or PaO_2 less than 50–60 mmHg for 2–12 hours despite maximum ventilator support.
  - Two values of oxygen index (OI) of >40 after one hour of conventional ventilation.
  - One value of OI ≥40 combined with cardiovascular instability.
  - OI >50–60 on HFV.
- *Cardiac failure*
  - Cardiomyopathy
  - Pulmonary hypertension
  - ECMO can be provided as a temporary or palliative measure for management of following severe conditions until definitive treatment is offered.
    1. Hypoplastic left heart syndrome
    2. Coarctation of the aorta
    3. Pulmonary atresia
    4. Total anomalous pulmonary venous return (TAPVR)
- Rapid-response ECMO (ECMO-cardiopulmonary resuscitation or ECMO-CPR)
  - In the setting of a witnessed cardiorespiratory arrest, ECMO can be offered in centers with a rapid response team.
- Ex-utero intrapartum treatment (EXIT) with ECMO procedure at birth.
  - The vessels are cannulated during a cesarean section while the neonate remains on placental support. Indications of ECMO at birth include severe congenital diaphragmatic hernia, lung tumors and obstructive airway lesions, such as large neck masses and mediastinal tumors.

Contraindications

- **Absolute**
  - Severe and irreversible brain injury
  - Grade 3 or 4 IVH
  - Severe and irreversible lung, liver or kidney disease (multi-organ failure)
  - Lethal congenital malformations
  - Severe coagulopathy
  - Progressive chronic lung disease
  - Continuous CPR for more than one hour
- **Relative**
  - Gestational age <34 weeks
  - Birth weight <2000 g
  - Infant on mechanical ventilation for more than 14 days
  - IVH Grades 1–2
  - Disease states associated with a high probability of a poor prognosis
  - Congenital diaphragmatic hernia if pre-ductal PaO_2 is persistently less than 70 mmHg or $PaCO_2$ more than 80–100 mmHg.

Preferred Initial Modes of Assisted Ventilation in Common Respiratory Conditions.

Respiratory distress syndrome (RDS). Start with CPAP and intubate to provide CMV if apneic or FiO_2 >0.4.

Persistent pulmonary hypertension (PPHN). CMV and iNO are effective, HFV may be required as it has been shown to significantly reduce the need for ECMO.

Meconium aspiration syndrome. Severe respiratory failure and hypoxemia may require HFV and iNO administration, followed by ECMO for those who fail to respond.

Pulmonary hemorrhage. The condition can be successfully treated by CMV employing extra PEEP and transfusion of fresh blood; occasionally HFV may be required.

Bronchopulmonary dysplasia. Avoid use of high PIPs, and prolonged ventilation, and ensure optimal weaning strategies.

Apnea. Nasal CPAP at 3 to 5 cm H_2O → NIPPV → CMV.

BIBLIOGRAPHY

Attar MA, Donn SM. Mechanisms of ventilator-induced lung injury in premature infants. *Semin neonatol* 2002; 7:353–60.

Bhandari V. Nasal intermittent positive pressure ventilation in the newborn: review of literature and evidence-based guidelines. *J Perinatol* 2010; 30:505–12.

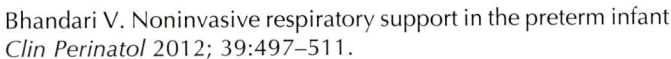

Bhandari V. Noninvasive respiratory support in the preterm infant. *Clin Perinatol* 2012; 39:497–511.

Bhandari V. The potential of non-invasive ventilation to decrease BPD. *Semin Perinatol* 2013; 37:108–14.

Cheifetz IM. Invasive and noninvasive pediatric mechanical ventilation. *Respiratory care* 2003; 48:442-53.

Cummings JJ, Polin RA. Committee on Fetus and Newborn. American Academy of Pediatrics. Noninvasive Respiratory Support. *Pediatrics* 2016; 137(1):1–11.

Dumpa V, Katz K, Northrup V, Bhandari V. SNIPPV vs NIPPV: does synchronization matter? *J Perinatol* 2012; 32:438–42.

Farley RC, Hough JL, Jardine LA. Strategies for the discontinuation of humidified high flow nasal cannula (HFNC) in preterm infants. *The Cochrane Database of Systematic Reviews* 2015; 6:CD011079.

Firestone KS, Fisher S, Reddy S, White DB, Stein HM. Effect of changing NAVA levels on peak inspiratory pressures and electrical activity of the diaphragm in premature neonates. *Perinatol* 2015; 35:612–6.

Gerstmann DR, deLemos RA, Clark RH. High-frequency ventilation: issues of strategy. *Clin Perinatol* 1991; 18:563–80.

Henderson-Smart DJ, Cools F, Bhuta T, Offringa M. Elective high frequency oscillatory ventilation versus conventional ventilation for acute pulmonary dysfunction in preterm infants. *The Cochrane Database of Systematic Reviews* 2007:CD000104.

Jasani B, Nanavati R, Kabra N, Rajdeo S, Bhandari V. Comparison of non-synchronized nasal intermittent positive pressure ventilation versus nasal continuous positive airway pressure as post-extubation respiratory support in preterm infants with respiratory distress syndrome: a randomized controlled trial. *J Maternal-Fetal Neonatal Medicine* 2016; 29:1546–51.

Keszler M. Update on Mechanical Ventilatory Strategies. http://neoreviews.aappublications.org/

Manley BJ, Owen LS. High-flow nasal cannula: Mechanisms, evidence and recommendations. *Semin Fetal Neonat Med* 2016; 21(3):139–45.

Mehta P, Berger J, Bucholz E, Bhandari V. Factors affecting nasal intermittent positive pressure ventilation failure and impact on bronchopulmonary dysplasia in neonates. *J Perinatol* 2014; 34:754–60

Meneses J, Bhandari V, Alves JG. Nasal intermittent positive-pressure ventilation vs nasal continuous positive airway pressure for preterm infants with respiratory distress syndrome: a systematic review and meta-analysis. *Arch Pediatr Adolesc Med* 2012; 166:372–6.

Papile LA, Polin RA, Carlo WA, et al. Committee on Fetus and Newborn. American Academy of Pediatrics. Respiratory support in preterm infants at birth. *Pediatrics* 2014 Jan, 133(1):171–4.

Pillow JJ. High-frequency oscillatory ventilation: mechanisms of gas exchange and lung mechanics. *Crit Care Med* 2005; 33: S135–S141.

Stein H, Beck J, Dunn M. Non-invasive ventilation with neurally adjusted ventilatory assist in newborns. *Semi Fetal Neonat Med* 2016; 21(3):154–61.

Stein H, Firestone K. Application of neurally adjusted ventilatory assist in neonates. *Semin Fetal Neonat Med* 2014; 19:60–9.

32

Follow-up of NICU Neonates

Meharban Singh

Background

There have been tremendous advances both in the understanding and the availability of technology for effective and rational management of high-risk newborn babies. The focus has also shifted from mere survival to intact survival and the quality of life among the survivors. The earlier passive nurse-dominated "hands off" approach in the care of premature babies has been replaced by more "aggressive" interventional strategies to enhance newborn survival. Technology-oriented approach, though beneficial in many situations, has lead to the emergence of a large number of potentially avoidable iatrogenic disorders. Over the years, the birth weight-specific survivals of newborn babies have considerably improved in the developed countries but there has been no reduction in the load of neuromotor disability and sensorineural handicaps to the society. Technology is being harnessed to save tiny babies with grossly immature organs whom nature never wanted them to survive ("unnatural survivors"). The concern is often expressed, is modern specialized obstetrical and neonatal care converting deaths into disabilities? Although over the years, the percentage of babies with neuromotor disability is lower in different birth weight groups but the load of neuro-motor disability to the society is unaltered because of higher number of newborn survivors among various birth weight groups.

The neonatal intensive care is highly cost and labor intensive. It is futile and unwise to have a concern on mere survival of the babies. *It is important to remember that the aim and goal of newborn care is not only to reduce neonatal mortality but more importantly to ensure their intact survival.* It is mandatory that every neonatal unit must establish adequate facilities and a program to follow-up the nursery graduates to assess their health related quality of life and contributions to the society. Infants with neuromotor disability should be provided with early stimulation and rehabilitation. Apart from developing an excellent infrastructural layout and availability of adequate tools for asessment, there is a need to have a dedicated team of specialists comprising of neonatologist, nutritionist, pediatric neurologist, developmental physician, child psycho-logist, dietician, audiologist, ophthalmologist, speech therapist, physiotherapist, occupational therapist, medical social worker and public health nurse.

INDICATIONS FOR FOLLOW-UP

For all practical purposes, all the nursey graduates should be followed up. The following infants are at a moderate to high-risk to develop neuromotor disability and must be followed in accordance with a set protocol.

- All infants with a birth weight of <1500 g or gestation of <32 weeks and grossly small-for-dates (<3rd centile) or large-for-dates (>97th centile) babies.
- Birth asphyxia with 5-minute Apgar score of 3 or less and/or hypoxic–ischemic encephalopathy (HIE) grade 2 and more.
- Babies on assisted ventilation.
- Babies with metabolic disorders
- Neonatal seizures due to any cause.
- Hyperbilirubinemia requiring exchange blood transfusion and infants with cholestasis.
- Neonatal sepsis with or without meningitis.
- Infants with major congenital malformations.
- Infants with major morbidities, like retinopathy of prematurity (ROP), chronic lung disease, necrotizing enterocolitis (NEC), intraventricular hemorrhage and periventricular leucomalacia.
- Infants of HIV-positive mother.

- Infants with abnormal neurological behavior during their NICU stay and at discharge.

Counseling and Documentation at Discharge

Discharge should be planned well in advance so that family can be adequately counseled. Mother should be given all the information and skills to look after the baby at home. Public health nurse should assess the home conditions before baby is discharged and medical social worker should coordinate to ensure timely follow-up and referral to various specialists. The need and importance of regular follow-up should be explained to the family. The following follow-up schedule and components of care of the baby after discharge should be explained to the parents.

- *Temperature control.* Proper clothing, cap, socks, mittens, kangaroo-mother care to ensure that trunk is warm and hands and feet are reasonably warm and pink.
- *Optimal feeding* with human milk and need for nutritional supplements. Avoidance of bottle feeding. Home-based complementary foods should be started at 6 months of corrected age.
- *Prevention of infections.* Handwashing, keeping the baby and mother in a room having adequate ventilation and exposure to sunlight.
- Schedule of follow-up visits with their timing and place of reporting.
- Consultation schedule with specialists to screen for ROP, hearing, cranial USG, non contrast CT or MRI brain, neuromotor development, early stimulation, physiotherapy, occupational therapy, speech therapy and special educators.
- *Immunization schedule.* In preterm babies vaccinations are given according to post-natal age or alternatively date of discharge can be considered as zero day of life.
- Danger signs, whom to contact and where to report when baby is sick.

The following parameters should be recorded in the discharge summary to serve as useful guidelines to the follow-up team for the "intensity or level of follow-up."

- Gestation at birth and discharge (postconceptional age).
- Anthropometric measurements, i.e. weight, length and head circumference at birth and discharge.
- Complete medical diagnosis, medications and transfusions received.
- Details regarding assisted ventilation and oxygen therapy.
- Results of various screening tests, like ROP screen, hearing screen (OAE), sonography of brain and metabolic screening.

- Details regarding feeding, nutritional supplements and hematological parameters.
- Immunization status.
- Family characteristics and dynamics.

Motivate and Ensure Compliance for Follow-up

The importance of follow-up, early stimulation and intervention should be explained to the parents when baby is discharged from the NICU. Elder members of the family, especially grandparents should be involved and motivated to ensure regular follow-up. It is desirable that a permanent round-the-clock telephone helpline is provided to the family to seek prompt guidance whenever child is unwell. A dedicated social worker should serve as a coordinator to handle all appointments and consultations with various experts. She should assess the family dynamics and home conditions of the baby by paying a visit to the family at the time of discharge or within 48–72 hours. The permanent and present address of the family along with their contact numbers should be maintained to send reminders if appointment for follow-up is missed. It is desirable to have easily accessible, hassle-free follow-up services under one roof to save time and assure satisfaction of the parents.

THE FOLLOW-UP SCHEDULE

The process of screening should begin during their stay in the NICU. Anthropometric measurements should be taken every week and recorded on the intrauterine-postnatal growth charts. Cranial ultrasound examination should be routinely conducted on day 3, 7 and 21 to identify intraventricular–periventricular hemorrhage, ventriculomegaly, periventricular leukomalacia and hydrocephalus. In infants with abnormal USG or neurological findings, CT scan, MRI and aEEG is advised at the corrected age of 3 months. The screening for ROP should be conducted as per the standard protocol. After discharge, physical growth, anthropometry and screening for systemic disorders should be conducted when infant reports for various immunizations. *Detailed neurological examination and neuromotor development is undertaken at the corrected ages of 4 months, 8 months, 12 months and then every 6 months till 5 years of age.* Medical social worker should establish a rapport with the family to ensure timely follow-up visits and help them to seek referral and appointment with various experts and specialists. Some neonatal centers follow their high-risk newborn population throughout childhood and adolescence to study their social integration and contribution towards society. During first 2 years of follow-up, the corrected age or

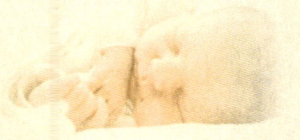

postconceptional age should be used for comparison with norms. Therefore, their chronological age should be calculated from the expected date of delivery rather than the actual date of birth. A separate follow-up file should be maintained for each baby and it could be color-coded, blue for boys and pink for girls.

Maintenance of Record

A separte file should be made on the day of registration of the infant in the High Risk Clinic (HRC). The case file should have a uniform format and include the following information for each infant.

- Demographic and contact details of the family.
- Detailed diagnosis and anthropometry at discharge including any special focus during follow-up.
- Anthropometry (weight, length and head circumference) at each visit.
- Any specific morbidities, issues and concerns reported by the parents.
- Feeding, nutritional details and supplements.
- Immunization details.
- Development screening chart.
- Neurological assessment proforma.
- Important investigations like complete blood count, cranial ultrasonography (CUS) and MRI brain.
- Reports of assessment of hearing and vision including ROP screening.
- Brief report of salient observations and advice given by the pediatrician.
- The date of next follow-up visit should be given.

PHYSICAL GROWTH

Anthropometric evaluation should be conducted at monthly intervals during first 6 months followed by every 3 months subsequently. The average growth velocity of various anthropometric parameters during first 3 years of life is shown in Table 32.1. There is a gradual reduction in the velocity of growth of various anthropometric parameters as the child grows. Most preterm babies remain below the expected weight (and

Table 32.1 Growth velocity of anthropometric parameters			
Age	Weight gain (g/day)	Length gain (cm/month)	Head circumference gain (cm/month)
0–3 months	30	3.0	2.0
3–6 months	20	2.0	1.0
6–9 months	15	1.5	0.5
9–12 months	12	1.2	0.5
1–3 years	8	0.5–1.0	0.25

occasionally for length and head circumference) during the first 2 years of life. Almost 20% of very LBW babies remain below 3rd percentile for weight at the age of 3 years. Infants with underlying systemic disorders, like bronchopulmonary dysplasia, necrotizing enterocolitis and severe CNS abnormalities are more likely to have physical stunting. Failure of normal growth of head circumference is a simple and reliable parameter of neuromotor development. Babies whose head circumference is below 2 standard deviations from the mean, or when head centile is less than the length centile of the baby, are at an increased risk of development of neurological abnormalities. Abnormalities of head shape, especially scaphocephaly or dolichocephaly, are common. The indices of physical growth, i.e. weight, length and head circumference should be charted on a (combined intrauterine-postnatal growth chart) (Wright's or Ehrenkranz charts) up to 40 weeks of postmenstrual age and gender specific WHO growth charts subsequently to serve as ready reckoner to identify any deviations. In preterm infants, the corrected or postconceptional age should be used while using these charts.

NEUROMOTOR DEVELOPMENT AND COGNITION

The pediatrician should be able to identify neurological abnormalities and early markers of neuromotor disability by clinical examination.

Assessment of muscle tone Evaluation of muscle tone is useful for early diagnosis of cerebral palsy. During fetal life, acquisition of muscle tone and motor functions evolve from lower extremities and spread upwards in the direction of head. Healthy term babies are hypertonic by adult standards. The process of muscle relaxation spreads cephalocaudally after birth. Thus the upper limbs begin to relax and acquire skills before the lower limbs. The head control appears first, followed by ability to sit, stand and finally walk by 12–18 months.

Amiel-Tison's method for assessment of muscle tone is useful for early diagnosis of cerebral diplegia. Table 32.2 gives the range of normal angles at various joints during the first year of life. Reduction of these angles occurs due to hypertonia and is suggestive of cerebral palsy. Indian babies are physiologically more hypotonic possibly due to higher incidence of intrauterine growth retardation and unsatisfactory postnatal nutrition.

There are some babies who develop transitory hypertonia during 3–6 months of age but they normalize by the age of 9 months–1 year. These infants may manifest with subtle neurological abnormalities and learning difficulties later in life.

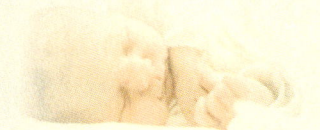

Table 32.2 Normal range of angles for assessment of muscle tone during infancy*

Age (months)	Adductor angle of thighs	Popliteal angle	Dorsiflexion angle of foot	Scarf sign
0–3	40°–80°	80°–100°	60°–70°	Elbow does not cross the midline
4–6	70°–110°	90°–120°	60°–70°	Elbow crosses midline
7–9	110°–140°	110°–160°	60°–70°	Elbow goes beyond anterior axillary line
10–12	140°–160°	150°–170°	60°–70°	—

*Adapted from Singh M, Pediatric Clinical Methods, *CBS Publishers and Distributors Pvt. Ltd., New Delhi,* 5th edition, 2015.

Table 32.3 Cardinal or target developmental milestones

Upper age limit* (months)	Motor	Fine motor	Language	Social
2	—	—	—	Social smile
4	Head control	Holds objects	Cooing, turns towards sound	Recognition of mother
8	Sits without support	Transfers objects from one hand to the other	Nonsense vocalization	Laughs
12	Stands without support	Pincer grasp	Babbles syllables	Plays interactive games
18	Walks independently	—	—	—

*Corrected or postconceptional age is used in preterm babies until 24 months age.

Development screening A number of monographs are available for detailed assessment of neuromotor development. Table 32.3 gives the upper age limits of some cardinal milestones which are useful to diagnose developmental delay. A development observation card (DOC) can be given to the parents for early identification of retardation of neuromotor development.

Early markers of cerebral palsy Neurological examination and developmental assessment by the pediatrician can readily identify the following early clinical markers of cerebral palsy. In experienced hands, they have a high degree of specificity and sensitivity as a screening tool.

- Episodes of inconsolable crying, chewing movements, and excessive sensitivity to light or sound.
- Persistent asymmetric neck tonic posture beyond 4 weeks.
- Clenched fists (cortical thumbs) beyond 8 weeks.
- Abnormalities in tone. Hypertonia in lower limbs and hypotonia in neck/upper limbs.
- Paucity or absence of fidgety, purposeless limb movements during 6–12 weeks of life.
- Persistence of automatic reflexes beyond 4–5 months.
- Slow head growth.

Formal Scales to Assess Neuromotor Development and Intelligence

A number of culture-specific tools have been developed to assess neuromotor development and cognition. The development is assessed in 4 domains, i.e. gross motor, fine motor, language and social. Bayley Scale of Infant Development (BSID) and Denver Development Screening Test (DDST) are widely used and have been simplified for use in our country as Baroda Development Screening Test (BDST) or Developmental Assessment Scale for Indian Infants (DASII) (22 motor items and 31 mental items), Denver Development Screening Test II (DDST II) and Trivandrum Development Screening Chart. DASII is the most reliable formal test for developmental assessment and should be performed on first birthday and repeated yearly till the age of 5 years. The Stanford Binet Intelligence Scale and McCarthy Scale of Children's Abilities can be used in children above 3 years of age to assess their intelligence. The Vineland Social Maturity Scale (Indian adaptation by Malins) is used to assess social competence, self-help skills and adaptive behavior from infancy to adulthood. These tests require the services of a trained psychologist, sound proof room and availability of formal kits. The results of formal tests can be used to calculate developmental and intelligence quotients (developmental or intelligence age/chronologic or corrected age × 100). Detailed psychological evaluation can be done to assess the behavior, personality and learning capabilities of the child. Additional tools like child behavior checklist language development survey (CBCL-LDS) and modified checklist of autism for toddlers (M-CHAT) are used for assessment of behavior and screening for autism spectrum disorder

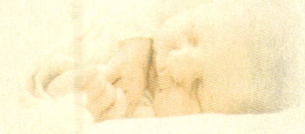

Table 32.4 Spectrum of neurological problems in VLBW and high-risk newborn babies

Severe neurological problems
- Cerebral palsy
- Seizures (around 1%)
- Hydrocephalus (1–2%) or microcephaly
- Visual handicaps
- Deafness
- Mental retardation (IQ <70)

Subtle, minor and common neurological problems
- Transient changes in muscle tone
- Strabismus
- Fine motor coordination difficulties and clumsiness
- Attention deficit hyperactivity disorder (ADHD)
- Learning and language disabilities
- Behavior problems

after the age of 18 months. Aptitude testing can help in providing occupational guidance keeping in mind the existence of other neuromotor and sensory disabilities.

The intact survival of NICU graduates depends upon the quality of neonatal care provided and vigilance and skills of health team providing the services. The incidence of CP among VLBW babies is usually reported to vary between 5 and 15%. Almost 30–50% of extremely LBW babies may require special educational resources. Table 32.4 gives the spectrum of neurological problems in VLBW and sick newborn babies. The incidence and severity of neurological handicaps are inversely related to the birth weight and gestational age of the babies.

VISION

The frequent use of assisted ventilation and improved survival of premature infants is associated with increased risk of retinopathy of prematurity (ROP) which may progress to blindness. The overall incidence of ROP varies between 25 and 55% in VLBW babies. The majority of cases resolve spontaneously but those with threshold disease can be effectively managed with cryotherapy or laser coagulation therapy. The details of protocol for monitoring and mangement of ROP are given in Figure 32.1.

Ophthalmologist should evaluate the baby for vision, squint, cataract and optic atrophy at 9 months corrected age. Ophalmoscopic examination is mandatory to look for red reflex and identify opacities in the visual axis (cornea and lens) including fundus examination for retinal abnormalities and retinoblastoma. Congenital blindness should be differentiated from global mental retardation. The blinking response to bright light, turning the head towards diffuse light or following a red moving ball or ring are suggestive of intact vision. Pupils may be dilated and fixed in infants with optic atrophy or retinal detachment while in cortical blindness pupillary responses are preserved. Roving nystagmoid eye movements, persistent squint beyond 6 months of age, absence of opticokinetic nystagmus (tested with a rotating striped drum), lack of blink response to bright light or to sudden movement of examiner's finger towards infant's eyes are suggestive of congenital blindness. The absence of visual evoked responses provide confirmatory evidence. A blind infant is usually extra-sensitive to sound and gets easily frightened by sudden noise. Visual acuity can be assessed at 9 months corrected age using the Teller Acuity Cards (TAC) and Cardiff Acuity Cards (CAC). Whenever indicated, the child should be provided with glasses, patching of normal eye (to stimulate the "lazy" or amblyopic eye) and corrective surgery without delay.

HEARING

The overall population based incidence of deafness is 2–4 per 1000 live births but 1.5 to 15.0% of LBW infants requiring neonatal intensive care are likely to develop some degree of sensorineural hearing loss.

Risk Factors

The spectrum of risk factors is so wide that almost every infant with a prolonged stay in the NICU should be screened for hearing. When risk-based approach is followed for hearing assessment, almost 40% of hearing impaired children may be missed. It is, therefore, recommended to follow the policy of universal screening for hearing.

- Family history of hearing loss in childhood. Almost 50% of hearing impairment in children is due to genetic or developmental causes.
- Birth weight <1500 g or gestation <32 weeks.
- CNS damage. Hypoxic-ischemic encephalopathy, intracranial hemorrhage, neonatal seizures, pyogenic meningitis, encephalitis, and sepsis.
- Otologic damage. Hyperbilirubinemia requiring exchange blood transfusion, assisted ventilation, ototoxic drugs (aminoglycoside, furosemide), TORCH infections (especially CMV, rubella), fetal alcohol syndrome and hyperventilation (PPHN, diaphragmatic hernia).
- Congenital malformations. Abnormalities of ear development and craniofacial anomalies.

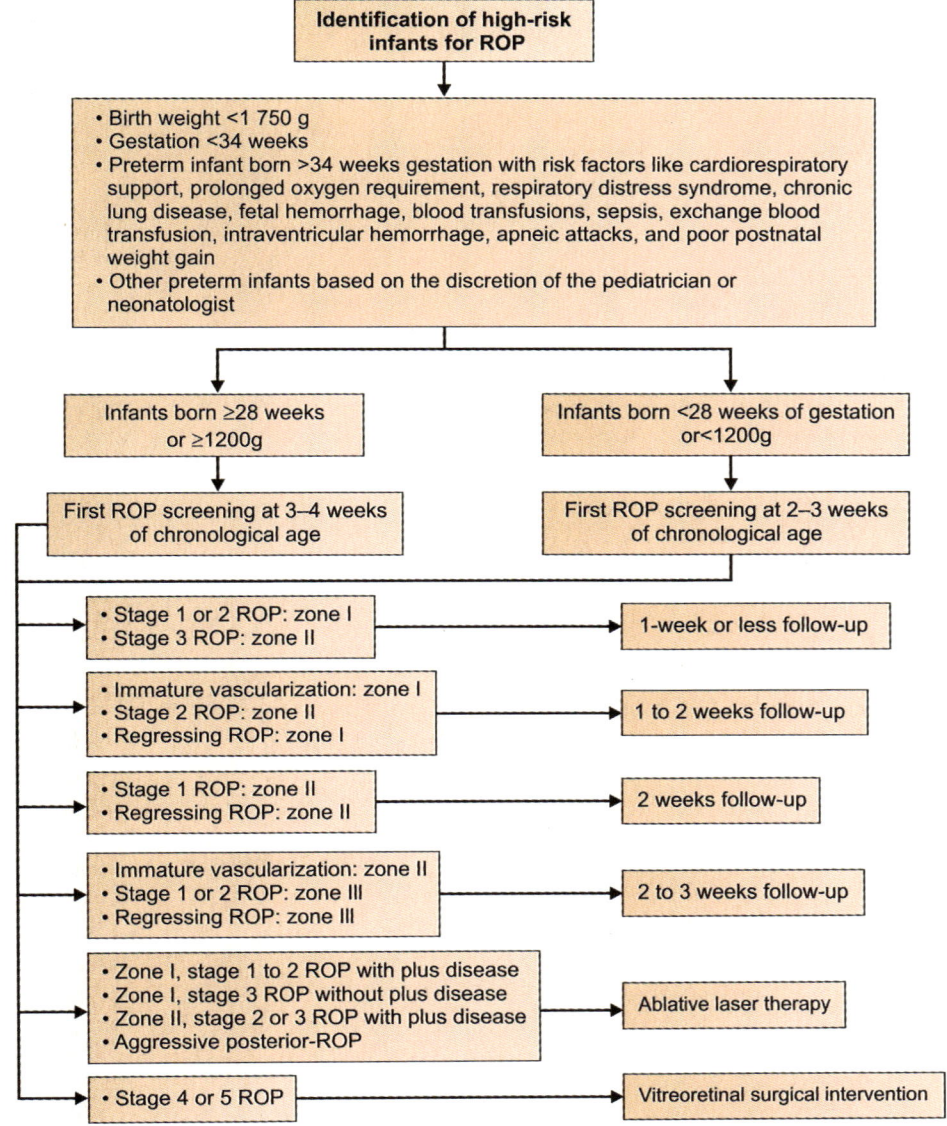

Figure 32.1 Algorithm for assessment and management of retinopathy of prematurity.

Screening Tests

Clinical evaluation The clinical examination for hearing in the newborn is not reliable. The baby is watched for several responses after giving a sound stimulus of a bell or 60 dB vocal sound. The sound stimulus should not be visible to the infant and it should not produce a whiff of air. The infant may give a startle response, blinking of eyes, sudden change in the activity with greater alertness, increase in breathing or heart rate. The positive response indicates that hearing is intact and there is no generalized neurological distubance while a negative response is of little significance because many variables may affect it. Many normal infants would turn towards the source of sound by the corrected age of 4 months.

Transient evoked otoacoustic emissions (TEOAEs) This test records acoustic "Feedback" or echoes from cochlea through the ossicles to the tympanic membrane and ear canal following a click stimulus. It evaluates the functioning of peripheral auditory system. The test is unreliable due to false-positive results and lack of gestation-related norms. However, it is highly cost-effective screening test and can be performed before baby is discharged from the NICU. It is not reliable before 34 weeks of postconceptional age.

Auditory brainstem responses (ABRs) The NICU graduates can be assessed by automated ABR (AABR) after 34 weeks of postconceptional maturity. The auditory threshold, the minimum intensity of sound click that produces a recognizable wave V, should be

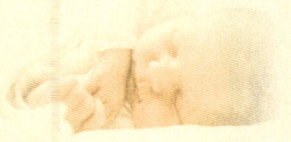

identified and compared with postconceptional age-adjusted norms. The AABR method produces a simple pass or fail result to a fixed 35 dB HL click without any need for interpretation and the test can be conducted even in the presence of background noise of NICU. In manual ABR, the intensity of stimuli is varied to determine the lowest level of sound that elicits a clear and repeatable response. Infants who fail AABR screening on two occasions in the NICU, are administered diagnostic brainstem evoked response audiometry (BERA) by an audiologist. The manual ABR testing allows the audiologist to determine the severity as well as nature of the hearing loss (sensorineural, conductive or neural) using both air and conduction stimuli. The hearing loss is classified into mild, moderate, severe and profound, based on lack of response to 30–40 dB, 41–70 dB, 71–90 dB and >90 dB, respectively.

Screening Protocol

All infants with abnormal AABR or EOAE at discharge from NICU should be reassessd at the corrected age of 3 months by ABR testing, auditory response cradle or Crib-o-Gram and tympanometry with a high frequency (1000 Hz) probe tone. Infants with history of neonatal seizures, perinatal viral infections and evidences of neurodevelopemental delay should be retested at 6 months of age irrespective of initial ABR results. Behavioral audiometry is best done at the age of one year. *The hearing aids should be provided by 6 months of age to improve congitive development and speech outcome.* Ideally a soundproof screening room with all the necessary tools should be available next to the NICU.

SYSTEMIC DISORDERS

Depending upon the diseases and complications encountered during their NICU stay, a number of systemic disorders may be encountered during follow-up (Table 32.5). During follow-up, the ongoing health problems and intercurrent illnesses should be identified and appropriately managed. Whenever indicated, the child should be admitted to the hospital on a priority basis. Bronchopulmonary dysplasia (BPD) or chronic lung disease (CLD) may lead to development of "irritable airways" and reactive airway disease with recurrent respiratory infections. Gastroesophageal reflux may lead to feeding difficulties and recurrent aspirations. Thickening of feeds, use of prokinetic agents and fundoplication may be required in some babies. NEC may lead to sequelae of short gut and bowel strictures with nutritional problems.

Table 32.5 Common non-neurologic systemic disorders in high-risk and VLBW babies

Pulmonary
- Bronchopulmonary dysplasia
- Reactive airway disease
- Recurrent respiratory infections
- Palatal grooves, enamel hypoplasia, and blocked nose
- Damage to vocal cords with speech disorder

Cardiovascular
- Systemic hypertension
- Cor pulmonale
- Pulmonary hypertension

Renal
- Nephrocalcinosis
- Renal dysfunction

Gastrointestinal
- Gastroesophageal reflux
- Feeding difficulties
- Short gut
- Nutritional disorders
- Umbilical and inguinal hernias

Reticuloendothelial
- Nutritional anemia
- Immunodeficiency

Miscellaneous conditions
- Rickets
- Amputation of digits due to thromboembolic complications
- Scars due to procedures, like heel punctures, chest drainage, intubation, etc.

EARLY INTERVENTION PROGRAM

Stimulation in the NICU

Neonates in the NICU should not be treated as "objects" but provided with developmentally supportive care. Babies should be protected against bright light, loud sounds and painful procedures. They should not be unnecessarily disturbed and allowed to have peaceful and quiet periods as long as feasible without compromising their care. The bonding with mother should be promoted through kangaroo-mother care. Preterm babies can be provided non-nutritive sucking on the empty breasts of the mother or with the help of a dummy nipple. Gentle touch, massage and passive movements of joints are useful to improve muscle tone and prevent contractures. Soothing music, taped voice or heart beats of mother can be played near the baby or through headphones. Rocking and oscillating water bed has been used to stimulate kinesthetic and vestibular senses.

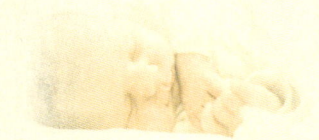
Stimulation at Home

Early recongnition of neuromotor handicaps should be followed by a home-based stimulation program. There is evidence to suggest that early stimulation is associated with improved functioning of synapses and even regeneration of neurons because of plasticity of the brain. Gentle inputs of visual, auditory and tactile stimuli promote the maturation and development of specific areas of brain. Soothing music, soft voice, gentle

---

Table 32.6 Guidelines for providing early stimulation to the infant by parents

0–2 months
Maintain eye-to-eye contact, talk and sing to the baby while doing daily chores, like bathing, dressing, feeding, nappy change, etc. Show bright light or object from the side, provide different sounds, like rattle, bell, and squeezing a sequeky toy. Place the baby on different surfaces and different positions and rock the baby gently while supporting the head.

2–4 months
Hold the baby at the shoulder, hang bright objects about 30 cm above the crib in an arc or semicircle, talk to the child and maintain an eye contact, show bright objets to encourage the child to reach out and grasp, cuddle and caress the child after placing him on different surfaces and positions.

4–6 months
Place the baby flat on the mattress and encourage him to roll over, make him sit in the lap, place hands under the child's feet to encourage him to press and make pedaling movements, show a toy to reach out, sound a bell from the side to make him turn towards the sound. Play soft instrumental music. Give a small rattle to hold.

6–8 months
Make the child to sit with support and place him in various positions, call him by name, encourage him to roll over by showing colorful toys from sides, give him pieces of paper to crumple and tear. Play peek-a-boo.

8–10 months
Encourage the child to stand with support, clap hands, look at a picture book and turn pages, drop objects into a box, place cubes one over the other.

10–12 months
Name the body parts while bathing, do simple tasks, like clapping, saying bye-bye, encourage him to pull to stand, make him stand with support, show him a mirror, let him play with other kids, show animals and birds in the park.

12–15 months
Give picture books and encourage him to turn the pages, ask him to put one cube over the other, hide a toy under a pillow and let him discover, encourage him to scribble on paper, observe him to hold small objects (strictly under observation), put objects in a box and retrieve them, encourage him to walk with support by holding on to a three-wheeled cart.

Note: The type of activities to be encouraged may be modified on the basis of developmental age of the child. Corrected or postconceptional ages are used.

---

touch and massage, rhythmic movements, eye-to-eye contact, caressing, cuddling and skin-to-skin contact provide useful sensory inputs to augment the process of neuromotor development. Most infants with CP are helped by passive stretching exercises and increasing the range of movements of limbs. *Massage is contraindicated as it may further increase the muscle tone.* Parents should be instructed about ideal or functional positioning of their baby to make most effective use of limited motor skills. At times, more intensive physiotherapy, occupational therapy, special shoes, braces or surgical intervention is required.

Mother is the best therapist for the child and she should be given the necessary guidance, skills and encouragement to stimulate the child at home. The stimulation is provided through various special senses, like touch (tactile, physical activities, kinesthetic), auditory and visual stimuli (Table 32.6). The stimulation should be done as matter of routine in the form of a play activity and not as a ritual. The interactive play activities that both the parents and the child enjoy, is the best way to stimulate sensory system and brain of the baby.

In addition, the infant should be provided specialized stimulation services including physiotherapy and occupational therapy by specially trained personnel with the help of dedicated protocols, like Bobath neurodevelopmental stimulation program. The aim of therapy is to reduce the pathologic muscle tone and facilitate the development of integrated righting and equilibrium functions of the brain. Massage is generally contraindicated because in most cases of cerebral palsy muscle tone is increased. Early intervention is likely to prevent atrophy of muscles and reduce fixity or contractures of joints and promote functional capabilities of the child.

'BIBLIOGRAPHY

American Academy of Pediatrics. Update on newborn screening and therapy for congenital hypothyroidism. *Pediatrics* 2006, 117(6):2290–303.

Bear LM. Early identification of infants at risk of development of disabilities. *Pediatr Clin North Am* 2004, 51:685–701.

Blauw-Hospers CH, Hadders AM. A systematic review of the effects of early intervention on motor development. *Dev Med Child Neurol* 2005, 47:421–32.

Clarke P, Iqbal M, Mitchell SA. A comparison of transient-evoked otoacoustic emissions and automated auditory brainstem responses for predischarge neonatal hearing screening. *Int J Audiol* 2003, 42:443–47.

Committee on Children with Disabilities. American Academy of Pediatrics. Developmental surveillance and screening of infants and young children. *Pediatrics* 2001, 108(1):192–95.

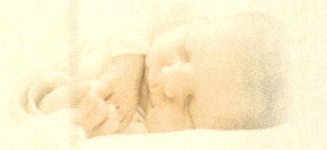

Costello D, Friedman H, Minich N, *et al.* Improved neuro-developmental outcomes for extremely low birth weight infants in 2000–2002. *Pediatrics* 2007, 119:37–45.

Downs MP, Yoshinag-Itano C. The efficacy of early identification and intervention for children with hearing impairment. *Pediatr Clin North Am* 1999, 46(1):79–87.

Garcia-Alix A, Sanz-de Pipaon M, *et al.* Ability of neonatal head circumference to predict long term neurodevelopmental outcome. *Rev Neurol* 2004, 39(6):548–54.

Hall JW, Smith SD, Popelka GR. Newborn hearing screening with combined otoacoustic emissions and auditory brain stem responses. *J Am Acad Audiol* 2004, 15(6):414–25.

Johnson S, Marlow N. Developmental screen or developmental testing? *Early Hum Develop* 2006, 82(3):173–83.

Lim G, Fortaleza K. Overcoming challenges in newborn hearing screening. *J Perinatol* 2000; 20:S138–S142.

Mwaniki MK, Atieno M, Lawn JE, Newton CR. Long-term neurodevelopmental outcome after intrauterine and neonatal insults: A systematic review. *Lancet* 2012, 379(9814):445–52.

Nagapoornima P, Romesh, A, Srilakshmi, Rao S, Patricia PL, Gore M, *et al.* Universal hearing screening. *Indian J Pediatr* 2007, 74(6): 545–49.

Nair MKC, Chacko DS, Paul MK, Nair L, George B, Kumar GS. Low birth weight babies: outcome at 13 years. *Indian Pediatr* 2009, 46(Suppl): 571–74.

Qui X, Lodha A, Shah PS, Sankaran K, Seshia MMK, et al. Neonatal outcomes of small-for-gestational age preterm infants in Canada. Canadian Neonatal Network. *Am J Perinatol* 2012, 29(2):87–94.

Sigiura T, Kouwaki M, Togawa Y, Koyama N. Neuro-developmental outcomes at 18 months corrected age of infants born at 22 weeks of gestation. *Neonatology* 2011, 100(3):228–32.

Spittle AJ, Orton J, Doyle LW, Boyd F. Early developmental intervention programs; posthospital discharge to prevent motor and cognitive impairments in preterm infants. *Cochrane Database Systematic Rev* 2007, Issue 2 Art. No. CD005495 DOI 10.1002/14651858.

US Joint Committee on Infant Hearing. Year 2007 position statement: Principles and guidelines for early hearing detection and intervention program. *Pediatrics* 2007, 120(4):898–921.

Vohr B, Wright LL, Hack M, *et al.* Follow-up care of high-risk infants. *Pediatrics* 2004, 114 (Suppl): 1377–97.

Ziviani J, Feeney R, Rodger S, Watter P. Systematic review of early intervention programs for children from birth to nine years who have a physical disability. *Aust Occup Ther J* 2010, 57:210–23.

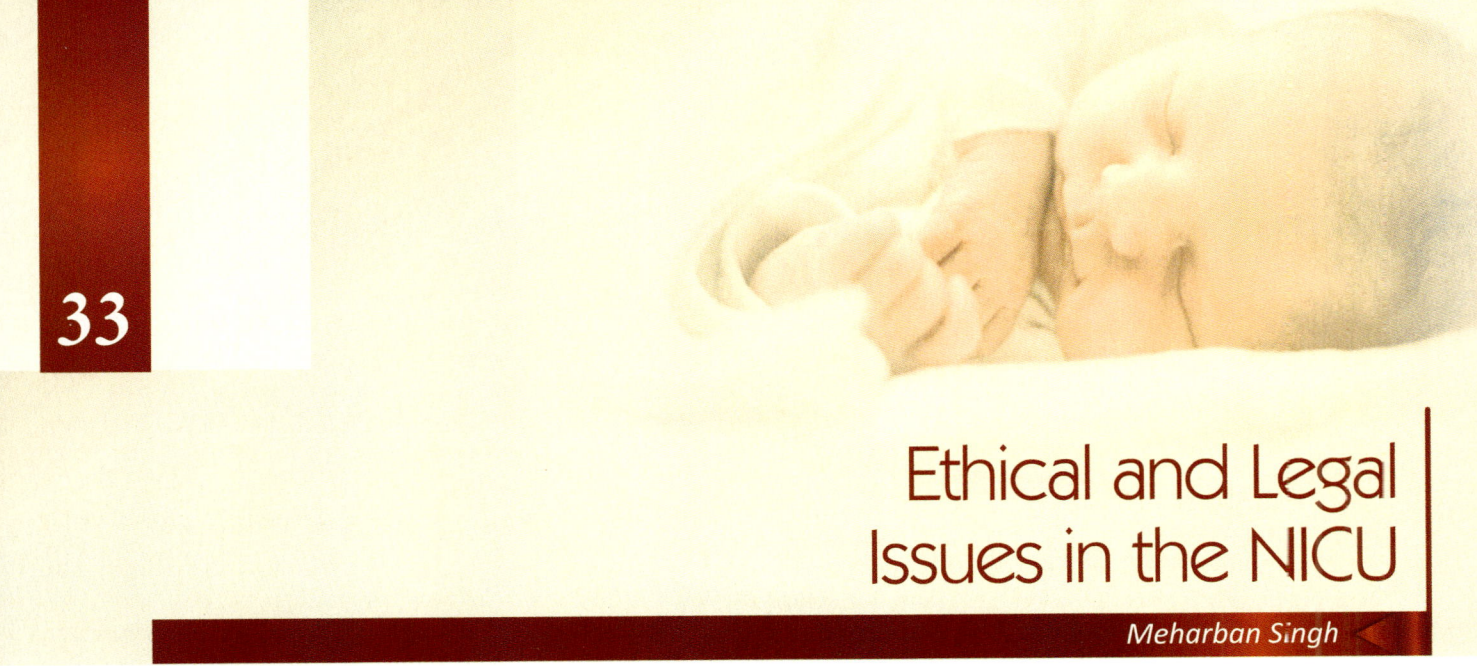

33

Ethical and Legal Issues in the NICU

Meharban Singh

Medicine is considered as a noble profession because physicians are charged with the supreme responsibility of maintaining health and preserving life of their fellow human beings. Physicians are both morally and legally accountable to the society. There is an age old trust and respect towards physicians in Indian culture. In our culture, especially among the masses, the doctor is viewed as a demigod and his advice and treatment is followed with full confidence without any questions or misgivings. The legendary bond of faith between the patient and doctor is aptly summed up by Charaka:

"No other gift is greater than the gift of life. The patient may doubt his relatives, his sons and even his parents, but he has full faith in his physician. He gives himself up in the doctor's hands and has no misgivings about him. Therefore, it is the physician's duty to look after him as his own…".

To maintain this trust and faith, which is essential to augment the process of healing, it is incumbent upon the physicians to be ethical, honest and up-to-date in their knowledge and skills to effectively and rationally manage the patients under their care. Despite growing commercialism in medical profession, in a survey conducted in UK, 80% people said that they still have faith and trust in their physicians while only 5% had trust in their politicians!

Ethics refers to moral principles or set of moral values which determine the code of conduct as stipulated by the medical profession. The ethical decisions are based upon a system of moral values that serve the best interests of society in a humane and caring way. The moral values are governed by the society and they extoll what is correct, righteous, virtuous, noble, desirable and acceptable. The physicians are both morally and legally accountable to the society. Due to tremendous advances in technology, the care of critically ill and tiny newborn babies has unfolded complex medical, social, ethical, fiscal, philosophical, moral and legal issues. Apart from tremendous financial cost of neonatal intensive care to the parents and society, there is incalculable cost in terms of pain, grief, frustration and guilt with survival of a severely handicapped child.

PRINCIPLES GOVERNING ETHICAL DECISIONS

Ethical decisions are based on the five principles of beneficence, non-maleficence, parental autonomy, correct medical facts and justice. Beneficence bequeaths that we should be the best advocates of our patients and ensure their best interests in accordance with the age old Hippocratic tradition. The physicians should be concerned with saving life and avoid doing any wilful harm to their patients, i.e. they should be non-maleficence in their therapeutic actions. Hippocrates epitomized the principle of *Primum non-nocere*—first do no harm. Florence Nightingale also said that the first dictum of patient care is *"Do No Harm"*. Almost 1000 years ago, according to Manu's code of conduct for the physicians, it was ordained that *"Dedicate yourself entirely for helping the sick, even though this may be at the cost of your own life. Never harm the sick, not even in thought or dream …… May the gods help you if you follow this rule. Otherwise may the gods be against you"*. This has been stipulated to maintain the sanctity and dignity of life so that doctor's professional capabilities are not abused which may erode doctor-patient relationship. The parental autonomy should be honored and they should be given the right and taken into confidence while making a decision regarding the medical care of their children.

We should assist parents to make an informed decision on the basis of available medical facts. The principle of justice demands that we seek the morally correct distribution of resources, ensure cost-effectiveness of therapeutic measures by balancing medical benefits and burdens to the family and society. The basic and essential perinatal services must be made available to all irrespective of their abode, socioeconomic status, religion, caste and creed.

The decision whether to treat aggressively or palliatively should be taken jointly after discussion with the concerned consultants and nurses and by taking parents into confidence. The resolutions should be taken jointly by weighing all pros and cons. There are several issues which have moral and ethical considerations. Should a newborn baby who is extremely tiny or grossly malformed resuscitated and admitted to the NICU or not? Is there any reasonable chance of survival of the infant with available technology? Whether to continue invasive and intensive care or replace active treatment with palliative care? Would quality of life be worth living if the child survives with aggressive management? Can family afford expensive NICU costs? What do parents want? How to ensure equitable distribution of neonatal intensive care? What are the principles and goals of neonatal intensive care? Should we be concerned with the best interests of the patient alone or global interests of the family, society and state? And there are cultural considerations, the fertility of the couple, the concept of destiny or will of God, the doctor-knows-the-best attitude, socioeconomic status, education of parents, social support system and national priorities. It is unfortunate but true that in a developing country, economic and social realities may outweigh and override ethical considerations.

The sound ethical decisions are based on correct medical facts. The ethical dilemma should be identified and analyzed in depth by all the specialists looking after the baby before a final decision is taken (Figure 33.1). The decision must be taken after taking the family into confidence. However, whatever the final decision, it must be based on facts and logic and the decision should be justified and recorded in the case file.

The Rights of Fetus and the Indian Law

Nearly 1000 years ago when there was no legal system, as per "Manusmriti", fetus was recognized to have the right to live and inherit property. According to Indian Penal Code, way back in 1860, it was recognized that fetus is a living being and any person causing intentional death of the fetus in the womb shall be accountable. However, if in the opinion of a doctor, termination of pregnancy was considered to be in the interest of the mother, it was legally permitted. The Medical Termination of Pregnancy Act (MTP) was enacted by the Parliament in 1971 further liberalizing abortion for family welfare purposes. According to the provisions of MTP Act, if pregnancy is less than 12 weeks of gestation, it can be terminated on the advice of one registered medical practitioner but if the pregnancy is more than 12 weeks but less than 20 weeks, the opinion of two medical practitioners is mandatory before undertaking abortion. However, selective abortion of female fetuses by antenatal determination of sex is highly unethical which has been legally banned throughout the country. Under section 5 of MTP Act, even if the duration of pregnancy is more than 20 weeks, the physician has the right to terminate pregnancy in order to save the life of mother. The physicians caring for the pregnant women are concerned with the welfare of two lives and of the two, the mother is considered as more precious than the fetus.

Can pregnancy beyond 20 weeks be legally terminated?

According to MTP Act, pregnancy beyond 20 weeks can be terminated for maternal and not for fetal reasons. The cut-off of 20 weeks has been kept possibly because fetus becomes viable at this gestation and the procedure of abortion at this stage of pregnancy is fraught with danger to the life of mother. However, premature induction of labor is routinely done for maternal and fetal indications (unfavorable maternal environment) without raising any ethical or legal issues. It is morally justified though illegal to abort a malformed fetus after 20 weeks if both of the following conditions are fulfilled:

  i. Fetus is afflicted with a condition that is incompatible with postnatal survival beyond a few weeks

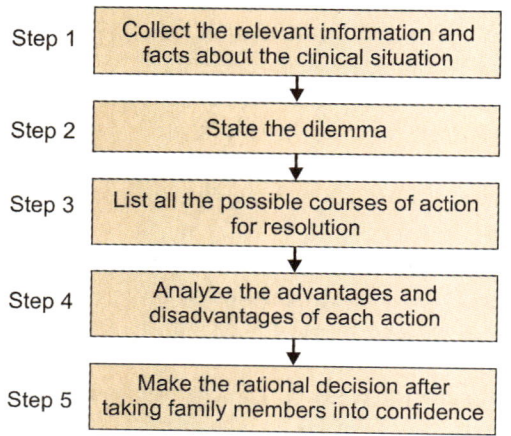

Step 1	Collect the relevant information and facts about the clinical situation
Step 2	State the dilemma
Step 3	List all the possible courses of action for resolution
Step 4	Analyze the advantages and disadvantages of each action
Step 5	Make the rational decision after taking family members into confidence

Figure 33.1 The ethical decision-making process.

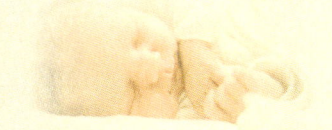

> **BOX 33.1** Lethal congenital malformations
>
> - Anencephaly
> - Hydranencephaly
> - Holoprosencephaly
> - Trisomy 13 and 18
> - Triploidy
> - Renal agenesis
> - Sirenomelia
> - Short-limb dwarfing syndromes
> - Miscellaneous conditions: Pterygium syndrome, Meckel-Gruber syndrome, Neu-Laxova syndrome

or survival is likely to be associated with total or virtual absence of cognitive functions later in life.

ii. Prenatal diagnosis of the condition is highly reliable.

These criteria are adequately met by the fetus having anencephaly. The other lethal congenital malformations which can be considered for abortion after 20 weeks are listed in Box 33.1. It must be kept in mind that medical uncertainty regarding correct diagnosis and prognosis in fetal medicine is profound. The decision for termination of pregnancy should, therefore, be taken after due consultations with a group of experts and by informed consent of parents.

There is certainly a need to revise the law to justify and legalize termination of pregnancy after 20 weeks of gestation. Life is life irrespective of gestation and the life is not smaller or lesser when a baby is small!

Is it Justified to Establish Neonatal Intensive Care Facilities in a Developing Country?

In a developing country like India, a large number of salvageable babies are dying in the community without receiving even basic or essential care. It is logical to ask should we waste our meager resources for a cost-intensive and cost-ineffective intensive care for critically sick and tiny newborn babies. According to the principle of justice and fairness, there is macro-allocation of resources by the society for various activities like defense, agriculture, industry, energy, education, health, etc. Allocation of budget for health competes with preventive, promotive and curative services at all age groups depending upon the national priorities. The neonatal care becomes one competing component of these multiple areas for "micro" allocation of resources. In view of the fact that about 70% of infant deaths are accounted by neonatal deaths, there is certainly a need to establish special care neonatal units to reduce neonatal mortality. However, the improvements in the neonatal care should not be

restricted to specialized neonatal units but globally distributed at all levels, i.e. home, sub-center, primary health center, community health center, district hospital, medical college hospital and private nursing homes or corporate hospitals. It is desirable to ensure equitable development of health care of neonates at all levels, be it at the grass roots or urban elites! There is an urgent need to introduce doable and sustainable strategies to provide essential perinatal services to the community which are highly cost-effective, evidence-based, and useful to the society to reduce infant mortality rate.

To ensure the effectiveness and credibility of the referral system, it is mandatory to establish specialized units of neonatal care where sick and small babies from the community health centers can be referred for optimal management. There is certainly a need to develop and establish NICU facilities in the country in a phased manner. It is unwise to establish intensive care and tertiary care facilities in a district hospital without first strengthening the crucial components of essential newborn care. In order to stabilize the population dynamics, there is a need to reduce infant mortality rate because enhanced survival of babies would discourage parents to produce more children. Moreover, saving the life of the newborn baby is more cost-effective for the society as it is associated with life-long productivity as opposed to saving a life due to cardiac or cerebral stroke and cancer in the elderly which is followed by survival for a short period of 2–5 years.

Withholding and Withdrawal of Life Support

According to the controversial and historical "Baby Doe" regulation, all newborns should receive maximal life prolonging treatment. However, this policy is not uniformly followed. In an infant who is inevitably destined to die or likely to survive with a profound risk of severe neuromotor disability, "selective non-treatment" is ethically and morally justified. These infants should be provided with a loving tender care comprising of warmth, nutrition and hydration without exploiting any heroic or aggressive therapeutic measures. They should be handled with compassion and provided comfort and relief from pain. This approach of withholding active treatment applies to all those conditions listed for termination of pregnancy after 20 weeks of gestation, infants with gross lethal congenital malformations and extremely tiny babies (<750 g or <26 weeks). Depending upon the level of expertise and available technology in the neonatal intensive care unit, different birth weight/gestation cut-offs can be used for providing neonatal intensive care.

Recent progress in neonatal care has significantly improved the prognosis and chances of survival of critically ill or extremely preterm neonates and has modified the limits of viability. It is unethical to deny admission to any baby in the NICU but we can specify the type and intensity of care to be provided to different babies. In view of the economic constraints, we should follow the philosophy of utilitarian ethics based on the concept of "value for money" and focus our efforts and resources for the care of salvageable babies. It is generally believed that duodenal atresia or cardiac malformation in an infant with Down syndrome should be operated and only developmental malforations worse than Down syndrome should be considered for non-treatment. However, in clinical practice the certainty of death (>90% chance of dying) and inevitability of cognitive or neuromotor disability after survival are extremely difficult to predict with accuracy. The decision for "selective non-treatment" should be recorded in the case file along with clinical justifications and parental consent. Every NICU should clearly define its policies for "selective non-treatment" to avoid guilt feelings and legal implications.

By and large the same reasons that justify with-holding the treatment, also hold true for stopping the treatment. The withdrawal of life support treatment like assisted ventilation is ethically acceptable, if infant is diagnosed to have brain death, likely to die regardless of any existing medical treatment, and should he live, he would have virtually no chance of leading a normal life. These conditions include extremely preterm baby with massive or grade 4 intraventricular hemorrhage, lethal CNS malformations, severe birth asphyxia with lack of breathing efforts for >30 min or HIE Sarnat stage 4 and persistent vegetative state. In these situations, death is considered as a more humane option than a life filled with suffering and misery. Moreover, in several cases the daily cost of NICU care may be more than the monthly salary of the family. The financial burden, misery and mental agony of looking after a child with extremely poor quality of life are profound especially in India where there is lack of social support system and inadequate facilities for management of children with serious neuromotor disabilities.

Communication as the Key to Enhance Doctor-Patient Relationship

"What we do not say and what we do say, how we say it and when we say it, makes all the difference between helping and not helping our patients."

John Apley

The all important communication link between a doctor and patient which is crucial to generate faith and trust, is being snapped by the technology boom. Most parental complaints in the NICU originate due to lack of communication or because of abrasive and unsympathetic attitude of the members of the health team rather than due to lack of skills or faulty technical management of the patient. It is an amazing fact that most parents are grateful even when we are unable to save the life of their baby especially if we showed concern, care and compassion and family members were made to perceive that whatever was humanely possible was done for the care of their infant. It is crucial to listen and talk with the parents at least twice a day in a relaxed unhurried manner.

Humility, concern, empathy and compassion are crucial to generate faith and provide emotional support to the family. The neonatologist should be careful and tactful not only in deciding "what to tell" to the parents but also "how to tell it". The parents should be told about the condition of their neonate in a simple language. It is important to establish an eye-to-eye contact while communicating and it is better to explain and talk with the parents at the cot-side. Efforts should be made to be pragmatic and honest to communicate prognosis to the family but you must try to keep the hope alive which has tremendous healing capabilities. Avoid creating confusion in the mind of parents due to conflicting messages given by different physicians. In a critically sick neonate, always give a guarded prognosis which can be tempered or mollified with hope and godly benevolence. The health team should not only try to do their best, but the family must perceive and appreciate that whatever was humanely possible in the circumstances was actually done for their child. The parents should be encouraged to touch and talk with their critically sick neonate because it transmits healing vibes. The religious faith of the family should be honored and if the parents wish they may be allowed to use any *mantras* or *charms* to enhance the process of healing through faith. By and large, efforts should be made to honor all the wishes of the parents of critically sick neonate if they are not obviously harmful or contrary to the recommended therapies in a specific situation.

Ethical Dilemmas

An opinion survey conducted by us among 103 pediatricians and obstetricians revealed that two-thirds of them faced ethical dilemmas in their professional work. The common and major ethical issues and dilemmas, include management of babies with severe birth asphyxia, lethal congenital malformations, extremely LBW or preterm babies, terminally sick neonates on life support and when parents are unable to afford the high-cost of intensive care. Due to profound economic disparities, there is lack of social justice and equitable health care in India. In developed countries, where medicare is supported by the social security system of the state or insurance companies, the parents want that everything possible on the earth must be done for their children. They demand initiation and continuation of intensive care with all the conceivable life support measures (including extracorporeal membrane oxygenation) even when the treating health team feels that it is futile to treat. On the other hand, unfortunately in developing countries, at times treatable conditions and salvageable babies are denied essential life-sustaining therapies either due to the non-availability of technology or because of its non-affordability by the parents.

Maurice King made the historical controversial ill conceived and unethical statement that to stabilize population dynamics in developing countries, "Health care activities including immunizations should be withdrawn so that nature is allowed to take its toll to eliminate the unwanted weaklings and weanlings from the society." It must be realized that in Indian society children are a source of social security to parents in their old age. When we are unable to provide assurance and confidence to parents that at least two or three children would survive the critical and vulnerable period of infancy, they have no motivation to adopt family planning measures. It is unethical and immoral on the part of any society to accept the Maurice doctrine which recommends "blatant neglect" of its children which constitute an asset and foundation of life.

In perinatal medicine it is often difficult and at times impossible to correctly prognosticate immediate survival and later neuromotor outcome. The "futility" issue often becomes controversial because as rightly said by Sir William Osler, *Medicine is a science of uncertainty and an art of probability*". At times it is difficult to know which interests are "best" for the baby; with-holding treatment or treating aggressively. Should we be concerned with the "best interests" of the child, family, society or the state? It is important that our concern should be the global interests of the family and society rather than the narrow interest of the child alone. Should NICU care be denied if family cannot afford it? It is not uncommon to be faced by the critically sick neonate whose parents have been monetarily drained off by the private nursing home and they are then referred to the government hospital when they are at the brink of bankruptcy and their child is near the threshold of death. In view of gloomy prognosis and outcome, both in terms of immediate survival and quality of life after survival, the economic drainage is often unbearable with profound adverse consequences to the family dynamics for many months and years.

Should a "brain dead" pregnant woman be maintained on the life support system for the sake of her unborn baby? It is morally desirable and ethical to do so if facilities are available and fetus is normal and viable. In view of our limited resources, should a poor risk extremely low birth weight baby be hooked off the ventilator to provide assisted ventilation to a more salvageable bigger baby? I think it is not morally justified. It must be decided beforehand, that based on the benefit-to-burden ratio, which babies should be provided high-tech care including assisted ventilation. And once that decision has been taken, it is not morally appropriate to take the baby off the ventilator, irrespective of the fact how appropriate and salvageable the next baby may be. It is desirable to take the family into confidence in the decision-making process but the physician should not succumb to the wishes of the family for continued life support facilities when it is felt with certainty and confidence that further treatment is futile. According to Christiaan Barnard, *"The prime goal of a doctor is to alleviate suffering and not to prolong life. And if your treatment does not alleviate suffering, but only prolongs life, that treatment should be stopped."* Humanistic teachings in general and philosophies of all the major religions of the world recognize that there comes a time in the care of every patient when it is appropriate for the doctor to stop further attempts to prolong unnecessarily the process of dying. *We must accept death as the ultimate truth because medicine can never achieve immortality.*

Ethics of Organ Transplantation

The enaction of Human Organ Transplant Act by the Indian Parliament in 1994 has opened opportunities for cadaveric transplant of organs. It is legally justified to remove organs from brain dead patients. However, the criteria for brain death are not well-defined in preterm babies and term neonates less than 7 days of age thus posing difficulties for donation of organs for transplantation (Box 33.2).

However, merely 1% of all perinatal deaths are due to brain death. Anencephalic infants are inevitably destined to die and logically should constitute good source of healthy and intact heart, liver and kidneys for transplantation. In Europe, physicians have removed organs from anencephalic infants without

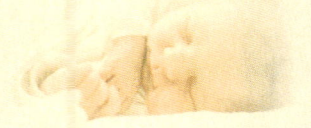

BOX 33.2   Criteria for the brain death in the newborn*
▪ Absent brainstem reflexes for more than 48 hr.
▪ Two EEGs 48 hr apart showing electrocerebral silence.
▪ Absence of cerebral blood flow for more than one hour on dynamic scan (133 Xenon isotopic scanning, PET).

*The observation period may be extended up to 72 hr in preterm babies <32 weeks.

waiting for their death on the ground that these infants are "brain absent". This approach is not generally approved and is illegal at present. If one waits for an anencephalic infant to die, most deaths occur due to cardiorespiratory failure thus compromising the perfusion and viability of organs required for transplantation. They would thus need a life-sustaining support and allowed to die by virtue of cessation of functioning of the brainstem. It is controversial though logical that a legislation should be enacted to consider all anencephalic infants as legally dead for purposes of organ donation. However, medical benefits are likely to be minimal due to low incidence of live born anencephalic infants and even lower incidence of infants whose lives could be prolonged by transplantation. There is a potential fear that such a law may lower the sanctity of life and organs may be surreptitiously removed from patients not fully brain dead.

Surrogate Motherhood

Due to technological advances, the well-to-do infertile couples are seeking parenthood by *in-vitro* fertilization with the help of various techniques like GIFT, ZIFT, TOT, etc. When the ovum and sperm of the prospective parents are harnessed it does not raise any ethical or legal issues. In other situations when a donor is used to provide a sperm or ovum, there is a need for maintaining strict confidentiality and there are risks of strained husband-wife relationship, neglect of the child, congenital malformations, issues of paternity, and right to property. Commercial hiring and subletting of a womb (surrogacy) for monetary gains raises ethical and legal issues akin to the sale of body organs and it should be discouraged. Impregnation of a hired womb through a sex act raises additional concerns regarding morality and its acceptability by the law and society. The government of India is considering to introduce a Bill in the near future to control the various assisted reproductive techniques (ARTs). The Indian Council of Medical Research (ICMR) has produced a draft ART (Regulation) Bill in 2014 which is awaiting approved by he Parliament. The Bill is likely to deny surrogacy option to a single man. The reality of genetic engineering and cloning capabilities in the near future is likely to provide unbelievable medical potentialities which is likely to unfold a variety of ethical, legal and moral concerns and issues.

Perinatal HIV Infection

Physicians are obliged to provide competent and humane care without any discrimination to all patients including those with HIV infection. The denial of appropriate care to any class of patients for any reason is unethical. In view of the increasing incidence of HIV, universal precautions should be followed in attending all deliveries. The risk of vertical transmission of HIV infection varies between 15 and 35%. The transmission rate can be reduced by treatment of the mother with antiretroviral therapy and delivering the baby by cesarean section. The definitive diagnosis of HIV infection at birth is difficult due to constraints of culturing the virus and unreliability of 1gM antibody assays. Early diagnosis is now feasible with HIV–DNA polymerase chain reaction and antigen detection by P24 analysis. There is a 10–15% chance of transmission of HIV infection through breastfeeding and mother is encouraged to make an informed decision whether to breastfeed her baby or not. There is a need for HIV screening of all mothers. The infected mother should be told about the risk of vertical transmission of HIV to her offspring and given the option for abortion on medical grounds. The confidentiality should be honored and maintained at all costs.

Handling End-of-life Situations and Neonatal Death

Despite all the technological advances, medicine can never achieve immortality. It is as natural to die, as to be born. According to Srimad Bhagavad Gita, *"Death is certain for the born and rebirth is inevitable for the dead. You should not, therefore, grieve over the inevitable"*. But these philosophical thoughts are very difficult to accept by the bereaved families. When a neonate is destined to die despite our best intentions and efforts or survival is likely to be associated with extremely poor quality of life or vegetative state, the family should be provided with emotional support. The news of adverse outcome should be communicated to both the parents simultaneously in a relaxed sitting in a quiet room with due concern and empathy. The family should be encouraged to talk and express their misgivings and doubts. In this session we should follow the well-known philosophy *"Talk less and listen more"* and that is why God has given us two ears and one mouth! The family should be made to understand that whatever was humanely possible has been done for the care of their baby. When decision has been taken to withdraw life support or deny life-saving measures, they should be introduced gradually keeping in mind the acceptance level of the family and comfort of the baby. The process of dying should be made as painless and comfortable for the baby as possible. The permission for autopsy or organ biopsies should be sought with extreme care and diplomacy with sole objective of helping the family to have normal babies in future and not for advancement of scientific knowledge or for the sake of ego satisfaction of knowing about the exact or correct diagnosis.

The coping of death of a neonate in the NICU is a challenging and traumatic experience both for the health care professionals and the families. Death deflates our ego and teaches us humility and provides strength to face and accept the greatest reality and truth of life with equanimity, peace and poise. The family's wishes for religious or spiritual support (like amulets, mantras, holy water, etc.) and presence of priest at bed side should be allowed. The parents should be encouraged to hold, embrace and cuddle their baby when he is leaving them. They should be allowed to take photographs of the baby with family members for future recollection and remembrance. The family should be emotionally and spiritually prepared before declaration of death. The news of death should be conveyed with utmost compassion but in no unmistakable terms that the baby has died despite our best efforts. The family should be assisted with due compassion and consideration to complete post death formalities without unnecessary delay. When autopsy has been conducted, the family must be provided the autopsy report and given guidance and counseling regarding subsequent pregnancies and newborn babies.

Conclusions and Recommendations

Ethical decisions in perinatal medicine are difficult and often complicated by profound medical uncertainty for making a correct diagnosis and prognosis in maternal, fetal and neonatal medicine. Ethical issues are indeed complex and often affected by economic and social realities, gender of the child and attitude of 'paternalism' by the pediatricians in a developing country. The narrow principle of 'best interest' of the baby should be replaced by global beneficence to the family, society and state. Medicine is enigmatic and many a times it is difficult to be certain which interest is the 'best'—withholding treatment or treating aggressively? Medicine is dynamic and neonatology is far more dynamic and therefore ethical perceptions and interventions cannot be static. Medical disorders

considered lethal in the past can be salvaged by newer technologies thus changing ethical perspectives and decisions. One should always put oneself in the situation of parents and ask "Would I want the child to live if it were mine"? We must take joint decisions within the legal framework after due consultations with a team of medical and nursing experts and by taking the family into confidence. Above all, we should neither ignore the parents nor give them unbridled autonomy to make decisions. We should evolve a rational process and sound mechanism to make correct ethical decisions. Bioethics Committees and Grievance Redressal Cells should be constituted in all hospitals who should serve as a watchdog to monitor and maintain the sanctity of all ethical decisions.

It is unfortunate that following the technology boom, the physicians are becoming more of technocrats and less of human beings. It is a pity that we are allowing technology to dehumanize neonatology. The revolution in technology is no substitute for trust and communication which indeed is the key for maintaining cordial doctor-patient or doctor-parent relationship. When practicing physicians are more considerate, cautious, honest and ethical in their dealings with their patients, there should be no fear of Consumer Forum or "legal eagles". The health personnel should exhibit exemplary humane behavior with compassion, tact and concern towards their patients and serve as role models to their students. The doctors should thus be imbued with the qualities and attributes as extolled in Charak Samhita; … *"Thou shalt behave and act without arrogance and with undistracted mind, humility and constant reflection, and thou shalt pray for the welfare of all creatures (not only your patients!) …"*. It is timely and mandatory that all medical and nursing schools in the country should initiate regular education programs in the field of behavioral sciences, communication techniques and medical ethics for the graduate and postgraduate medical and nursing students. The physicians should make concerted efforts to resurrect and master the sublime art of medicine and acquire the divine gift of healing. And we must treat babies and their families under our care not only with our brains but also with our hearts!

BIBLIOGRAPHY

AAP Committee on Fetus and Newborn: Noninitiation or withdrawal of intensive care for high-risk newborns. *Pediatrics* 2007; 19(2):401–403.

American Academy of Pediatrics, Committee on Bioethics. Ethical issues with genetic testing in pediatrics. *Pediatrics* 2009; 123:(5):1421–22, doi: 10–1542/peds. 2009–0405.

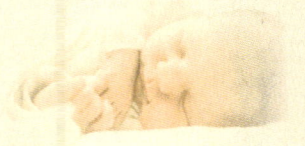

American Academy of Pediatrics: Bioethics Committee. Infants with anencephaly as organ sources: Ethical considerations. *Pediatrics* 1992; 89:1116–19.

Ashwal S. Brain death in the newborn. *Clin Perinatol* 1989; 16:501–18.

Bonkovsky FO. Ethical issues in perinatal HIV. *Clin Perinatol* 1994; 21:15–29.

Byrne S, Szyld E, Kattwinkel J. The ethics of delivery room resuscitation. *Semin Fetal Neonat Med* 2006; 117(5):e978–88.

Chervenak FA, Farley MA, Walters LR, *et al*. When is termination of pregnancy during the third trimester morally justifiable? *N Engl J Med* 1984; 310:501–504.

Doyal L, Wilsher D. Towards guidelines for withholding and withdrawal of life prolonging treatment in neonatal medicine. *Arch Dis Child* 1994; 70:66–70.

Doyal L, Wilsher D. Withholding cardiopulmonary resuscitation: Proposals for formal guidelines. *Brit Med J* 1993; 306:1593–96.

Fost N. Removing organs from anencephalic infants: Ethical and legal considerations. *Clin Perinatol* 1989; 16:331–37.

Gale G, Brooks A. Implementing a palliative care protocol in a newborn intensive care unit. *Adv Neonatal Care* 2006; 6(1):7–53.

Goldworth A, Silverman W, Stevenson DK, *et al*. Ethics and Perinatalogy. *Oxford University Press New York*, 1995.

King M. Human entrapment in India. *Natl Med J India* 1991; 4:196–201.

Kopelman LM, Irons TG, Kopelman AE. Neonatologists judge the "Baby Doe" regulations. *N Engl J Med* 1988; 318:677–83.

Leuthner SR. Decisions regarding resuscitation of the extremely premature infant and models of best interest. *J Perinatol* 2001; 21:1–6.

Meadow W, Lantos J. Moral reflections on neonatal intensive care. *Pediatrics* 2009; 123(2):595–97.

Nakagawa IA, Ashwal S, Mathur M, Mysore M. Guidelines for the determination of brain death in infants and children: An update of the 1987 Task Force Recommendations: Executive Summary. *Ann Neurol* 2012; 71:573–85.

Nolan K. Ethical issues in caring for pregnant women and newborn at risk for human immunodeficiency virus infection. *Semin Perinatol* 1989; 13:55–65.

Pellegrino ED. The metamorphosis of medical ethics. *JAMA* 1993; 269:1158–62.

Perkins H. Teaching medical ethics during residency programme. *Acad Med* 1989; 64:262–66.

Sauer PJJ. Ethical decisions in neonatal intensive care units: The Dutch experience. *Pediatrics* 1992; 90:729–32.

Sekar KC. Brain death in the newborn. *J Perinatol* 2007, 27 (suppl): S59–S62.

Singh J, Lantos J, Meadow W. End-of-life after birth: death not dying in a neonatal intensive care unit. *Pediatrics* 2004; 114(6):1620–26.

Singh M, Kumar S, Mittal S, *et al*. Ethical issues in perinatology (Panel discussion). *Natl Med J India* 1996; 9:32–37.

Singh M. Communication as a bridge to build a sound doctor-patient/parent relationship. *Indian J Pediatr* 2016, 83(1):33–37.

Singh M. Ethical and social issues in the care of newborn babies. *Indian J Pediatr* 2003; 70(5):417–20.

Singh M. Ethical issues and dilemmas in the care of newborn babies in the developing world. *Semin Neonatol* 1999; 4:151–57.

Singh M. The art, science and philosophy of newborn care. *Indian J Pediatr* 2014, 81(6): 552–59.

Stahlamn M. Ethical issues in the nursery: Priorities versus limits. *J Pediatr* 1990; 116:167–170.

Tomlinson T, Brody H. Ethics and communication in do-not-resuscitate orders. *N Engl J Med* 1988; 318:43–46.

Tyson JE, Stoll BJ. Evidence-based ethics and the care and outcome of extremely premature infants. *Clin Perinatol* 2003; 30(2): 365–87.

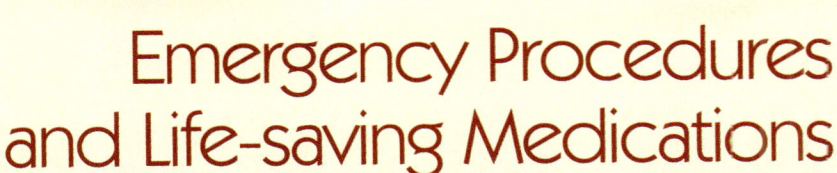

34

Emergency Procedures and Life-saving Medications

Sindhu Sivanandan, Ramesh Agarwal and Meharban Singh

GENERAL CONSIDERATIONS

Informed Consent

Preterm birth or admission of a neonate to the neonatal intensive care unit (NICU) is stressful for the parents. Informed consent is a process of communication between the physician and the parents, who are the surrogate decision-makers for their children. At the time of admission to the NICU, hospitals generally obtain a 'blanket consent' from parents for consenting to treatment and routine interventions or procedures which are part of care of the neonate like blood pressure monitoring, checking sugar by heel prick, vene-puncture, insertion of peripheral intravenous line, intubation, extubation, imaging studies, etc. The interventions and procedures considered routine vary between hospitals and these are not enumerated in the consent form. Obtaining consent for each of these routine interventions would place unnecessary burden on the health care system and at the same time increases parental anxiety and causes significant delay in patient care.

At certain times during patient management, a diagnostic or therapeutic procedure may need to be done which is not without risks to the patient. This includes all surgical procedures and major interventions like insertion of a central venous catheter, bone marrow examination, lumbar puncture, aspiration of body fluids etc. for which informed parental consent is required. Each hospital has its own policy regarding informed consent and usually has a list of surgeries, procedures, or situations where a specific informed consent is needed. An exception to the requirement for informed consent may occur in an emergency when the procedure or intervention becomes life-saving (e.g. endotracheal intubation in the setting of acute respiratory failure, insertion of umbilical catheters during delivery room resuscitation, paracentesis or thoracocentesis during resuscitation of a hydropic neonate) and delaying the procedure in order to obtain informed consent would pose a serious risk of imminent harm (e.g. death or severe disability) to the neonate.

Informed consent should be obtained by the treating physician or the physician who would perform the intervention. The parents should be explained the following facts in simple terms and in a language that they can understand.

1. The diagnosis or disease of the infant and the need for the proposed procedure.
2. The risks and benefits of the proposed procedure.
3. The alternatives to the procedure if any (regardless of costs) and its risks/benefits.
4. The risks and benefits of not undergoing the procedure.

During the process of informed consent, the physician should also ensure that the parents have an adequate understanding of the information and that the consent is given voluntarily. At times parents cannot give an informed decision because they do not understand the choices available or the potential consequences of their decisions. In such scenarios, the physicians should participate in a joint deliberation with parents and give their unbiased opinion regarding the proper course of action. The physicians should carefully document all informed consent discussions and keep the duly signed consents in the patient's medical record.

Aseptic Preparation for Procedures

It is mandatory of follow appropriate aseptic precautions for all procedures performed in neonates. The following are some general guidelines for ensuring asepsis.

1. *Hand hygiene* Remove rings, wrist-watch, bangles and religious wrist threads before surgical hand preparation. Nails should be cut short and artificial nails should not be worn. If hands are visibly soiled, wash them with plain soap and water. Surgical hand antisepsis should be ensured by using either an antimicrobial soap or a suitable alcohol-based hand-rub. One should scrub hands and forearms up to elbows for 2–5 minutes. Sinks should be sufficiently deep to avoid the risk of water splash and the taps should be elbow or foot operated.

2. *Standard or universal precautions* These are a set of precautions designed to prevent transmission of HIV, hepatitis B virus (HBV), hepatitis C virus (HCV), and other bloodborne pathogens when providing health care. Under standard precautions, blood and certain body fluids of all patients are considered potentially infectious for HIV, HBV, HCV and other bloodborne pathogens. The major components of standard precautions include the use of gloves when touching blood or body fluids, use of gown or a plastic apron, a mask and eye protection where splashing of blood or body fluids is likely (Figure 34.1). Take extreme care in handling sharps and dispose them in puncture proof containers.

3. *Sterile supplies* Sterile trays or kits received from the CSSD (central sterile supplies department) should be kept dry. Check that the seal and outside covering of the package is intact.

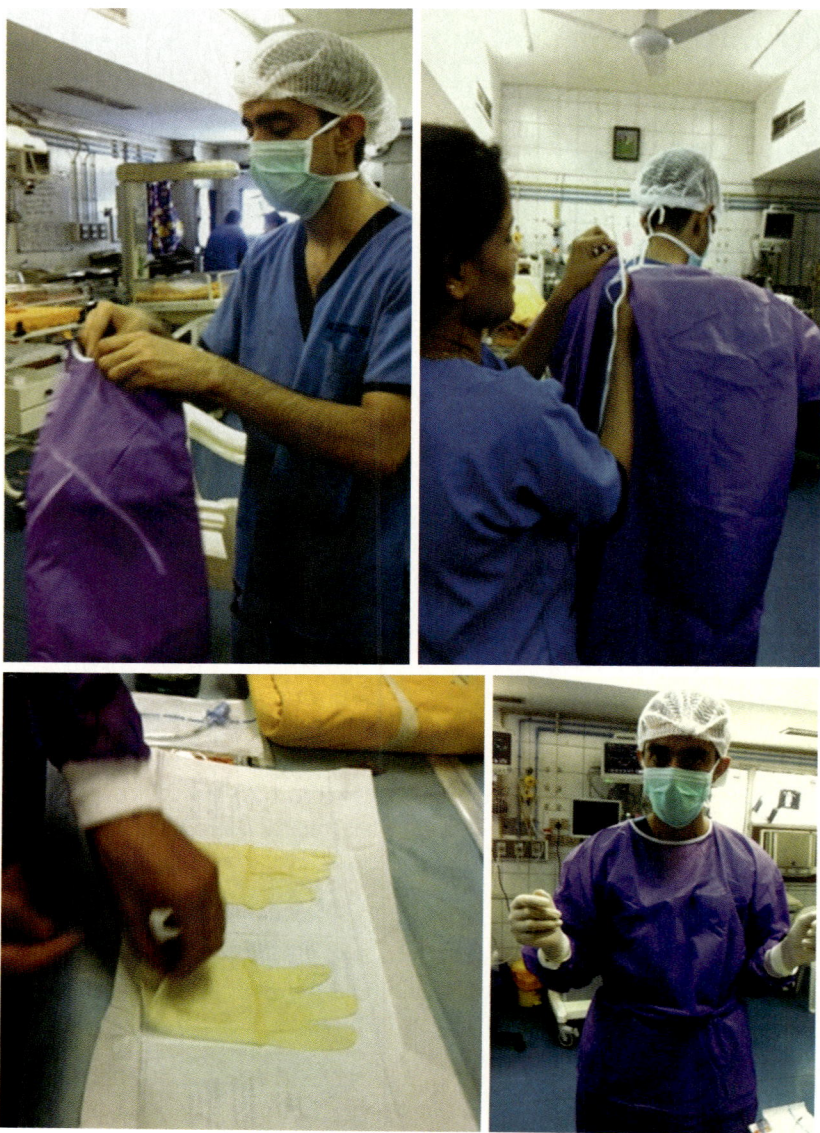

Figure 34.1 Operator is being helped to gown by an assistant. Operator wears a mask and sterile gloves and is ready for the procedure.

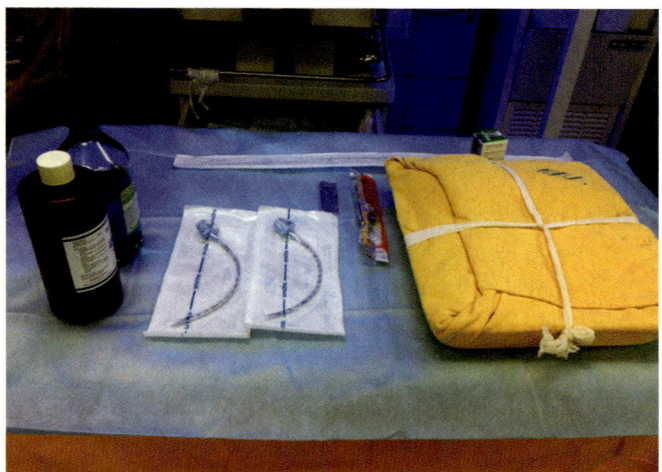

Figure 34.2 Setting up the sterile supplies for administration of surfactant.

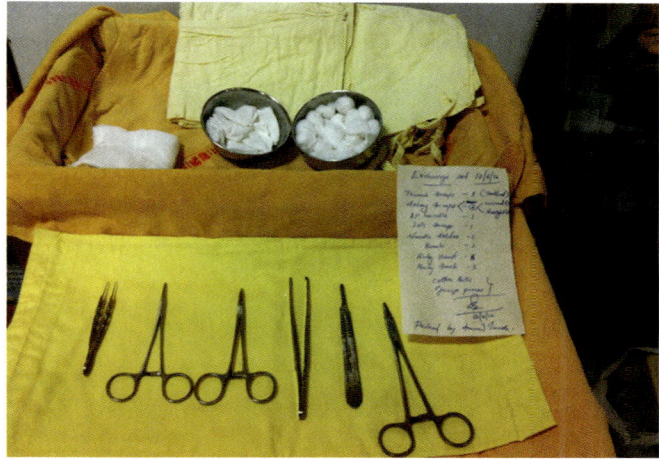

Figure 34.3 Contents of the major procedure pack for umbilical vessel catheterization or PICC insertion.

4. Use a mobile table or trolley that can be conveniently placed near the patient's bedside to keep the sterile sets. Clean the surface of the table with disinfectant spray or wash with soap and water. Make sure that the surface or table is dry before the sterile supplies are kept on it. Figure 34.2 shows the setting up of a sterile set and equipments on a mobile table for a procedure.

5. *Opening the sterile sets* Let the assistant help you to open the first flap of the kit after appropriate hand hygiene. Do not sneeze, cough or reach over the supplies. None other than the operator who has done hand hygiene and has worn sterile gown and gloves should touch the inside of the procedure kit. In case an item needs to be added to the sterile kit (for example a blade, syringes, catheters or suture materials), peel the flaps of the package and drop the item in the center of the kit. Avoid touching the sterile field with the package wrapper. The kit or tray contents are sterile and the wrapper (cloth or paper) is also sterile except for about 1 inch around the edge.

The Contents of Sterile Procedure Sets

In NICUs when commercially available sterile procedure trays are not used, one can prepare the tray with a minimum set of instruments that can be used for most procedures after getting it sterilized by the hospital CSSD department. In our NICU, we have 2 types of sterile trays, a major one and a minor one. A major set is used for central line insertions, umbilical catheter insertions while a minor one is used for lumbar puncture, wound dressing, urethral catheterization etc. (Figure 34.3).

The contents of the major set are listed below:
1. Steel tray = 1
2. Steel bowl = 1
3. Measuring scale = 1
4. Iris forceps = 1
5. Mayo scissors = 1
6. Needle holder = 1
7. BP handle = 1
8. Straight artery forceps = 1
9. Curved artery forceps = 1
10. Thumb forceps = 1

The contents of the minor set include:
1. Steel tray
2. Steel bowls = 2
3. Artery forceps = 1
4. Small glass bottles with caps = 3

A cut-down set has dissecting forceps, single hook and Allis forceps in addition to the instruments in the major set and is used for venous cut-down or muscle biopsy.

Skin Preparation for Procedures

An ideal antiseptic for skin preparation in neonates should be capable of destroying and inhibiting growth of microorganisms on the skin, without harming the neonate, and should have a sufficiently long duration of action. The three commonly used antiseptics in neonates are chlorhexidine, alcohols and idophores. Chlorhexidine has broad-spectrum bactericidal activity and also kills yeasts, but is ineffective against mycoplasma and bacterial spores. It causes cell membrane lysis and coagulation of cellular components. Its wide antimicrobial activity and sustained topical action makes it desirable for skin asepsis prior to invasive procedures. Ethanol, isopropanol, and n-propanol are the most commonly used alcoholic antiseptics. Alcohol causes bacterial cell membrane lysis and protein denaturation. Alcohol is active against most bacteria, fungi, and viruses, but is ineffective against spores. Iodophores are halogen-releasing compounds and povidone iodine is the most commonly used agent. They have cidal properties against bacteria, fungi, mycobacteria, viruses and spores. They cause denaturation of cell proteins, nucleotides and fatty acids.

General recommendations for skin preparation in neonates There is little evidence to support the preferential use of any specific antiseptic for skin preparation in the NICU. Irrespective of preferred antiseptic agent, the following are some general recommendations regarding skin disinfection:

1. Before skin preparation, ensure that the skin is free of visible soiling or dirt. If visibly soiled, clean the area with sterile water or saline and allow it to dry before applying antiseptic.
2. Ensure that the antiseptic agent is compatible with the site to be prepared. Avoid the use of betadine or alcohol solution over the genitalia and eyes and avoid the use of chlorhexidine for lumbar puncture or ventricular tap.
3. Always prepare the site of intervention from center to periphery, taking care not to track back the same site with the same sponge after cleaning another area. Do not double dip the contaminated sponge into the antiseptic solution. Use dedicated swab containers (Figure 34.4) or disposable pre-packed swabs for each neonate.

4. The prepared area should be liberal and extend to accommodate potential shifting of the drape.
5. Allow the antiseptic to dry completely before the procedure.
6. Topical antiseptics can cause irritation and skin erythema in neonates. We avoid using povidone iodine solutions in extremely low birth weight neonates. Antiseptic skin burns have been reported with iodophores (Figure 34.5), 0.5% chlorhexidine with 70% isopropyl alcohol and both alcoholic and aqueous-based 2% chlorhexidine. Most cases result from excessive application of antiseptic solution with consequent pooling of the antiseptic and prolonged direct contact with the skin. Some workers recommend

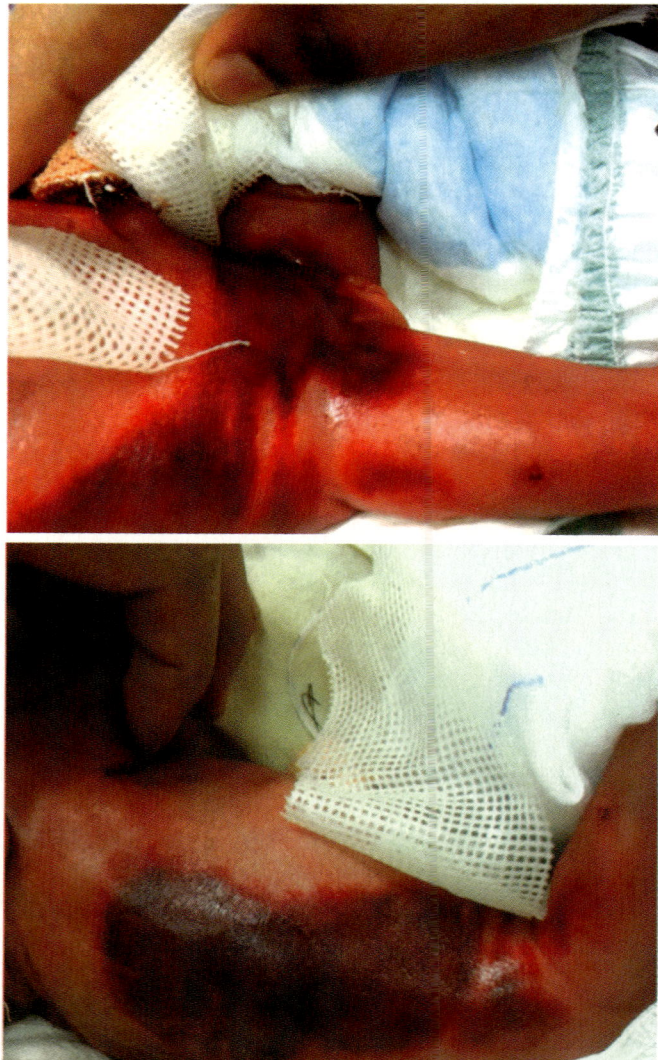

Figure 34.5 Povidone iodine burn in an extremely preterm neonate. The distribution of the injury is typical of excessive dripping of antiseptic over the dependent sites.

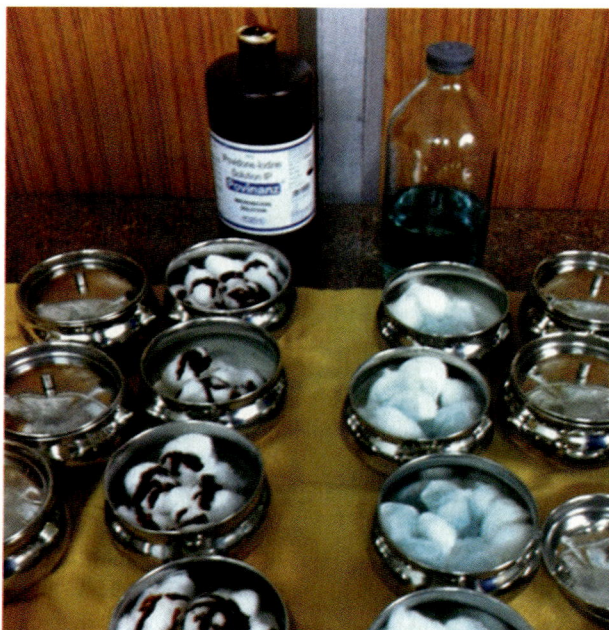

Figure 34.4 Swab containers containing cotton balls soaked in 70% alcohol and povidone iodine for skin disinfection.

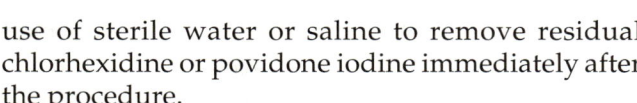

use of sterile water or saline to remove residual chlorhexidine or povidone iodine immediately after the procedure.

7. Povidone iodine can be absorbed through the skin of neonates especially preterm and can cause thyroid dysfunction. Similarly, chlorhexidine can be absorbed through the skin after topical application. Preterm neonates demonstrate higher serum concentrations of chlorhexidine after topical application. The studies have not documented any neurotoxic effects of chlorhexidine in term neonates, its effects in preterm neonates need to be studied.

Pain Management

Optimum pain relief is essential for any intervention or procedure which is likely to be painful. In general, for a mildly painful procedure, one can use non-pharmacological approaches like oral sucrose or swaddling, topical anesthesia like EMLA cream (eutectic mixture of lignocaine and prilocaine). For more painful procedures opioid analgesics are preferred. Table 34.1 lists pain control measures for common neonatal procedures.

Thoracentesis and Chest Tube Placement (Thoracostomy)

Pneumothorax, pleural effusion and empyema are life-threatening and may need emergency drainage in neonates. Drainage of air or fluid accumulation in the pleural cavity is an important and necessary skill and is often performed urgently if there is tension pneumothorax or associated with respiratory distress.

Indications for chest tube drainage include; (i) drainage of a pneumothorax and (ii) drainage of a moderate to large pleural fluid collection like chylothorax, empyema or hemothorax.

According to the British Thoracic Society, the size of a pneumothorax should be categorized according to the amount of air visible between the lung edge and chest wall.

- Small pneumothorax: <2 cm rim present between the lung edge and chest wall.
- Large pneumothorax: ≥2 cm rim present between the lung edge and chest wall.

This helps in clinical management, because a small pneumothorax in a non-ventilated neonate or in those without lung disease is usually reabsorbed spontaneously in 24–48 hours. Moderate or large pneumothoraces are usually symptomatic and require drainage.

Table 34.1 Recommended pain control measures for common neonatal procedures

Procedure	Suggested pain control measures
Heel lance	- Sucrose (concentration 12–24%) or breastfeed given 2 minutes before the procedure - Swaddling, containment or facilitated tucking or skin-to-skin contact with the mother - Avoid squeezing the heel for blood collection
Peripheral venous cannulation Peripheral arterial insertion Venepuncture	- Use a pacifier with sucrose - Use swaddling, containment, or facilitated tucking - Apply EMLA (eutectic mixture of lignocaine and prilocaine) cream to the local site at least 30 minutes prior to the procedure especially if it is non-urgent
Umbilical catheter insertion and central venous catheter insertion Lumbar puncture	- Consider administration of opioid if intravenous access is available and airway is not an issue - Use a pacifier with sucrose. - Apply EMLA to the site 30 minutes prior to the procedure - Careful handling during the procedure without compromising the airway
Endotracheal intubation	Pre-medication is recommended for all intubations other than those conducted in the delivery room Several combinations of premedication drugs can be considered - Use a combination of atropine sulfate and ketamine hydrochloride - A combination of atropine, thiopental sodium and succinylcholine chloride - Coadministration of atropine, morphine, or fentanyl, and non-depolarizing muscle relaxant (pancuronium bromide, vercuronium bromide, rorcurcnium bromide)
Chest tube insertion	- Anticipate the need for intubation and ventilation in neonates breathing spontaneously - Use a pacifier with sucrose - Consider subcutaneous infiltration of lidocaine - Low dose intravenous opioids

Needle thoracentesis A tension pneumothorax is life-threatening as it obstructs venous return to the heart and needs to be drained immediately (Figure 34.6). A needle thoracentesis can offer temporary relief while arrangements are made for thoracostomy. A butterfly needle or an intravenous cannula is inserted into the pleural space aseptically and air or fluid is aspirated. This procedure is life-saving with prompt relief of symptoms and re-expansion of the lungs. The equipment needed for thoracentesis are listed in Box 34.1.

Procedure

1. Before needling a suspected pneumothorax, perform auscultation of the chest and transillumination to confirm the side of air leak. Sometimes, a pneumothorax or an effusion is identified on skiagram of chest.

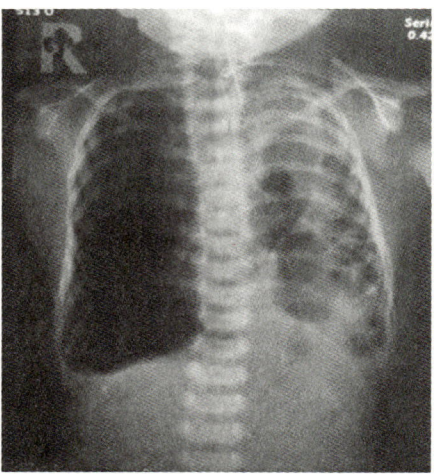

Figure 34.6 Tension pneumothorax on the right side in an intubated neonate with congenital diaphragmatic hernia. Needling of the chest can be done while arrangements are made for chest tube insertion.

BOX 34.1 Equipment for needle thoracentesis

- Choose a 23–25 G butterfly needle or 22–24 G IV catheter with needle
- A sterile tray with linen and bowls
- Antiseptic solution (e.g. povidone-iodine and 70% isopropyl alcohol or 2% chlorhexidine)
- 3-way stopcock
- Pressure line or IV tubing
- 10–20 mL syringe
- Analgesia: Topical 1% lidocaine (0.5% mL/kg/dose to a maximum of 5 mL/single injection) or intravenous opioid analgesic in intubated neonates
- Bottle of sterile water
- Sterile rolled towels and limb restraints

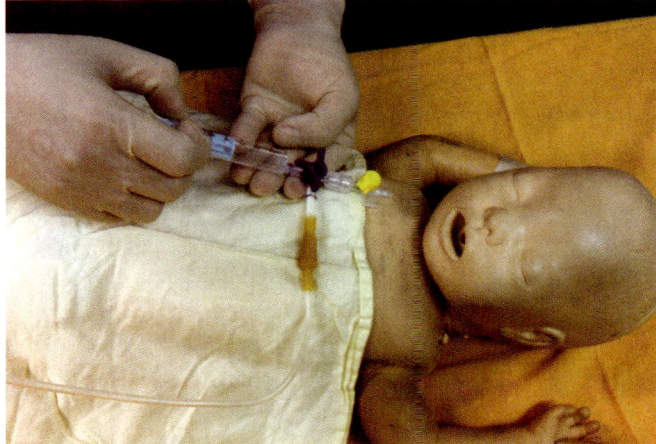

Figure 34.7 The procedure of thoracentesis on a mannequin.

2. Prepare the equipments. Attach the 3-way stopcock to a 10–20 mL syringe on the outer end side and an IV tube on the chest side (Figure 34.7). Open a bottle of sterile saline and place it below the level of the neonate.
3. Prepare the skin with antiseptic solution. Clean and drape the site of procedure, i.e. second intercostal space in the mid-clavicular line on the superior aspect of the lower rib.
4. Insert the needle or IV cannula 3–5 mm into the chest wall in the second intercostal space in the mid-clavicular line above the superior border of the third rib. Once the pleural space is entered, a "give way" or loss of resistance is felt. Remove the stylet of the IV cannula and attach the 3-way stop cock fitted with a syringe and tubing to its outer end. The draining end of the IV tubing is dipped in the sterile water bottle held below the level of the patient.
5. Aspirate through the syringe and drain the air or effusion into the underwater tubing. The suction can be repeated several times until no more fluid or air comes out. The IV cannula can be left *in situ* after closing its end if further accumulation of air or fluid is anticipated. After recovery, the needle or cannula can be removed and dry gauze placed at the insertion site and taped with a small Tegaderm.

Chest Tube Insertion

Indications

1. To evacuate a moderate and large pleural effusion or pneumothorax.
2. To evacuate an empyema, hemothorax or chylothorax.
3. Evacuation of recurrent effusions secondary to a tumor.
4. Post-operatively after thoracic surgeries, e.g. esophageal repair, and repair of congenital diaphragmatic hernia.

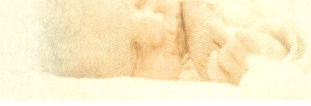
Equipments
- In addition to the sterile tray, and antiseptics for skin preparation, the additional equipment needed include 8, 10 or 12 Fr chest tube depending on the size of the infant
- Sterile underwater seal container

Procedure

Position infant supine and slightly elevate the affected side 45–60 degrees off the bed by placing a towel under the back. In case of pneumothorax this helps the air to rise anteriorly and facilitates the correct anterior insertion of the chest tube.

- Use appropriate local anesthesia or opioid analgesia for pain relief.
- Prepare and drape the area of tube insertion on the involved side of the chest.
- The usual site of chest tube insertion is the mid-axillary line in the 6th intercostal space.
- A small 0.5–1 cm incision is made with a Bard-Parker knife through the skin at this point on the superior aspect of the 7th rib. Using a small curved forceps, separate the tissues up to the pleura.
- Grasp the end of the chest tube with the tips of curved forceps and apply pressure until the pleural space is entered at the level of 4th ICS. Do not use the trocar.
- Direct the chest tube toward the apex of thorax (mid-clavicle) and advance it to ensure that the side holes are within thorax. Observe for vapor or misting in the chest tube to verify the intra-pleural location. The chest tube should be inserted 2–3 cm for a small preterm infant and 3–4 cm for a term infant.
- Connect the distal end of the chest tube to an under-water seal system. If using a commercially available system such as a PleurX® system, apply a negative pressure of 10–20 cm H_2O. If multiple chest tubes are placed, each should be connected to it's own dedicated water seal system and suction source.
- Secure the chest tube to skin with a suture and cover incision site with a sterile dressing.
- Confirm the position of chest tube on AP and lateral view of X-ray chest.
- Prior to removal, the chest tube should be clamped for 2–4 hours or longer. If there is no re-accumulation of air, or effusion, the chest tube can be removed.

Site of chest tube placement The site of insertion of chest tube depends on whether fluid or air or both needs to be evacuated. Commonly, a chest tube is inserted at the mid axillary line between the 4th and 5th ribs. If air needs to be evacuated, the tube is placed anteriorly near the apex of the lung (second intercostal space) and in case of pleural effusion the tube is placed posteriorly near the base of the lung (fifth or sixth intercostal space).

When both air and fluid are present, a chest tube may be placed at either the base or at the apex.

Complications

- Bleeding at the site of insertion of tube
- Infection of the lung and pleura
- Malpositioned chest tube
- Tension pneumothorax
- Subcutaneous emphysema
- *Trauma*
  - lung laceration or perforation
  - bronchopleural fistula
  - injury to major blood vessels like axillary, inter-costals or internal mammary vessels
  - injury to the liver on the right side
  - accidental entry into peritoneal cavity or damage to abdominal organs

Care of a Neonate with a Chest Tube

The nurses and the physicians caring for a neonate with a chest drain should pay attention to the following parameters:

1. Vital signs every 1–2 hourly.
2. Observe the drain insertion site for signs of infection or leak, check whether the dressing is clean and intact and whether the tube is fixed at the correct position or not.
3. Observe the connection tubing and under water seal system. The outer end of the tube should be below the chest level of the infant to facilitate drainage and the underwater seal (UWS) should be kept upright at the ground level. The tubing should be airtight and have no kinks or obstructions. In the neonatal ICU, we fix the tubing with an adhesive paper to the radiant warmer bed so that it is not accidentally pulled or removed (Figure 34.8).
4. The volume of drainage into the UWS is documented in the nursing sheet at regular intervals. Change in color or consistency or volume of drainage fluid merits physician's attention. If a catheter stops draining or is bubbling excessively, it must be informed to the physician immediately. Milking the draining tube creates a high negative pressure that can cause pain, tissue damage and bleeding.
5. Sometimes a slow negative suction is applied through the UWS. Indications for chest drain suction include a non-resolving pneumothorax, assisted drainage of empyema or following thoracic surgery. If suction is to be used, it must be at high volume and low negative pressure. Usual suction force recommended in neonates is 10 to 20 cm H_2O. The

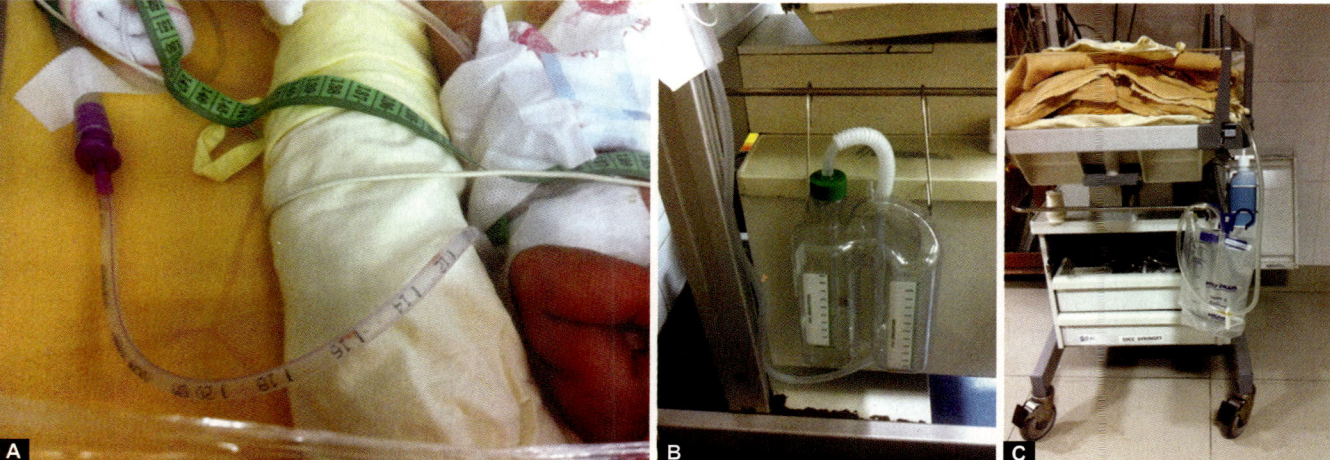

Figure 34.8 A. The chest tube should be attached to the baby bed by an adhesive tape to prevent accidental displacement. B. A dual chamber container for drainage. C. Single chamber drainage. Note that the drainage system is fixed below the chest level of the neonate.

standard or conventional wall suction is a high volume, high-pressure unit and should not be used for this purpose.

6. Observe for bubbling in the UWS and swinging of the water column in the tubing. A bubbling in the UWS will be noticed when a pneumothorax is being drained. It usually occurs during expiration and as the pneumothorax resolves, the bubbling also ceases. Swinging of the water column in the chest tube with each breath is a normal phenomenon seen due to the changes in pressure during respiration. The column rises during inspiration and falls during expiration. This "swing" is useful in assessing tube patency and confirms the position of the tube in the pleural cavity. An unexpected cessation of swinging may indicate that the tube is blocked or kinked. On the contrary, in a neonate who develops worsening of distress or pneumothorax, sudden loss of bubbling may point to a blocked chest tube. A continuous vigorous bubbling indicates a possible bronchopleural fistula.

Care of Chest Tube

1. Dressing should be changed if it is soiled or loose or soaked with secretions. There is no need for routine change of dressing.

2. The underwater seal drain is changed when significant drain is collected, or it is leaking or damaged or routinely after 48 hours. When instead of a glass container, a plastic bag or pouch is used for drainage, it should be changed every 24 hours. The tube is temporarily clamped while changing UWS.

3. A neonate with a chest tube can be transported safely. A nurse or physician should accompany the neonate during transport. The tubings should be kept below the level of the infant, the bottle upright and the tube should not be clamped.

Removing the chest tube There are no clear indications for chest tube removal but the basic premise is that the lung should have re-expanded and the chest tube is no longer draining any gas or fluid. It is necessary that there should be no tube air leak for at least 24 hours before removing the chest tube. A chest X-ray is usually obtained to confirm that the air leak has resolved and the lung has re-expanded. We do not routinely clamp chest tube prior to removal but clamping for a short period of 6–8 hours prior to removal can be considered in infants on mechanical ventilation and if the initial air leak was severe or in infants with a higher risk of recurrence of air leak like congenital diaphragmatic hernia with associated lung hypoplasia or traumatic air leaks. Chest tubes can be removed in neonates who continue to be on mechanical ventilation if the underlying condition necessitating insertion of chest tube has resolved. A skiagram of chest must be taken prior to and after removal of tube in babies on mechanical ventilation.

Abdominal Paracentesis

Indications

1. *Diagnostic* To determine the etiology of ascites. Ascitic fluid could be transudate or an exudate. Ascitic fluid analysis can help in differentiating the various etiologies of ascites. Ascitic tap can also help in diagnosing spontaneous or post-NEC bacterial peritonitis.

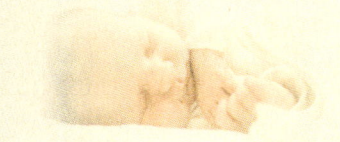
2. *Therapeutic* To relieve respiratory distress or other symptoms because of massive ascites.

Contraindications

There are no absolute contraindications for paracentesis. Coagulopathy should be corrected if there is active bleeding or if thrombocytopenia is severe ($<50,000/mm^3$). Consider arranging or transfusing platelets or fresh frozen plasma before the procedure.

> **Equipments needed**
> 1. Sterile tray with bowls, artery forceps and sterile drapes
> 2. Sterile gown, gloves and antiseptic solution
> 3. 22–24 G intravenous cannula
> 4. 3-way stop cock, 5 and 10 mL syringes, IV tubing

Procedure

1. Place gentle restraints or swaddle the infant while exposing the abdomen. The right or left lower quadrant is the usual site for paracentesis. The chosen site is prepared and sterile drapes are placed.

2. Mark the point for introduction of the cannula. A small wheal is raised at this point with 1% xylocaine with a tuberculin syringe and it is then infiltrated through the muscle and peritoneum.

3. Use the Z-track technique for introduction of cannula, wherein the operator retracts the skin of the abdominal wall with non-dominant hand while inserting the cannula. This ensures that the entry sites in the skin and peritoneum are not aligned to each other and it minimizes the risk of ascitic fluid leakage. The usual site of insertion of cannula is the point joining outer one-third with inner two-thirds of line joining anterior superior iliac spine with the umbilicus.

4. With the stylet in place, the cannula is introduced slowly. A distinct loss of resistance will be felt once the peritoneal cavity is reached. When cannula has entered the peritoneal cavity, the stylet is removed, a syringe is attached, and an attempt is made to aspirate the fluid.

5. If a large amount of ascitic fluid needs to be drained, attach a 3-way stopcock with one end attached to a 5–10 mL syringe and the other end to an IV tubing for drainage. Removal of large volumes in a neonate (>15 mL/kg) within a short time period can lead to hemodynamic instability. In such cases, it is better to leave the cannula *in situ* for repeated aspirations of smaller volumes and consider intravenous fluid replacement of crystalloids or fresh frozen plasma. Apply minimal continuous negative pressure for drainage because excessive pressure can lead to bowel or omentum getting trapped in the cannula.

6. Document the color and turbidity of fluid and send it for cell count, differential count, biochemistry (sugar, protein, albumin), Gram stain and culture. Special studies can be ordered (amylase, malignant cell cytology and mycobacterial studies) when indicated.

Complications

1. Bleeding due to injury to the blood vessels of anterior abdominal wall.
2. Injury to the liver or intestines leading to hemorrhage or perforation.
3. Injury to the bladder.
4. Ascitic fluid leakage from the skin wound.
5. Excessive removal of fluid within a short time can cause hemodynamic instability.

Pericardiocentesis

Indications

Diagnostic Isolated pericardial effusion with or without concomitant signs of pericarditis. Fluid analysis can differentiate between infectious, inflammatory and malignant disorders.

Therapeutic To relieve the hemodynamic compromise due to cardiac tamponade. Patients with pus in the pericardium (pyopericardium) are often toxic and they require early intervention either by closed needle aspiration or more effectively by open surgical drainage.

Echocardiography guided pericardiocentesis

Bedside echocardiogram or ultrasound is crucial in confirming the diagnosis of pericardial effusion and cardiac tamponade and it is advisable to do it in all patients before subjecting them to pericardiocentesis. The exception being the rare situation where there is a delay in arranging the echo scan and the child is critically ill and the clinical diagnosis of pericardial effusion with tamponade is obvious (hypotension, pulsus paradoxus, elevated venous pressures and muffled heart sounds). Echocardiogram helps in ruling out the presence of adhesions that may compartmentalize the pericardial space and adversely affect the success of closed needle aspiration.

Bedside echocardiography is extremely useful to guide the puncture site and confirm the presence of needle in the pericardial space. It can also monitor the reduction of pericardial fluid volume during the aspiration and confirming the dry tap at the end of procedure.

Table 34.2 Technique for pericardiocentesis			
Approach	Technique	Advantages	Disadvantages
Sub-xiphoid is most common approach	Needle is inserted between xiphisternum and left costal margin at a 45° angle relative to the transverse plane. Needle is directed towards left shoulder	Provides the safest approach in emergent situation. It can be attempted without echo/USG guidance. Needle enters the pericardium where it is in direct contact with diaphragm, and there is less risk of pleural injury	Risk of injury to liver, colon and stomach if needle orientation is not correct

Procedure

Procedure can be done safely at the bedside with proper aseptic precautions by effective antiseptic cleaning and draping the skin. Availability of equipment for cardiopulmonary resuscitation is mandatory before attempting the procedure and adequate peripheral/central venous access ensured for administration of life-saving drugs. A blood sample for cross-matching should be sent. Antibiotic prophylaxis is not required. The sub-xiphoid approach to pericardiocentesis is attempted as shown in Table 34.2.

Technique

1. The sub-xiphoid approach is used for emergency procedure (Figure 34.9). Adequate pain control measures should be undertaken. Neonate is positioned supine with head raised 30–40 degrees with a support under the shoulders. Assemble the needle or cannula, syringe and three-way stopcock so that the stopcock is open both to the needle and the syringe but closed to the draining port. After skin preparation with antiseptics and draping, insert the cannula and advance it slowly with constant negative pressure at about 45-degree angle beneath the xiphoid process with needle directed towards left shoulder. Careful monitoring for arrhythmias on a vital signs monitor is mandatory. As soon as the needle pierces the pericardium, a give way feel is experienced followed by entry of fluid into the syringe. At this point, the entry of needle in the pericardium can be confirmed by echo/ultrasound.

2. Gently remove the stylet by keeping cannula in position and aspirate the fluid If there is air in the pericardium, one can use an underwater drain as described for aspiration of pneumothorax. In cases of tamponade, hemodynamic improvement can be noticed after removal of fluid. If a large volume of fluid is removed, one can replace intravascular volume with fluid boluses.

Complications

The procedure may be associated with several complications if the direction of needle is erroneous. There is risk of injury to coronary vessels, damage to myocardium and life-threatening arrhythmias. Infectious pericarditis, septicemia, injury to neighboring vital organs like pleura with risk of pneumothorax, liver and bowel injury are other potential major complications. Minor complications include local pain and bleeding.

Umbilical Venous and Arterial Catheterization

Indications for Umbilical Venous Cannulation

1. For emergency venous access to administer medications or fluids during neonatal resuscitation.
2. To obtain central venous access in neonates in the first 14 days of life to administer intravenous fluids, parenteral nutrition and medications.
3. To perform exchange or partial exchange blood transfusion in neonates with jaundice, anemia, sepsis and hydrops fetalis.
4. To monitor central venous pressure in critically sick neonates.

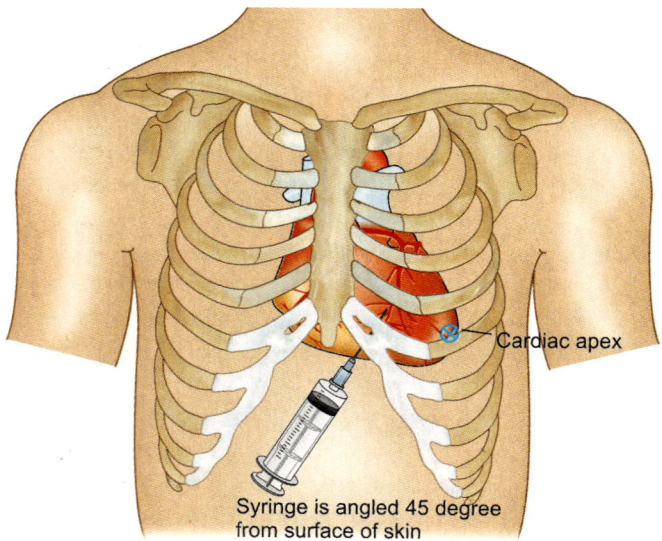

Cardiac apex

Syringe is angled 45 degree from surface of skin

Figure 34.9 Sub-xiphoid approach for pericardiocentesis.

Indications for Umbilical Arterial Access

1. Invasive blood pressure monitoring.
2. Frequent need for blood sampling for arterial blood gases.
3. Iso-volumetric exchange transfusion when both umbilical artery and vein are cannulated.

Contraindications

1. Abdominal surgery that requires an incision above the umbilicus
2. Omphalitis
3. Peritonitis or necrotizing enterocolitis
4. Anterior abdominal wall defects like omphalocele, and gastroschisis
5. In preterm neonates with antenatal diagnosis of absent or reversed end diastolic flow, we prefer cannulation of peripheral arterial line instead of umbilical artery.

Relevant anatomy and position of catheters The umbilical vein passes cephalad through the falciform ligament and to the right. After giving off several large intra-hepatic branches, it joins the left branch of the portal vein. The ductus venosus arises from the point where the umbilical vein joins the left portal vein. The ideal catheter tip position of UVC is at the junction of the ductus venosus and the inferior vena cava just above or at the level of the diaphragm and outside the heart opposite T9–T10 vertebrae. Umbilical artery is a branch of internal iliac artery. The umbilical artery catheter tip is positioned in the aorta between the T6 and T9 vertebrae (high position) or between the L3 and L4 vertebrae (low position). A high UAC position is associated with significantly lesser risk of clinical vascular compromise and aortic thrombus formation. The exact positions for umbilical venous and arterial catheters can be determined by using a formula or by using a chart.

a. *Using the formula* Desired UVC length in cm = (1.5 × birth weight in kg) + 5.5 cm. Desired UAV length in cm = (4 × birth weight in kg) + 7 cm.

b. *Shoulder-umbilical length* Measure the distance between the umbilicus and an imaginary line passing through the shoulders. Use this length against the standard charts to obtain the UVC and UAC insertion distance.

The formula and chart based measurements may over estimate the required length and location of the catheter which should be cross checked with an X-ray abdomen. The size of catheter depends upon the birth weight of the baby, 3.5 Fr for <1500 g, 5.0 Fr for 1500–3000 g and 6.0 Fr for infants >3000 g.

Analgesia/Sedation

No specific analgesia is needed, as the umbilical cord has no pain sensation; however oral sucrose can be given if no other contraindications exist. Swaddling the lower limbs may help to pacify the baby.

Equipment Needed

1. Umbilical vessel catheterization set that is autoclaved. The contents of the set should include the following:
   - Three sterile sheets including a holed sterile drape
   - Two small bowls to contain betadine and spirit solutions
   - Sterile cotton balls and cut gauze pieces
   - Bard-Parker knife holder
   - Straight artery and a small curved artery forceps
   - Sponge holder
   - Needle holder
   - Umbilical cord tie
2. Additional equipment
   - Sterile gown and gloves
   - Silk suture with curved needle
   - Umbilical arterial catheter size 3.5–4 Fr
   - Umbilical venous catheter 3.5–6 Fr double lumen or single lumen
   - 2 × 5 or 10 mL syringes
   - 0.9% saline bottle
   - 2 × 3-way stopcocks
   - Fixation adhesive tape.

Procedure

1. *Preparation* Intravenous fluids to be used may be prepared prior to the procedure under sterile technique. Each catheter will require an infusion rate of a minimum of 0.5 mL per hour. The infant is placed supine under the radiant warmer and gently restrained by using soft tapes tied to the lower limbs. Sucrose or breast milk or a soother can be used to offer comfort and pain relief. The infant's vital signs are monitored throughout the procedure. The temperature probe of the radiant warmer is placed on the thighs or upper abdomen away from the procedure site to allow cleaning and preventing it from getting soiled. The bedside nurse should remain with the infant during the procedure for assistance and monitoring.

2. *Arranging the equipment* Clean a freshly opened normal saline bottle with spirit-betadine-spirit. Draw 5 mL saline in two syringes. Attach 3-way stopcock to the outer end of each UVC lumen and prime the tap and lumen with saline and take care to exclude air bubbles within the system.

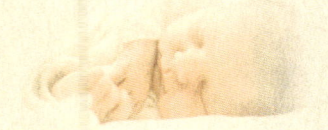

3. **Cord cleaning and cutting the stump** Let the assistant hold the cord clamp with a long artery or sponge holding forceps clear of the abdomen. The operator should then clean the cord and an area of abdomen around the cord with spirit-betadine-spirit. In preterm neonates <1000 g we avoid the use of betadine as it can cause skin burns. Place a cord tie at the base of the cord and cut the stump with a blade so that no more than 0.5–1 cm of stump is left. The cord tie should be tied loosely around the base of the cord to prevent brisk arterial hemorrhage and slow ooze from the umbilical vein. Too much of a pull on the cord before cutting can lead to umbilical arteries getting coiled within the stump. Place sterile drapes around the cord.

4. **Identification of vessel** The umbilical vein is a single vessel that is thin walled and located at 6 o'clock and often gaping. The umbilical arteries are two in number and are thick walled and often constricted.

5. **Insertion of the UVC** Stabilize the umbilical stump by holding the Wharton's jelly with two artery forceps with gentle upward traction at 3 and 9 o'clock, grasping the edge of the cord. Remove clots and dilate the vein gently with iris forceps. Grasp the catheter approximately 0.5 cm above the tip with the iris forceps and gently insert the tip into the vessel lumen. Push the catheter gradually in 1 cm increments and gently advance the catheter into the umbilical vein up to the measured distance. Avoid excessive pressure or repeated probing.

6. **Difficulties encountered during UVC insertion** It may be difficult to negotiate the catheter through the ductus venosus. There are some maneuvers that can assist in placement of the catheter. One can pull the catheter back to about 4–5 cm, then advance the catheter whilst rotating it clockwise. The other technique is to insert another catheter along the already mal-placed catheter. The second catheter may be pass through the ductus venosus. As the umbilical vessels are thin walled and lack support because of the surrounding Wharton's jelly, it is very easy to false track between the vessel intima and vessel wall. Do not exert excessive pressure or frequently manipulate the vessels with iris forceps. The vessel lumen can be crushed if the vessels and not the Wharton's jelly are held by the forceps. A catheter should never be forced if resistance is encountered.

7. **Difficulties encountered during UAC insertion** The initial step of identification and arterial dilatation is very important and great care should be taken as it is very easy to create a false track in the adventitia of the artery. During advancement of the catheter, one may feel resistance at a distance of 1–2 cm where the umbilical arteries turn suddenly downwards. This can usually be overcome by pulling the umbilical stump upwards towards the baby's face and applying steady gentle pressure on the catheter. A second site where resistance is encountered again is at a distance of 5–6 cm, where the artery arises from the iliac vessels. Again, gentle sustained pressure to the catheter is enough to by pass the obstruction. Once 6–10 cm of catheter is inserted, one can freely aspirate blood in the syringe. Advance the catheter to the desired calculated length

8. **Securing the umbilical catheters** Take one bite of the suture through the umbilical cord and tie a loose purse-string knot. Place one end of the suture parallel to the UVC and pass the other end around the UVC and end of the first suture and return through the loop created. Repeat this action by placing the "second" end parallel to the UVC and pass the "first" end around the UVC and return through the loop created. Repeat this procedure 1 cm above the first set of ties.

9. **Obtain hemostasis** If hemostasis is not achieved, place a purse-string suture (using 3 small bites) around the cord without piercing the skin and secure it with a knot.

Confirm the position of catheter Confirm that the position of the UVC is correct with an antero-posterior and lateral X-ray of chest and abdomen (Figure 34.10). This must be done prior to using the UVC except when UVC is inserted for resuscitation at birth. If there is a delay in obtaining the skiagram, intermittently flush the line with 0.9% saline to keep it patent. The tip of the UVC should lie between T9–T10 at junction of IVC and heart and never inside the heart. The UVC may be withdrawn but never advanced to correct its position.

Complications

1. Infection
2. UA cannulation is associated with risk of thrombo-embolism which may involve femoral artery (lower limb ischemia), renal artery (hypertension, hematuria, renal failure), and mesenteric artery (gut ischemia, NEC).
3. Thrombophlebitis of hepatic or portal vein.
4. Portal vein obstruction which can later lead to portal hypertension.
5. Blood loss from umbilical stump or accidental disconnection.
6. Hematoma or abscess in the liver, and hepatic necrosis.

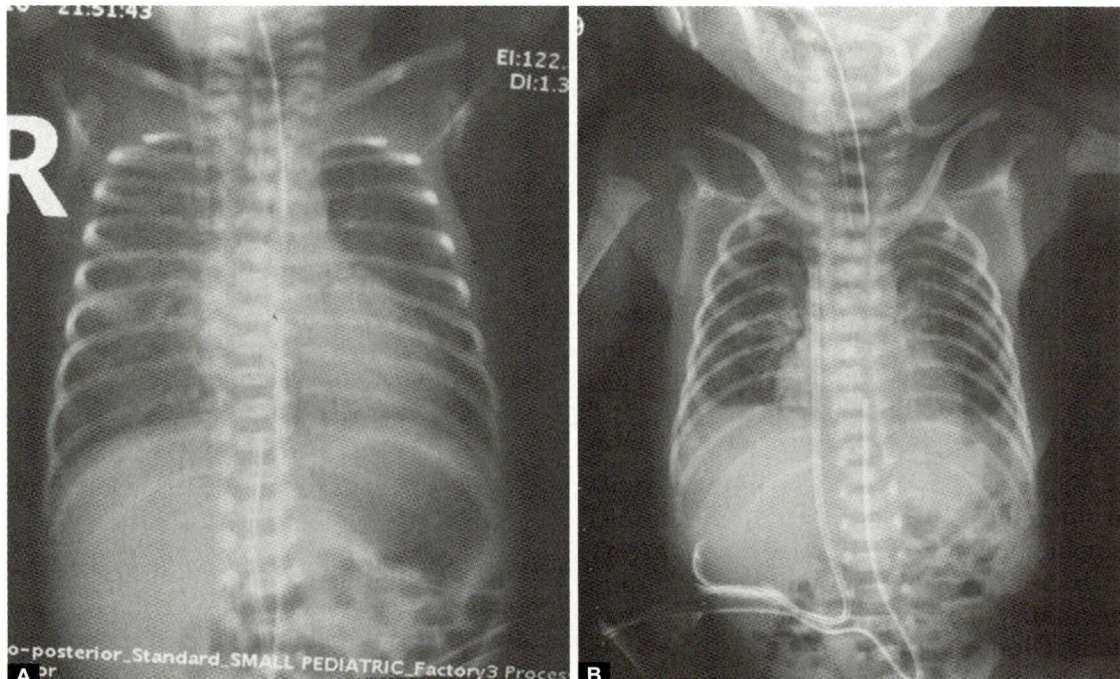

Figure 34.10 The first X-ray done for confirmation of position of umbilical catheter should include the pelvis so that the lines can be traced. UAC makes a downward dip before ascending upwards into the aorta (umbilical artery is a branch of internal iliac artery). The umbilical venous line ascends without the downward dip. It travels through the ductus venosus before entering the inferior vena cava. A. unsatisfactory skiagram. B. Correct X-ray to see the course of lines (UVC is too high and needs to be pulled out; UAC is correctly placed).

7. Complications secondary to malposition of catheters include
   - Malposition in the heart and great vessels
   - Pericardial effusion/cardiac tamponade
   - Cardiac arrhythmia
   - Pleural effusion or hydrothorax
   - UVC malposition in portal system may lead to portal hypertension.

When to remove the catheter? Umbilical artery catheter should be removed as soon as possible when no longer needed or whenever any complication related to its use is noted. According to CDC (Center for Disease Control) recommendations, an UAC should not be left in place for more than 5 days. In case of difficult vascular access we have sometimes used UACs for up to 7 days. Umbilical venous catheters should also be removed as soon as possible when no longer needed, but can be used up to 14 days. If a long term access is needed we use peripherally inserted central catheters or by using another central access.

How to remove the catheter? Turn off infusion pump. Remove the suture from stump. Apply a purse-string cord tie at the base of the cord if a stump is still visible or hold the base of the cord firmly with a gauze to prevent oozing of blood. Withdraw the UVC with continued traction slowly. When removing the UAC exert gentle traction in a slow continuous motion to promote vasoconstriction. Sudden removal can lead to torrential bleed from a patent artery that may at times be difficult to control. Check whether the catheter is removed intact. Continuous local pressure should be applied for a minimum of 5 minutes. Ensure that the peripheries stay pink and well perfused. Observe the site carefully for bleeding over the next hour. If bleeding does occur, press firmly just above the umbilicus or pinch the remainder of stump between thumb and forefinger.

Complications

Complications can occur in about 10% of umbilical catheter insertions. Hemorrhage during insertion or secondary to slipping of purse string suture is common. Arterial obstruction can occur in 6% of cases with the limb becoming pale or blue with feeble pulses (Figure 34.11). In a majority of cases, the vasospasm responds promptly to removal of the catheter.

Usually umbilical arterial catheters are used for blood pressure monitoring, blood sampling and infusion of fluids, electrolytes and nutrients. Infusion of hypertonic solutions (25% or 50% dextrose) can lead to vasospasm, thrombosis or vessel wall damage.

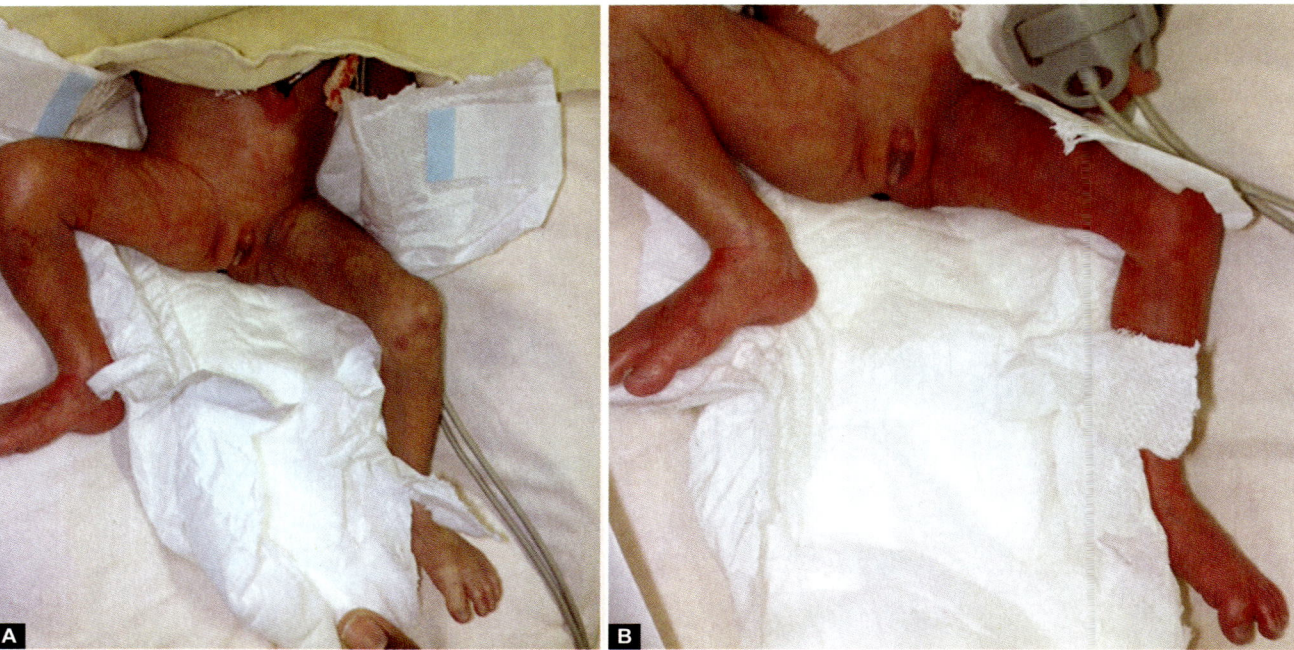

Figure 34.11 A. Limb is mottled and pale. There is an umbilical artery catheter in place. B. Return of limb perfusion after removal of catheter.

Management of Complications Related to Umbilical Catheters

1. In most cases, the vasospasm is transient. If you notice, mild blanching or cyanosis of an extremity, the catheter can be left *in situ*. It is useful to warm opposite limb. In order to warm the contralateral foot, apply warm water-soaked disposable diaper whose temperature should not exceed 40°C. The rationale for this intervention is to induce reflex vasodilatation of the affected extremity. If the cyanosis or vasospasm resolves, the catheter may be left in place.

2. Another intervention that has been tried in catheter related vasospasm that persists after catheter removal is topical application of nitroglycerine. Nitroglycerine ointment is easily absorbed through the thin neonatal skin and is converted intracellularly to nitric oxide, a potent vasodilator. The dosage used is 4 mm/kg of 2% nitroglycerine ointment that is applied as a thin film to the affected extremity. The ointment is applied sparingly to the affected extremity, approximately 1 cm proximal to the line of pallor. The improvement in color and perfusion is likely to occur within 30–45 minutes but at times it may take 3–8 hours. The subsequent doses of nitroglycerine ointment are applied every 8 hours approximately 1 cm proximal to the site of ischemia along the anatomic course of the arterial supply. The pharmacokinetics of cutaneously applied nitroglycerine and its duration of action are not well-known in neonates and there are reports of hypotension as a side effect.

3. In a neonate who has persistent vasospasm in the form of cyanosed, pale, cold or pulseless extremity, an urgent Doppler ultrasound of the aorta and renal arteries should be performed to look for thrombo-emboli. The management depends on the severity of thrombosis. For example, if the thrombus involves a unilateral renal vein without extension to the inferior vena cava (IVC) and there are no signs of renal failure, supportive care with close monitoring may suffice. Alternatively, anticoagulation therapy with heparin may be considered. If the thrombus involves bilateral renal vein or if the thrombus extends to the IVC, treatment with heparin is recommended. Thrombolytic therapy is reserved for life- or limb-threatening thrombus and can be considered in neonates with bilateral renal vein thrombosis and impending renal failure.

4. Anticoagulation should be individualized and hematologist and cardiologist should be involved when such a decision is made. There are absolute (major surgery within the last 10 days and evidence of major intracranial, pulmonary, or gastrointestinal bleeding) and relative contraindications (thrombo-cytopenia, a fibrinogenemia, hypertension and severe coagulation deficiency) for the use of anticoagulation in neonates which should be kept in mind before initiating it.

Intraosseus Access

The establishment of an intravenous access in cases of shock, injury or burns can be challenging and sometimes impossible. Intraosseus infusion is the establishment of an intravenous line through the bone. This technique helps in rapid establishment of vascular access within a few minutes and delivery of fluid bolus, emergency medications and blood products. Intraosseus access is recommended in all children after two failed attempts at IV access or during circulatory collapse. The American Heart Association recommends intraosseus-access if venous access cannot be quickly and reliably established. During neonatal resuscitation, if the resuscitators have little experience with umbilical venous access, they should use intraosseus access as it can be rapidly and safely initiated.

Anatomy The long bones contain medullary cavities within which lies a vast network of blood vessels that run both vertically and horizontally. This vascular network drains via emissary veins into the general circulation. The fluids and medications injected into these marrow cavities are rapidly carried into the central circulation. The intraosseous network of vessels do not collapse during shock.

Indications for Intraosseus Infusion

An intraosseus access is indicated after 2 failed attempts to establish an intravenous access in an infant requiring immediate cardiopulmonary resuscitation due to following clinical situations:

- Delivery room resuscitation
- Shock secondary to sepsis, hypovolemia or cardiac failure
- Cardiopulmonary resuscitation
- Severe dehydration
- Status epilepticus
- Massive trauma
- Burns
- Edema or obesity in small children
- Anaphylaxis
- As an emergency access before central line is established.

Contraindications

- Bony fracture suspected at the planned site of insertion
- Infection or osteomyelitis at the planned site
- Absence of adequate anatomical landmarks
- Previous orthopedic procedure at the proposed site

- If a site had been used earlier, one has to wait for at least 48 hours before accessing the same site again.

Sites for Insertion of Intraosseus Needle

The two most commonly preferred sites are proximal end of tibia and distal end of femur. Other sites include sternum, medial and lateral malleoli, os calcis, and the anterior superior iliac spine. The intraosseus line offers vascular access for about 12 hours and one should establish another central access that can be used for a long-term after fluid resuscitation of the infant.

In children younger than 6 years, choose either the proximal tibia or the distal femur for IO insertion (Figure 34.12A). The tibial site is located in the proximal flat-broad tibial plateau, 1 to 2 finger breadths below the tibial tubercle on the antero-medial surface. The femoral site is located in the distal femur, 2 to 3 cm above the external condyles in the midline. The bony cortex is easy to penetrate in children up to 6 years of age. In both the sites, the epiphysis or the growth plate is located at the end of the long bones and care must be taken to avoid damage to the epiphyseal plates.

Equipment

1. Sterile tray containing bowls to hold antiseptics, sterile drape and instruments.
2. Prepare intravenous fluids or medications to be administered in a sterile manner.
3. *Choice of intraosseus needle and insertion device* A variety of needles have been used for IO access including those specifically designed for that purpose and ordinary needles. The specific intraosseus needles are wide bored (16–18 G), with a short rigid shaft, a special handle for easy insertion and also contain a stylet that prevent occlusion of needle by bony spicules. Commercially available IO systems include Bone Injection Gun (BIG), Cook Disposable OI infusion needle (Sur-Fast Needle), EX-IO infusion system, First Access for Shock and Trauma (FASTI) IO infusion system and the Jamshidi IO needle (Figure 34.12B). When specific IO needles are not available in an emergency situation, butterfly needles, spinal needles, standard metal IV needles, and bone marrow biopsy needles have been used. The use of needles without stylets is associated with a higher incidence of obstruction by bony spicules.
4. *Manual versus automated devices for insertion* The IO needle can be inserted manually or with the help of automated insertion devices or drills. The EZ-IO (Vidacare, San Antonio, TX) device is battery operated whose beveled tip can be inserted up to preset depth. The needle that accompanies this

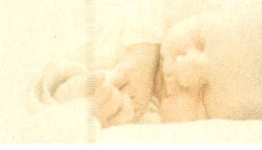

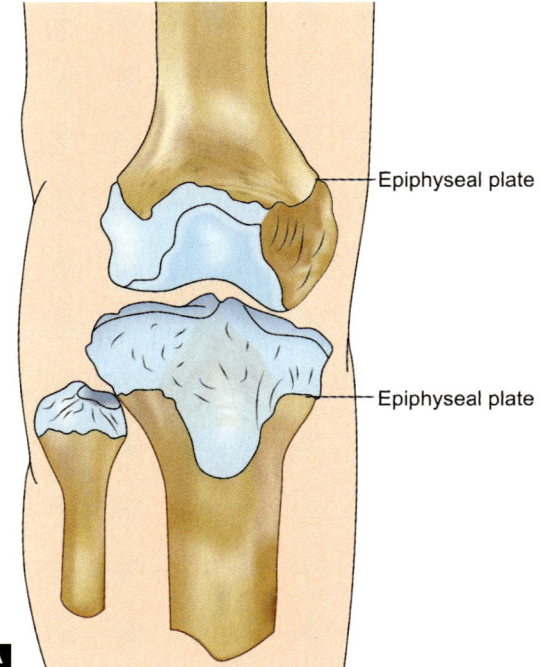

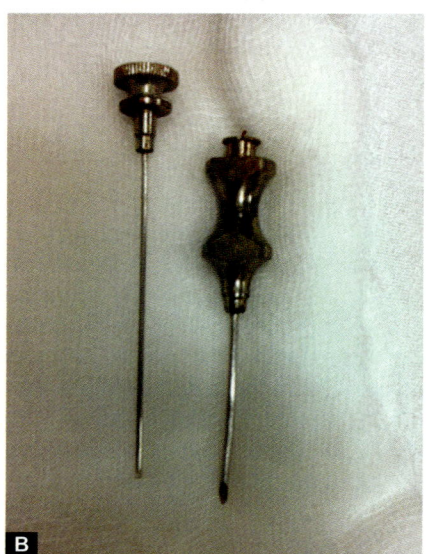

Figure 34.12 A. Sites in the lower limb where an intraosseous needle can be inserted. B. Jamshedi bone marrow needle.

device is 15 gauge and there are 3 different lengths for different weight categories (15 mm for children weighing 3–39 kg, 25 mm for patients weighing >40 kg, and a 45-mm length for patients with significant tissue edema overlying the bone). Once the needle enters the IO space by the drilling motion, a "give way" feel is felt, the drilling is stopped and the stylet is withdrawn and the metal IO needle is left in place. The Bone Injection Gun uses a spring loaded mechanism that pushes the IO needle by triggering a button.

5. *Manual procedure* Position the leg with the knee slightly bent and semi-externally rotated. Place a sandbag or towel roll under the leg for support. Stabilize the extremity and point the IO needle at a 90° angle to the center of the bone directing it towards the diaphysis. Place the hub of the intraosseus needle handle in the palm of your hand and place your index finger on the shaft. Insert it firmly through the skin overlying the tibia. Push the needle tip through the skin until the tip rests against the bone. Advance the needle through the bone with a gentle rotating to-and fro action. Once the medullary cavity is entered a "pop" or "give way" sensation is felt. The IO catheter that is placed in marrow cavity should be firmly located in the bone and should allow blood/bone marrow to be aspirated. Flush the IO catheter with normal saline and connect the intravenous fluids.

7. The IO needle should be snugly fixed in position so that it can be used for at least next 12 hours or until definite venous access is obtained.

Uses of Intraosseus Access

1. A variety of fluids and medications can be infused into the medullary cavity including crystalloids, colloids, blood, and blood products and medications such as calcium, glucose, atropine, sodium bicarbonate, epinephrine, diazepam, dopamine/dobutamine, and anesthetic agents. Both bolus as well as slow infusions can be administered. Boluses take 15 seconds or less to reach the central circulation. The rate of flow through IO route is slow compared to a peripheral vein and can be helped with the use of infusion pumps or syringes.

2. Blood samples taken from the intraosseus access is similar to mixed venous blood and can be used to measure hemoglobin, electrolytes, blood cultures, blood gases, blood type and cross matching. However, the primary purpose for this procedure is to get IV access and not for sampling. The IO samples correlate well with blood samples when obtained immediately after needle placement.

Removal

When an intravenous access is obtained; the IO needle can be removed. Place sterile gauze over the site and apply pressure for 5 minutes. Do not reuse the same site for next 48 hours.

Complications

The risk of complications increase when IO access is used for a prolonged period. The common complications are listed below.

- Cellulitis or subcutaneous abscess
- Osteomyelitis and periosteitis

- Extravasation of fluid into the subcutaneous space
- Fat embolism
- Epiphyseal injury in children
- Bone marrow damage

Exchange Blood Transfusion

The procedure was first performed by Hart in 1925 for infants affected by erythroblastosis fetalis. In that procedure, blood was removed from the sagittal sinus via the anterior fontanel and donor blood was transfused through the internal saphenous vein. Later in 1946, Louis K. Diamond pioneered the use of a polyethylene catheter to cannulate the umbilical vein (UV), a major milestone in neonatal medicine.

Indications

1. Severe hyperbilirubinemia
2. Non-immune hydrops fetalis
3. Polycythemia
4. Disseminated intravascular coagulation
5. Sickle cell disease
6. Reye syndrome, drug overdose, and hyperammonemia
7. Neonatal sepsis.

Neonatal jaundice is the most common indication for exchange blood transfusion where in a double volume exchange transfusion is done. Besides the bilirubin level, it is recommended that any jaundiced infant who has features of acute bilirubin induced neurological dysfunction (BIND) like high pitched cry, hypertonia, arching, retrocollis, fever, opisthotonos should undergo immediate exchange transfusion since many of the acute changes related to bilirubin toxicity are reversible. Partial exchange transfusion in which blood is removed and replaced with saline or albumin to normalize hematocrit has been used to treat hyperviscosity and high hematocrit due to polycythemia.

Contraindications

1. Omphalitis
2. Malformations of the cord, as seen in gastroschisis or omphalocele
3. Gastrointestinal complications like necrotizing enterocolitis or intestinal perforation.

In older infants, the umbilical cord may be shriveled or fallen off precluding access. In the first week of life, application of warm moist saline gauze to the umbilical stump can help in cannulation.

Equipments needed

The following equipments are needed for the procedure of exchange transfusion:

1. *Exchange transfusion tray* The tray for exchange transfusion should contain the following instruments:
   a. Three sterile sheets including a holed sterile drape
   b. Two small bowls with betadine and spirit solutions
   c. Sterile cotton balls and cut gauze pieces
   d. Bard-Parker knife holder
   e. Straight artery and a small curved artery forceps
   f. Sponge holder
   g. Needle holder
   h. Umbilical cord tie
2. Additional equipment
   a. Umbilical catheters (5 Fr, 6 Fr)
   b. Two Luer-Lock syringes, two extension tubing sets, two 3-way stopcocks
   c. Small bottle of normal saline and one waste bag
   d. It is desirable to have a blood warmer to warm donor blood.
3. During exchange transfusion the infant should be continuously monitored with the help of an electronic vital sign monitor and pulse oximeter. Emergency medications like epinephrine, calcium gluconate (10%), and normal saline bolus should be readily available at the bedside.
4. Exchange transfusion monitoring sheet should be maintained.

Donor Blood

The following considerations should be kept in mind during selection of donor blood for exchange transfusion:

1. Typically blood banks store red blood cells and plasma separately and reconstitute blood to a hematocrit level ranging between 55–65% just before it is used. However, if whole blood is to be used (due to nonavailability of packed red cells and plasma), then fresh (<5 days old) blood is preferred, as older blood may have higher potassium values and lower pH. All blood products used in neonatal period should be leukoreduced and irradiated if possible to reduce the risk of graft versus host disease.
2. Typing and cross-matching of blood:
   a. *Rh incompatibility* If the blood is arranged before the baby's birth, O Rh negative packed red blood cells (RBCs) reconstituted in AB plasma should be used and cross-matched against the mother. If the blood is arranged after the birth of the baby,

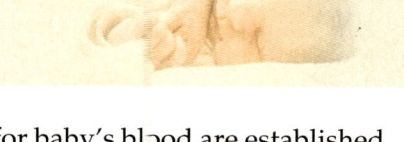

Rh negative RBCs of the infant's blood group should be arranged and cross-matched both against the mother and the infant's sample. If the baby has received intrauterine transfusion, then O Rh negative RBCs in AB plasma should be used for postnatal exchanges.

b. *ABO incompatibility* Rh identical matched O group blood cross-matched with mother is recommended.

c. In minor blood group incompatibility (i.e. anti-Kell, anti-E, anti-Duffy, anti-RhC), the donor blood should be cross-matched with the mother's blood after removing the offending antigen

d. *Jaundice not related to isoimmune disorders* Donor blood must always be cross-matched against both infant's and mother's serum to safeguard against unrecognized minor blood group incompatibilities.

3. *Volume of donor blood* For a double volume exchange transfusion, one should arrange 2 times the blood volume of a neonate. For example, for a 3 kg infant with expected blood volume of 90 mL/kg, the total blood volume required is 3 × 90 × 2 = 540 mL. Of this 70% is the volume of packed RBCs and 30% is the volume of fresh frozen plasma. As a rule of thumb, in emergencies when charts for blood volume are not available, one can consider the blood volume to be approximately 80 mL/kg in a term infant and 100 mL/kg in a preterm infant. A single volume exchange replaces 63% of the infant's blood, whereas a double volume exchange is likely to replace 86% of the infant's blood.

Procedure

1. The neonate is started on intensive phototherapy while arrangements are being made for exchange transfusion. The infant is kept nil per oral during and for at least 2–4 hours post-transfusion. The neonate is gently restrained and non-pharmacological methods like oral sucrose or breast milk is used to alleviate pain and provide comfort during the procedure.

2. *Single-catheter pull push technique* Under aseptic precautions catheterize the umbilical vein with an appropriate size umbilical catheter. The depth of insertion is usually 3 cm in preterm and 5 cm in term babies. A low position is preferable as a greater depth of insertion can sometimes lead to the catheter being placed in hepatic sinusoids or in the cardiac chambers.

3. The connections between the umbilical catheter, 3- way stopcocks and the inlet tubing for donor blood

and the exit tubing for baby's blood are established. It is essential that the catheter and the connections are flushed with normal saline to prevent infusion of air bubbles.

4. Each aliquot of exchange is generally kept between 5–8% of estimated blood volume of the infant. Aliquots smaller than 2 mL, are likely to make the procedure ineffective as the proportion of dead space increases. In preterm and sicker infants, the aliquots of smaller volume can be used (5 mL/kg). The procedure should generally be completed within 60–90 min with the help of 35–40 cycles.

5. *Monitoring during the procedure* Monitor heart rate, respiratory rate, SpO$_2$ continuously during the procedure. Blood pressure should be monitored every 15–30 minutes by a noninvasive method. In a sick neonate, it is advisable to have continuous invasive blood pressure monitoring. The bedside nurse should make a note of each cycle of the exchange transfusion, the aliquot volume and the vital parameters in the transfusion record.

6. The first "out" sample from the neonate should be preserved for baseline investigations like hemogram, bilirubin, electrolytes, blood culture if indicated and G6PD enzyme test. Similarly, the last "out" sample can be sent for post procedure serum bilirubin, electrolytes and can be preserved for repeat cross-match for subsequent exchanges.

7. *Double catheter push-pull technique* In this technique, both umbilical vein and artery are catheterized. Blood is withdrawn from the umbilical artery and simultaneously an equal volume of donor blood is infused through the umbilical vein. The procedure is conducted by two operators and it achieves isovolumetric exchange transfusion.

Don'ts

1. Do not apply strong suction pressure to the syringe. The excessive negative force can lead to collapse of the vessel at the tip of the catheter leading to dry blood return. Avoid infusing the blood rapidly with force because it can lead to trauma to internal organs like liver, hemodynamic instability and air embolism.

2. Do not allow disconnection in the system or leave 3-way system open to the atmosphere to prevent risk of air embolism.

3. Do not perform exchange transfusion with cold blood. It can lead to hypothermia or cardiac arrhythmias. Blood should always be warmed to body temperature by wrapping in a warm towel or by the use of blood warmers.

4. Antibiotic prophylaxis is not routinely given during exchange transfusion. However, if the procedure was messy or asepsis was compromised, one can consider administration of antibiotics after taking blood cultures.

5. Some centers administer vitamin K after the procedure in infants with severe Rh isoimmunization because of the liver involvement and coagulation abnormalities.

6. If the infant is on antibiotics or anticonvulsants, their dose must be repeated after the exchange transfusion.

Complications of Exchange Transfusion

1. *Electrolyte imbalance* Hyperkalemia may occur if blood used for exchange transfusion is old (>7 days). Hypocalcemia and hypomagnesemia can occur because of citrate in the blood that binds ionic calcium and magnesium. However, routine calcium or magnesium supplements are not indicated during exchange transfusion unless there are laboratory or clinical evidences of hypocalcemia.

2. *Hypoglycemia* Usually occurs 1–2 hours after the exchange transfusion due to rebound increase in insulin secretion stimulated by the higher concentration of glucose in the CPD (citrate phosphate dextrose) blood.

3. *Acid-base disturbances* Both metabolic acidosis and alkalosis can complicate exchange transfusion. Acidosis is due to inability to metabolize citric acid in the blood by a sick neonate and alkalosis may occur because of conversion of citrate to bicarbonate in the liver.

4. *Hemodynamic disturbances* Rapid exchanges or large volume aliquot exchanges in a sick neonate can lead to volume overload, hypotension, tachycardia and cardiac arrest. Infusion of cold blood can lead to arrhythmias. Injury to liver, umbilical vessels and hepatic vein thrombosis may occur.

5. Thrombocytopenia and coagulopathy can lead to decrease in platelets and deficiency of coagulation factors after exchange transfusion.

6. Infection, hemolysis, graft versus host disease, transfusion related reactions, temperature instability and necrotizing enterocolitis are other recognized complications of exchange transfusion.

Peritoneal Dialysis

In neonates, peritoneal dialysis is preferred over hemodialysis because the procedure is technically easy and allows adequate removal of excess water and solutes without the need for systemic anticoagulation. The indications for peritoneal dialysis are listed below.

1. Renal failure with severe electrolyte disturbances
   a. Hyperkalemia refractory to medical management
   b. Hyponatremia
   c. Volume overload (pulmonary edema, severe hypertension)
   d. Severe metabolic acidosis not responding to medical management
   e. Hypocalcemia/ hyperphosphatemia refractory to therapy
   f. Inability to provide adequate nutrition due to fluid restriction

2. Removal of toxic metabolites associated with inborn errors of metabolism for example removal of ammonia in urea cycle disorders.

Contraindications

1. Peritonitis or intestinal perforation
2. Anterior abdominal wall defects
3. Surgical abdomen
4. Diaphragmatic hernia

Equipment Needed

1. Sterile peritoneal dialysis set
2. Mask, sterile drapes, gowns
3. Local anesthetic (lignocaine)
4. 22 gauge intravenous cannula
5. Burette set, intravenous sets, 3-way stopcock
6. *Peritoneal dialysis (PD) catheter* Peritoneal access in most institutes is achieved by a stiff catheter and trocar. Risk of infection and visceral injury is less with soft PD catheters made of silicone. Most of the catheters have side holes that allow for easy ingress and egress of fluid. The catheters for prolonged use are provided with cuffs.
7. *Dialysis fluid* The dialysis fluid used for peritoneal dialysis contains 1.7% dextrose with lactate. When higher solute gradient is required as in case of fluid overload, 3% dextrose solution can be used. This can be prepared by adding 25 mL of 50% dextrose to one liter of 1.7% PD fluid. In case of liver failure as in asphyxia, lactate free bicarbonate containing fluid should be used as these neonates may be unable to metabolize lactate. If hypokalemia is noted during the procedure, one can add one mL of potassium chloride to one liter of dialysate fluid.

Procedure

1. *Preparation for the procedure* Obtain informed consent. After a thorough surgical scrub, gowning and gloving, the operator should prepare the anterior abdominal wall area for the procedure. The stomach

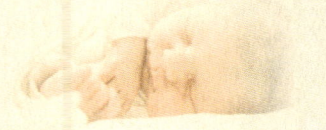

should be decompressed by inserting an orogastric tube and the bladder is emptied by catheterization prior to the procedure.

2. The first step involves creating a fluid filled reservoir by infusing 20–30 mL/kg dialysate into the peritoneum using a cannula.

3. After this, the catheter is inserted into the peritoneal cavity and connected to a three way cannula. The common sites of insertion are in the midline below the umbilicus, right or left lower quadrant of the abdomen.

4. The dialysate fluid is connected to a pediatric burette set and its terminal end is connected to one of the ports of three-way cannula. The remaining port of the three-way is connected to an intravenous (IV) set, the end of which is allowed to drain into a sterile container (empty IV fluid bottle).

5. The abdomen is filled with 20–30 mL/kg of dialysis fluid infused over 10 min. A dwell time of 20–30 min is used before draining the fluid over 10 min. The dwell time can be reduced in case of respiratory compromise.

6. A total of 20–40 cycles can be used or the procedure should be continued till the desired effect is obtained.

7. Blood sugar, serum electrolytes and blood gases should be monitored every 6 hourly and serum creatinine every 24 hours. At the end of the procedure, the catheter should be removed and the effluent fluid is sent for culture.

Complications

Peritoneal dialysis is an invasive procedure and the following complications can occur:

1. Peritonitis

2. *Catheter related complications*. Dislodgement of catheter, bleeding, catheter malfunction, leakage from exit site, extravasation of dialysis fluid into anterior abdominal wall, perforation of abdominal viscera, adhesion of catheter tip to omentum.

3. *Metabolic derangements*. Hyperglycemia can occur when a higher concentration of dextrose is used, hypokalemia , hyponatremia, and lactic acidosis.

4. Abdominal distension secondary to instillation of dialysis fluid can cause respiratory compromise. This may be circumvented with smaller volume cycles.

5. Hypothermia must be prevented by using pre-warmed dialysis fluid, and procedure should be conducted under a radiant warmer.

6. PD will be less effective when there is poor cardiac output or hypoperfusion of gut.

Surfactant Replacement Therapy

The indications for prophylactic and rescue surfactant therapy are variable and one should follow the unit policy. In our unit, we administer prophylactic surfactant if the neonate is <25 weeks of gestation or less than 28 weeks but has incomplete antenatal steroid cover or needs positive pressure ventilation in the delivery room for more than one minute. In preterm neonates <32 weeks of gestation who do not satisfy these criteria, are put on nasal CPAP with ≥40% oxygen or mechanical ventilator with ≥35% oxygen.

Pre-requisites

- Physician and a nurse experienced in surfactant administration should be available
- The neonate should be attached to a pulse oximeter or a multipara monitor for continuous monitoring of vital signs
- Surfactant vial (dosing based on the type of surfactant used; see manufacturer's instructions)
- Orogastric and endotracheal tubes of appropriate size
- Sterile surgical blade
- Laryngoscope with blades
- Tapes for fixation of endotracheal tube and Tegaderm

Steps for Surfactant Administration

1. Strict aseptic precautions should be observed during administration of surfactant.

2. Surfactant should be warmed prior to administration (for 8 minutes if the vial is held in the palm of the hand or for 20 minutes at room temperature.) The vial should not be heated. Shaking the vial to mix surfactant should be avoided.

3. The baby should be intubated with an appropriate sized endotracheal tube. If intubated for the purpose of surfactant administration, endotracheal tube position should be confirmed clinically by auscultation. It is preferable to use an endotracheal tube with a side port.

4. Oxygen saturation and heart rate of the neonate should be monitored continuously with a pulse oximeter during the procedure.

5. Measure the length of the endotracheal tube to be inserted, from tip till the adapter. Prepare the appropriate sized endotracheal tube by cutting the redundant length. Now, use this endotracheal tube to measure appropriate length of orogastric tube to be used for instillation of surfactant. The length of orogastric tube should be such that its tip should protrude 1.0 mm beyond the length of the endotracheal tube.

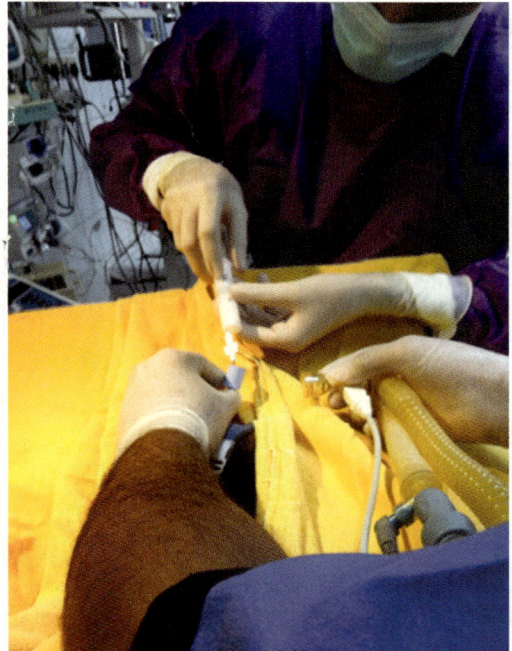
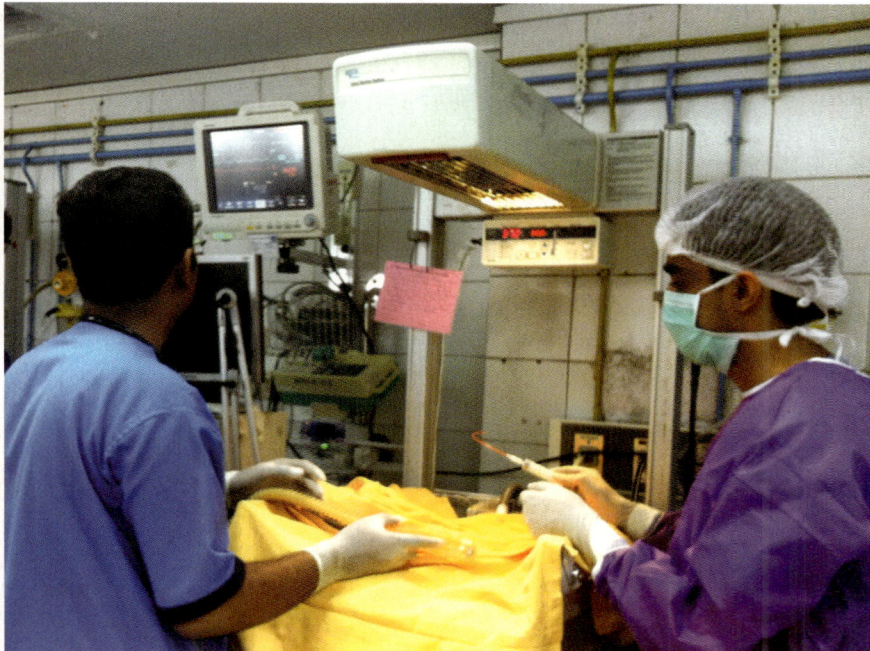

Figure 34.13 Administration of surfactant. The neonate is momentarily disconnected from the ventilator while instilling surfactant. The physician monitors the vital signs of the neonate and makes necessary changes in ventilator settings. We avoid the use of a resuscitation bag during instillation of surfactant to reduce the risk of barotrauma.

6. Clean the surfactant vial and load the appropriate volume into a syringe. Charge the orogastric tube with the surfactant so that the exact calculated dose to be infused remains within the syringe and tube.

7. The neonate should preferably be connected to the ventilator during surfactant administration. One can also use a T-piece device with blended oxygen. We avoid the use of self-inflating bag as inadvertent use of high peak inspiratory pressures can lead to barotrauma. Surfactant is administered through the feeding tube inserted in the ET tube or through the side port of the ET tube.

8. Surfactant is administered as a bolus in three to four aliquots. The neonate should be kept supine with head in midline. The position of the neonate should not be changed during administration of surfactant. Keep the disconnection from the ventilator brief. One may have to increase the PIP on the ventilator transiently if the surfactant is noted to be still in the tubing. Surfactant administration can cause transient desaturation and bradycardia. The clinician should remain at the bedside to monitor the neonate clinically and to adjust the ventilator settings and FiO_2 appropriately (Figure 34.13).

9. Suctioning of the endotracheal tube should be avoided for at least 4 hours after surfactant administration. It is preferable to suction the endotracheal tube prior to administration of surfactant.

10. During the administration of surfactant, if bradycardia or desaturation is significant, the dosing procedure should be interrupted and appropriate measures should be taken to stabilize the infant before the procedure is resumed.

11. After surfactant administration, the neonate can be extubated and put back on nasal CPAP ('InSurE'—Intubation, Surfactant and Extubation) if baby is hemodynamically stable, has a good respiratory drive and maintaining saturation between 90–95%. Mechanical ventilation should be continued if the baby does not have good spontaneous respiratory efforts or if the baby has hemodynamic instability or if the clinician feels that the baby is unlikely to tolerate extubation.

LIFE-SAVING MEDICATIONS

The ability of the newborn to deal with drugs depends upon his functional maturity which is related to conjugatory ability of the liver and excretory capacity of the kidneys. Due to hepatic and renal immaturity, the half-life of the drug in the newborn is prolonged so that administration of drugs every 12 or 8 hours is satisfactory. The poor detoxification and clearance of drugs in the newborn predisposes the infant to develop toxic effects unless due caution is exercised during their use. In addition to above factors, absorption handicaps,

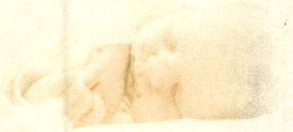

Table 34.3 Commonly used drugs in the newborn

Agent	Dose	Route of administration	Comments
I. Antibiotics			
Amikacin	10 mg/kg loading dose, 7.5 mg/kg/dose	IM, IV (over 20–30 min)	Maintain serum levels between 10 and 25 mg/mL. Furosemide and vancomycin enhance ototoxicity and nephrotoxicity
Ampicillin	25–50 mg/kg/dose	Oral, IM, IV	Solution is stable only for 4 hours. The dose is doubled in meningitis
Benzyl penicillin	25,000 units/kg/dose	IM, IV	Use 5 to 10 times this dose for serious infections and meningitis
Carbenicillin	100 mg/kg/dose, 5 mg per intrathecal dose	IM, IV	Should not be mixed with gentamicin and watch for hypokalemia
Cefazoline sodium	20 mg/kg/dose	IM, IV	Does not penetrate cerebrospinal fluid space
Cefepime	50 mg/kg/dose	IV	Its antipseudomonal activity is similar to ceftazidime
Cefotaxime sodium	50 mg/kg/dose	IM, IV	Readily crosses blood-brain barrier
Ceftazidime	50 mg/kg/dose	IM, IV	Excellent for *Pseudomonas aeruginosa*
Ceftriaxone sodium	50–75 mg/kg single dose daily	IV	For meningitis, use higher dose twice a day. Avoid in neonates with severe jaundice. Drug of choice for gonococci resistent to penicillin
Cefuroxime	100 mg followed by 50 mg after 3 days q 8 hr	IM, IV	
Chloramphenicol	25 mg/kg/dose up to 2 weeks q 24 hr, 15–30 d q 12 hr, later q 6–8 hr 10 and 25 mg/mL	Oral, IM, IV	Gray baby syndrome. Do not exceed 75 mg/kg/day during first week in term and two weeks in preterm babies. Maintain serum levels between 10 and 25 µg/mL
Cloxacillin	25–50 mg/kg/dose	IM, IV	
Colistin sulfate	10–15 mg q 6–8 hr	deep IM, oral	
Erythromycin	25–50 mg q 6–8 hr	Oral, IM, IV	Antibacterial resistance develops fast.
Gentamicin sulfate	2.5 mg/kg/dose, 4 mg/kg single dose daily, 1.0 mg per intrathecal dose and 1–2 mg/kg per intra-ventricular dose	IM, IV	Use pediatric dosage vial (10 mg/mL). For IV use, concentration should not exceed 1.0 mg/mL. Nephro- and ototoxic. Serum levels should be monitored and maintained between 4 and 8 mg/mL
Imipenem/cilastin	20 mg/kg/dose	IM, IV	im formulation cannot be given iv
Kanamycin sulfate	2.5–5.0 mg/kg/dose	IM, IV slow drip	For iv use, concentration should not exceed 2.5 mg/mL. Nephro- and ototoxic. Serum levels should be maintained between 15 and 25 mg/mL
Methicillin sodium	25 mg/kg/dose	IM, IV slow infusion	Give double the dose for meningitis
Metronidazole	15 mg/kg loading dose followed 24 hours later by 7.5 mg/kg dose every 12 hours	IV, PO	Anerobic infections and necrotizing enterocolitis. Reddish-brown discoloration of urine may occur
Moxalactam disodium	50 mg/kg/dose	IV	
Nafcillin	25 mg/kg/dose	IV	Good CSF penetration
Neomycin sulfate	12.5 mg/kg/dose	Oral	
Netilmicin sulfate	2.5–3.0 mg/kg/dose	IM, IV	
Piperacillin sodium	50–75 mg/kg/dose	IM, IV	May cause neuromuscular irritability and seizures

The lower dose is used in a preterm baby. Administer every 12 hr for all infants between 0 and 7 days and every 8 hr for infants >7 days

In preterm infants up to 7 days administer every 12 hr, term infants up to 7 days and preterm infants >7 days administer every 8 hr, and term infants after 7 days every 6 hr.

(contd.)

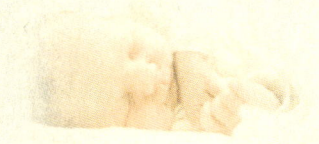

Table 34.3 Commonly used drugs in the newborn (*Contd...*)

Agent	Dose	Route of administration	Comments
▪ Polymyxin B sulfate	2.5 mg/kg/dose	Oral, IM, IV	Does not cross the blood-brain barrier
▪ Ticarcillin sodium	75 mg/kg/dose	IM, IV	
▪ Tobramycin	2.5 mg/kg/dose	IM, IV	
▪ Trimethoprim sulfamethoxazole (cotrimoxazole)	TMP 2 mg/kg loading dose followed by TMP 1.2 mg/kg every 12 hours	IV, oral	Diluted in 5% dextrose in a ratio of 1:20 and given in 10 minutes. Readily crosses blood-brain barrier
▪ Vancomycin hydrochloride	15 mg/kg/dose q 8–12 hr Oral dose is 40–50 mg q 6 hr for colitis in a concentration of 5 mg/mL	oral, IV slowly over 30 min	For oral use dilute with water to a concentration of 5 mg/mL. "Red man syndrome" occurs if given as a bolus. Diphenhydramine provides relief
II. Anticonvulsants and sedatives			
▪ Chloral hydrate	25–50 mg/kg per dose	Oral	Avoid in hepatic and renal impairment
▪ Chlorpromazine	0.5–2.0 mg/kg per dose	Oral, IM, IV	
▪ Diazepam	0.1–0.3 mg/kg/dose q 15–30 min. Maximum dose 2–5 mg	IM, IV, PR	Avoid if infant is jaundiced because it contains sodium benzoate as a preservative
▪ Fentanyl citrate	2–4 mg/kg/dose q 2–4 hr continuous infusion @ 1–5 mg/kg/hr	IV slowly over 3–5 min	Watch for respiratory depression, ileus and muscle rigidity. Naloxone is a useful antidote.
▪ Lorazepam	0.05–0.10 mg/kg/dose q 10–15 min to a maximum of 4 mg	IV over 2–3 min	Dilute with equal volume of normal saline. Flumazenil 5–10 mg/kg/dose iv is effective antidote
▪ Magnesium sulfate	0.2 mL/kg per dose as 50% solution q 6 hr for 4 days	IM	Useful for treatment of refractory hypocalcemia
▪ Midazolam	0.1–0.2 mg/ kg/ dose every 2–4 hours or continuous iv infusion @ 0.4–0.6 mg/kg/min	IM, IV over 2–5 min	Give after dilution as it contains 1% benzyl alcohol
▪ Morphine sulfate	0.05 mg/kg per dose. Continuous iv infusion 0.01–0.02 mg/kg/hr	SC, IV	Keep watch on respiration
▪ Paraldehyde	0.2 mL/kg per dose	IM, per rectum in oil or liquid paraffin	Use ampoules. May decompose into acetic acid and cause necrosis
▪ Pethidine	1 mg/kg per dose	IM, IV	
▪ Phenobarbitone sodium	20 mg/kg loading dose followed by 5–8 mg/kg/d q 12 hr	Oral, IM, IV	Induces maturation of glucuronyl transferase and Y-acceptor protein. Do not give along with diazepam. Optimal serum levels range between 20 and 30 mg/mL
▪ Phenytoin sodium	20 mg/kg loading dose followed by 5–8 mg/kg/day q 12 hr	Oral, IV	Watch bradycardia, arrhythmia, hypotension. Optimal serum therapeutic level is 10–20 mg/mL
▪ Pyridoxine	50–100 mg/dose Maintenenace 50–100 mg oral daily	IV	Give under EEG control
▪ Triclofos sodium	10–20 mg/kg per dose	Oral	

The lower dose is used in a preterm baby. Administer every 12 hr for all infants between 0 and 7 days and every 8 hr for infants >7 days

In preterm infants up to 7 days administer every 12 hr, term infants up to 7 days and preterm infants >7 days every 8 hr, and term infants after 7 days every 6 hr.

(contd.)

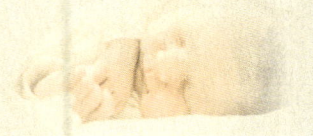

Table 34.3 Commonly used drugs in the newborn (*Contd...*)

Agent	Dose	Route of administration	Comments
III. Antifungal agents			
▪ Amphotericin-B	Initial dose 0.25–0.5 mg/kg. Dose is increased daily by 0.25 mg till the maximum daily dose of 1.0 mg/kg. Total dose 30–35 mg/ kg over 2–4 weeks	IV slow drip over 2 hr	Disseminated fungal infection. Maximum concentration limited to 1.0 mg/10 mL of 5% dextrose. It is incompatible with sodium chloride. Watch renal and hematologic toxicity and hypokalemia. Protect from light
▪ Amphotericin-B liposome (ambisome)	5 mg/kg q 24 hr infused over 2 hr in a maximum concentration of 2 mg/mL. Average duration of therapy is 2–4 weeks	IV slow infusion	Avoid concurrent use of corticosteroids and nephrotoxic drugs
▪ Fluconazole	Loading dose 12 mg/kg followed by 6 mg/kg/ dose q 24–48 hr	Oral or IV over 30 minutes	Good CSF penetration, monitor renal and liver functions
▪ Flucytocine	25–50 mg/kg/dose q 6 hr	Oral, IV	Combined with amphotericin B for severe or CNS fungal infections
▪ Ketoconazole	1–2 mg/kg/dose q 12 hr	Oral	Avoid in infants with hepatic dysfunction
▪ Nystatin	0.5–1.0 mL of 100,000 U/mL q 6 hr	Oral and topical	Continue therapy for 3 more days after recovery
IV. Antiviral agents			
▪ Acyclovir	20 mg/kg/dose q 8–12 hr for 10–21 d	IV infusion in a concentration of 5 mg/mL over 1–3 hr	Monitor renal and hepatic function.
▪ Ganciclovir	10–15 mg/kg/day q 12 hr for 3–6 weeks. For long term suppression 10 mg/kg 3 days in a week for 3 months	IV slow over one hour	Monitor hematologic, renal and hepatic functions. Avoid contact with skin and mucous membranes because it is cytotoxic. It has been shown to cause testicular atrophy in experimental animals
▪ Vidarabine	15–30 mg in a concentration of 0.5 mg/mL	IV infusion over 12 hr	It has been replaced by acyclovir
▪ Zidovudine	1.5–2.0 mg/kg/dose q 6 hr for 6 weeks	Oral, IV infusion over 1 hr	Monitor hematologic, renal and hepatic side effects
V. Corticosteroids			
▪ Aldosterone	1 mg per dose	IM, IV	Salt-losing adrenal crisis
▪ Cortisone acetate	5–10 mg/kg/d	IM, IV, oral	Maintenance for congenital adrenal hyperplasia.
▪ Dexamethasone	0.1–0.25 mg/kg/ dose q 6 hr	Oral, IM, IV	For cerebral edema, raised intracranial tension, airway edema and BPD. There is increased risk of neuromotor disability and cerebral palsy on long-term follow-up
▪ Fludrocortisone	0.1–0.2 mg/day	Oral single dose	Adrenogenital syndrome

The lower dose is used in a preterm baby. During the first week, parenteral medications are administered 12-hourly in preterm babies and 8-hourly in term babies.

(contd.)

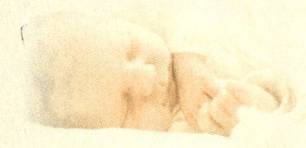
Table 34.3 Commonly used drugs in the newborn (*Contd...*)

Agent	Dose	Route of administration	Comments
▪ Hydrocortisone	5–10 mg q 8 hr. For shock 50–150 mg q 6 hr	IM, IV	Solution is stable for few hours only. Indicated in endotoxic shock, sclerema, adrenal hemorrhage and laryngeal edema following intubation
VI. Decongestive and cardiotonic drugs			
▪ Captopril	0.05–0.5 mg/kg/dose 8–12 hr	Oral empty stomach	May cause oliguria, hyperkalemia, renal failure, jaundice
▪ Digoxin	0.03–0.05 mg, 1/2 stat, 1/4 after 8 hours and 1/4 after 12–16 hours	Oral, IM, IV	IV should be preferred in seriously sick infants. 1/4 of total digitalizing dose should be given as maintenance dose in two divided doses. Blood levels should be maintained between 3 and 4 ng/mL
▪ Dobutamine*	5–25 mg/kg/min	IV through infusion pump	Do not mix with sodium bicarbonate. It does not compromise renal perfusion and is useful alternative, if dopamine administration is associated with tachycardia
▪ Dopamine*	2.5–25 mg/kg/min	IV through infusion pump	Low dose infusion is useful to promote renal perfusion. Administration of high dose (>25 mg/kg/min) is associated with tachycardia, increase in pulmonary artery pressure and reduction of renal blood flow
▪ Epinephrine 1:10,000 (0.1 mg/mL)	0.1–0.3 mL/kg q 3–5 min. Repeat same dose of 1:1000 solution in an unresponsive case. For nebulization, 0.5 mL/kg of 1:1000 soution diluted in 3 mL normal saline	IV push, intratracheal dose is 0.3–1.0 mL/kg	Avoid intracardiac. Indicated in asystole, shock and anaphylaxis
▪ Furosemide	1–2 mg/kg/dose, maximum 6 mg/kg/dose	Oral, IM, IV	May cause deafness
▪ Hydralazine	0.15 mg/kg/dose every 6 hourly. Increase by 0.1 mg/kg every 6 hours till desired effect is achieved or up to maximum dose of 2 mg/kg	Oral, IV	
▪ Methyldopa	10 mg/kg/dose	IV, Oral	
▪ Nifedipine	0.2 mg/kg/dose	Sublingual, Oral	Sparingly used in neonates
▪ Nitroprusside sodium	0.2–6.0 mg/kg/min	IV through infusion pump	Thiocyanate toxicity causes hyperreflexia, seizures and coma
▪ Propranolol	0.2–0.4 mg/kg/dose, 2 mg/kg/day q 6–8 hr	IV, Oral	Paroxysmal atrial tachycardia, neonatal thyrotoxicosis and asymmetric septal hypertrophy
▪ Tolazoline	1–2 mg/kg bolus followed by continuous infusion at 1–2 mg/kg per hr	IV	Persistent fetal circulation

The lower dose is used in a preterm baby. During the first week, parenteral medications are administered 12-hourly in preterm babies and 8-hourly in term babies.

$$*\text{mg dobutamine/dopamine per 100 mL solution} = \frac{[6 \times \text{infant's weight (kg)} \times \text{desired dose (µg/kg/min)}]}{\text{Desired infusion rate (mL/hr)}}$$

(contd.)

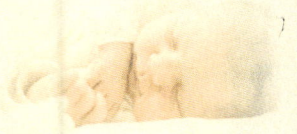

Table 34.3 Commonly used drugs in the newborn (*Contd...*)

Agent	Dose	Route of administration	Comments
VII. Miscellaneous drugs			
■ Acetaminophen	10–15 mg/kg/dose q 6-8 hr	Oral	Use formulation dispensed as drops
■ Acetazolamide	10–25 mg/kg/dose q 8 hr	Oral	Hydrocephalus unassociated with Arnold-Chiari malformation. Watch for hyperchloremic metabolic acidosis
■ Acetyl cysteine	10 mL of 10% solution every 6 hr	Oral, PR	Used for treatment of meconium ileus and hepatic failure
■ Albumin-salt free (25%)	0.5 to 1.0 g/kg per dose. Maximum dose 6 g/kg/d	IV slowly over one hour	Half an hour before exchange transfusion. Dilute with saline to 5% solution.
■ Atropine sulfate	0.02 mg/kg/dose q 10–15 min	SC, IV	
■ Caffeine citrate	20 mg/kg stat, 5–10 mg/kg per dose in 1–2 doses daily for maintenance	IV over 30 minutes. Do not give iv bolus push, give oral for maintenance therapy	Recurrent apnea of prematurity. Risk of kernicterus and seizures.
■ Calcium gluconate 10%	100–200 mg/kg/dose (1–2 mL/kg/dose) followed by 200–800 mg/kg/day for maintenance	IV slowly over 10 min, stop if heart rate <100 bpm	Do not mix with sodium bicarbonate solution. Dilute with equal volume of distilled water and watch for bradycardia. Avoid in digitalized infants
■ Carbimazole	2.5 mg per dose	Oral	Congenital thyrotoxicosis
■ Cardioversion	0.5 J/kg, double the dose each time for a total of 3 attempts	The paddle diameter should be 4.5 cm, apply one paddle to the apex of the heart and the other to the right sternal border	Correct acidosis, sedate with IV midazolam Administer IV adenosine 0.05–2.0 mg/kg/dose bolus before cardioversion
■ Carnitine	50–100 mg/kg/d q 24 hr	Oral, IV	Diarrhea is a common side effect
■ Cisapride	0.1–0.3 mg/kg/dose q 8–12 hr	Oral	It is contraindicated, if QTC interval is more than 0.44. It should not be co-administered with erythromycin and antifungal drugs which are known to increase QTC interval
■ Diazoxide	8–15 mg q 8–12 hr	Oral, IV	For glucose-refractory hyperinsulinemic hypoglycemia
■ Doxapram hydrochloride	2.5 mg/kg/stat, infusion rate 1–2 mg/kg/hr	IV	The margin of safety is low. Hypertension, IVH and seizures may occur
■ Edrophonium bromide (tensilon)	1 mg stat	IM, IV	For diagnosis of transient neonatal myasthenia gravis
■ Ephedrine saline nose drops (0.25%)	One drop 15 minutes before feed for local use		Do not use more than 2–3 times per day. Jitteriness, excessive crying and fever may occur
■ Ferrous sulfate	Prophylaxis 2 mg elemental iron q 24 hr. Therapeutic dose 4–6 mg q 12 hr	Oral	Give in-between feeds
■ Gentian violet (0.5%)	One drop after each feed under the tongue	Oral thrush	
■ Glucagon	0.1–0.3 mg/kg/dose up to maximum of 1 mg	IM, IV bolus	Use in macrosomic babies with hypoglycemia

The lower dose is used in a preterm baby. During the first week, parenteral medications are administered 12-hourly in preterm babies and 8-hourly in term babies.

(contd.)

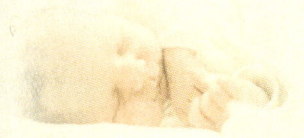

Table 34.3 Commonly used drugs in the newborn (*Contd...*)

Agent	Dose	Route of administration	Comments
▪ Heparin	100 units/kg/dose every 4 hourly, 10 units/mL for rinsing syringes and catheters	IM, IV	To maintain clotting time of 20–30 minutes or 2–3 times of pretherapy clotting time
▪ Hepatitis B immune globulins	0.5 mL/dose (0.16 mL/kg) at birth or alternatively 2.0 mL pooled gamma globulins	IM	Given if mother is carrier of hepatitis B virus
▪ Ibuprofen	10 mg/kg stat followed by 5 mg/kg at 24 hr and 48 hr	IV, Oral	Pharmacologic closure of ductus arteriosus
▪ Immune gamma globulins	0.15 mL/kg stat for HAV prophylaxis, 500–750 mg/kg IV over 2–6 hr stat for prevention and treatment of sepsis, 400 mg/kg/d for 3–5 days for immune thrombocytopenia	IM, IV	The role in prophylaxis and treatment of sepsis is controversial
▪ Indomethacin	0.2 mg/kg/dose q 12 hr for 3 doses	Oral, IV over 30 min	Avoid if there is bleeding, renal dysfunction
▪ Isoniazid	5–10 mg/kg q 24 hr	Oral	For chemoprophylaxis and congenital tuberculosis Always combine it with pyridoxine
▪ Lomodex (10%)	1–2 g/kg/dose	IV	
▪ Lugol's iodine	One drop q 8 hr	Oral	
▪ Magnesium sulfate (50%)	25–50 mg/kg/dose q 6 hr for 4 doses	IM	Calcium gluconate 10% is useful antidote
▪ Mannitol (20%)	1.0 g/kg/dose q 8 hr for 3 doses	IV over 30 min	For relief of raised intracranial tension.
▪ Metoclopramide	0.2–0.3 mg/kg/dose q 6–8 hr	Oral	May cause hypertrophy of breast tissue
▪ Methylene blue	0.1–0.2 mg/kg as 1% solution	IV	Given for methemoglobinemia. Blue-green discoloration of urine occurs.
▪ Nalorphine	0.2 mg/kg/dose	IV, IM, SC, intratracheal	If mother had received pethidine or morphine 4 to 6 hours before delivery.
▪ Naloxone	0.1 to 0.2 mg/kg/dose q 3–5 min	IV, IM, SC, intratracheal	Do not administer to newborns of narcotic-dependent mothers
▪ Neostigmine methyl sulfate	0.05 to 0.1 mg/kg stat	IM, IV, Oral	Give atropine before administeration of prostigmine
▪ Omeprazole	0.5–1.5 mg/kg single or two doses daily	Oral through NG tube	Monitor hepatic transaminases
▪ Pancuronium bromide	0.05–0.1 mg/kg loading dose q 5–10 min twice. 0.03–0.1 mg/kg/dose q 1–4 hr for maintenance or continuous infusion @ 0.05–0.2 mg/kg/hr	IV bolus or through infusion pump	Neostigmine 0.025 mg/kg IV with atropine (0.02 mg/kg) is effective antidote
▪ Prostaglandin E$_1$	0.05–0.4 mg/kg/ min	IV infusion @ 0.05 µg/min	Adjust the dose on the basis of improved oxygenation versus side effects. The side effects include apnea, bradycardia, flushing, hypotension, seizure-like activity, hypocalcemia, hypoglycemia, diarrhea and inhibition of platelet aggregation

The lower dose is used in a preterm baby. During the first week, parenteral medications are administered 12-hourly in preterm babies and 8-hourly in term babies.

(contd.)

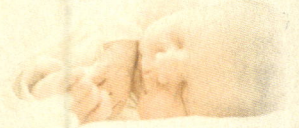

Table 34.3 Commonly used drugs in the newborn (*Contd...*)

Agent	Dose	Route of administration	Comments
■ Protamine sulfate	1 mg for every mg (100 units) of heparin taken during past 4 hours	IM, IV	Antidote for heparin
■ Pyrimethamine	1 mg for 3 days, then 0.5 mg for one month	Oral	Folinic acid 5 mg should be given twice weekly.
■ Ranitidine	1–2 mg/kg/dose q 8–12 hr 0.5–1.0 mg/kg/dose q 6–8 hr	Oral IV	Use in VLBW infants is associated with increased risk of NEC
■ Rifampicin	10 mg/kg/dose q 24 hr	Oral	Causes red discoloration of urine and body secretions
■ Salbutamol	0.1–0.3 mg/kg/dose q 8 hr 0.5 mg/kg/dose with 1.5 mL normal saline q 2–6 hr	Oral and nebulization	Stop if heart rate goes >180 bpm. Look for hypokalemia
■ Sodium bicarbonate 7.5%	2–4 mL/kg	IV slowly over 15 min	Never infuse till adequate ventilation is established. Avoid rapid bolus administration due to risk of IVH and pulmonary hemorrhage
■ Sodium polystyrene sulfonate	1g/kg/dose q 6 hr. For rectal administration use 20–25% sorbitol q 2–6 hr	Oral, PR	Constipation and fecal impaction may occur
■ Sulfadiazine	100–150 mg q 8 hr	Oral	Toxoplasmosis and urinary tract infection. Avoid during first week of life
■ Tetanus human immunoglobulins	30–300 units/kg	IV	Neonatal tetanus
■ Theophylline	5 mg/kg stat, 1–2 mg/kg/ dose in 3 doses daily for maintenance	IV, oral	For recurrent apneic attacks. Single dose to neonates with birth asphyxia to reduce the risk of acute kidney injury
■ Thyroxine	10–15 mg/kg/day single dose. Adjust the dose by increments of 12.5 mg every month.	Oral empty stomach	Maintain T4 between 10 and 15 mg/dL and TSH less than 10 mU/L
■ Tromethamine (THAM)	Loading dose (mL) of 0.3 M solution = wt (kg) x 1.1 x base deficit (mEq/L). Maintenance 3 mL/kg/hr	IV	Infuse through a peripheral vessel
■ Urokinase	Loading dose 4000 IU/kg followed by constant infusion @ 4000–6000 iu/kg/hr	IV over 20 min as bolus	Watch for bleeding
■ Vitamin E	25 units per day	IM, Oral	Give to all infants weighing less than 1500 g at birth
■ Vitamin K₁ Prophylactic Therapeutic dose	0.5–1.0 mg single 2.0 mg	Oral, IM, IV	Lower dose is given to infants <1500 g
■ Zinc acetate	0.5–1.0 mg/kg/day	Oral	Absorption interfered by concomitant adminis-tration of iron

The lower dose is used in a preterm baby. During the first week, parenteral medications are administered 12-hourly in preterm babies and 8-hourly in term babies.

altered distribution due to membrane permeability, specific protein binding of drugs, deficiency of certain enzymes, such as G-6-PD, pseudocholinesterase and methemoglobin reductase and end organ sensitivity may determine and modify the response of drugs in the newborn. Table 34.3 outlines the dosage schedule, route of administration, indications and salient side effects of commonly used drugs in the newborn.

Drugs in the newborn should be used when absolutely indicated and only those agents which have been well tried in the newborn period should be prescribed. As far as possible, oral and intravenous routes should be used because absorption through intramuscular route is erratic. For oral medications, formulation in drops should be preferred over syrup for ease of administration and reduced osmolar load.

Over dosage by accidental use of vials (vitamin K and nalorphine) intended for use in the mother must be avoided. It is desirable to use insulin (40 unit marks/mL) or tuberculin syringes for ease and accuracy of administration. The amount of diluent used for administration of intravenous medications should be recorded and subtracted from the recommended daily fluid requirements. The proprietary combinations should be avoided due to risk of inadvertent over-dosage of one of the agents.

Chloramphenicol when administered in a dose of 100 mg/kg per day has been shown to result in "gray baby syndrome" which is characterized by abdominal distension, vomiting, hypothermia, shallow and irregular breathing, grayish circumoral cyanosis and circulatory collapse. There is unexplained metabolic acidosis and hyperammonemia. Streptomycin, neomycin, kanamycin and colistin may cause respiratory paralysis by blockage of muscle endplate when applied locally over large raw surface areas or after intraperitoneal instillation. Tetracyclines have been shown to cause growth retardation and brownish staining of teeth by virtue of their chelation with calcium. Hyperbilirubinemia and/or kernicterus may occur at relatively lower serum bilirubin levels during administration of large doses of synthetic vitamin K, long-acting sulfonamides, salicylates, caffeine, lobeline, cedalinid, novobiocin and gentamicin.

It must be remembered that preservatives and vehicles contained in certain drug formulations, which are safe in adults, may be toxic and sometimes dangerous in newborn babies. Sodium benzoate used as a preservative for diazepam is associated with the risk of bilirubin brain damage at relatively lower serum bilirubin levels by blocking bilirubin binding sites in albumin. Propylene glycol (1, 2-propanediol) used as a vehicle in several parenteral drug formulations, such as multivitamins, digoxin, cotrimoxazole, phenobarbitol, phenytoin, diazepam and hydralazine, is fraught with dangers of hyperosmolality. It is desirable that these hyperosmolar medications (including sodium bicarbonate 7.5% and potassium chloride 15%) should be administered slowly after adequate dilution to prevent capillary damage and tissue anoxia. Benzyl alcohol is widely used as a preservative in flush solutions and multiple-dose vials of medications and parenteral electrolyte-containing fluids. It is potentially unsafe in very low birth weight babies and can cause severe metabolic acidosis, encephalopathy and respiratory depression. Benzyl alcohol is oxidized to benzoic acid, conjugated with glycine in the liver and excreted as hippuric acid. This metabolic pathway may not be functional in premature infants and may allow accumulation of benzoic acid and perhaps unmetabolized benzyl alcohol with resultant metabolic acidosis and toxicity.

Hexachlorophene skin applications, without effective rinsing, may result in diarrhea, dehydration, shock, seizures and neuromuscular disturbances. Boric acid applications on large raw areas or accidental oral ingestion may lead to diarrhea, vomiting, generalized skin rash, hepatic necrosis and renal failure. Boric acid must never be stored in the nursery as it is devoid of any therapeutic utility. Lead poisoning may occur following use of lead acetate ointment and lead nipple shields for cracked nipples by the mother.

BIBLIOGRAPHY

Butler-O'Hara M, Buzzard CJ, Reubens L, McDermott MP, DiGrazio W, D'Angio CT. A randomized trial comparing long-term and short-term use of umbilical venous catheters in premature infants with birth weights of less than 1251 grams. *Pediatrics* 2006; 118(1):e25–35.

Committee on Fetus and Newborn, Section on Pain Management. Prevention and management of procedural pain in the neonate: An update. *Pediatrics* 2016; 137(2):e20154271.

Deorari AK, Paul VK, McMillan DD, Scotland J, Singhal N (Eds.). Practical Procedures for the Newborn Nursery. A Manual for Physicians and Nurses. *Sagar Publications, New Delhi*, 3rd Edition, 2010.

Engle WA. Intraosseous access for administration of medications in neonates. *Clin Perinatol* 2006; 33(1):161–8.

Grady C. Enduring and emerging challenges of informed consent. *N Engl J Med* 2015; 372(22):2172.

Henry M, Arnold T, Harvey J, Pleural Diseases Group SoCCBTS. BTS guidelines for the management of spontaneous pneumothorax. *Thorax* 2003; 58 (Suppl 2):39–52.

Moghal NE, Embleton ND. Management of acute renal failure in the newborn. *Semin Fetal Neonatal Med* 2006; 11(3):207–13.

Murki S, Kumar P. Blood exchange transfusion for infants with severe neonatal hyperbilirubinemia. *Semin Perinatol* 2011; 35(3):175–84.

Sathiyamurthy S, Banerjee J, Godambe SV. Antiseptic use in the neonatal intensive care unit—a dilemma in clinical practice: An evidence based review. *World J Clin Pediatr* 2016; 5(2):159–71.

Singh M. Deorari AK. Drug Dosages in Children. *CBS Publishers & Distributors Pvt Ltd, New Delhi*, 9th Edition, 2015.

Singh M, Procedures. In: Care of the Newborn. *CBS Publishers & Distributors Pvt Ltd, New Delhi*, 8th Edition, 2017; pp 600–624.

Strutt J, Kharbanda A. Pediatric chest tubes and pigtails: An evidence-based approach to the management of pleural space diseases. *Pediatr Emerg Med Pract* 2015; 12(11):1–24; quiz 0–1.

Tomek S, Asch S. Umbilical vein catheterization in the critical newborn: a review of anatomy and technique. *EMS World* 2013; 42(2):50–2.

Tsang TS, Oh JK, Seward JB. Diagnosis and management of cardiac tamponade in the era of echocardiography. *Clin Cardiol* 1999; 22(7):446–52.

Vasquez P, Burd A, Mehta R, Hiatt M, Hegyi T. Resolution of peripheral artery catheter: induced ischemic injury following prolonged treatment with topical nitroglycerin ointment in a newborn: a case report. *J Perinatol* 2003; 23(4):348–50.

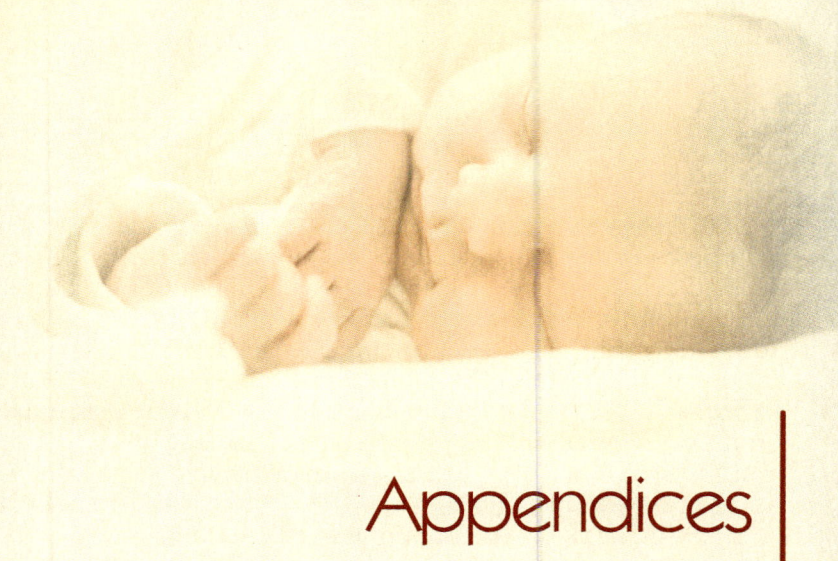

Appendices

APPENDIX 1. Weight, length and volume conversion tables

Weight equivalents		Height and weight conversion factors	
Apothecary	*Metric*	*To convert*	*Multiply by*
1 grain	60 mg or 0.05 g	Inches to centimeters	2.54
15 grain	1000 mg or 1.0 g	Inches to meters	0.0254
60 grain (1 dram)	4 g	Feet to meters	0.3048
8 dram (1 oz)	30 g	Pounds to kilograms	0.4535
1 pound (16 oz)	480 g	Kilograms to pounds	2.2
2.2 pounds	1 kg		

Liquid measures				
Apothecary	*Exact*	*Metric*	*Approx*	*Household measures**
1 minim (drop)	—	0.06 mL	Teaspoon	5 mL
15 minims	—	1.0 mL	Tablespoon	15 mL
60 minims (1 fl dram)	—	3.7 mL	Cup or katori	150 mL
8 fl dram (1 fl oz)	29.6 ml	30.0 mL	Glass	250 mL
16 fl oz (1 pint)	473.2 ml	500.0 mL		
32 fl oz (1 quart)	946.4 ml	1000.0 mL		
1 gallon	—	4 quarts		

*They are not standard in size and may vary widely in their volume

APPENDIX 2. Temperature equivalents

Celsius	Fahrenheit	Celsius	Fahrenheit
35.0	95.0	38.6	101.4
35.4	95.7	39.0	102.2
35.8	96.4	39.4	102.9
36.0	96.8	39.8	103.6
36.4	97.5	40.2	104.3
36.8	98.2	40.6	105.1
37.0	98.6	41.0	105.8
37.4	99.3	41.4	106.5
37.8	100.0	41.8	107.2
38.2	100.7	42.0	107.6

The normal body temperature of 98.4°F corresponds to 36.9°C. To convert Fahrenheit to Celsius subtract 32 and divide by 1.8 To convert Celsius to Fahrenheit multiply by 1.8 and add 32.

APPENDIX 3. Mean hematologic values in preterm and term newborns

Determination	Preterm		Term				
	28 wks	34 wks	Cord blood	Day 1	Day 3	Day 7	Day 14
Hemoglobin (gm/dL)	14.5	15.0	16.8	18.4	17.8	17.0	16.8
Hematocrit (%)	45.0	47.0	53.0	58.0	55.0	54.0	52.0
Red blood cells (mm^3)	4.0	4.4	5.2	5.8	5.6	5.2	5.1
MCV (m^3)	120.0	118.0	107.0	108.0	99.0	98.0	96.0
MCH (pg/cell)	40.0	38.0	34.0	35.0	33.0	32.5	31.5
MCHC (%)	31.0	32.0	31.7	32.5	33.0	33.0	33.0
Reticulocytes (%)	5–10	3–10	3–7	3–7	1–3	0–1	0–1
Nucleated RBCs	—	—	500.0	200.0	0.5	0	C

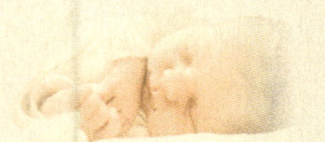

APPENDIX 4. Total and differential white blood cell count in term and preterm newborns

Term newborn	Total leukocytes			Neutrophils			Lymphocytes		Eosinophils		Basophils		Monocytes	
	Mean	Range (× 10³)	Total (mean)	Seg.	Band	B/N	Total (mean)	%	Total (mean)	%	Total (mean)	%	Total (mean)	%
Birth	18,100	9–30	11,000	9,400	1,600	0.14	5,500	31	400	2.2	100	0.6	1,050	5.8
12 hours	22,800	13–38	15,500	—	—	0.14	5,500	24	500	2	—	—	1,200	5.0
24 hours	18,990	9.4–34	11,500	—	—	0.14	5,800	31	500	2	—	—	1,100	6.0
7th day	12,200	5–12	5,500	4,700	730	0.14	5,000	41	500	4.1	50	0.4	1,100	9.1
14th day	11,400	5–20	4,500	3,900	6.30	0.14	5,500	48	350	3	50	0.4	1,000	8.8
Preterm newborn <1500 gm														
Day 7	16,800	61–32.8	10,240	9,000	1,700	0.11	5,000	30	330	2	168	1	1,000	6
Day 14	15,400	10.4–21.3	8,000	7,100	900	0.11	5,400	35	450	3	150	1	1,550	10
1500–2000 gm														
Day 7	13,000	6.7–14.7	8,200	7,200	1,050	0.13	4,000	29	260	2	130	1	650	5
Day 14	10,000	7.0–14.1	5,100	4,300	800	0.15	3,600	36	300	3	100	1	900	9

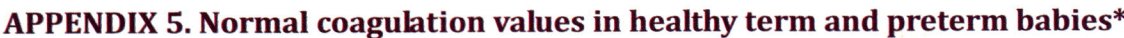

APPENDIX 5. Normal coagulation values in healthy term and preterm babies*

Procoagulants	Synonyms	Term	Preterm	
			32–36 weeks	28–31 weeks
Factor I (mg/dL)	Fibrinogen	246 ± 55	244 ± 55	270 ± 85
Factor II+ (%)	Prothrombin	45 ± 15	35 ± 12	30 ± 10
Factor V (%)	Proaccelerin, labile factor	*100 ± 5	*80 ± 9	*76 ± 7
Factor VII+ (%)	Proconvertin, stable factor	56 ± 16	40 ± 15	38 ± 14
Factor VIII (%)	Antihemophiliac factor (AHF)	105 ± 34	98 ± 40	70 ± 30
Factor IX+ (%)	Plasma thromboplastin component (PTC), Christmas factor	28 ± 8	NA	27 ± 10
Factor X+ (%)	Stuart Prower factor	56 ± 16	40 ± 15	38 ± 14
Factor XI (%)	Plasma thromboplastin antecedent (PTA)	29 ± 70	NA	5 ± 13
Factor XII (%)	Hageman factor	25 ± 70	30–100	NA
Factor XIII (%)	Fibrin stabilizing factor	100	100	100
Prekallikrein (PK)	Fletcher factor	33 ± 6	NA	27
High molecular weight kininogen (HMWK)	Williams, Fitzgerald, Flaujac factor	56 ± 12	NA	28
Platelet count (#mm³)	Thrombocytes	150–400	150–400	100–400
PT (seconds)	Prothrombin time	13–20	12–21	23
APPT (seconds)	Activated partial prothrombin time	55 ± 10	70	NA
FSP (mg/mL)	Fibrin split products	55	48	33 ± 9
Thrombin time (seconds)		10–16	11–17	16–28

* These values may differ depending on the methodology of each laboratory
+ Vitamin K-dependent protein

APPENDIX 6. Normal blood chemistry values in cord blood and capillary blood of full term infants

Determination			Infant's blood							
	Cord blood		1–12 hr		12–24 hr		24–48 hr		48–72 hr	
	Mean	Range	Mean	Range	Mean	Range	Mean	Range	Mean	Range
Sodium (mEq/L)	147	126–166	143	124–156	145	132–159	148	136–160	149	139–162
Potassium (mEq/L)	7.8	5.6–12	6.4	5.3–7.3	6.3	5.3–8.9	6.0	5.2–7.3	5.9	5.0–7.7
Calcium (mg/dL)	9.3	5.2–11.2	8.4	7.3–9.2	7.8	6.9–9.4	8.0	6.1–9.9	7.9	5.9–9.7
Phosphorus (mg/dL)	5.6	3.7–8.1	6.1	3.5–8.6	5.7	2.9–8.1	5.9	3.0–8.7	5.8	2.8–7.6
Blood urea (mg/dL)	29	21–40	27	8–34	33	8–63	32	13–77	31	13–63
Total proteins (gm/dL)	6.1	4.8–7.3	6.6	5.6–8.5	6.6	5.8–8.2	6.9	5.9–8.2	7.2	6.0–8.5
Blood sugar (mg/dL)	73	45–96	63	40–97	63	42–104	56	30–91	59	40–90
Lactic acid (mg/dL)	19.5	11–30	14.6	11–24	140	11–23	14.3	9–22	13.5	7–21

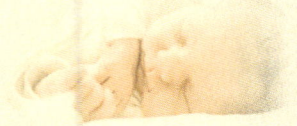

APPENDIX 7. Blood chemistry values in premature infants (birth weight 1500–1700 gm)

Determination	1 week		3 weeks		5 weeks		7 weeks	
	Mean	Range	Mean	Range	Mean	Range	Mean	Range
Sodium (mEq/L)	139.6	133–146	136.3	129–142	136.8	133–148	137.2	133–142
Potassium (mEq/L)	5.6	4.6–6.7	5.8	4.5–7.1	5.5	4.5–6.6	5.7	4.6–7.1
Calcium (mg/dL)	9.2	6.1–11.6	9.6	8.1–1.0	9.4	8.6–10.5	9.5	8.6–10.8
Phosphorus (mg/dL)	7.6	5.4–10.9	7.5	6.2–8.7	7.0	5.6–7.9	6.8	4.2–8.2
Blood urea (mg/dL)	18.6	6.2–51	26.6	4.2–62.8	26.6	4.0–53	26.8	5.0–61.0
Total proteins (gm/dL)	5.49	4.40–6.26	5.38	4.28–6.7	4.98	4.14–6.9	4.93	4.02–5.86
Blood sugar (mg/dL)	45	28–61	56	23–98	52	18–77	48	22–83

APPENDIX 8. Normal blood chemistry values of healthy neonates

Component	Age	Values	
Alanine aminotransferase or glutamic-pyruvic transaminase (ALT or SGPT)		5–28 iu/L	
Alkaline phosphatase		20–225 iu/L	
Ammonia nitrogen	Term newborn		
	At birth	90–150 µg/dL	
	0–2 wks	79–129 µg/dL	
Amylase		5–65 u/L	
Aspartate aminotransferase or glutamic-oxaloacetic transaminase (AST or SGOT)		5–40 iu/L	
Bilirubin (Total)		Premature (mg/dL)	Full term (mg/dL)
	Cord	2	2
	0–1 day	8	6
	3–5 days	15	12
Bilirubin (Direct)		0.0–0.2 mg/dL	
C-Reactive protein		10–350 mg/mL	
Calcium		See Appendices 5 and 6	
Ceruloplasmin		1–30 mg/dL	
Cholesterol			
	Cord	45–100 mg/dL	
	Newborn	53–135 mg/dL	
	3 days–1 year	69–174 mg/dL	
Complement C3		88.4 ± 1.7 mg/dL	
		99.5 ± 17.4 mg/dL	
Cortisol		1–24 µg/dL	
Creatinine			
	Cord	0.6–1.2 mg/dL	
	Newborn	0.3–1.0 mg/dL	
Creatinine phosphokinase			
	Premature	0–210 iu/L	
	Birth–3 weeks	22–267 iu/L	
	3 weeks onwards	15–134 iu/L	
Ferritin		25–200 ng/dL	
Fetal hemoglobin (% HbF)			
	1st day	77.0 ± 7.3	
	5th day	76.8 ± 5.8	
	3rd week	70.0 ± 7.3	
	6–9 weeks	52.9 ± 11.0	

(contd.)

(contd.)

Component	Age	Values
Fibrinogen		See Appendix 5
Galactose		0–20 mg/dL
Glucose		See Appendices 6 and 7
Growth hormone		
	Cord	10–15 ng/mL
	Newborn	10–40 ng/mL
Haptoglobin		5–48 mg/dL
Hematocrit (capillary)		
	1st day	48–69%
	2nd day	48–75%
	3rd day	44–72%
	After 3rd day	28–42%
Immunoglobulins (mg/dL)		

Age	IgG	IgA	IgM
Newborn	631–1431	up to 8	1–21
6 days–4 weeks	400–1250	4–36	20–80	1–2 months
200–950	5–64	20–142	Iron	100–250 µg/dL

Component	Age	Values
Osmolality		275–295 mOsmol/kg
Phospholipids (Total)		75–170 mg/dL
Phosphorus (mg/dL)		See Appendices 5 and 6
T4 (µg/mL)	Birth	6.9–16.7
	1–3 days	11–23
	1 week–1 month	9–18
Transferrin		130–275 mg/dL
Triglycerides		10–98 mg/dL
TSH (µIU/mL)	Birth	3–22
	24 hours	17.1 ± 3
	48 hours	12.8 ± 1.9
	2 weeks	<10
Uric acid		2.0–6.2 mg/dL

APPENDIX 9. Normal blood gas and acid–base parameters in newborn babies

Determination	Arterial blood	Venous blood
pH	7.30–7.40	7.35–7.45
PaO_2 (mmHg)	90–100	45–50
$PaCO_2$ (mmHg)	35–45	40–45
HCO_3^- (mmol/L)	20–22	20–22
Base excess	–3 to –7	–3 to –7
Oxygen saturation (%)	92–95	—

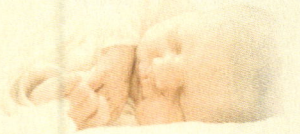

APPENDIX 10. Cerebrospinal Fluid in Healthy Term and Preterm Newborns

Determination	Premature	Term infant		
		0–24 hours	*Day 1*	*Day 7*
Color	Xanthochromic	Clear or xanthochromic	Clear or xanthochromic	Clear or xanthochromic
Pressure (mm CSF)	—	50–80	50–80	50–80
Red blood cells (per mm³)	—	9 (0–1070)	23 (0–620)	3 (0–48)
Polymorphs (per mm³)	—	3 (0–70)	7 (0–26)	2 (0–5)
Lymphocytes (per mm³)	—	2 (0–20)	5 (0–16)	1 (0–4)
Protein (mg/dL)	100 (50–180)	63 (32–240)	73 (40–148)	47 (27–65)
Sugar (mg/dL)	50 (30–70)	51 (32–78)	48 (38–64)	55 (48–62)
Chloride (mg/dL)	—	720 (680–760)	720 (680–760)	740 (720–760)
LDH (iu/L)	—	1.5–50.0	—	—

APPENDIX 11. Average systolic, diastolic and mean blood pressures (mm Hg) during first twelve hours of life in normal newborn according to birth weight

Birth weight	Blood pressure (mmHg)	Age in hours											
		1	2	3	4	5	6	7	8	9	10	11	12
1001 to 2000 gm	Systolic	49	49	51	52	53	52	52	52	51	51	49	50
	Diastolic	26	27	28	29	31	31	31	31	31	30	29	30
	Mean	35	36	37	39	40	40	39	39	38	37	37	38
2001 to 3000 gm	Systolic	59	57	60	60	61	58	64	60	63	61	60	59
	Diastolic	32	32	32	32	33	34	37	34	38	35	35	35
	Mean	43	41	43	43	44	43	45	43	44	44	43	42
Over 3000 gm	Systolic	70	67	65	65	66	66	67	67	68	70	66	66
	Diastolic	44	41	39	41	40	41	41	41	44	43	41	41
	Mean	53	51	50	50	51	50	50	51	53	54	51	50

Note: The mean arterial pressure is 30–35 mmHg in a 1000 g infant and increases approximately by 1.0 mmHg for every 100 gm increase in birth weight. The mean arterial blood pressure corresponds to the gestational age in weeks. Mean arterial blood pressure (MAP) is calculated by formula: Diastolic pressure + 1/3 pulse pressure. The pulse pressure is difference between systolic and diastolic blood pressure.

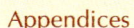

APPENDIX 12. Normal electrocardiographic values in newborn babies

Parameter	Age		
	0–24 hours	1–7 days	8–30 days
Heart rate	119 (85–145)	133 (100–175)	163 (115–190)
P-R interval	0.10 (0.07–0.13)	0.09 (0.05–0.13)	0.09 (0.07–0.13)
P duration	0.051 (0.040–0.075)	0.046 (0.035–0.065)	0.048 (0.040–0.065)
QRS duration	0.065 (0.05–0.09)	0.056 (0.04–0.08)	0.057 (0.04–0.08)
P amplitude in lead II	1.5 (0.5–2.6)	1.6 (0.5–2.8)	1.6 (0.5–2.7)
QRS axis	135 (160–180)	125 (60–180)	110 (0–180)
T axis	70 (–20–180)	25 (–40–100)	35 (–20–120)
T amplitude in V4	4.3 (8.5)*	4.4 (8.5)*	5.3 (8.5)*
T amplitude in V6	2.4 (4.5)*	2.9 (4.5)*	3.5 (7.5)*
Age	30 hours	30 days	
R amplitude in V4R	8.6 (3.5–15.0)	6.3 (3.0–12.0)	
R in V1	11.9 (5.0–30.0)	11.1 (4.0–20.0)	
R in V5	9.4 (2.0–20.0)	15.0 (3.8–30.0)	
R in V6	5.4 (1.5–15.0)	10.8 (1.0–22.0)	
S in V4R	3.8 (0–12.0)	1.8 (0–9.0)	
S in V1	9.7 (0–26.0)	6.1 (0–15)	
S in V5	9.5 (5.0–22.0)	8.3 (0–30)	
S in V6	5.6 (0.2–20.0)	4.8 (0–18.0)	

* maximum value

BIBLIOGRAPHY

Abdollahi A, Sheikhbahaei S, Mohdaviani B. Hemostatic profile in healthy premature neonates. Does birth weight affect the coagulation profile? *J Clin Neonatal* 2014 Apr-Jun 3(2):89–92.

Acharya PT, Wayne WW. Blood chemistry of normal full term infants in the first 48 hours of life. *Arch Dis Child* 1965, 40:430.

Altman PL, Dittmer DS. Blood and other body fluids. *Washington DC. Federation of American Societies for Experimental Biology*, 1961.

Avery ME, Norman ICS. Respiratory physiology in the newborn infant. *Anesthesiology* 1965, 26:510.

Cockburn F, Drillien MC. Neonatal Medicine. *Blackwell Scientific Publications* 1974, p. 802–805.

Hastreiter AR, Abella JB. The electrocardiogram in the newborn period. *J Pediatr* 1971, 78:147.

Hathaway WE, Bonnar J. Perinatal Coagulation. *Grune and Stratton, New York*, 1978.

Kiterman JA, Phibbs RH, Tooley WH. Aortic blood pressure in normal newborn infants during first 12 hours of life. *Pediatrics* 1969, 44:959.

Majumdar A, Jana A, Bannerjee S. Importance of normal values of CSF parameters in term versus preterm neonates. *J Clin Neonatol* 2013, Oct-Dec, 2(4):166–68.

Naidoo T. The cerebrospinal fluid in the healthy newborn infant. *South Africa Med J* 1968, 42:933.

Oski FA, Naiman JL. Hematologic Problems in the Newborn. *WB Saunders and Co.*, 1972, p.13.

Otilo E. Studies on the cerebrspinal fluid in premature infants. *Acta Paediatr Scand* 1984, 35: (suppl.) 9.

Pramanik AK. The bleeding neonate. In Medical Emergencies in Children. Singh M (Ed), *CBS Publishers & Distributors Pvt Ltd, New Delhi*, Revised 5th edition, 2016, pp. 306–336.

Samanta M, Mondal R, Ray S, et al. Normative blood pressure data for Indian neonates. *Indian J Pediatr* 2015, Aug, 52:669–72.

Schaffer AJ. Diseases of the Newborn. *WB Saunders and Co., Phila*, 3rd edition, 1971.

Schwartz PJ, Garson A Jr, Paul T, Strama-Badiale M, Vetter VL, Villain E, Wren C. Guidelines for the interpretation of the neonatal electrocardiogram. A Task Force of the European Society of Cardiology. *Eur Heart J* 2002, 23:1329–44.

Thomas JL and Reichelderfer T. Premature infarts: Analysis of serum during the first seven weeks. *Clin Chem* 1968, 14:272.

Tietz NW. In: Fundamentals of Clinical Chemistry, *WB Saunders and Co., Phila*, 3rd edition, 1987, p. 975.

Wolf H and Hoepffner L. The cerebrospinal fluid in the newborn and premature infant. *World Neurol* 1961, 2:871.

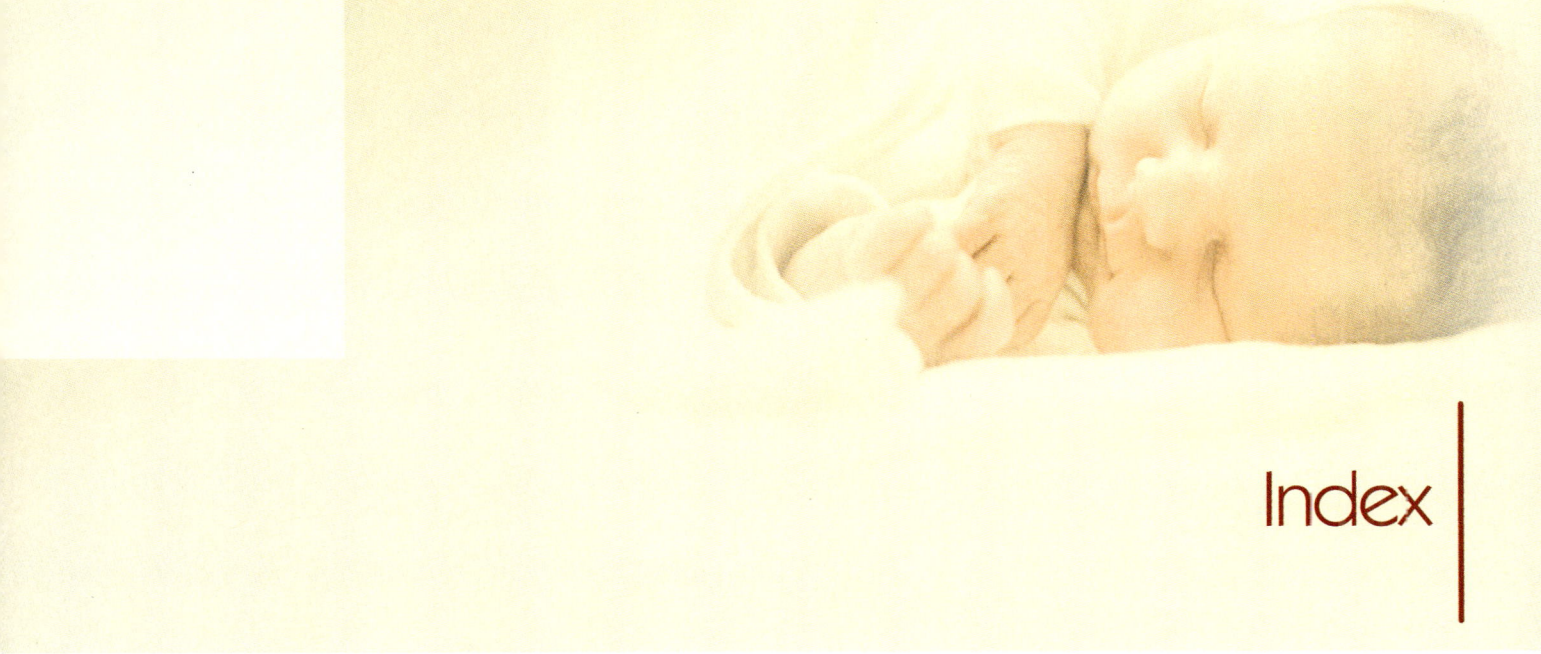

Index

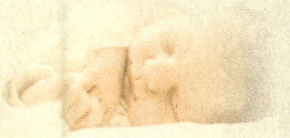

C

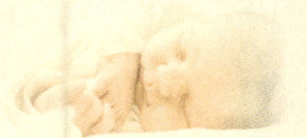

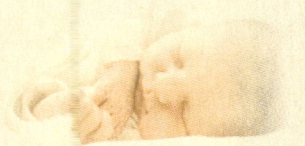

O

P

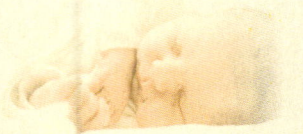